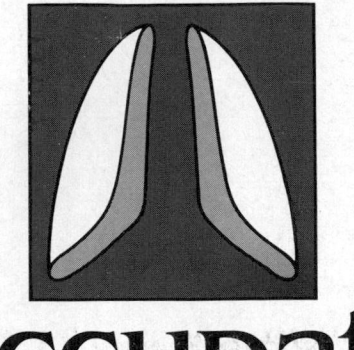

Occupational
Lung Diseases
SECOND EDITION

W. Keith C. Morgan, M.D. (Sheff.), F.R.C.P. (Ed.), F.R.C.P. (C.), F.A.C.P.

Director, Sir Adam Beck Chest Unit,
University Hospital, London
Professor of Medicine,
University of Western Ontario,
Ontario, Canada

Anthony Seaton, M.D. (Cantab.), F.R.C.P. (Lond.), F.F.O.M.

Director, Institute of Occupational Medicine, Edinburgh,
Honorary Senior Lecturer in Medicine,
Universities of Edinburgh and Dundee, Scotland

1984
W. B. Saunders Company
Philadelphia London Toronto Mexico City Rio de Janeiro Sydney Tokyo

W. B. Saunders Company: West Washington Square
Philadelphia, PA   19105

1 St. Anne's Road
Eastbourne, East Sussex BN21 3UN, England

1 Goldthorne Avenue
Toronto, Ontario M8Z 5T9, Canada

Apartado 26370—Cedro 512
Mexico 4, D.F., Mexico

Rua Coronel Cabrita, 8
Sao Cristovao Caixa Postal 21176
Rio de Janeiro, Brazil

9 Waltham Street
Artarmon, N.S.W. 2064, Australia

Ichibancho, Central Bldg., 22-1 Ichibancho
Chiyoda-Ku, Tokyo 102, Japan

Library of Congress Cataloging in Publication Data

Morgan, W. Keith C.

Occupational lung diseases.

1. Lungs—Dust diseases.   2. Lungs—Diseases.   3. Occupational diseases.   I. Seaton, Anthony.   II. Title. [DNLM:
1. Lung diseases.   2. Occupational disease. WF 600 M849o]

RC773.M67 1984   616.2′4   83–18960

ISBN 0-7216-6556-X

Occupational Lung Diseases   ISBN   0-7216-6556-X

Last digit is the print number: 9   8   7   6   5   4   3   2   1

Dedication of the First Edition

To our wives, who have of necessity had to remain almost completely silent for the past two years, and who in the end came to share Carlyle's belief that "Under all speech that is good for anything there lies a silence that is better."

Dedication

To our wives, without whose constant presence this book would have appeared two years earlier.

Contributors

BRIAN BOEHLECKE, M.D., M.P.H.
Associate Professor of Medicine, University of North Carolina School of Medicine, Chapel Hill, North Carolina

ROBERT BURRELL, Ph.D.
Professor of Microbiology, West Virginia University School of Medicine, Morgantown, West Virginia

JIM DODGSON, B.Sc., F.R.M.S.
Head of Environmental Branch, Institute of Occupational Medicine, Edinburgh, Scotland

J. BERNARD L. GEE, M.D., F.R.C.P.
Professor of Medicine, Yale University School of Medicine, New Haven, Connecticut

A. R. GIBBS, M.D., M.R.C.Path.
Senior Lecturer in Pathology, University Hospital of Wales, Cardiff, South Wales

JAMSON LWEBUGA-MUKASA, M.D., Ph.D.
Assistant Professor of Medicine, Yale University School of Medicine, New Haven, Connecticut

R. M. E. SEAL, M.B., F.R.C.P., F.R.C.Path.
Consultant Pathologist, South Glamorgan Area Health Authority, Glamorgan, South Wales

DOUGLAS SEATON, M.D., M.R.C.P.
Consultant Physician, Department of Respiratory Medicine, Ipswich Hospital, Ipswich, England

J. C. WAGNER, M.D., F.R.C.Path.
Senior Scientific Officer, Medical Research Council Pneumoconiosis Unit, Llandough Hospital, Penarth, South Wales

Preface
to the Second Edition

Since the first edition there has been increasing interest in occupational lung disease, both within the profession and indeed among laymen. Moreover, many new advances in understanding have occurred. These two facts are our justification for producing an almost entirely rewritten second edition. In doing so, we have tried to take account of a number of comments on the first edition by reviewers and others, in order to satisfy the needs of a wide range of readers within the profession. Several new chapters have been added, and we are indebted to our colleagues Dr. Bernard Gee, Dr. Brian Boehlecke, and Mr. Jim Dodgson for help with these. In addition, Drs. Chris Wagner, Roger Seal, Alan Gibbs, Robert Burrell, and Douglas Seaton have assisted in the rewriting of other chapters. Many other friends have helped with advice, but we should like to mention especially Mr. Bob Boothby and Mrs. Brenda McGovern for photographic and source-tracing help; our long-suffering secretaries, Mrs. Joan Blamires and Mrs. Betty Crolla, without whom the work would not have been possible; and Miss Janet Bronwen Morgan, who compiled the index. We are also indebted to the secretaries of our colleagues, but since so many have been involved, we hope that they will forgive us if we do not name them individually. Once again, Ms. Suzanne Boyd and the staff of W. B. Saunders have proved endlessly patient and helpful in getting our manuscript ready for publication. In spite of all this help, some faults will remain, and for these we must accept responsibility.

W. KEITH C. MORGAN
ANTHONY SEATON

Glossary

Proper Names

ATP	Adenosine triphosphate
CWP	Coal workers' pneumoconiosis
IgA, IgE, IgG, IgM	Immunoglobulins A, E, G, and M
ILO	International Labor Organization
PMF	Progressive massive fibrosis
SRS–A	Slow-reactive substance A
TMA	Trimellitic anhydride
UICC	Union Internationale Contre le Cancer
ALFORD	Appalachian Laboratory for Occupational Respiratory Disease

Physiological Measurements

$(A\text{-}a)O_2$	Alveolo-arterial oxygen gradient
$(A\text{-}a)CO_2$	Alveolo-arterial carbon dioxide gradient
$(a\text{-}v)O_2$	Arteriovenous oxygen difference
ATPS	Ambient temperature and pressure, saturated with water vapor
BTPS	Body temperature and pressure, saturated with water vapor
Cdyn	Dynamic compliance
Cstat	Static compliance
CV	Closing volume
DL	Diffusing capacity
DL_{CO}	Diffusing capacity for carbon monoxide
DM	Membrane diffusion coefficient
ERV	Expiratory reserve volume
f	Frequency
$FE(O_2, CO_2, \text{etc.})$	Fractional concentration of expired gas
FEF_{25} ($\dot{V}max_{25}$)	Forced expiratory flow rate at 25 per cent of forced vital capacity

FEF_{50}, FEF_{75}, FEF_{90}	Forced expiratory flow rates at 50, 75, and 90 per cent of forced vital capacity
FEF_{25-75} (MMF)	Forced expiratory flow rate between 25 and 75 per cent of forced vital capacity
$FEV_{0.75}$	Forced expiratory volume exhaled in 0.75 second
FEV_1	Forced expiratory volume exhaled in one second
FEV_3	Forced expiratory volume exhaled in three seconds
FI (CO_2, O_2, etc.)	Fractional concentration of inspired gas
FRC	Functional residual capacity
FVC	Forced vital capacity
IC	Inspiratory capacity
MEFV	Maximal expiratory flow volume curve
METS	Multiple of resting metabolic state. (If resting O_2 consumption is 250 ml, an O_2 consumption of 1 L is 4 METS)
MV	Minute volume
P	Pressure
PA_{O2}, PA_{CO2}	Alveolar partial pressure for oxygen, carbon dioxide, etc.
Pa_{O2}, Pa_{CO2}	Arterial partial pressure for oxygen, carbon dioxide, etc.
PF	Peak flow
Pst	Elastic recoil
$\dot{Q}$	Flow in unit time (blood)
Raw	Airways resistance
RQ	Respiratory quotient
TLC	Total lung capacity
$\dot{V}$	Volume flow of gas per unit of time
$\dot{V}A/Q$ ($\dot{V}/Q$)	Ratio between ventilation and perfusion, with each expressed in the same units
VC	Pulmonary capillary blood volume
VD_A	Anatomical dead space
VD_P	Physiological dead space
VD/VT	Ratio of dead space to tidal volume
VE	Pulmonary ventilation
$\dot{V}_{O2}$(max)	Maximal oxygen uptake
VT	Tidal volume
$\dot{V}$iso $\dot{V}$ (PIF)	Point of identical flow on MEFV curve

Preface
to the First Edition

Almost all physicians, pathologists, and radiologists at some time encounter the problem of occupational lung disease, and not uncommonly difficulties arise in the course of investigation and diagnosis. Descriptions of the classical features of such diseases are hidden in a multitude of early publications, yet often the disease has been modifed by changes in the industrial processes and hygiene. Moreover, new diseases are being described with increasing frequency as modern methods of investigation are brought to bear on new industrial processes and the workers concerned in them. It has become relatively difficult for the practicing clinician to keep in touch with the changes in this expanding field, and this book has been written with the needs of such clinicians primarily in mind. While it is intended especially for those engaged in the practice of internal medicine and the subspecialties of respiratory and occupational medicine, it is hoped that it will be of use also to radiologists and pathologists who may be called upon to assist in the investigation of patients with occupational lung disease.

The preliminary chapters, for two of which we are indebted to our colleagues Drs. Chris Wagner, Roger Seal, and Robert Burrell, are intended more as an outline of current work in the basic subjects of physiology, pathology, immunology, and epidemiology as applied to occupational lung diseases than as a comprehensive review of those subjects. It is hoped, however, that these chapters illustrate the expanding nature of the subject and the number of different resources that are now being applied to the study of this one increasingly important aspect of the general problem of pollution.

Several other friends and colleagues have contributed to the book. We are particularly grateful to Dr. N. LeRoy Lapp, who contributed the chapter on Industrial Bronchitis, and to Drs. E. P. Pendergrass and C. Dundon for advice, criticism, and help throughout. Drs. D. A. Williams, H. M. Foreman, and J. Lyons also gave help and encouragement. The burden of typing was borne by Mrs. D. Thomas and Miss P. Edwards, to whom we are very much indebted. Many other friends have helped at various stages and to all we extend our thanks.

W. KEITH C. MORGAN
ANTHONY SEATON

Contents

1

HISTORICAL AND LEGAL ASPECTS OF INDUSTRIAL DISEASE

W. Keith C. Morgan

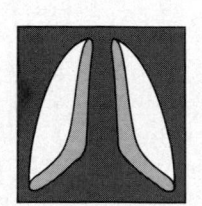

Throughout antiquity and the Middle Ages manual labor was frowned on as unworthy of a gentleman, and the worker in the mechanical arts was felt to be socially inferior. This philosophy prevailed even in the Hellenic civilization. Xenophon in his treatise "Economicus" quotes Socrates as saying the mechanical arts carry a social stigma. It was not until the days of Rousseau, Carlyle, and Marx that manual work became accepted as a respectable vocation. Consequently, diseases peculiar to the working classes attracted little attention until the Renaissance, and it was not until the middle of the sixteenth century that the first attempt was made to relate disease to specific trades.

In the Ertz mountains of Silesia and Bohemia, silver and gold were discovered around A.D. 1000 and mining in this area became the main occupation for the next several centuries. It was in these metal mines that the first observations were made that led to the recognition of dust as an industrial hazard. The earliest account of metal mining was published by George Bauer, commonly known as Georgius Agricola. A Saxon by birth, he was born two years after Columbus rediscovered America. He attended the Universities of Bologna and Venice and in 1526 took up the practice of medicine at Joachimstal. He died in 1555 and it was not until the following year that *De re metallica* was published.[1] This work dealt with all aspects of the mining and smelting of gold and silver. The mining machinery used, the type of ventilation, and the manner in which drainage was effected were all described by him, as were the diseases and accidents to which miners were prone. He was aware of the dangers of inadequate ventilation, and death by suffocation was correctly attributed by him to this cause. Agricola described the harmful effects of dust in these words: "On the other hand, some mines are so dry that they are entirely devoid of water and this dryness causeth the workmen even greater harm, for

1

the dust, which is stirred and beaten up by digging, penetrates into the windpipe and lungs and produces difficulty in breathing and the disease the Greeks call asthma. If the dust has corrosive qualities, it eats away the lungs and implants consumption in the body. In the Carpathian mines, women are found who have married seven husbands, all of whom this terrible consumption has carried away." To avert the unpleasant effects of dust, Agricola recommended the use of ventilating machines.

Some ten or so years after the publication of *De re metallica,* a further monograph appeared devoted to the occupational diseases of gold and silver miners. The author of this was Aureolus Theophrastus Bombastus von Hohenheim, who fortunately was, and is, known by the sobriquet "Paracelsus." This contentious but gifted person studied medicine in Ferrara. In 1515 he was awarded his medical degree and spent the next ten years roaming Europe, enlisting in various armies and living a life of lechery and debauchery. In 1527 he returned to Basle University as a lecturer. A dyed-in-the-wool iconoclast, Paracelsus wrote in German rather than Latin.[2] His lectures were characterized by mordant wit and irreverence; he was daring enough to burn the works of Galen in public and to question the rituals of alchemy. Paracelsus was the first person to realize the benefits of mercury for syphilis and perhaps was the originator of the aphorism, "One night with Venus is followed by seven years with mercury." In 1528 he was compelled to leave Basle and he resumed his nomadic life. He found refuge in 1536 in Salzburg, where he enjoyed the patronage of Prince Ernst of Bavaria. Unfortunately, he met his end in a tavern brawl five years later.

As an astute observer he noticed that cough, shortness of breath, and wasting diseases were more prevalent in certain mines. He attributed these symptoms to either "vapors," "The Heavenly Bodies," or "The Workings of the Gods" rather than dust inhalation. Nonetheless, on other occasions he was more discerning and gave the first good description of erethism, recognizing, moreover, that the disease was produced by the ingestion of mercury.

About a century after Agricola made the first observations concerning the relationship of occupation to disease, Bernardino Ramazzini was born. He was destined to become the Father of Occupational Medicine and lived for over 80 years (1633–1714). He owes his reputation to his treatise *De morbis artificum diatriba,* which was published in 1700.[3] This work is to occupational medicine as Harvey's *De motu cordis* is to physiology.

Ramazzini studied medicine at the University of Parma, where he qualified in 1659. After several years in practice in Rome, he became Professor of Medicine at the University of Modena. He held this position for eighteen years and continued on in Modena for a further twelve years. His researches there were an inspired blend of public health and epidemiology and he wrote extensively on malaria and lathyrism.

In 1700 he moved to Padua as Professor of Medicine. By this time he was known throughout Europe. Over the next few years his eyesight

failed and in 1707 he asked to retire. He was successfully dissuaded, and as a token of the esteem in which he was held was elected President of the Venetian College. He died in 1714 of a stroke.

During his life he looked into the health problems and conditions of workers in numerous occupations, including potters, metal miners, apothecaries, and sulfur workers. It was through his efforts that the vital question "What is your job?" became part of the medical history.

From the time of Ramazzini there has been a gradual increase in the awareness of the dangers of certain occupations, but until Victorian times preventive measures were largely voluntary and depended mainly on the conscience of the employer. With the advent of the Industrial Revolution, the problem of industrial injury and disease increased tenfold. It became obvious that the health of the worker had to be safeguarded and, moreover, that this could be effected only by legislation. The hideous conditions in which the British laboring class worked and lived remained largely unknown and ignored until reformers such as Shaftesbury, Owen, Chadwick, and Simon called them to the attention of the government and people. Dickens' graphic descriptions of mill and factory working life disposed the growing middle class to the need for social and industrial reform. Without adequate morbidity and mortality statistics, truly appalling death rates in certain industries were known only to a few persons. In Sheffield, cutlery trade workers were dying of silicosis with as little as five years' exposure. The condition became known as "grinders' rot." Because of the horrific conditions which prevailed in many factories in which children were employed, a series of acts concerned with the medical supervision of industrial workers were passed. The first of these was the Factory Act of 1844, which made provision for the appointment of factory surgeons to certify that children and other young persons employed in the factories were physically capable of working and were not incapacitated by disease. This was followed by the Factory Act of 1891, which introduced special rules and regulations to protect the health of workers in those industries where dangerous materials were in production or being handled. A detailed and excellent account of the various social and industrial reforms which took place in nineteenth-century Britain and slightly later in America is to be found in Donald Hunter's book *The Diseases of Occupations*.[4]

WORKMEN'S COMPENSATION

In the nineteenth century the only recourse open to a workman who was injured while at work was to bring a common law action against his employer. Since he had neither the understanding nor the money to finance such litigation, successful actions were rare. To help the workmen, Employer's Liability Statutes came into effect. These made provision for financial compensation in the case of industrial disease or injury, but the

employer had three powerful defenses against such actions. Thus, an employer was not held responsible (1) if he could show either that another worker was wholly or partly responsible for the injury, (2) if the injury occurred as a result of the worker's own negligence, or (3) if the workman knew of or should have known that such injury or illness was an inherent risk in his occupation. With such defenses available to the employer, it was indeed unusual for a worker to win his case.

In 1907, industrial injury was responsible for over 7000 deaths among coal miners and railroad workers in the United States, yet very few if any of the workers' families received compensation. Although recompense was in theory available, for the reasons given above, the worker's family seldom received compensation and was usually forced to rely on charity for its subsistence. Compensation under common law for industrially acquired injuries evolved for the most part during a period when most businesses were family concerns with a strictly limited number of employees. When an accident occurred, the employer saw to it that the injured party's medical and financial needs were cared for. Common-law suits attracted little attention and still less sympathy, and the courts were for the most part unconcerned or passive concerning industrial injury.

In the first few years of the twentieth century a series of workmen's compensation acts were put into effect in Britain and slightly later in the United States and Canada. While in Britain the acts applied to the whole country, in the United States and Canada each state or province enacted its own laws. The prime purpose of the workmen's compensation laws was to provide adequate benefits while limiting the employer's liability to workmen's compensation payments. These payments or premiums were to be predetermined so as to avoid uncertainty for the injured worker and the employer. Appropriate medical care was to be provided and costly litigation avoided. Most important of all was the establishment of the principle of liability without fault; the cost of the compensation was to be assigned to the employer, not because he was always culpable, but because of the inherent risks of industrial employment. Thus, assent was given to the concept that awards for industrial injury and sickness were part of the cost of production. The introduction of workmen's compensation was a tremendous social advance, but even so, in the United States obligations for industrial injury and sickness were sometimes inadequate and occasionally evaded, and in addition there were and still are large disparities in compensation between the various states. From 1932 to 1934 over 400 workmen were reported to have died from acute silicosis after working on the Gauley Bridge tunnel in southern West Virginia.[5,6] The bodies were buried in secret so that exhumation was impossible, thereby preventing legal action based on autopsy evidence. Not a single worker received compensation for the illness he contracted, and the families were equally unfortunate. These happenings occurred despite the existence of the state's workmen's compensation laws.

It has become apparent over the years that many other inadequacies

exist in the United States system, and as a result a National Commission was appointed by the President to study the effectiveness and operation of workmen's compensation laws. The Commission published its report in 1972 and detailed three major deficiencies in the present system,[7] including the following:

1. *The number of employees covered by workmen's compensation.* At present only 85 per cent of employees in the United States are covered by state and federal programs. In certain areas and in certain states, barely 50 per cent of the work force is covered. Those excluded from such social programs are usually the lowest paid and the most in need, namely, farm workers, employees of small firms, and temporary laborers. In this regard some states still permit elective coverage.

2. *The variation in injury and diseases covered.* There is little uniformity from state to state as to which diseases or injuries are regarded as occupationally related. Thus, some states do not recognize byssinosis or farmer's lung. Some states recognize only total disability, while others make provision for partial disability. Furthermore, benefits for the same degree of disability differ widely from state to state and in some instances are inadequate. There is a regrettable but easily understood tendency for industry to move to those states where workmen's compensation laws are less liberal. In addition, certain industries have their own federally mandated programs, as, for example, coal miners, whose Federal Coal Mine Health and Safety Act provides infinitely more generous compensation than is available to other workers. Currently, the United States taxpayer is paying $1.5 billion a year for black lung benefits, 40 per cent or more of the total sum disbursed for all industrial injury and illness. Yet there are only 160,000 working coal miners, and probably about twice the number who are retired, as compared to the 80 million other workers covered by workmen's compensation. Thus, 40 per cent of the total awards for injury and illness is going to 1/300th of the working population.

3. *The provision of medical care and rehabilitation services.* The workmen's compensation system provides reasonable cover for medical care; however, only 25 per cent of the beneficiaries receive any form of vocational rehabilitation.

The National Commission published its report in 1972 and made many recommendations, few of which have been put into effect. For the most part they continued to recommend that each state continue with its own set of laws, failing to realize that the present system guarantees that inequities will persist and that uniformity will not be achieved. In Britain, in contrast to the United States and Canada, workmen's compensation laws apply to the whole country, benefits are uniform, and there are no regional differences in the administration of workmen's compensation laws.

Aside from workmen's compensation, workmen have the right to bring a law suit against a company if they consider that the company or

employer has been negligent and has not conformed to the legislated rules and regulations. In Canada such an option is not available in most provinces, and once the worker has been awarded compensation, he forfeits the right to sue his employer. In the United States, however, many lawyers take cases on a contingency basis, and as such their fee is related to whether they win the suit and on the extent of the damages that the particular claimant is awarded—all of which are strong incentives to enter into litigation. There is little doubt that in the United States at the present time an attempt is being made to relate virtually all naturally occurring disease to occupational exposure, and suits for all types of so-called occupational injury and illness are two a penny.[8, 9] The present system has done much to undermine the public's faith in the legal and medical professions, but since vast sums of money are involved, it is likely to persist. Under such circumstances one cannot but sympathize with Jonathan Swift when he defined lawyers as a "breed of men bred from their youth in the art of proving by words that white is black and black is white, according as they are paid."

TORT AND CIVIL LIABILITY

In Britain the issue of tort has been the subject of much discussion, and in 1973 a Royal Commission on civil liability and compensation was set up. The stimulus to the appointment of the Commission was the Report of the Robens Committee on Safety and Health at Work. The charge given to the Commission was to consider to what extent, under what circumstances, and by what means compensation should be payable for death or injuries suffered under the following five circumstances:

1. In the course of employment.
2. During the use of a motor vehicle or other means of transportation.
3. Through the manufacture, supply, or use of goods or services.
4. On property belonging to or occupied by another party.
5. Otherwise through an act of omission by another person where compensation is recoverable only on proof of fault or under rules of strict liability.

In more simple terms the Commission was charged with producing a report which would recommend the first steps to be taken towards the introduction of an unified system that would deal with all injuries and would apply to the whole country. In time the system would be extended so that provision would be made to compensate all disabled persons irrespective of cause, that is to say, whether the disability was the result of injury or of acquired or congenital disease.

The recommendations of the Commission were eventually published in what has become known as the Pearson Report.[10] Some of the more radical suggestions relate to modifications of the laws of tort, namely,

those actions arising from private or civil wrongs. While not recommending the complete abolition of tort, the report did seek to limit its role as a means of obtaining redress for injury. The Commission suggested putting an end to double compensation, e.g., by offsetting Social Security payments against tort damages. It also recommended that compensation awards should be indexed so that the payments did not decrease with inflation. Other suggestions related to the elimination of certain minor claims and changes in the method of assessment of damages. The Pearson Report can be regarded as a landmark and a first step towards achieving a comprehensive and equitable compensation for all forms of disability.[11] It proposes and supports the concept of no-fault, and suggests that those who are disabled should be compensated because of their needs rather than because of another's fault.

Inherent in any civilized society is the tenet that such a society should provide its disabled members with sufficient financial support for the necessities of life. Ethically and morally it matters little whether the disability is industrially acquired or not. If this doctrine is accepted, the same impairment and the same disability should receive the same compensation. The present tort laws suggest that the person who loses a leg in an industrial injury is somehow worthy of greater compensation than the man who through no fault of his own loses a leg in a car accident. In the United States it is clear that the only way of establishing equal compensation for equal disability is through a federal workmen's compensation system administered in the same fashion as Social Security.[12] This would necessitate a actuarial calculation of the frequency of industrial injury and disease throughout the nation. Based on these data, every employee would pay a premium into a centrally administered fund. Also being paid into the same fund would be that portion of each Social Security payment that is applied towards premature retirement and permanent disability awards. Such a system would ensure that the employer would be compelled to assume financial responsibility for industrial injury and disease, and premiums could be weighted according to the health and safety record of the company concerned. Impairment would then be determined by a panel of physicians with wide experience in disability assessment, rather than being left to the whims of a sympathetic but partial jury and the cupidity of a financially involved lawyer.[12]

With the passage of time, more and more industrial hazards are being recognized. In the last few years, the hazards of exposure to asbestos, detergent enzymes, and polyurethane foams have been described. Inevitably there is a delay in the introduction of measures designed to prevent or control such diseases, and it is usually even longer before the legislative action that gives them official recognition comes into effect. There is little doubt that with advancing technology, new industrial hazards will develop and as such, their initial recognition will depend on somebody asking the time-honored question "What is your job?"

References

1. Agricola, G., De re metallica, 1556. Hoover, H. C., and Hoover, L. H., translators, The Mining Magazine (London), 1912.
2. Paracelsus, T., Von der Bergsucht, Dilinger, 1567.
3. Ramazzini, B., De morbis artificum diatriba, Geneva, 1713. Wright, W. C., translator, Chicago, University of Chicago Press, 1940.
4. Hunter, D., The Diseases of Occupations, 6th ed. London, English Universities Press. 1978.
5. Skidmore, H., Hawk's Nest, West Virginia Heritage *4*, 1, 1970.
6. Subcommittee of the Committee of Labor, House of Representatives, An investigation relating to health conditions of workers employed in construction and maintenance of public utilities, 74th Congress, H. J. Res. *449*, 2603, 1936.
7. Report of the National Commission on State Workmen's Compensation Laws. Washington, D.C., Government Printing Office, 1972.
8. Morgan, W. K. C., On disability, demagoguery, and dialectic. Forum XIV, *3*, 473, 1979. Published by the American Bar Association.
9. Morgan, W. K. C., Compensation for industrial injury and disease. Am. Rev. Respir. Dis. *114*, 1047, 1976.
10. The Report of the Royal Commission on Civil Liability, Compensation for Personal Injury, Vol. 1. London, Her Majesty's Stationery Office, 1978.
11. Collinson, J. M., The Pearson report. Br. J. Ind. Med. *36*, 263, 1979.
12. Morgan, W. K. C., The adversary system: cui bono? Ann. Int. Med. *97*, 919, 1982.

2

THE CLINICAL APPROACH

Anthony Seaton

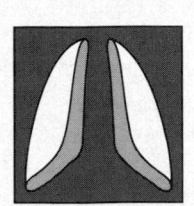

Understanding of occupational lung diseases has come from two different but complementary approaches, clinical and epidemiological. It is usual for the initial suspicion of a hazard to arise from an observation by a clinician and then for the inter-relationships between the hazardous material and the lung's reaction to it to be investigated by the epidemiologist. The clinician may be a physician investigating an obscure lung disease, as was the case with farmer's lung[1]; a pathologist, as when Wagner noted a high prevalence of mesothelioma in parts of South Africa[2]; or a radiologist noticing an unusual radiographic abnormality, as when stannosis was described.[3] In all such cases, the key factor has been the clinician's awareness that pulmonary disease may have an external cause and that the cause may be related to the occupation of the patient.

The increasing complexity of industry, and particularly the newer aspects of the chemical and plastics industries, means that workers may be exposed to respiratory hazards of which they and often management are unaware. Perhaps the greatest increase in pulmonary hazards over the last few years has been in the occupational allergic disorders, asthma and allergic alveolitis, where new sensitizing agents are being described with alarming frequency. It is therefore particularly important that physicians, especially those specializing in internal, respiratory, and occupational medicine, be aware that many lung diseases have an external cause and understand how to investigate such patients to confirm or deny the suspicion of such a cause.

THE HISTORY

The essential question to ask is "What is your work?" Since this often elicits an incomprehensible reply (filler, sagger-maker's, bottom knocker, fettler, and so on), it is necessary to ask the patient for supplementary details. Most patients warm to this task and a genuine interest shown by the physician is an excellent way of establishing rapport. In some cases,

9

especially if the patient has only been in his present job for a short time, it is necessary to inquire about previous jobs, and it is always wise to ask specifically if the patient has worked with asbestos or in any particularly dusty jobs. It is also well to remember that some patients may have a part-time occupation, such as running a small farm or pigeon breeding, that could harm their lungs. In finding out a patient's job it is also important to establish how long he has done it and the relationship of symptoms to time in the job. In general, mineral pneumoconioses such as silicosis or asbestosis require regular exposure to dust over many years before symptoms develop, whereas allergic alveolitis may start after as little as one year of exposure but once it has developed may be provoked by minute, sometimes undetectable doses of the sensitizer. Byssinosis can only be diagnosed by a careful history[4] that describes the characteristic exacerbations which initially occur in the early part of the week and later extend throughout the week. Similarly, the disease called humidifier fever[5] may present with symptoms of chills and cough on Mondays and is very likely to be misdiagnosed if its regular relationship to the work week is not discovered.

The importance of a careful occupational history is illustrated by the following case report, in which the patient's job superficially sounded quite harmless:

Mrs. F had worked for the same company in a clerical post for 30 years. She described her present occupation as a camera operator. She presented to the chest clinic with progressive breathlessness due to upper lobe fibrosis. Inquiry as to details of her work revealed that she operated a dry industrial camera in a confined space and that she used a dusting powder to clean off the plates when they had been exposed. She described her work as dusty, the powder lying about the room and even being thought responsible for jamming another machine in the same room. A sample of the powder showed it to be diatomaceous earth, 100 per cent silica, a fact of which her employers were unaware. Though the discovery was made too late to help the patient, it did prevent other people from suffering the same fate.

Sometimes the patient's knowledge of his or her work and of possible hazards is incomplete, and in such cases if there is a strong suspicion of work-associated disease, further information may be obtained from the company physician or from the patient's trade union.

Mr. B was a laborer in a factory producing electrical domestic apparatus. He had developed asthma, which he did not relate to his work, but his wife was quite sure that he was better at weekends and on vacation. Her suspicion was confirmed by peak flow rate recordings. The local trade union official provided a list of substances which were

used in the factory and this list included isocyanates. Subsequent challenge testing confirmed his sensitivity to toluene diisocyanate and redeployment within the company allowed him to cease exposure and be relieved of his asthma.

In addition to giving clues to the etiology of lung disease, the clinical history should include an assessment of the patient's disability. This is not only essential in medicolegal cases (see Chapter 3) but is also a most important part of making the diagnosis. Abnormal shortness of breath is almost always the result either of cardiac disease or of obstructive or restrictive lung disease. If one of these is not present, psychoneurosis or simple lead-swinging is likely to be the cause. The physiological patterns of different occupational lung diseases are for the most part well described, and the physician is therefore able to fit a suspected diagnosis with the symptoms appropriate to the known physiological effects of that condition. For example, paroxysmal episodes of wheeze and nocturnal breathlessness are wholly consistent with exposure to flour in a bakery and bakers' asthma, while progressively increasing exertional dyspnea is similarly consistent with asbestosis in an insulation worker. Equally important, exertional dyspnea is not consistent with the sole diagnosis of simple coal workers' pneumoconiosis or stannosis, and in such cases an alternative cause should be sought.

Mr. L, a nonsmoker, had worked for 35 years at the coal face, having retired on health grounds three years before being referred to the chest clinic. His symptoms were increasing shortness of breath on exertion and dry cough, and for the past year he had been too breathless to leave his house. His breathing was worse in the mornings and frequently woke him in the small hours. A chest radiograph three years previously had shown category 3 simple pneumoconiosis and he had been told that his symptoms were due to that disease and that nothing could be done.

Knowledge that simple pneumoconiosis is not a cause of respiratory disability prompted further investigation. His disability was found to be the result of airways obstruction, which responded to corticosteroids, and once the asthma was controlled he was able to return to a fully active life.

THE PHYSICAL EXAMINATION

The most striking finding in most patients with occupational lung diseases is the relative absence of physical signs. Certain conditions are nonetheless associated with physical signs, and the alert physician will note both their absence when a disease in which they should occur is suspected as well as their presence when the suspected disease is not usually

associated with signs. Either finding should give rise to the consideration of an alternative diagnosis.

Clubbing of the digits is a physical sign that is easy to recognize when advanced and equally easy to exclude when the finger ends are completely normal. It should be noted that there are many situations in which it is not possible to be sure. Gross clubbing has also passed through a stage of transformation from normal to abnormal, and many normal nails are in a permanent shape suggestive of this stage of transformation. Repeated injury to the fingers often causes deformity resembling clubbing. It is the author's practice to grade clubbing as present, absent, or "don't know." In the latter cases, a tracing of the finger end on the patient's chart or a photograph allows later assessment of any change.

Clubbing occurs in asbestosis and usually appears after other evidence of the disease has become apparent. It does not normally occur in other mineral pneumoconioses or allergic alveolitis, and if it is present when one of these is suspected, it is wise to assume that the diagnosis is wrong or that the patient has an additional disease. The most common nonoccupational causes of clubbing are bronchial carcinoma and cryptogenic pulmonary fibrosis. Other diseases with which it is occasionally associated include hepatic cirrhosis, coeliac disease, bronchiectasis, chronic pulmonary tuberculosis, and lung abscess.

Bilateral, repetitive basal crackles are heard in asbestosis and in acute and chronic allergic alveolitis. They are not heard in silicosis or coal workers' pneumoconiosis. However, the same types of crackles are heard in many nonoccupational diseases, for example, cryptogenic pulmonary fibrosis, bronchiectasis, left ventricular failure, and pneumonia. Similar crackles that clear after a few deep breaths are commonly heard at the lung bases in patients on first waking and in the obese. For this reason it is important to make the patient take a few deep breaths and cough before listening carefully over the lower parts of the lungs for such crackles. If then they are heard to recur on several breaths, organic lung disease can be assumed to be present.

Distinction must be drawn between the crackles typical of pulmonary fibrosis, allergic alveolitis, and left ventricular failure, which occur in the middle and towards the end of inspiration and are always maximal in the dependent parts of the lung, and those due to bronchiectasis and pneumonia, which occur over the affected site. Moreover, repetitive crackles occurring in early inspiration occur in conditions associated with severe airways obstruction. Mid- and late inspiratory crackles are believed to be generated by delayed opening of small airways, each crackle characteristically occurring at the same transpulmonary pressure in each respiratory cycle.[6, 7] Such crackles are an important finding in suspected asbestosis, their presence in association with an appropriate exposure history considerably increasing the likelihood of the diagnosis. The more advanced the disease, the further up the lung from the bases they are heard. In allergic alveolitis, crackles may be the only physical sign and, again in the presence

of an appropriate exposure history, considerable weight should be attached to this finding.

Mrs. W worked in a pet shop. For the past year she had complained of exertional dyspnea, varying from day to day with no obvious pattern. Bilateral basal crackles were heard at the ends of inspiration. Her chest radiograph and spirometry were within normal limits and precipitating antibodies to parakeet serum, droppings, and feathers were absent from her serum. In view of the crackles, further investigation was carried out. A slightly reduced lung diffusing capacity was found and percutaneous lung biopsy showed evidence of extrinsic allergic alveolitis. Finally a challenge test with parakeet extract produced a rise in temperature and a further fall in transfer factor after 4 hours, confirming the diagnosis. A short course of corticosteroids and avoidance of further exposure prevented further symptoms.

Other physical signs are of less importance in occupational lung diseases. Intermittent wheezing may alert the occupational physician to work-related asthma, and the overinflation, quiet breath sounds, and hyper-resonance associated with advanced emphysema may be found in a proportion of patients with either chronic allergic alveolitis or progressive massive fibrosis. The newly described technique of auscultatory percussion[8] may be an aid to the detection of masses in the latter condition, though the general availability of chest radiographs has allowed physicians to manage without this technique.

It should be remembered that physical examination of the chest, though traditionally emphasizing anatomical abnormalities, also gives considerable insight into pulmonary function. Measurement of chest expansion and diaphragmatic excursion gives a good indication of vital capacity; forced expiratory time is the best clinical test of airways obstruction[9] and noisy breathing at the mouth denotes narrowing of the large airways[7]; while the relative intensity of breath sounds heard over the chest relates to regional ventilation.[10] Moreover, a simple exercise test, such as the 12-minute walking distance, is a useful indicator of exercise tolerance. These clinical tests should be among the techniques that a physician can deploy in the assessment of pulmonary disorders.

CLINICAL INVESTIGATION

In most patients in whom an occupational lung disease is suspected, relatively little investigation is required beyond the history and physical examination. A chest radiograph is of course essential, and is regarded by most chest physicians as a part of the examination. Some occupational lung diseases, for example, coal workers' pneumoconiosis and silicosis, are

in practice only diagnosed on their radiological appearances. In others, such as asbestosis, serious doubts are cast on the diagnosis in the absence of an abnormal radiograph. However, contrary to the belief of some lawyers and even some of their medical witnesses, the chest radiograph is not an infallible guide to diagnosis. A normal radiograph is, of course, to be expected in occupational asthma and byssinosis, but it is not infrequent to find no abnormality in allergic alveolitis, where even quite extensive interstitial pneumonitis can exist in spite of a film regarded as within normal limits. Conversely, small irregular shadows are frequently seen on radiographs of the elderly, especially those with chronic bronchitis, in the absence of dust exposure. Such age-related changes are indistinguishable from the early signs of asbestosis. Moreover, the interpretation of radiographic appearances is subject to wide inter- and intraobserver differences, and the sensible clinician in investigating suspected occupational lung disease will *record* changes seen and only attempt to *interpret* those changes in the light of other evidence from history, lung-function testing, and so on. The uncertainties and variability attendant upon radiographic interpretation may be a considerable source of problems in epidemiological studies, and great care has to be taken in designing such studies to overcome this. The use of a standard set of radiographs,[11] several readers, and multiple readings has gone a long way towards solving these problems. However, uncertainty in the interpretation of a radiograph is reduced more by looking elsewhere for evidence than by comparison with standard films.

The other investigation most likely to be helpful is pulmonary function testing. Here the tests should be determined by the suspected diagnosis. To the nonphysiologist, a bewildering array of tests is available, but, fortunately, in clinical practice only a few of these are helpful and these are all relatively simple. Any organic pulmonary disorder causing disability must be associated with a functional abnormality either of airways caliber or of gas transfer and/or lung volumes. Fixed airways obstruction, as in chronic byssinosis and emphysema, is best demonstrated by simple spirometry, while variable obstruction such as that which occurs in occupational asthma is best diagnosed by asking the patient to record frequent peak flow rates with a portable meter—a process infinitely cheaper and more valuable than body plethysmography. Diseases such as asbestosis and silicosis, which cause pulmonary fibrosis, are best assessed by measurement of vital capacity, lung volumes, and diffusing capacity. Exercise testing is of value in assessing exercise tolerance, and the more complicated exercise tests with arterial gas analysis are useful in excluding the presence of any organic cause for respiratory disability. Measurement of compliance, closing volumes, flow-volume loops, and airways resistance are fun for the physiologist but are of little additional clinical value, and physicians dealing with occupational lung diseases should think twice, or preferably more often, before putting their patients through the expense of undergoing them.

Blood tests make less contribution to the diagnosis of occupational

lung diseases than in many other areas of medicine. Positive diagnostic help may be obtained in allergic alveolitis, in those instances in which precipitating antibody may be found, and in some cases of occupational asthma in which specific IgE antibody may be demonstrated by radioallergosorbent test (RAST). Tests for rheumatoid factors may help in the diagnosis of Caplan's syndrome and very occasionally measurements of blood or urine levels may help in the diagnosis of acute toxic pneumonitis. In most occupational lung diseases, however, the hazard is known, and the diagnostic problem is to demonstrate whether the disease is present.

The most difficult decisions to make in the investigation of occupational lung disease are whether or not to perform challenge tests or lung biopsy. In general, since both these procedures entail a small hazard, they should not be performed unless there is serious doubt about the diagnosis. Challenge testing needs to be done in occasional cases of allergic alveolitis or asthma in which the diagnosis or the allergen is in doubt. A test approximating most closely the environment of the patient's work (and that may mean a test done at the patient's place of work) is probably the safest, but close medical supervision is always necessary. A proper question for the physician to ask before performing such a test is whether the result, whatever it is, will alter the management of the patient. It is not ethically justifiable to subject one's patient to such procedures for medicolegal reasons.

Lung biopsy is potentially more hazardous than challenge testing and rarely needs to be done when an occupational cause is seriously suspected. In the author's practice, biopsies on patients with occupational lung disease have usually been performed when a cause other than occupational was seriously considered and management depended on knowing which condition the patient had. If lung biopsy is considered necessary, the choice should depend on the physician's experience. Probably the most generally used technique since fiberoptic bronchoscopy was introduced has been transbronchial biopsy. This has the disadvantage of producing such small fragments that the pathologist is often unable to narrow the differential diagnosis. Open lung biopsy provides excellent specimens for the pathologist, though it is much more uncomfortable for the patient. For diffuse disease, which occupational disease usually is, a cutting needle is traumatic and can cause serious hemorrhage. Use of the Steel high-speed drill[12] is less likely to tear the lung and is the technique that the author favors; it usually produces a good core of lung. If the patient breathes oxygen for a few minutes beforehand, pneumothorax is rarely troublesome, though death from hemorrhage has been reported from this as well as from all other pulmonary and bronchial biopsy procedures. None of these tests should be embarked upon lightly.

MANAGEMENT

An interest in occupational lung disease often extends only to diagnosis of the conditions. The clinician, however, also has the problem of

management of the patient once the diagnosis has been made. Management can be divided into assessment of the disability, prognosis, treatment, and advice.

Assessment of disability is essential to making a reasonable prognosis and advising the patient on such matters as future employment prospects. Disability is a measurement of the patient's inability to perform normal daily tasks, and therefore is more than just a measure of lung function. Its assessment has to take account of lung function, the patient's work requirements, and his psychological reaction to the illness. Prognosis is based on knowledge of the natural history of the patient's illness, information that this book is intended to provide, and of the stage of physiological deterioration that the clinical examination and testing have revealed. Armed with this information, the physician can plan the treatment in order to attempt to alter the course of the disease or palliate its symptoms.

In many cases of occupational lung disease therapeutics has little part to play, and treatment usually consists of advice on avoiding future exposure to dust or fumes at work. It should not be forgotten, however, that some diseases may be affected by corticosteroids. Berylliosis and, probably, acute toxic pneumonitis respond to these drugs, and allergic alveolitis may require such treatment in addition to avoidance of further exposure. The mineral pneumoconioses in general do not respond to therapy, but they vary considerably in their natural histories; due account of this should be taken in advising the patient. For example, a coal miner developing the early signs of pneumoconiosis five years before he is due to retire would be well advised to continue at work, since he is unlikely to progress to massive fibrosis at that stage of his life. Similarly, radiological shadowing in a welder or foundryman need not cause concern unless it is felt to be due to a nonoccupational cause, as siderosis is a benign condition. However, pneumoconiosis in a 40-year-old coal miner or asbestosis at any age are indications to cease further dust exposure, since both entail a serious risk of progression to crippling disease.

The most difficult aspect of the management of patients with occupational lung disease is giving sensible advice. The usual explanations of causation, treatment, and prognosis need to be amplified by advice on employment. More harm may be done by well-intentioned but incorrect advice on future employment, based on an imperfect knowledge of the disease, than by the disease itself. Furthermore, the knowledge that his disease was caused by his occupation not infrequently gives rise to resentment in the patient and, with a little help from legal advisers and union officials, to thoughts of compensation. Society inevitably has to accept some cost in human health for the benefits of industry's productivity, and while in a just society all ill health should attract appropriate compensation whatever its cause, regrettably Utopia is not yet with us. Compensation laws and their interpretation differ from country to country and from state to state, and benefits are often inequitable or inadequate.

In such a situation common law claims for injury due to an employer's negligence are an understandable and frequent outcome of the diagnosis of occupational lung disease. The clinician may well be asked by the patient whether or not to pursue such a claim. In such circumstances he should confine himself to advising on diagnosis, causation, and management and leave legal advice, particularly on matters of liability and negligence, to lawyers. Here, as in other fields, medicolegal considerations can be a dangerous distraction from objectivity in doing one's best for one's patient.

The chest physician is in the unusual position of dealing with an organ of which the diseases are largely caused by outside agents, be they bacteria, allergens, cigarette smoke, or other pollutants. The pollutants to which man is exposed in his occupation are an important source of lung diseases and constitute a challenge to the alert physician. The physician who bears this in mind will not only help his or her patients but will also lead the way in preventing disease in others. The key to this is still, as in the time of Ramazzini, the question "What is your job?"

References

1. Campbell, J. M., Acute symptoms following work with hay. Br. Med. J., 2, 1143, 1932.
2. Wagner, J. C., Sleggs, C. A., and Marchand, P., Diffuse pleural mesothelioma and asbestos exposure in the North-West Cape Province. Br. J. Ind. Med., 17, 260, 1960.
3. Pendergrass, E. P., and Pryde, A. W., Benign pneumoconiosis due to tin oxide: a case report with experimental investigation of the radiographic density of the tin oxide dust. J. Ind. Hyg., 30, 119, 1948.
4. Lee, W. R., Clinical diagnosis of byssinosis. Thorax, 34, 287, 1979.
5. MRC Symposium. Humidifier fever. Thorax, 32, 653, 1977.
6. Nath, A. R., and Capel, L. H., Inspiratory crackles and mechanical events of breathing. Thorax, 29, 695, 1974.
7. Forgacs, P., Lung Sounds. London, Baillière Tindall, 1978.
8. Guarino, J. R., Auscultatory percussion of the chest. Lancet, 1, 1332, 1980.
9. Macdonald, J. B., Cole, T. J., and Seaton, A., Forced expiratory time—its reliability as a lung function test. Thorax, 30, 554, 1975.
10. Leblanc, P., Macklem, P. T., and Ross, W. R. D., Breath sounds and the distribution of pulmonary ventilation. Am. Rev. Resp. Dis., 102, 10, 1970.
11. ILO/UC international classification of radiographs of pneumoconioses. Occupational Safety and Health, Series 22. Geneva, International Labor Organization, 1972.
12. Steel, S. J., and Winstanley, D. P., Lung biopsy with a high-speed air drill. Thorax, 22, 286, 1967.

3

PULMONARY PHYSIOLOGY— Its Application to the Determination of Respiratory Impairment and Disability in Industrial Lung Disease*

W. Keith C. Morgan and Douglas Seaton

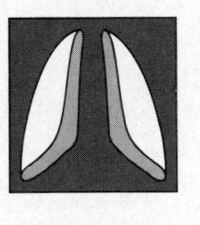

The primary purpose of the lungs is to maintain the oxygen and carbon dioxide content of the arterial blood within a relatively narrow range. This has to be effected despite the fact that both oxygen needs and carbon dioxide production are constantly changing with the degree of activity and metabolic rate of the subject. The lungs achieve this homeostasis by allowing venous blood to come into contact with the alveolar gases; such contact taking place over an enormous surface area, the alveolocapillary bed. Three basic mechanisms are involved in gas exchange, namely, (1) ventilation, or, as it is often known, the bellows function of the lungs, (2) diffusion, or the transfer of gas from the alveolus to the capillary, and (3) perfusion, or pulmonary blood flow.

VENTILATION

The ventilatory capacity of the lungs depends first on the size of the lungs (lung volumes), second, on the resistance to flow present in the

*Portions of this chapter also appear in W. Keith C. Morgan and D. Seaton, Pulmonary ventilation and blood gas exchange, in W. A. Sodeman, Jr., and T. M. Sodeman, Pathologic Physiology, 7th ed. Philadelphia, W. B. Saunders Co., 1984.

airways, and third, on the elastic properties or compliance of the lungs and the chest wall. Movement of air in and out of the lungs can be compared to the action of a pair of bellows, and is dependent on the pressure difference between the mouth and the alveoli at various phases of breathing. At times of no flow, alveolar and mouth pressure are equal. During inspiration, the thorax enlarges, the diaphragm descends, and as a result the chest cage increases in volume, as do the lungs. In contrast, expiration is largely passive and depends on the elastic recoil of the chest wall and lungs. The pressure that acts upon the lungs and causes them to expand during inspiration is that which exists in the pleural cavity. Intrapleural pressure is negative as compared to the atmospheric pressure, and during normal breathing varies between -5 and -9 cm of water. Much larger pressure changes occur during forced expiratory and inspiratory maneuvers; for example, at total lung capacity, the intrapleural pressure is -35 to -40 cm of water, while at residual volume, the pressure may become slightly positive, especially at the lung bases. A detailed description of the mechanical events involved in inspiration is beyond the scope of this chapter but can be found in *The Respiratory Muscles.*[1]

At this stage it is necessary to point out there is a gradient in pleural pressure from the top to the bottom of the lung. This gradient is largely gravity dependent and is thought to be related to the weight of the lung. Pleural pressure increases from the apex to the base; there being a gradient of around 7 to 8 cm of water from top to bottom of the lung. This gradient has profound effects on regional ventilation and perfusion and will be discussed in more detail later in the chapter.

Static Lung Volumes

Certain lung volumes can be measured with a spirometer; however, others require more complicated apparatus. The volume of each breath exhaled during quiet respiration is known as the tidal volume (V_T). The total volume of air that the lungs and bronchial tree contain after maximal inspiration is known as the total lung capacity (TLC). If the subject then exhales as much air as he can, the volume of air remaining in the lungs after the expiration is known as the residual volume (RV), while that which has been expelled is known as the vital capacity (VC). It must be stressed that during the measurement of VC, the patient is permitted to take as long as he likes to complete the maneuver. If after maximal inspiration, he exhales as rapidly and as forcibly as possible, then the measurement obtained is known as the forced vital capacity (FVC). In normal persons the FVC and the VC are not significantly different; however, in certain types of airways obstruction, e.g., emphysema, the FVC may be considerably less than the VC as a result of collapse of the smaller airways during forced expiration; this is a phenomenon known as air trapping. The volume of air remaining in the lung at the end of a

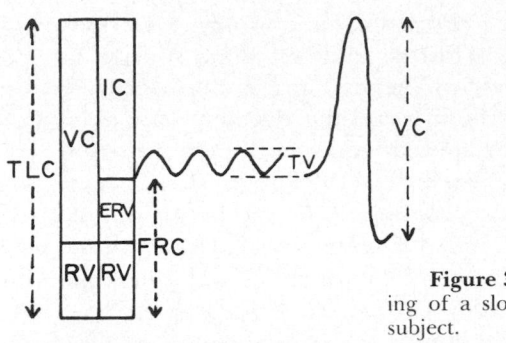

Figure 3–1. Lung volumes and spirometric tracing of a slow vital capacity maneuver in a normal subject.

normal tidal expiration is known as the functional residual capacity (FRC), whereas the volume that can be exhaled from FRC is known as the expiratory reserve volume (ERV). Similarly, the volume of air that can be taken in from FRC is known as the inspiratory capacity (IC) and, needless to say, the sum of the ERV and IC equals the VC (Fig. 3–1). The VC, ERV, and IC can be measured with a spirometer; TLC and its derivatives, FRC and RV, require other means, namely, closed-circuit helium equilibration, the nitrogen washout, a radiographic method, or plethysmography. The helium equilibration method depends on the subject rebreathing a known volume of helium in a closed circuit until equilibration is reached. The carbon dioxide produced during the rebreathing is absorbed. If the volume of the helium reservoir is known, and if the initial and final concentrations of the helium in the system are known, it is therefore possible to calculate the FRC. The nitrogen washout depends on giving the subject 100 per cent oxygen, and collecting all the expired air in a large spirometer. When the nitrogen has been completely washed out from the lungs and collected along with the expired air in a Tissot spirometer, the volume of the expirate and the nitrogen concentration are measured. Since the concentration of nitrogen in the lungs at the start of the maneuver is known, it is therefore possible to calculate the volume of nitrogen present in the lungs and hence the FRC.

The plethysmographic method is probably the best and most accurate way of determining lung volumes, since it measures all the gas in the thoracic cage. In contrast, the helium equilibration and nitrogen washout methods do not include regions of poorly ventilated lung that contain trapped gas, e.g., bullae, and thus falsely low estimates are obtained. A body plethysmograph consists of an air-tight box, in which the subject sits. As the subject breathes in and out, the pressure inside the box changes and is recorded by sensitive transducers. If the change in lung volume with each breath is also known, then by simple application of Boyle's law it is possible to calculate the intrathoracic gas volume.

Total lung capacity can also be accurately determined from the chest film. Barnhard and his colleagues have described a method which utilizes anteroposterior and lateral films.[2] The method depends on treating the

lungs as a series of elliptical cylindroids and calculating the volume of each. Allowance is made for heart size, pulmonary blood volume, the spine, and domes of the diaphragm. The method has been simplified by Reger and his co-workers,[3] is accurate, and has application to epidemiological surveys. If the VC is determined by spirometry, it then becomes possible to measure the RV and hence the RV/TLC.

In a healthy young adult, the residual volume (RV) is around 20 per cent of the total lung capacity (TLC). As the subject grows older, the RV slowly increases so that by the age of 60 it may constitute up to 40 per cent of the TLC. The increase in RV is related to the fact that with increasing age the lung loses some of its elasticity. The decreased elastic recoil of the older person is opposed by an unchanged but relatively greater intrapleural pressure which maintains the lungs at a higher level of inflation than present previously when the subject was younger. The increased lung volumes and associated increased radiographic translucency that occurs with age used to be known as senile emphysema; however, since there is neither airways obstruction nor disruption of the alveolocapillary surface, the term is a misnomer.

In obstructive airways disease and emphysema, the RV/TLC is increased and in many instances the RV may be well over 50 per cent of the TLC (Fig. 3–2). An increased RV/TLC is an almost invariable finding in air flow obstruction but lesser increases in the ratio are sometimes seen in diffuse fibrosis, such as occurs in fibrosing alveolitis or asbestosis. Such increases are often more apparent than real, and are often related either to inadequacies in the predicted values for RV and TLC or sometimes to an appreciable decrease in TLC with the RV being less affected. In most subjects with emphysema, the TLC is increased above the predicted figure owing to a decrease in the elastic recoil of the lungs; however, the increase in TLC is not as dramatic as the increase in RV. In the diffuse fibroses all the lung volumes tend to be smaller than the predicted figure, and this is particularly true of the VC and TLC (Fig. 3–3). In contrast, and for the reasons mentioned above, changes in RV are sometimes less spectacular in pulmonary fibrosis. Thus in an individual subject, small increases in the RV/TLC are not necessarily diagnostic of any particular type of

Figure 3–2. Lung volumes and spirometric tracing of a slow vital capacity maneuver in a subject with airways obstruction. The hatched area represents predicted values.

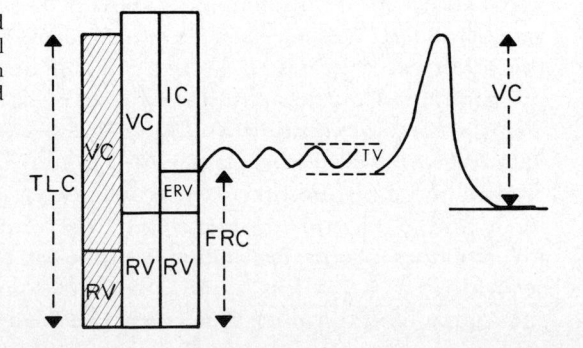

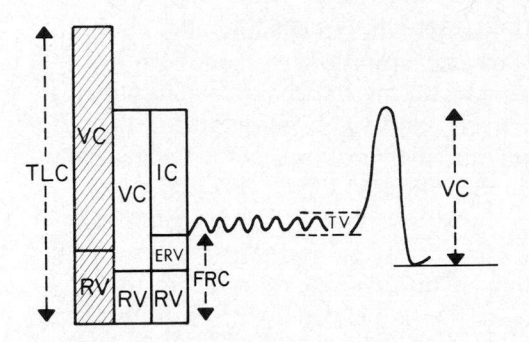

Figure 3–3. Lung volumes and spirometric tracing of a slow vital capacity in a subject with diffuse fibrosis. The hatched area represents predicted values.

physiological impairment, and in many subjects there is a mixed effect, the subject having some degree of airways obstruction and then subsequently contracting another disease which produces stiff and smaller lungs. In epidemiological studies a knowledge of the RV/TLC in large groups of persons is much more useful than it is in the individual. Thus the demonstration in a particular group of subjects that the sample as a whole has an increased RV/TLC as compared to a comparable control group indicates a higher prevalence of airways obstruction or emphysema.

Dynamic Lung Volumes

Ventilatory capacity also depends to a large extent on the resistance to air flow in the bronchial tree. If a normal young subject is asked to take in as big a breath as he can, and then to blow it out as rapidly and as forcibly as possible, he should be able to get out 80 per cent of his FVC in 1 second (FEV_1) and 95 per cent in 3 seconds. While this is true for the young subject, there is a fall in the FEV_1/FVC ratio with age, and by the time the subject is 55 or over, the ratio will often be around 65 to 70 per cent. Expiratory flows are most rapid early in the forced expiratory volume maneuver, but as the subject begins to approach RV, there is a marked slowing. This is most evident once the subject gets below his FRC, and when RV is reached flow ceases entirely (Fig. 3–4). Subjects with airways obstruction, that is to say, those who have an increased resistance to airflow in and out of their lungs, namely, asthmatics, chronic bronchitics, and those with emphysema, all show a flatter curve with decreased flow rates. In some instances, there is also a loss of VC. In asthma, but not in the other two conditions, the use of bronchodilators such as isoproterenol or salbutamol by nebulization will appreciably lessen the obstruction so that the forced expiratory volume curve becomes steeper and more closely resembles that of a normal person. As indices of obstruction, both the 1-second and 3-second timed vital capacity tests (percentage of FVC exhaled in 1 and 3 seconds respectively) are frequently used. A minority of investigators prefer the actual volume of air exhaled in the first 0.75 second ($FEV_{0.75}$). A less popular but still commonly used measurement is the maximal expiratory flow rate (MEFR), this being the rate of flow

between 200 and 1200 ml on a forced expiratory volume tracing. Another index which has its advocates is the FEF_{25-75} (MMF), or the maximal expiratory flow over the midhalf of a forced expiratory spirogram. The latter measurement may be more sensitive but it is also more variable, and if the forced expiratory volume maneuver is not recorded for long enough, spurious results are frequently obtained. All of these indices have their proponents, but there are valid reasons for preferring the FEV_1.

An additional method by which the ventilatory capacity can be assessed is the maximal breathing capacity (MBC). This should preferably be known as the maximal voluntary ventilation (MVV) and is the maximal volume of air that is breathed over one minute. As the test is very tiring to subjects with airways obstruction, the volume is usually measured over a period of 15 to 20 seconds and the result multiplied by the necessary factor. This test is effort dependent and has little advantage over the single breath tests. To help those physicians who were brought up on this measurement, the simple expedient of multiplying the FEV_1 by 40 yields an excellent approximation to the measured MVV.

The normal respiratory rate (f) of a young adult is around 12 per minute. With increasing age there is an increase to 14 or 16. Since the tidal volume is normally around 500 ml, the minute ventilation is 12×500 ml $= 6L$ ($V_T \times f$). Not all of every breath reaches the alveoli, since some air remains in the nose, nasopharynx, and bronchi and therefore does not come into contact with the alveolocapillary surface. The non-gas–exchanging part of the respiratory system is known as the anatomical dead space (V_{D_A}) and is normally around 150 ml. In a normal subject the volume of gas reaching the alveoli with each breath is $500 - 150$ ml $= 350$ ml ($V_t - V_{D_A}$). Alveolar ventilation per minute therefore equals 350 ml $\times 12 = 4.2$ L. The anatomical dead space has to be distinguished from the physiological dead space (V_{D_P}), which consists of the anatomical dead space plus the fraction of each breath which is wasted, either to ventilate underperfused alveolar units or to overventilate alveolar units relative to perfusion. In a normal subject the anatomical and physiological dead spaces are approximately the same, but with mismatching of ventilation and perfusion, the V_{D_P} increases. Lung volumes are generally expressed at the subject's body temperature, saturated with water vapor,

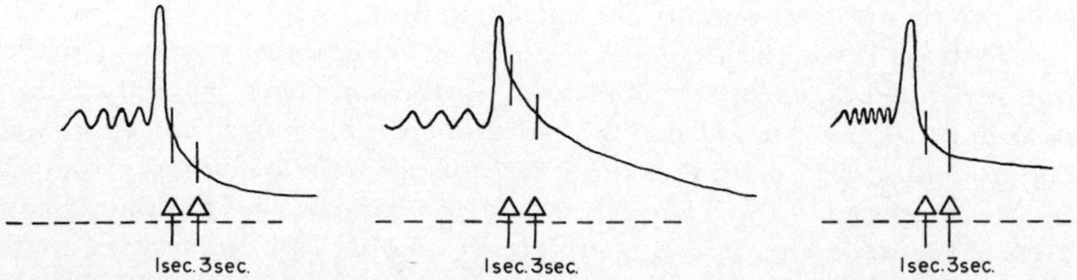

Figure 3–4. Forced expiratory volume maneuvers in a normal subject and in subjects with obstructive and restrictive impairment.

and at 760 mm Hg (BTPS). When expressed at BTPS, the various indices represent the actual volume in the lungs.

Air Flow Resistance

During quiet breathing, most of the respiratory effort goes towards overcoming the compliance of the lungs and chest wall. By comparison, the work necessary to overcome air flow resistance is small, but when breathing becomes deeper and more rapid, the work expended overcoming airways resistance increases rapidly. When the airways are narrowed or obstructed by mucus, there may be a huge increase in both the airways resistance and the work of breathing, especially at low lung volumes at which the lumina of the airways are significantly narrowed.

Gas flow in the airways is governed by the same factors that regulate the flow of fluid in tubes or, if it comes to that, the flow of the electricity in a conductor. Ohm's law ($C = E/R$, where C is the current or flow, E the voltage or pressure gradient, and R the resistance) applies equally well to the flow of gas in the airways. Air flow may be either turbulent or laminar. When flow is turbulent, the pressure gradient necessary to produce a certain flow rate is appreciably higher. With laminar flow, the pressure gradient necessary to produce a certain flow is directly proportional to the viscosity of the gas. In contrast, during turbulent flow, the viscosity of the gas is less important and the density more important. Under normal circumstances, flow in the larger airways tends to be turbulent, and in addition, at the bifurcation of the airways, eddy currents are set up. In contrast in the smaller airways, that is to say from the 12th generation and down, flow is mainly laminar. Thus, flow in the central airways is mainly density dependent, while in the smaller airways it is related more to the viscosity of the gases present. Poiseuille's law ($P = K_1V$, where P is driving pressure, V is flow, and K_1 is a constant that depends on the viscosity of the gas) applies only to laminar flow in a straight line in a tube whose cross-sectional diameter is not changing. Clearly this situation does not apply in lungs, where the cross-sectional diameter is constantly changing, where the airways are repeatedly dividing, and where, due to disease, the diameter of the airways may be either narrowed and distorted or occasionally dilated. Nonetheless, despite all these variables, the concept of airways resistance and the basic physical laws can be applied to many clinical situations.

Airways resistance depends not only on the number of patent airways but on the total cross-sectional area of the airways. The intrathoracic resistance of the airways may be partitioned into central and peripheral components. The central component includes the resistance from the trachea to roughly the 11th generation of bronchi. The peripheral component is made up of the resistance from the 12th generation to the alveoli. Central resistance in normal subjects makes up 85 to 90 per cent of the total airways resistance (Raw). Thus the peripheral resistance

constitutes only 10 to 15 per cent of the total resistance and, moreover, at high lung volumes is negligible (Fig. 3–5). It is, therefore, possible for a subject to have diffuse disease of the small airways and yet have a normal airways resistance and normal spirometry. When the resistance in the peripheral airways is increased, the lungs become less distensible, although total resistance may still be within normal limits. The peripheral airways are usually not uniformly and diffusely affected; rather the pathological processes producing small airways disease tend to lead to patchy or regional involvement. Airways resistance is normally expressed at FRC. This is related to the fact that the cross-sectional diameter of the airways varies greatly with lung volume. Thus at TLC the airways are widely patent and with expiration there is a fairly minor decrease in a cross-sectional diameter until FRC is approached, at which time the airways start to narrow rapidly. For this reason, Raw remains relatively unchanged until FRC, at which time it starts to rise geometrically. It is also important to remember that in airways obstruction both the Raw and FRC are likely to increase, although not always to the same extent.

Airways resistance can be measured directly in several ways, including the body plethysmograph, the simultaneous recording of alveolar pressure and flow using an esophageal balloon, the interrupter technique, and also the oscillator method. A description of these various techniques is beyond the scope of the present chapter; however, suffice it to say, the plethysmographic method is the preferred, since it is most accurate in the clinical situation. There is little doubt that measurement of Raw in many instances adds little and is not as useful as spirometry in most clinical situations.

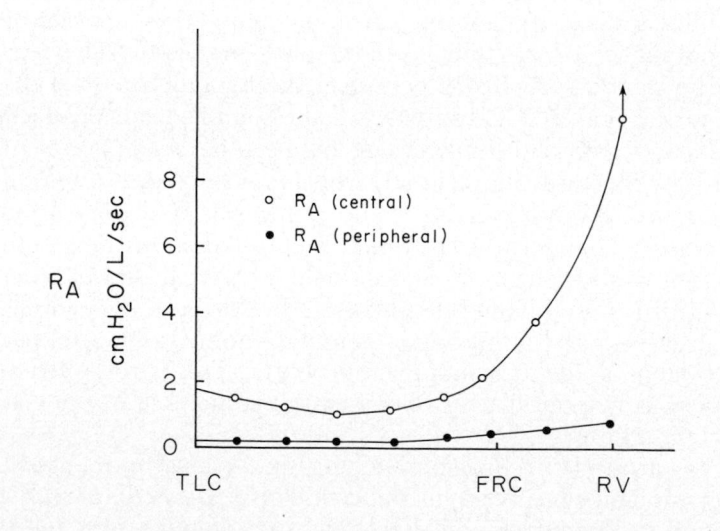

Figure 3–5. Relationship of central and peripheral airways resistance to lung volumes. (From Sodeman, W. A., Jr., and Sodeman, T. M.: Pathologic Physiology. 7th ed. Philadelphia, W. B. Saunders Co., 1984.)

However, determination of Raw can be most useful in challenge tests and in the assessment of various bronchodilator drugs. Under the latter circumstances, objective measurements of resistance may be preferable to spirometry.

The normal airways resistance is around 1.5 cm H_2O/L/sec. In comparison, the nasal air flow resistance is two to three times as high. In bronchitis and emphysema the airways are irreversibly obstructed, and Raw may be increased four- to six-fold, under which circumstances most of the increased resistance is located in the respiratory bronchioles and smaller airways. In asthma, even greater increases in Raw occur, but here the obstruction is usually located in both small and large airways.

Compliance of the Lungs

Ventilation also depends on the compliance of the lungs. This is a measurement of the distensibility of the lungs, and is expressed as the change in lung volume that occurs when the pressure gradient between the pleura and the alveoli is changed by 1 cm of water. It may be measured during breath-holding (static compliance) or during regular breathing (dynamic compliance). If the increase in volume were directly proportional to the pressure change through the range of inflation and deflation, then a single value for static compliance would describe the elastic properties of the lungs. In reality this is not the case; the lungs becoming less compliant at high lung volumes and only in the tidal volume range is the relationship approximately linear. Lung compliance also depends on lung size, and the larger the lungs the more compliant they are. Thus an infant's lung is less compliant than an adult's and likewise there is disparity in the compliance of the lungs of large and small men. The reason for this can be clearly seen if one considers the hypothetical case of a man whose vital capacity is 5 L and whose static compliance is 0.2 L/cm H_2O. Under such circumstances increasing his negative intrapleural pressure by 1 cm H_2O increases the volume of his lungs by 200 ml. Were he then to have one lung removed, this would reduce his vital capacity to 2.5 L and a pressure change of 1 cm would then increase his lung volume by only 100 ml. In short, his compliance would be halved, although the elastic properties of his lung would be unchanged. This is an oversimplification of the problem, since following pneumonectomy some compensatory overdistension of the remaining lung occurs. The latter phenomenon, nonetheless, is responsible for only a marginal increase in the volume of the remaining lung.

To get around the problem of lung size, a measurement known as specific compliance has been introduced. This relates compliance to lung volume and is obtained by dividing the static compliance by the FRC. If the lungs become stiff and fibrotic, as frequently occurs in asbestosis, sarcoidosis, berylliosis, and certain other diffuse fibroses, the compliance is markedly reduced and values of 0.04 L/cm H_2O and less may be found.

In subjects who have a marked reduction of compliance the vital capacity is usually concomitantly decreased. In conditions in which the lung has lost elasticity, a small change of pressure may produce a large increase in lung volume (Fig. 3–6). Under such circumstances, the lungs are said to be more compliant than normal. This is the usual state of affairs in emphysema and conditions associated with loss of recoil. Measurement of compliance is usually carried out by relating intrapleural pressure changes as reflected by changes in esophageal pressure to volume change in the lungs. Esophageal pressure is recorded by placing a cylindrical balloon attached to a fine plastic tube in the lower third of the esophagus. The measurement of compliance is objective, but care must be taken to see that the balloon is situated correctly.

Dynamic compliance may be defined as the ratio of tidal volume to the difference between pressure at end inspiration and end expiration at points of no flow during breathing. In normal subjects, measurement of dynamic compliance gives similar values to the static compliance; however, when airways resistance is increased an appreciable difference is often present. This is best explained by considering a state of affairs in which there is partial obstruction of a lobe or lung. In the unobstructed region, flow is maximal and there is an appropriate increase in flow volume for this area. In contrast, the flow of gases into the region with the increased airways resistance takes place more slowly, thereby causing a smaller increase in volume per head of pressure.

Surfactant

The compliance of the lungs is also dependent on the presence of surfactant. The latter is a substance that lines the alveoli and respiratory bronchioles and tends to prevent their collapse. Radford first demonstrated that the lungs of an animal that had been filled with saline distend more easily than they did with air.[4] This phenomenon suggests that saline

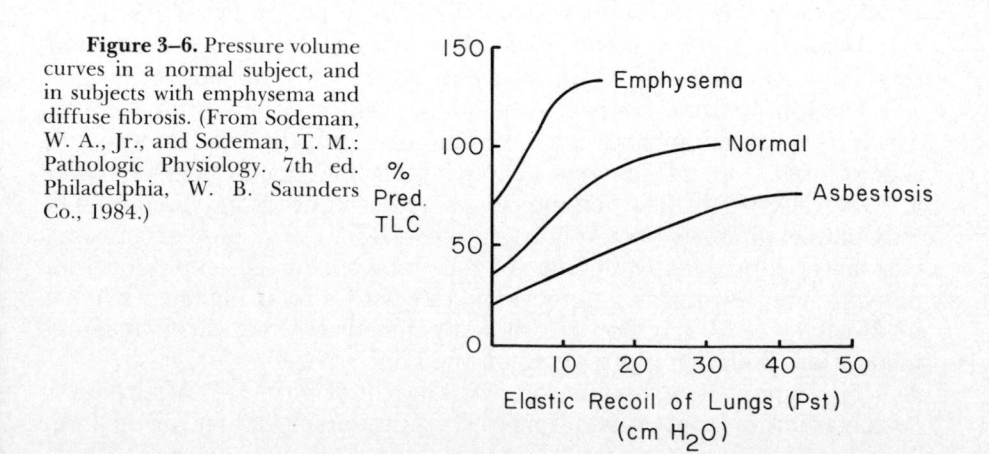

Figure 3–6. Pressure volume curves in a normal subject, and in subjects with emphysema and diffuse fibrosis. (From Sodeman, W. A., Jr., and Sodeman, T. M.: Pathologic Physiology. 7th ed. Philadelphia, W. B. Saunders Co., 1984.)

either removed or rendered noneffective a substance which regulates the surface tension of the gas-tissue interface. Pattle subsequently showed that pulmonary edema fluid has a much lower surface tension than does plasma, an observation that suggests there is a substance lining the alveoli and influencing surface tension.[5] Subsequently, Clements and his colleagues demonstrated that the surface retractive forces are appreciable during lung expansion, but that during deflation of the lungs and as the surface area contracts these forces decrease.[6]

In normal subjects, there is a difference between the inspiratory and expiratory limbs of a pressure volume curve; a phenomenon usually referred to as hysteresis. By way of contrast, the saline-filled lung fails to show hysteresis, which suggests that the difference in the inspiratory and expiratory limbs in the normal subject is a consequence of a substance which regulates surface tension at the air-liquid interface. This substance has been shown to be surfactant and is a complex of dipalmitoyl-lecithin with protein. It can be extracted from minced lungs or by washing the lungs out with saline. It appears to be secreted by the type II alveolar cells and it has been shown to be present in decreased amounts in hyaline membrane disease, in conditions in which the blood flow to the lungs is decreased, and in sundry other conditions including the prolonged inhalation of 100 per cent oxygen.

Impairment of the Small Airways Function

The detection of changes in air flow resistance and function in the small airways is a challenge to the ingenuity of the physiologist, but several techniques have been devised which can be used to this end. Moreover, in many subjects such changes have been shown to be reversible, and it has therefore been suggested that if the abnormalities are detected early before there are accompanying spirometric abnormalities and if further exposure to the responsible agent is avoided, irreversible disease may be avoided. Whether such tests will prove useful in prognosticating whether a particular subject is going to develop irreversible airways obstruction remains undecided. Three approaches are presently popular.

1. Flow Volume Loop. The standard method of recording a forced expiratory volume maneuver plots volume against time. In contrast, the flow volume loop, as the name suggests, plots flow against volume. There are several types of flow volume curves and each needs a definition. The maximal expiratory flow volume curve (MEFV) is a plot of maximal expiratory flow (Vmax) against volume during a forced, expiratory maneuver. The term flow volume loop refers to a loop obtained when a maximal forced expiration is followed immediately by forced maximal inspiration, both being presented on the same tracing.

The typical flow volume loop is shown in Figure 3–7. Peak flow is largely effort dependent and is mainly a reflection of the state of the large

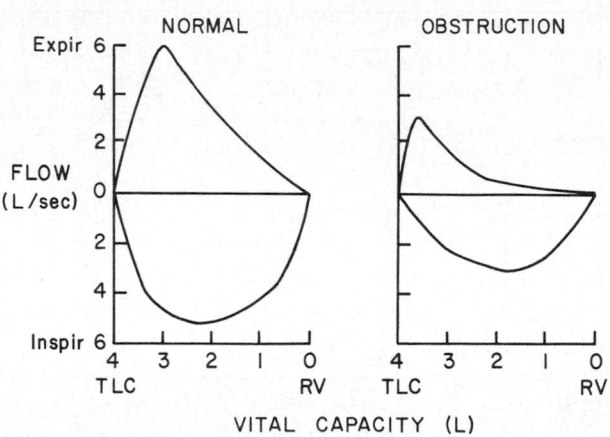

Figure 3–7. Flow volume loops of a normal subject and of a subject with airways obstruction. (From Sodeman, W. A., Jr., and Sodeman, T. M.: Pathologic Physiology. 7th ed. Philadelphia, W. B. Saunders Co., 1984.)

airways. Flow at 50 per cent of vital capacity (FEF_{50}) reflects both large and small airways function with the former probably predominating. The latter part of the curve is felt to represent flow in the smaller airways. Also shown in Figure 3–7 is the curve of a subject with airways obstruction.

Figure 3–8 shows a series of curves with different efforts. Although the peak flow varies, it can be seen that eventually the latter part of the curve blends with that of the MEFV, in short, there is a final common pathway. These phenomena stimulated Hyatt to construct iso-volume pressure flow curves (IVPF), in which he measured transpulmonary pressure showing that as driving pressure increased, flow concomitantly increased until a maximal value was attained, after which further increases

Figure 3–8. Series of flow volume curves showing graded respiratory efforts and different inspiratory volumes. (From Sodeman, W. A., Jr., and Sodeman, T. M.: Pathologic Physiology. 7th ed. Philadelphia, W. B. Saunders Co., 1984.)

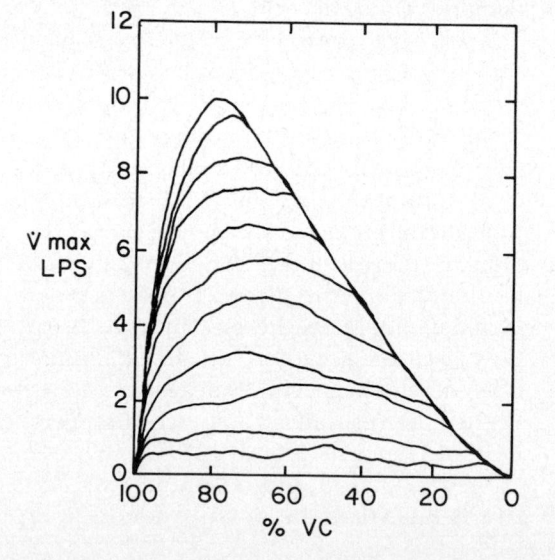

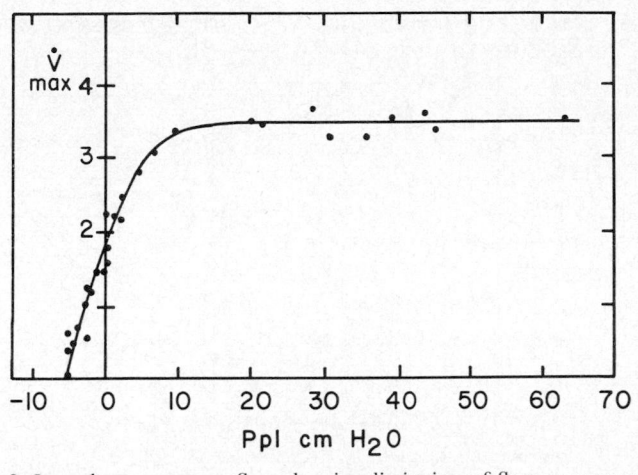

Figure 3–9. Iso-volume pressure flow showing limitation of flow at pressure of 15 cm/ H_2O. (From Sodeman, W. A., Jr., and Sodeman, T. M.: Pathologic Physiology. 7th ed. Philadelphia, W. B. Saunders Co., 1984.)

in pressure produced no further increase in flow (Fig. 3–9).[7] Although flow is usually expressed as a percentage of vital capacity, it is preferable to relate it to total lung capacity (TLC) for the following reasons. When the MEFV is being used to evaluate bronchodilator drugs or to assess changes in air flow resistance over a relatively short period, e.g., during challenge tests or when subjects may have been exposed to cotton dust or agents likely to produce an acute change in the airways, in some instances, not only do the flow rates decrease, but in addition VC may likewise show a decrease. Thus it is possible for a "before and after" challenge FEV_{50} when expressed as a percentage of VC to remain relatively unchanged; however, were the FEF_{50} related to TLC, a marked difference would become apparent.

In large airways because flow is partly turbulent, the pressure necessary to produce a particular flow rate increases with gas density. In contrast, flow in the peripheral airways is for the most part laminar and is therefore independent of gas density. If one measures airways resistance (Raw) when the subject is breathing a helium and oxygen mixture (4:1), it is found that the Raw is substantially decreased. If a subject with peripheral airways obstruction alone breathes a helium oxygen mixture (HeO_2), there is little change in Raw, since flow in small airways is mainly laminar. Since the effective pressure necessary to produce maximal flow is independent of the gas mixture breathed and since the difference in flow between breathing air and helium oxygen mixture is determined by how much the peripheral airways contribute to the total resistance, the higher the resistance to flow in the peripheral airways, the less will be the helium response (Fig. 3–10).

At a particular lung volume, the flows on HeO_2 and air coincide, and this is known as the point of identical flow (PIF, or Viso $\dot{V}$). It is usually

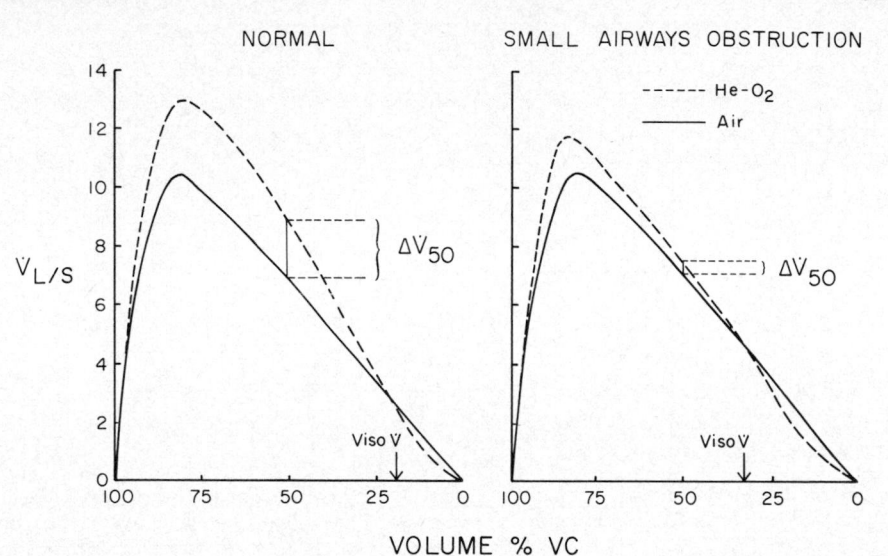

Figure 3–10. Helium oxygen and air flow volume curves in a normal subject and a subject with small airways obstruction. Note the point of identical flow (Viso $\dot{V}$) is farther from RV in the subject with small airways obstruction. (From Sodeman, W. A., Jr., and Sodeman, T. M.: Pathologic Physiology. 7th ed. Philadelphia, W. B. Saunders Co., 1984.)

expressed as a percentage of vital capacity. In normal subjects it varies from 0 to 6 per cent and is rarely elevated above 10 per cent. In small airways obstruction it may be elevated to around 30 per cent (Fig. 3–10).

The flow volume curve is also useful in detecting obstructing lesions of the right and left main bronchi, the trachea, and larynx. Figures 3–11,

Figure 3–11. Flow volume showing variable extra-thoracic obstruction. (From Sodeman, W. A. Jr., and Sodeman, T. M.: Pathologic Physiology. 7th ed. Philadelphia, W. B. Saunders Co., 1984.)

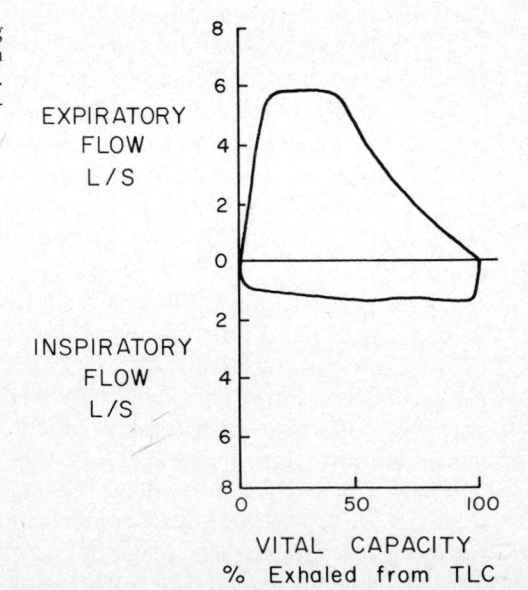

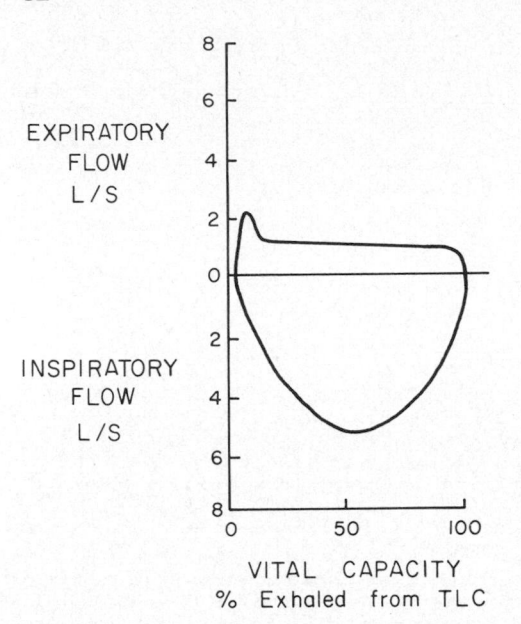

Figure 3–12. Flow volume curve showing variable intra-thoracic obstruction. (From Sodeman, W. A., Jr., and Sodeman, T. M.: Pathologic Physiology. 7th ed. Philadelphia, W. B. Saunders Co., 1984.)

3–12, and 3–13 show typical examples of the major airways obstruction. Figure 3–11 is a tracing from a subject with a variable extrathoracic obstruction, namely, bilateral vocal cord paralysis. It is obviously apparent that inspiratory flows are more affected than expiratory flows. A variable intrathoracic obstruction, e.g., a tracheal cylindroma, is represented in the tracing shown in Figure 3–12. Expiratory flows are worse affected since the trachea is compressed during exhalation. Figure 3–13 shows a fixed (extrathoracic) obstructive lesion in which inspiration and expiration are both affected, e.g., stenosis of the larynx following surgery or injury.

2. Closing Volume. It has been shown that small airways start to close somewhere between functional residual capacity (FRC) and residual volume (RV). Closure depends on the pressure difference acting on the wall of the airway and on the elastic properties of the small airways. If the lumina of peripheral airways are narrowed by mucus or some pathological process, or if concentration of surfactant is reduced, the surface forces acting on the airways become greater and a tendency to collapse occurs.

Fowler originally observed that when a person exhaled to residual volume, and then took a breath of oxygen and achieved total lung capacity (TLC), during a subsequent slow expiratory maneuver, a tracing of the percentage of nitrogen exhaled showed four distinct phases (Fig. 3–14). In phase 1 there is an absence of nitrogen owing to the fact that the dead space contains pure oxygen.[8] Phase 2 begins as the subject starts to exhale a mixture of gas from the dead space and alveoli, and is characterized by a sharp increase in the concentration of expired nitrogen. Phase 2 is followed by an alveolar plateau known as phase 3. Finally there is an abrupt increase in the concentration of nitrogen (phase 4). The junction

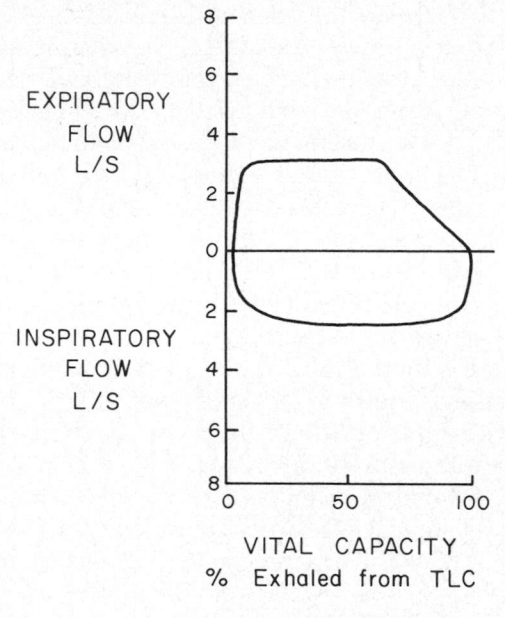

EXPIRATORY
FLOW
L/S

INSPIRATORY
FLOW
L/S

VITAL CAPACITY
% Exhaled from TLC

Figure 3–13. Flow volume curve showing fixed extra-thoracic obstruction. (From Sodeman, W. A., Jr., and Sodeman, T. M.: Pathologic Physiology. 7th ed. Philadelphia, W. B. Saunders Co., 1984.)

of phases 3 and 4 is thought to be the volume at which the basal airways close, and the volume between the junction of phases 3 and 4 and RV is known as closing volume (CV). CV plus RV is known as closing capacity (CC). The upward inflection at the end of phase 3 is best explained by the effects of gravity on the distribution of inspired gas. In a normal subject there is a gradient of transpulmonary pressure from the top to the bottom of the lung. When a sitting or standing subject takes a breath from RV, the first portion of the breath is distributed to the apices, while the latter portions are distributed to the lower lobes. During a subsequent

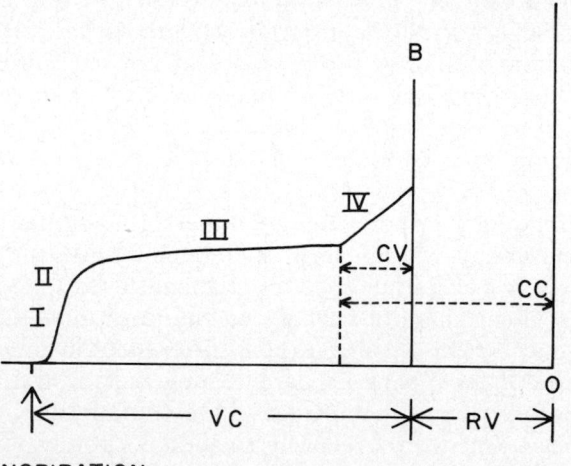

FULL INSPIRATION

Figure 3–14. Single breath oxygen test showing the four phases, along with closing volume and closing capacity. (From Sodeman, W. A., Jr., and Sodeman, T. M.: Pathologic Physiology. 7th ed. Philadelphia, W. B. Saunders Co., 1984.)

exhalation the air that is exhaled first comes from the upper and lower zones, but towards the end of the breath small airways in the lower zones close and the upper zones make a relatively greater contribution. This principle has been aptly named "First In—Last Out."[9]

Measurement of closing volume can be carried out in several ways. The most simple is the resident nitrogen method in which the subject takes a breath of 100 per cent oxygen. The nitrogen remaining in the airways forms a bolus of tracer gas. Other methods involve labeling the inspired air with a foreign gas such as argon, xenon, or helium. Differences in measurement of closing volume in the same subject have been noted according to the method used. A normal closing volume implies that the distribution of inspired gases is mainly dependent on gravity and that the lungs empty relatively homogenously. When filling and emptying become discordant, the principle of "First In—Last Out" is broken and a closing volume may not be apparent on the tracing. Phase 3 represents gas coming from alveoli, and as such the alveoli must contain different concentrations of nitrogen in order to account for the slope. The steepness of the slope is therefore an indication of abnormal distribution, since the concentration of nitrogen in each alveolus after a breath of oxygen depends on how much oxygen enters each alveolus.

Measurement of CV is influenced by the rate at which the inspired breath is taken, by expiratory flow, and by prolonged breath-holding, which leads to a greater percentage of oxygen being absorbed. Expiratory flow should be regulated to between 0.4 and 0.5 L/sec. CV, CV/VC%, and CC/TLC% all have higher coefficients of variation than do the FEV_1 and FVC. In this regard, CV and CV/VC% are the most variable, viz., 20 to 25 per cent. Moreover, while intelligent subjects have no difficulty in carrying out the CV maneuver, its applicability in field studies is severely limited by the inability of a substantial proportion of the less well-educated population to carry out the respiratory maneuvers in a satisfactory fashion. Abnormalities of CV, in the presence of normal spirometry, have been reported in obesity, cigarette smokers, asthmatics in remission, and coal miners and in skeletal deformities such as kyphosis. As such, an elevated CV is thought to indicate early disease; nonetheless, the prognostic significance of CV remains sub judice.

3. Frequency Dependence of Dynamic Compliance. The history of the development of this technique begins with the mechanical time constant theory elaborated by Otis et al. and used to explain the relationship between mechanical factors and the intrapulmonary distribution of inspired gas.[10] Theory suggests that differences in time constants (resistance × compliance) between parallel lung units would be associated with a decrease in dynamic compliance as breathing frequency increased. This would mean that a progressively smaller portion of the lung would be ventilated as breathing frequency increased.

Macklem and Mead reported that the time constants of the distal lung units (airways smaller than about 2 mm) were in the order of 0.01 second.[11]

They concluded that a fourfold difference in these time constants would cause dynamic compliance to fall with any increase in respiratory frequency because there would be less time for air to enter and leave the affected regions. Thus an increased resistance to flow in the smaller airways should lead to a fall in dynamic compliance at faster rates of breathing. This raised the possibility that the frequency dependence of dynamic compliance could be used as a test of obstruction in peripheral airways.

For widespread time constant discrepancies to occur the obstruction must be unevenly distributed; that is, airways must remain patent while others are narrowed. Other criteria are necessary before it can be assumed that frequency-dependent dynamic compliance is a consequence of peripheral airways narrowing rather than of lesions in large airways or other parts of the lung. If the static pressure/volume (compliance) curve of the lung is normal, then it is not likely that frequency-dependent dynamic compliance is due to abnormal elastic properties of the lung. It has been assumed that regional differences in elastic properties sufficient to cause a detectable fall in dynamic compliance at rapid respiratory rates should result in an abnormal static compliance curve. Thus, if a patient has normal pulmonary resistance, spirometry, and static pressure/volume curve, any fall in dynamic compliance with increased frequency of respiration (frequency-dependent compliance) is assumed to be due to peripheral airways obstruction. The time constants and ventilation of peripheral gas-exchanging units of the lung will be affected by:

1. Regional obstruction due to bronchiolar narrowing or obstruction by mucus.

2. Regional increases in elastic recoil produced by interstitial fibrosis; for example, in asbestosis and berylliosis.

3. Regional loss of elastic recoil with airways collapse; for example, in centrilobular emphysema and the focal emphysema of coalworkers' pneumoconiosis (CWP).

All three of these pathological processes may lead to unequal time constants in the lung, and hence an uneven distribution of ventilation that is more pronounced at faster rates of ventilation, and all should produce a fall in dynamic compliance at higher respiratory rates.

The detection of frequency-dependent dynamic compliance involves measuring dynamic compliance at various rates of respiration, e.g., 20, 40, 60, and 80 breaths/minute. The dynamic changes in volume are obtained using a pneumotachograph, while the intrapleural pressure changes are measured with an esophageal balloon.

Work of Breathing

A certain amount of energy is expended with each breath we take. Part of the energy expenditure is related to moving air in and out of the

lungs, and part to moving the thoracic cage and diaphragm. Normal values for the work of breathing are 0.5 kg/m^2/min at rest and up to 250 kg/m^2/min with a maximal voluntary ventilation maneuver. In asthma and emphysema, the main increase in the work of breathing is related to overcoming the increased air flow resistance, while in pulmonary fibrosis the additional work is necessary to overcome the stiffness of the lungs. The respiratory muscles under normal circumstances use about 2 to 4 per cent of the energy requirements at rest, but in diseased subjects this may rise to 35 to 40 per cent.

REGIONAL DISTRIBUTION OF VENTILATION AND PERFUSION

Ventilation

Quantitative studies of the regional distribution of gas over large zones of excised lung using radioactive xenon have shown relatively even distribution of inspired gas per unit lung volume. The situation in life, with the lungs suspended within the chest wall, is very different in that the intrapleural pressure is no longer uniform as in the isolated preparation. Instead, in the erect posture there is a vertical gradient of intrapleural pressure, with a progressive reduction in pressure from the base to the apex of the lung.[12] As the static transpleural pressure (i.e., pressure difference between pleural surface and atmosphere, during breath-holding with the glottis open) is more negative at the apex, the upper zone alveoli tend to be more expanded than those in the lower zones. An analogy is a loosely coiled spring which, when suspended by its uppermost coil, becomes progressively more expanded by its own weight from bottom to top (Fig. 3–15). The pleural pressure gradient in the chest always occurs in the direction of gravitational pull; thus in a supine subject the differences in alveolar expansion occur dorsoventrally.[13] Because of these regional differences in alveolar expansion, the static lung compliance of the more stretched upper zones is less than that of the lower zones in the erect posture, and during tidal breathing at low flow rates, basal ventilation therefore tends to exceed that of the apices.[14] As inspiratory flow rate increases, regional airways resistance is thought to become more influential than compliance in determining regional ventilation, which is then more evenly distributed. It is of note that in elderly normal subjects, particularly in the supine posture, regional ventilation may be altered by small airways closure occurring in dependent lung zones during tidal breathing, and that this may result in a reduction in arterial oxygen tension.[15]

Perfusion

Studies using a variety of different radioactive tracer techniques have also demonstrated that pulmonary perfusion is not uniformly distributed and that there is a vertical gradient of increasing pulmonary perfusion

per unit lung volume from apex to base in the erect posture, apart from some reduction over the most dependent 6 to 10 cm of lung. West and Hughes have explained these regional differences in terms of the interaction of pulmonary arterial, venous, alveolar, and interstitial pressures in the lungs (Fig. 3–16).[15, 16] In zone one of the upright lung there is no pulmonary arterial perfusion because pericapillary lung pressure, which under static conditions can be thought of as "alveolar" pressure, exceeds pulmonary arterial pressure at this level, and alveolar vessels therefore collapse. The junction of zones one and two, at which pulmonary arterial perfusion commences, is represented by the height of a column of blood in an open manometer tube connected to the pulmonary artery. Below this level, pulmonary arterial pressure exceeds atmospheric pressure and can therefore open the vessels, perfusion increasing down this zone as the hydrostatic pressure of the column of pulmonary arterial blood rises. The amount of perfusion at any level in this zone is determined by the difference between the pulmonary arterial and alveolar pressure which still exceeds pulmonary venous pressure. In the third zone, pulmonary venous pressure now also exceeds alveolar pressure. Here there is a

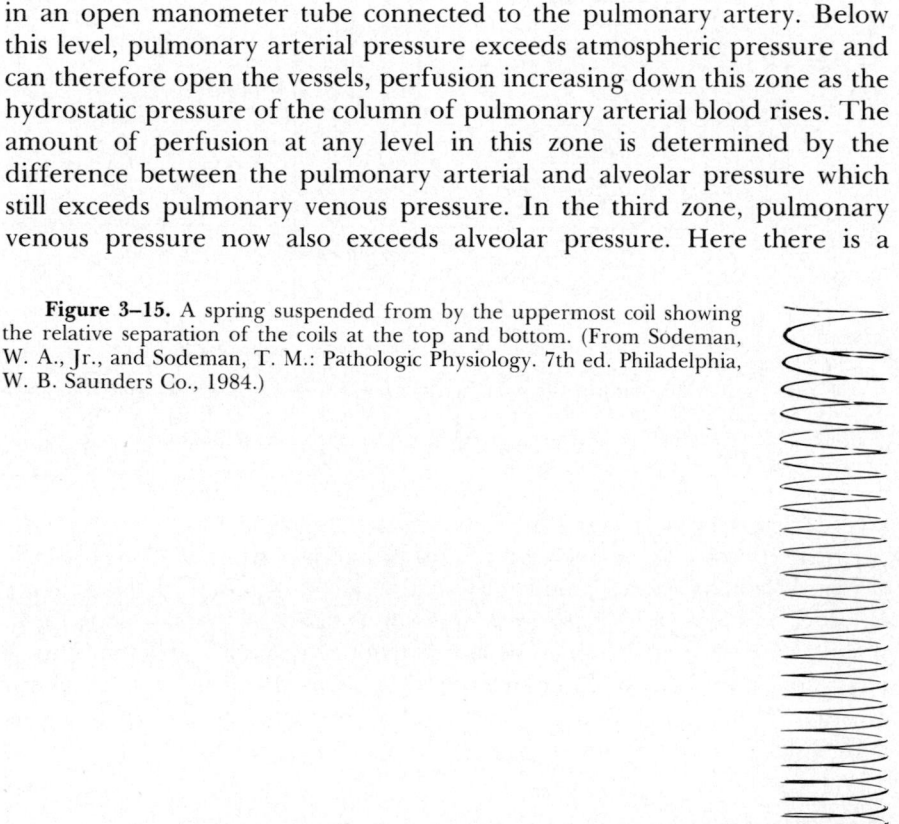

Figure 3–15. A spring suspended from by the uppermost coil showing the relative separation of the coils at the top and bottom. (From Sodeman, W. A., Jr., and Sodeman, T. M.: Pathologic Physiology. 7th ed. Philadelphia, W. B. Saunders Co., 1984.)

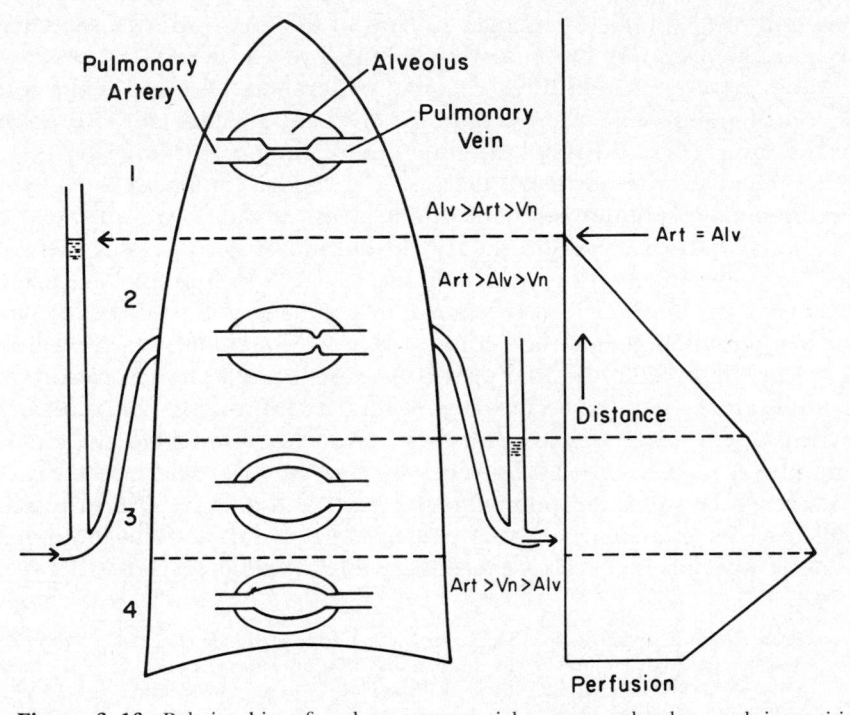

Figure 3–16. Relationship of pulmonary arterial, venous, alveolar, and interstitial pressures in the various zones of the lung (based on West). (From Sodeman, W. A., Jr., and Sodeman, T. M.: Pathologic Physiology. 7th ed. Philadelphia, W. B. Saunders Co., 1984.)

continued slower increase in perfusion probably due to distension of intra-alveolar vessels as a result of a continued increase in the hydrostatic pressure in both pulmonary artery and pulmonary vein, whereas alveolar pressure remains atmospheric. A fourth zone was added to this scheme when it was observed that there was some fall-off of basal blood flow, particularly at lung volumes below functional residual capacity. This is attributed to a lung volume–related change in the resistance of extra-alveolar pulmonary vessels, whose calibre is related to changes in surrounding interstitial pressure rather than alveolar pressure.

Regional Variation in the Matching of Ventilation and Perfusion

Although in the normal lung both alveolar ventilation ($\dot{V}A$) and perfusion ($\dot{Q}$) vary regionally in the same direction according to vertical gravity-dependent gradients, the rate of increase of perfusion from apex to base is steeper than that for ventilation. Consequently the regional matching of $\dot{V}A$ to $\dot{Q}$, which may be conveniently expressed as $\dot{V}A/\dot{Q}$ ratios, is not uniform, but decreases down the length of the lung. The total $\dot{V}A/\dot{Q}$ ratio for a normal upright lung with cardiac output of approximately 6 L per minute and alveolar ventilation of 5 L per minute

lies between 0.8 and 0.9; however, regional $\dot{V}A/\dot{Q}$ ratios vary considerably from about 3.3 at the apex to 0.6 at the lung base.[16] The predilection of post-primary pulmonary tuberculosis for the lung apices has been attributed to the high apical $\dot{V}A/\dot{Q}$ ratio, which results in an alveolar oxygen tension and hence tissue tension over 40 mm Hg higher than that at the lung base. This idea is supported by observations of a higher incidence of this disease in patients with pulmonary stenosis whose apical perfusion is still further reduced. Conversely, tuberculosis usually affects the lung *bases* in bats, since they hang upside down. Regional alterations in the normal pattern of $\dot{V}A/\dot{Q}$ matching are important as they determine the overall efficiency of the lung in its principal function as a gas-exchanger. Exercise and the assumption of the supine position even out the regional differences. In disease, most abnormalities of gas exchange result from mismatching of ventilation and perfusion and these inequalities may be expressed in terms of wasted blood flow or ventilation.

(a) **Wasted Perfusion.** If an alveolus is totally unventilated but remains perfused ($\dot{V}A/\dot{Q} = 0$), then the distal end of the capillary supplying it will still contain blood of venous composition, and perfusion will have been useless and is often referred to as a "true shunt." Suppose the supply of fresh air to the alveolus is not completely interrupted, but merely reduced disproportionately to its blood supply. It may be felt intuitively that some of the perfusion is still surplus to the requirements of that alveolus. We can imagine that the reduced amount of inspired gas will be totally accommodated by some fraction of the same volume of perfusing blood, and the rest will remain venous. In both these situations "venous" blood will mix with arterialized blood, reducing its oxygen content and increasing its carbon dioxide content. This process, which is called "shunting" or "venous admixture," may, if sufficient alveoli are involved, produce measurable changes in the gas tensions of arterial blood. It should be noted that both oxygen and carbon dioxide transfer are impaired in shunting; however, usually the respiratory center responds to hypercarbia by increasing ventilation, which lowers the P_{CO_2} of ventilated alveoli.[17] Since the carbon dioxide dissociation curve is nearly linear (Fig. 3–17), this will be accompanied by an approximately equal fall in CO_2 content for a given fall in P_{CO_2} over the physiological range, and, as a result, in shunts a normal arterial P_{CO_2} can usually be maintained. In the absence of a hyperventilatory response carbon dioxide retention would occur. Arterial oxygen content is less easily maintained because increasing the P_{O_2} of relatively well-ventilated alveoli on the flat part of the nonlinear oxyhemoglobin dissociation curve (Figs. 3–15 to 3–18) will produce only minimal improvement in the oxygen saturation of the blood perfusing these units, which cannot therefore compensate for unventilated units. The arterial blood gas abnormality most commonly found in significant shunts is a lowered arterial P_{O_2} in the presence of a normal or low arterial P_{CO_2}.

The direct passage of blood from the arterial to the venous side of

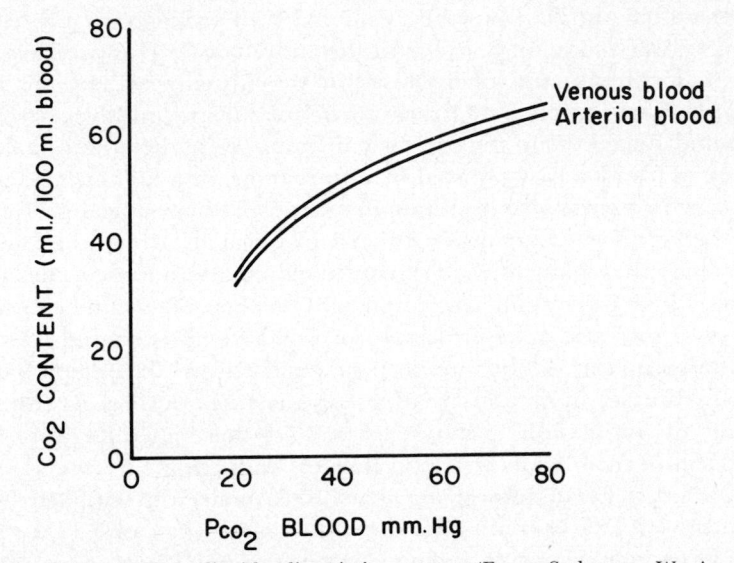

Figure 3–17. Carbon dioxide dissociation curve. (From Sodeman, W. A., Jr., and Sodeman, T. M.: Pathologic Physiology. 7th ed. Philadelphia, W. B. Saunders Co., 1984.)

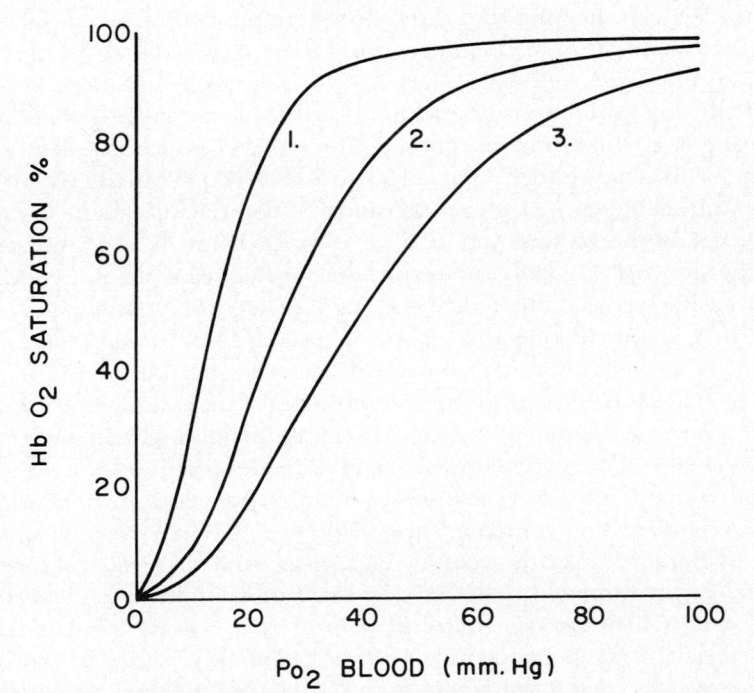

Figure 3–18. Oxygen dissociation curves showing right and left shifts (see text for explanation). (From Sodeman, W. A., Jr., and Sodeman, T. M.: Pathologic Physiology. 7th ed. Philadelphia, W. B. Saunders Co., 1984.)

the pulmonary circulation without any contact with ventilated alveoli is called true shunting, and is physiologically indistinguishable from the small amount of anatomical shunting that occurs in normal individuals through the bronchial circulation and Thebesian veins in the heart. Any remaining shunt is due to alveoli with low $\dot{V}A/\dot{Q}$ ratios and is really a shunt-like effect or physiological shunt. Total shunt in a resting normal individual does not usually exceed 5 per cent of the cardiac output, of which true shunt comprises about 2 per cent.[18]

(b) **Wasted Ventilation.** Now consider the opposite situation of a normally ventilated alveolus receiving no perfusion ($\dot{V}A/\dot{Q}$ ratio = infinity). This alveolus will act as an extra space in which air is moved to and fro without participating in gas exchange, and is therefore dead space or wasted ventilation. In terms of function, this dead space produces the same effect as an enlargement of the anatomical dead space, which comprises the whole of the nonalveolated respiratory tract from the mouth and nose to the respiratory bronchioles. If the perfusion of the alveolus is not completely interrupted but only reduced disproportionately to its ventilation, then a fraction of that ventilation will now be sufficient to meet the gas-exchanging potential of the reduced blood flow, and the remaining ventilation is therefore useless. This process will also contribute to alveolar dead space. Alveolar dead space is therefore the volume of inspired gas entering alveoli, but not taking part in gas exchange due to local $\dot{V}A/\dot{Q}$ imbalance and is more conceptual and less tangible than anatomical dead space, which, as it is a volume contained within a physical structure, is easier to picture. Alveolar and anatomical dead space together are conventionally referred to as physiological dead space. The measured physiological dead space in health is usually not more than 30 per cent of the tidal volume.

If anatomical dead space is increased artificially, for example, by mouth breathing through a length of tube, and if the rate and depth of breathing are unaltered, then less fresh air will reach the alveoli with each inspiration. It follows that alveolar PO_2 will fall and alveolar PCO_2 rise, with consequent hypoxemia and hypercapnia. Suppose now alveolar dead space is increased by relative underperfusion of a group of normally ventilated alveoli, and that the rate and depth of breathing and overall pulmonary perfusion remain unaltered. Although the oxygen tension of the reduced volume of blood perfusing these alveoli will be increased, it will be insufficient to compensate for a greater reduction of oxygen tension in blood coming from other normally ventilated alveoli, which are now overperfused as they receive additional blood which would normally have been directed to the first group of alveoli. The result will be a reduction in arterial oxygen tension. Even though overall alveolar ventilation may remain normal, wasted regional ventilation will also reduce carbon dioxide exchange, tending to produce a raised arterial carbon dioxide tension.[17] In disease this tendency is often corrected by compensatory hyperventilation, although hypoxemia often persists.

Alveoloarterial Oxygen Gradient [(A-a)O$_2$]

Were the matching of ventilation and perfusion perfect and assuming gas diffusion occurred across the alveolocapillary membrane to equilibrium, then arterial and alveolar oxygen tensions would be equal. When mismatching occurs, an alveoloarterial oxygen tension difference [(A-a)O$_2$] will develop. The measurement of arterial oxygen tension is easy, but that of average alveolar oxygen tension presents problems. Although end-expiratory samples of alveolar gas may not be contaminated by dead space air in normal subjects, in pulmonary disease some lung units may take much longer to empty than others, so that end-expiratory PO$_2$ measured at the mouth changes continually, and spot sampling introduces error. Consequently for clinical purposes "ideal" alveolar PO$_2$ is estimated indirectly.[19] This is the alveolar PO$_2$ that would be found in a given subject if, for the same overall rate of consumption of oxygen and production of carbon dioxide, ventilation and perfusion were to become perfectly matched throughout the lung. The calculation requires the analysis of an expired air and arterial blood sample. A simplified version of the ideal alveolar gas equation is:

$$\text{ideal } PA_{O_2} = PI_{O_2} - \frac{Pa_{CO_2}}{R}$$

where PI_{O_2} is the inspired oxygen tension, Pa_{CO_2} is the arterial carbon dioxide tension, and R is the respiratory quotient (rate of production of carbon dioxide divided by the rate of uptake of oxygen, which is usually 0.8). The ideal (A-a)O$_2$ underestimates true (A-a)O$_2$ because it fails to account for alveoli with a raised PO$_2$ due to high $\dot{V}A/\dot{Q}$ ratios. It is used as a nonspecific indicator of impaired gas exchange due to diffusion or distribution abnormalities. It remains normal (4 to 15 mm Hg) in patients with overall alveolar hypoventilation, and is increased by hyperventilation, whether voluntary or induced by anxiety (Table 3–1).

Estimation of Shunt

Physiological shunt (anatomical plus alveolar shunt) may be estimated using the following equation:

$$\frac{\dot{Q}s}{\dot{Q}} = \frac{Ci_{O_2} - Ca_{O_2}}{Ci_{O_2} - C\bar{v}_{O_2}}$$

where $\dot{Q}s/\dot{Q}$ is the proportion of total pulmonary flow taking part in the shunt, Ca_{O_2} and $C\bar{v}_{O_2}$ are the arterial and mixed venous oxygen contents, and Ci_{O_2} is the ideal arterial oxygen content (that which would result from an arterial PO$_2$ equal to the ideal alveolar PO$_2$) which can be obtained from a knowledge of the ideal alveolar PO$_2$, using the oxyhemoglobin dissociation curve. True shunt (anatomical shunt plus shunt through totally unventilated alveoli) may be separated from shunt-like effects (alveoli with

Table 3–1. CHANGES IN ARTERIAL BLOOD GASES AND (A-a)O$_2$ GRADIENT IN VARIOUS PHYSIOLOGICAL IMPAIRMENTS*

	Po$_2$	Pco$_2$	(A-a)O$_2$
Regional $\dot{V}/\dot{Q}$ mismatching	↓	↑ or N or ↓	↑
"Pure" diffusion block	↓	N or ↓	↑
Overall alveolar hypoventilation	↓	↑	N
Overall alveolar hyperventilation	N or ↑	↓	↑

*From Morgan, W. K. C., and Seaton, D.: Pulmonary ventilation and blood gas exchange. *In* Sodeman, W. A., Jr., and Sodeman, T. M., eds.: Pathologic Physiology, 7th ed. Philadelphia, W. B. Saunders Co., 1984.

low $\dot{V}A/\dot{Q}$ ratios) by the administration of 100 per cent oxygen for 20 minutes. This washes out all alveolar nitrogen and fully oxygenates even poorly ventilated alveoli (alveolar Po$_2$ approximately 670 mm Hg), thereby abolishing shunt-like effects. The only possible cause for persisting hypoxemia in this situation is a true shunt, where venous blood unexposed to ventilated alveoli continues to dilute oxygenated blood. It should be noted that the arterial Po$_2$ will rise to some extent in true shunts due to the increased alveolar Po$_2$, and only in large shunts (greater than 25 per cent of the cardiac output) will the blood remain desaturated. A widened (A-a) O$_2$ will persist in true shunts but not in shunt-like effects.

Estimation of Physiological Dead Space and Effective Alveolar Ventilation

Physiological dead space (anatomical dead space plus alveolar dead space) may be estimated using Bohr's equation in terms of alveolar and mixed expired Pco$_2$:

$$V_{D_P} = V_T \frac{(P_{A_{CO_2}} - P\bar{E}_{CO_2})}{P_{A_{CO_2}}}$$

The difficulties inherent in measuring average alveolar Pco$_2$ are avoided by equating it to arterial Pco$_2$ (equals ideal alveolar Pco$_2$). The proportion of the tidal volume (V_T) made up by the physiological dead space V_{D_P} may now be given by:

$$\frac{V_{D_P}}{V_T} = \frac{Pa_{CO_2} - P\bar{E}_{CO_2}}{Pa_{CO_2}}$$

Alveolar ventilation has already been defined in terms of anatomical dead space and minute ventilation. If the physiological dead space is known, it is possible to estimate the effective alveolar ventilation, this being the proportion of total ventilation being used effectively in carbon dioxide exchange according to the equation:

$$\underset{\text{ml/min}}{V_A(\text{eff})} = \underset{\text{breaths/min}}{f} \times \underset{\text{ml}}{(V_T - V_{D_A})}$$

In clinical practice, however, arterial P_{CO_2} alone is generally taken as a reliable and readily available indicator of the level of effective alveolar ventilation. Hypoventilation, by reducing the delivery of fresh air to gas exchanging areas, inevitably reduces arterial P_{O_2} and increases arterial P_{CO_2}. The resultant hypoxemia may be eliminated by the administration of a high concentration of oxygen, but the raised arterial P_{CO_2} cannot be corrected unless the level of alveolar ventilation is increased. Conversely, conditions that result in effective alveolar hyperventilation are associated with a lowered arterial P_{CO_2}. This may be seen in hysterical overbreathing, and occasionally following the hyperventilatory response to hypoxemia due to a diffusion impairment or ventilation-perfusion mismatch in which sufficient normal lung tissue remains to eliminate carbon dioxide.

THE TRANSPORT OF GASES BY THE BLOOD

In a mixture of different gases, the pressure exerted by each of the constituents, commonly referred to as the partial pressure (P), is the product of its fractional concentration by volume and the total pressure of the mixture. For inspired air which contains 20.93 per cent oxygen, 0.03 per cent carbon dioxide and 79 per cent nitrogen, and other inert gases, whose total pressure is 760 mm Hg (barometric pressure at sea level) and whose water vapor pressure is 10 mm Hg, the P_{O_2} will be:

$$\frac{20.93}{100} \times (760 - 10) = 157 \text{ mm Hg}$$

Water vapor pressure is subtracted as the volumes of gases are conventionally estimated dry. Similarly the atmospheric P_{CO_2} will be 0.2 mm Hg and the P_{N_2} 592 mm Hg. If a mixture of gases is brought into contact with a fluid, the constituent gases will continue to diffuse into it until their partial pressures in solution are equal to those of the gas phase. At this point equilibration is said to have occurred. The partial pressure of a gas in fluid is often referred to as its tension.

The content of a gas in a fluid is derived from the product of the gas's solubility coefficient (α) and its partial pressure, and is expressed in ml gas measured at standard temperature and pressure dry (STPD) per 100 ml of liquid or in volumes percent. The solubility coefficient of oxygen is 0.003 ml/dl/mm Hg and its average partial pressure in the alveoli is approximately 100 mm Hg. This is less than that of atmospheric air because of mixing with oxygen-depleted and carbon dioxide–rich gas already present in the lung, and since it also becomes saturated with water vapor during its passage to the gas exchanging surfaces; the saturated water vapor pressure at 37° C being 47 mm Hg. The average content of dissolved oxygen in pulmonary capillary plasma at equilibrium with alveolar air will therefore be $0.003 \times 100 = 0.3$ ml/dl.

A normal resting subject's oxygen requirement is around 300 ml/min, and were all dissolved oxygen in the plasma removed by the tissues on each complete circuit, the minimum cardiac output necessary to support life would be 60 L/min, a level that is impossible to sustain. This difficulty is overcome by the reversible binding of most oxygen to hemoglobin, of which whole blood contains approximately 15 gm/dl. Hemoglobin is a tetramer formed by a globulin molecule bound to four heme molecules, each of which may react with a single oxygen molecule. This complex structure is capable of binding 1.34 ml of oxygen/dl and the hemoglobin capacity is therefore $1.34 \times 15 = 20.1$ ml/dl. Percentage saturation is the oxygen content, which may be measured by Van Slyke's method, and expressed as a percentage of the blood oxygen carrying capacity.

Oxyhemoglobin Dissociation Curve

The content of a gas dissolved in fluid, expressed in volumes per cent, is related to its partial pressure in a linear fashion (Henry's law). This contrasts markedly with the S-shaped relationship of blood oxygen tension to saturation that results from the presence of hemoglobin (Fig. 3–18). The curve owes its distinctive shape to the so-called heme-heme reaction, in which the oxygenation of each heme molecule in the tetramer in turn affects the oxygen affinity of the other subunits, so that the molecule as a whole has four successive equilibrium constants.[20] Notice that the upper part of the curve is relatively flat, so that a drop in oxygen tension from 100 to 60 mm Hg is associated with a relatively small fall in oxygen saturation. As a result persons who live at an altitude of 10,000 feet, at which the alveolar Po_2 is about 60 mm Hg, still maintain an oxygen saturation of about 90 per cent, which is clearly to their advantage. Conversely, a rise in the Po_2 of arterial blood in this range produces only a minimal increase in oxygen saturation. Consequently hyperventilation of normal lung tissue may be unable to compensate for hypoxemia resulting from areas of impaired gas exchange elsewhere. The lower, steeper part of the curve is also physiologically important as a small fall in the Po_2 of blood is associated with a relatively large change in its oxygen content. Thus the transfer of oxygen from blood to metabolically active tissues is facilitated.

Factors Affecting the Oxyhemoglobin Dissociation Curve

The relationship of the Po_2 of blood to hemoglobin saturation may be altered by a number of factors that are capable of causing a "shift" of the oxyhemoglobin dissociation curve to either the right or the left, so that the flat part of the curve corresponding to high hemoglobin saturations is either expanded or contracted (Fig. 3–18). The most important of these factors are: pH, Pco_2, 2,3-diphosphoglycerate level (2,3 DPG), and temperature. These shifts may be defined in terms of the Po_2 of blood at

which hemoglobin is half saturated (P_{50}). If the oxyhemoglobin dissociation curve shifts to the right, the P_{50} rises, and with a shift to the left, it falls. Although it might at first seem that a raised P_{50} would be disadvantageous, since a smaller amount of oxygen is being transported for the given Po_2, careful examination of the diagram shows that as a result of the shape of curve 3, a raised P_{50} implies that for a given reduction in arterial Po_2 in the physiological range, a greater amount of oxygen becomes available to the tissues. If on passing through the systemic capillaries the Po_2 of arterial blood falls from 90 to 40 mm Hg (arteriovenous O_2 difference), then according to curve 2 the oxygen saturation would fall by only 20 per cent, whereas if curve 3 is applied, the fall would be 40 per cent.

When hemoglobin is oxygenated, hydrogen ions are released from the molecule. If the pH of the red cell, which is linearly related to that of the plasma, is reduced by the addition of hydrogen ions, then by the principle of mass action, this process tends to reverse, hemoglobin reverting to its deoxygenated state with the release of oxygen. In practice metabolically active tissues constitute a more acid environment for the blood perfusing them as a result of the local production of CO_2 and lactic acid, and this low pH therefore assists the transfer of more oxygen to the tissues for the same arteriovenous fall in Po_2. In other words, a fall in pH results in an increase in P_{50}, or shift of the oxyhemoglobin dissociation curve to the right. This is known as the Bohr effect. It might be thought that the reduced oxygen affinity of venous blood which is more acid would be detrimental to the uptake of oxygen in the lungs; however, at a higher Po_2, the dissociation curves come closer together and oxygen uptake is little affected. P_{50} may be altered by a change of either pH or Pco_2, for the shift to the right will still occur if pH is kept constant and Pco_2 increased, showing the latter has an effect independent of pH.

The organic phosphate 2,3 DPG is an intermediate in erythrocyte carbohydrate metabolism, and constitutes most of the phosphate in red cells. If the concentration of 2,3 DPG is increased, it competes with oxygen for binding sites on deoxygenated hemoglobin, thereby reducing its oxygen affinity, shifting the oxyhemoglobin dissociation curve to the right. The level of 2,3 DPG is regulated by erythrocyte enzyme systems which are pH dependent, so that acidity or alkalinity tend to suppress or stimulate its production respectively. We have seen that a fall in plasma pH causes an immediate shift of the curve to the right, thereby reducing the affinity of hemoglobin for oxygen. If this fall in pH persists for several hours, 2,3 DPG production is reduced, exerting a counterbalancing effect on the pH-mediated right shift. Consequently, when long-standing acidosis is quickly corrected with bicarbonate, a persisting low 2,3 DPG level may have a deleterious "overshoot effect" by increasing the oxygen affinity of hemoglobin and reducing its supply to the tissues. Deoxygenated hemoglobin, which is a weaker acid and therefore relatively alkaline, stimulates 2,3 DPG production, reducing the affinity of hemoglobin for oxygen and causing the shift to the right that is associated with long-standing hypox-

emic conditions such as cyanotic heart disease or chronic bronchitis.[21] Similarly, the rise in plasma alkalinity that occurs at high altitudes causes a shift to the left with increased hemoglobin-oxygen affinity, and also stimulates 2,3 DPG production which has a counteraction. Other situations in which 2,3 DPG may be depleted with a reduction in blood oxygen transferring efficiency include the storage of transfusable blood, hypophosphatemia, certain congenital hemoglobinopathies, and the raised blood levels of carboxyhemoglobin associated with cigarette smoking.

A rise in the temperature of blood reduces the oxygen affinity of hemoglobin and facilitates its removal by metabolizing tissues, the temperature of which is slightly higher than that of the lungs.

Carbon Dioxide Transport

The partial pressure gradient between metabolizing tissues and the capillaries perfusing them results in the diffusion of carbon dioxide into the blood in which it is carried in three forms: (1) in solution in plasma, (2) combined with hemoglobin, and (3) as bicarbonate (Fig. 3–19). Plasma alone is an inefficient carrier of carbon dioxide and only 5 per cent of total carbon dioxide is carried in this way. Although the volume of dissolved carbon dioxide is linearly related to the PCO_2 of blood, the slope of this relationship is not steep enough to enable the elimination of sufficient carbon dioxide by the lungs to keep pace with its production by the tissues. A small proportion of dissolved carbon dioxide in the plasma reacts with water to form carbonic acid which then ionizes according to the equation:

$$CO_2 + H_2O \rightleftharpoons H_2CO_3 \rightleftharpoons H^+ + HCO_3^- \qquad \text{(Equation 1)}$$

Carbon dioxide also diffuses into red blood cells and here the above reaction proceeds rapidly as a result of the action of the enzyme carbonic anhydrase. This results in a concentration gradient of bicarbonate between the erythrocyte and the plasma, so that bicarbonate diffuses out of the cell in exchange for chloride which passes in to maintain electrical neutrality, a process known as the chloride shift. The hydrogen ions are largely buffered by hemoglobin, although venous blood is rendered slightly more acid than arterial blood. Ninety per cent of total blood carbon dioxide is carried as bicarbonate in this way. The remaining 5 per cent combines reversibly with NH_2 on deoxygenated hemoglobin to form hemoglobin carbamate:

$$HbNH_2 + CO_2 \rightleftharpoons HbNHCOOH \rightleftharpoons HbNHCOO^- + H^+$$

When venous blood in the lungs comes into contact with alveolar gas, carbon dioxide in the plasma diffuses into the air spaces, causing the equations illustrated in Figure 3–19 to proceed in the opposite direction.

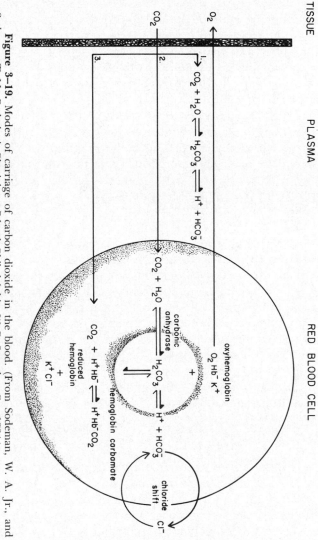

Figure 3–19. Modes of carriage of carbon dioxide in the blood. (From Sodeman, W. A. Jr., and Sodeman, T. M.: Pathologic Physiology. 7th ed. Philadelphia, W. B. Saunders Co., 1984.)

It is clear that the red blood cell is essential for not only oxygen, but also for carbon dioxide transport.

ACID–BASE BALANCE

The acidity or alkalinity of blood is expressed as pH, which is the negative logarithm of the hydrogen ion concentration $[H^+]$. If an acid is added to water (pH 7), it dissociates and the hydrogen ion concentration increases, producing a fall in pH.

$$HCl \rightleftharpoons H^+ + Cl^-$$

The addition of a base has the opposite effect reducing hydrogen ion concentration and therefore increasing pH:

$$NaOH + H^+ \rightleftharpoons Na^+ + H_2O$$

There is a constant tendency for the body to increase its acidity, by the production of both gaseous and nongaseous acid metabolites. This tendency is controlled by the excretion of hydrogen ions indirectly by the lungs and by the kidneys, and involves a number of chemical buffering systems. These mechanisms are normally able to maintain the pH in a narrow range between 7.36 and 7.44; a departure above or below these limits being referred to as alkalosis or acidosis, respectively.

A buffer solution is one whose pH is relatively unchanged following the addition of an acid or alkali. In general buffers are effective only over a certain range of pH. An example of such a buffer system is a solution containing a weak acid, by which is meant one that does not completely dissociate in solution, and a salt of that acid. A buffer system substitutes the stronger, more dissociable acid with one that is weaker and less dissociable, therefore reducing the hydrogen ion concentration. In man there are a number of buffers, the most important of which is the carbonic acid/bicarbonate system, which buffers nongaseous acidic metabolites such as lactic and pyruvic acids. Thus, sodium bicarbonate reacts with lactic acid to produce carbonic acid and sodium lactate:

$$NaHCO_3 + HLac \rightleftharpoons NaLac + H_2CO_3$$

Since carbonic acid is a weaker acid it is less dissociated than lactic acid and fewer hydrogen ions are released into solution. The buffer system has therefore "mopped up" a number of hydrogen ions that would otherwise have been released were lactic acid alone dissociated in solution.

In addition to nongaseous tissue metabolites, it can be seen from Equation 1 that the continual production of carbon dioxide also has an extremely important influence on pH, in that each molecule of carbon

dioxide produced releases one hydrogen ion. We have seen (Fig. 3–19) how this is buffered by reduced hemoglobin and its neutral salt:

$$H_2CO_3 + KHb \rightleftharpoons HHb + KHCO_3 \xrightarrow{\text{chloride shift}} Cl^-$$

Reduced hemoglobin is an even weaker, less dissociable acid than carbonic acid, and necessarily reduces hydrogen ion concentration, thereby preventing acidemia. Although the role of hemoglobin in buffering tissue carbon dioxide is important, the overall level of carbon dioxide retained in the body depends upon the rate at which it can be eliminated from the blood, and this in turn is dependent upon the level of alveolar ventilation. If alveolar ventilation is reduced disproportionately to the rate of carbon dioxide production, then Equation 1 moves to the right, with a consequent fall in pH.

The ability of these buffer systems to maintain pH within a given range is related to the readiness or otherwise with which the weak acid dissociates. This may be expressed mathematically:

$$K' = \frac{[H^+] \times [A^-]}{[HA]} \qquad \text{(Equation 2)}$$

where K' is the dissociation constant of HA, which is a weak acid; the brackets denoting concentration. The higher the value of the dissociation constant, the more readily the acid dissociates. Just as hydrogen ion concentration is for convenience expressed as the logarithm of its reciprocal: $-\log_{10} [H^+]$ or pH, so the dissociation constant is conventionally written as: $-\log_{10} K'$ or pK'. Equation 2 may therefore be rewritten:

$$-\log K' = -\log[H^+] - \log \frac{[A^-]}{[HA]}$$

or:

$$pK' = pH - \log \frac{[A^-]}{[HA]}$$

By adding the last term to both sides of this equation we obtain:

$$pH = pK' + \log \frac{[A^-]}{[HA]} \qquad \text{(Equation 3)}$$

The relationship of the pH of blood to its carbon dioxide content and tension may be derived by substituting carbonic acid from Equation 1 as the weak acid in Equation 3:

$$pH = pK' + \log \frac{[HCO_3^-]}{[H_2CO_3]} \qquad \text{(Equation 4)}$$

This is the Henderson-Hasselbalch equation. The dissociation constant of carbonic acid at 37°C is 6.10, and measurement of the remaining two factors will allow the pH to be calculated. In practice the concentration of carbonic acid in plasma is about 700 times lower than that of dissolved CO_2, as the reaction in equation 1 is driven to the left by HCO_3^- ions derived from sodium and potassium salts.

$$NaHCO_3 \rightleftharpoons Na^+ + HCO_3^- \qquad \text{(Equation 5)}$$

Dissolved CO_2 also bears a constant relationship to carbonic acid concentration and it can therefore be substituted for it in Equation 4:

$$pH = pK' + \log \frac{[HCO_3^-]}{[CO_2]} \qquad \text{(Equation 6)}$$

The quantity of CO_2 in solution is the product of its solubility coefficient (α = 0.03) and partial pressure and the latter can be measured directly with a CO_2 electrode. Carbonic acid contributes insignificantly to the plasma concentration of HCO_3^- ions which are largely accounted for by the reaction shown in Equation 5. The plasma bicarbonate of arterial blood may be derived by subtracting dissolved from total carbon dioxide content and is normally 24 mM/L. Substituting these values in Equation 6:

$$pH = 6.10 + \log \frac{24}{40 \times 0.03}$$
$$= 7.4$$

The practical importance of the Henderson-Hasselbalch equation is that in order for pH to remain constant, any change in bicarbonate (the numerator) has to be matched by a proportional change in CO_2 (the denominator). If this ratio, which is normally 20:1, is altered, a change in pH is inevitable. Disturbances of pH primarily due to alteration in CO_2 are referred to as respiratory, and those primarily due to alteration in HCO_3^- are called metabolic. Any primary change in one component of the HCO_3^-/CO_2 ratio leads to a similar change in the other component in an attempt to maintain normal pH. If for some reason the lungs are unable to remove CO_2 as fast as it is produced, arterial P_{CO_2} will rise and pH will fall. In order to correct this respiratory acidosis, the kidneys act by conserving HCO_3^- and excreting H^+ ions; leading to a compensatory rise in HCO_3^-. In disturbances of acid-base balance the compensatory change in HCO_3^- or CO_2 is less than the primary change and is also usually insufficient to return the pH to the normal range. The following analyses of arterial blood samples will illustrate this.

Example One: P_{CO_2} = 60 mm Hg, plasma bicarbonate = 26 mM/L

Here the rise in P_{CO_2} is greater than that of bicarbonate and is therefore likely to reflect respiratory acidosis rather than a metabolic alkalosis. The pH of 7.29 confirms this. Normally a rise in P_{CO_2} leads to an increase in output of the medullary respiratory center resulting in increased ventilation which "blows off" CO_2. A failure of this homeostatic mechanism to compensate can commonly occur with widespread airways obstruction producing ventilation-perfusion mismatching as seen in chronic bronchitis, or with failure of the bellows function due to muscle weakness as in myasthenia gravis or depression of the respiratory center by drugs.

Example Two: P_{CO_2} = 50 mm Hg, plasma bicarbonate = 40 mM/L

Here the greatest rise has occurred in bicarbonate with a smaller compensatory rise in P_{CO_2} and is therefore likely to result from a metabolic alkalosis rather than a respiratory acidosis. This is confirmed by the pH of 7.53. This situation might follow the excessive ingestion of alkali or after repeated vomiting, and may also occur in hypokalemia in which depleted intracellular potassium is replaced by hydrogen ions resulting in extracellular alkalosis.

Example Three: P_{CO_2} = 30 mm Hg, plasma bicarbonate = 12 mM/L

Here the major fall is in bicarbonate with a smaller compensatory fall in P_{CO_2}. This is therefore likely to be a nonrespiratory or metabolic acidosis rather than a respiratory alkalosis. This is confirmed by the pH of 7.24. This situation is commonly seen in renal failure and in diabetic ketoacidosis, in which the excretion of hydrogen ions fails to keep pace with the production of nongaseous acid metabolites.

Example Four: P_{CO_2} = 25 mm Hg, bicarbonate = 20 mM/L

Here the major change is in P_{CO_2} with only a small fall in bicarbonate and the fact that this is a respiratory alkalosis is confirmed by the pH of 7.53. This picture may be seen in hysterical hyperventilation, or with overbreathing due to other causes such as salicylate poisoning or diffusion defects.

GAS TRANSFER

Diffusing Capacity

The rate of diffusion of a gas in a gaseous medium is inversely proportional to the square root of its density (Graham's law). Thus in such a medium CO_2 diffuses less easily than does oxygen; however, diffusion in the lungs involves a gaseous phase and a liquid phase. For this reason the solubility of the gas in the liquid is an important factor and is governed in this instance by Henry's law. This law states that the

volume of the gas that dissolves in a given volume of a liquid is directly proportional to the partial pressure of that gas. CO_2 being 24 times more soluble than oxygen, it has a greater rate of diffusion.

Factors Influencing the Diffusing Capacity of the Lungs[22]
(Table 3–2)

1. The Pressure Gradient Between the Alveoli and the Capillary Blood. Under normal circumstances blood remains in the pulmonary capillaries for 0.75 second. Even this short time is more than enough to allow equilibrium to take place; the latter being reached in 0.3 second in a normal subject breathing ambient air at sea level. Under these conditions the alveolar PO_2 is around 100 mm Hg. With moderate impairment of diffusion, equilibration takes longer to occur, but even so, it is still achieved in less than 0.75 second. Only when alveolocapillary block is severe does hypoxemia result. During exercise, however, the time the blood remains in the capillaries is shortened, so although the subject may not be hypoxemic at rest, he may become so with exercise. The pressure difference responsible for the diffusion of oxygen is not as might be expected the initial alveolo-arterial gradient ($100 - 40 = 60$ mm) nor the end capillary gradient ($100 - 99.9 = .01$ mm), but is an integrated mean value that depends on a variety of complex factors including the time oxygen takes to traverse the membrane and combine with hemoglobin.

2. The Length of the Pathway of Diffusion. Before an oxygen molecule can combine with hemoglobin it must traverse the following:
   a. Surfactant lining of alveoli
   b. The alveolar membrane
   c. The capillary endothelium
   d. The plasma in the capillary
   e. The RBC membrane
   f. The intracellular RBC fluid

The distance across the membrane is usually about 0.2 microns. In certain disease states this distance may be increased by edema fluid, fibrous tissue, or the presence of additional alveolar cells.

3. The Surface Area Available for Diffusion. The area available for diffusion depends on the number of functioning alveoli rather than the total number of alveoli present in the lungs. In man, it is approximately 70 square meters. Thus, loss of diffusing surface occurs in emphysema, following resection, and in a fibrothorax with compression of the adjacent lung. Owing to the fact that in exercise many nonfunctioning alveoli open up, the diffusing capacity increases with exercise.

4. The Number and Character of the Red Blood Cells Available to Accept Diffused Oxygen. Anemia reduces the diffusing capacity since there are less red blood cells to take up the diffused gas. In addition, were the red cells affected in some anatomical or physiological way which impaired the acceptance of diffused oxygen, then the diffusing capacity would likewise be reduced. The latter is mainly a theoretical concept.

Measurement of Diffusing Capacity

To measure the diffusing capacity it is necessary that the gas used be more soluble in blood than in the alveolocapillary membrane and in the tissue fluid. Both oxygen and carbon monoxide fulfill this criterion because they combine with hemoglobin. Other gases such as N_2O are equally soluble in tissues and blood and therefore can be used to measure pulmonary capillary blood flow. They are not, however, suitable for the management of the diffusing capacity.

The equation for measurement of the diffusing capacity for oxygen is expressed thus:

$$Do_2 = \frac{ml/O_2 \text{ taken up by capillaries/min}}{\text{Alveolar } Po_2 - \text{Pulmonary capillary } Po_2} = ml\ O_2/min/mm\ Hg$$

To measure Do_2 necessitates a knowledge of the Po_2 of mixed venous blood, since this datum is necessary in order to calculate the alveolocapillary gradient. In addition, since the capillary Po_2 rises as the blood traverses the capillary, the gradient and hence rate of diffusion falls. To calculate the Do_2 requires that a knowledge of the Pao_2 is available at every moment as the blood traverses the capillary. Although these data can be derived mathematically, the calculations are tedious and many assumptions are made. Thus for the most part persons seldom measure the diffusing capacity of the lungs for oxygen. In this regard CO is far more convenient and is almost exclusively used now. The advantages of the use of CO are that the Pco in mixed venous blood is zero except in the case of heavy smokers and hence need not be measured. In addition, CO has 210 times the affinity for hemoglobin and consequently only very low concentrations of inhaled CO (0.3 per cent) are necessary to measure the DL_{CO}.

There are a number of methods for obtaining DL_{CO}, of which the most commonly used is the single breath technique.[23] This requires the subject to make a vital capacity inspiration of a mixture containing 0.3 per cent carbon monoxide, 10 per cent helium, and 21 per cent oxygen, and to breath-hold at total lung capacity for 10 seconds, so that some of the carbon monoxide diffuses into the blood. A forced expiratory volume maneuver is then made, and once dead space gas has been displaced, an "alveolar" sample is taken and is analyzed for the final carbon monoxide concentration (FE_{CO}). The carbon monoxide concentration that was present in the alveolar gas before transfer had taken place is estimated from the dilution of inspired helium (He) according to the equation:

$$\underset{\text{(initial CO concentration in alveolar gas)}}{FIN_{CO}} = \frac{FE_{He} \times FI_{CO}}{FI_{He}}$$

where:
FE_{He} = He concentration in expired alveolar sample
Fi_{He} = Inspired He concentration
Fi_{CO} = Inspired CO concentration

The change in carbon monoxide concentration during breath holding is now known and so DL_{CO} can be calculated according to Krogh's equation:

$$DL_{CO} \text{ (ml/min/mm Hg)} = \frac{\text{Alveolar Volume (L)} \times 160}{\text{Time (secs)}} \times \log 10 \frac{FIN_{CO}}{FE_{CO}}$$

Alveolar volume in this equation may be taken either as the sum of the inspired volume and the residual volume (measured separately), or the "effective" alveolar volume (VA_{eff}) may be calculated from the dilution of helium contained in the mixture according to the equation:

$$VA_{eff} = \frac{FI_{He}}{FE_{He}} \times (VI - VD_A) \times 1.05$$

where:
VI = inspired volume
VD_A = anatomical dead space
1.05 = correction for CO_2 absorbed before analysis of expired gas.

The effective alveolar volume tends to give a lower value for DL_{CO} in obstructive lung disease than does the former method.

DL_{CO} may also be measured by a steady state technique in which the subject rebreathes a mixture containing a small concentration of carbon monoxide in air, during which the rate of removal of the gas is measured.[24] This method has the advantage that it may be used during exercise, however, errors may occur in the estimation of alveolar PCO, particularly at rest when the tidal volume is small and dead space gas may not be entirely flushed out when sampling is made.

DL is analogous to an electrical conductance and its reciprocal is therefore comparable to a resistance. Resistances arranged in series may be added to give the overall resistance, and so in the lungs:

$$\frac{1}{DL} = \frac{1}{D \text{ alveolar walls}} + \frac{1}{D \text{ capillary walls}} + \frac{1}{D \text{ plasma}} + \frac{1}{D \text{ red cells}}$$

Although it is not possible to estimate each of these smaller values separately, they may be incorporated into two measurable terms to give:

$$\frac{1}{DL} = \frac{1}{DM} + \frac{1}{\theta VC}$$

where D_M is the diffusing capacity of the alveolocapillary membrane and θV_C is the diffusing capacity of the blood (V_C being the volume of alveolocapillary blood to which the gas is exposed in the lungs, and θ being the rate of reaction of the gas with hemoglobin in ml/min).[25] $D_{L_{CO}}$ falls following oxygen breathing because the value of θ, which can be determined *in vitro,* depends upon the degree of saturation of hemoglobin, which in turn determines the number of binding sites available for carbon monoxide. If two measurements of $D_{L_{CO}}$ are made after breathing first room air and then oxygen, and θ is known for each level, then simultaneous equations may be solved for the two unknowns D_M and V_{Cc}. The membrane component (D_M) falls in diseases in which the surface area available for diffusion is reduced, e.g., emphysema or following lung resection. It is also reduced in conditions causing abnormal thickening of the alveolocapillary membrane such as fibrosing alveolitis or sarcoidosis. The alveolocapillary blood volume (V_C) is labile as the pulmonary circulation has a large reserve capacity and it may not fall until pulmonary disease is advanced. It tends to increase in normal subjects when they exercise or lie flat. It is also increased in patients with left to right cardiac shunts. In mitral stenosis $D_{L_{CO}}$ may be initially raised due to an elevation of V_C (Table 3–2). This may later fall owing to "pruning" of the lungs' vasculature as a result of pulmonary hypertension. The picture may be further complicated by pulmonary edema, which leads to a reduction of D_M. θ is lowered in anemia and raised in polycythemia and $D_{L_{CO}}$ may be corrected for hemoglobin concentration by the equation:

$$D_{L,C} = D_{L,O} (14.6a + Hb) \div (1 + a)Hb$$

where $D_{L,C}$ and $D_{L,O}$ are corrected and observed $D_{L_{CO}}$ respectively, Hb is the hemoglobin concentration and a is the D_M/V_C ratio, which is assumed to be 0.7.

In bronchial asthma the $D_{L_{CO}}$ is normal, which is a useful point in distinguishing this condition from irreversible air flow obstruction due to emphysema. The measurement of D_M, V_C, and θ are laborious, and for clinical purposes, the simpler measurement of $D_{L_{CO}}$ usually suffices. It should be clear that this is influenced by a variety of factors other than thickening of the alveolocapillary membrane as was once thought, and it is therefore sometimes called the gas transfer factor ($T_{L_{CO}}$).

Carbon Dioxide

Because of its solubility, carbon dioxide diffuses from the pulmonary capillaries to the alveoli about 20 times more rapidly than oxygen. For this reason diffuse pulmonary fibrotic or granulomatous diseases such as asbestosis or sarcoidosis, which are associated with impaired diffusion of oxygen, do not affect the diffusion of carbon dioxide sufficiently to cause a rise in arterial P_{CO_2}. By the time that this stage is reached, the arterial

**Table 3–2. PHYSIOLOGICAL FACTORS AND DISEASE PROCESSES
AFFECTING THE DIFFUSING CAPACITY***

	DL_{CO}	Principal Determinants
Loss of lung tissue e.g., emphysema, lung resection	↓	D_M
Diffuse infiltrations e.g., asbestosis, sarcoid, scleroderma	↓	D_M/V_C
Altered pulmonary blood volume		
Mitral stenosis	↑ or ↓	D_M/V_C
left to right cardiac shunt	↑	
exercise	↑	V_C
supine posture	↑	
Valsalva maneuver	↓	
Altered Hb binding capacity		
anemia	↓	
polycythemia	↑	θ
reduced PaO_2	↑	
increased PaO_2	↓	

*From Morgan, W. K. C., and Seaton, D.: Pulmonary ventilation and blood gas exchange. *In* Sodeman, W. A., Jr., and Sodeman, T. M., eds., Pathologic Physiology, 7th ed. Philadelphia, W. B. Saunders Co., 1984.

PO_2 is too low to support life. A raised arterial PCO_2 usually indicates alveolar hypoventilation.

Control of Respiration

The regulation of ventilation, by which the arterial PO_2 and PCO_2 are maintained within a fairly narrow range, is complex and incompletely understood. The involuntary rhythmic nature of breathing depends primarily upon the integrity of collections of inter-related, reciprocally acting, inspiratory and expiratory neuronal pathways contained in the reticular formation of the medulla oblongata. These are known as the medullary respiratory centers, although they have no distinct anatomical boundaries. Their output to the respiratory neurons in the spinal cord is modified by cortical and pontine activity, by the aortic and carotid body chemoreceptors, and by vagus-mediated signals from the lungs and chest wall. They are extremely sensitive to the arterial PCO_2 level, and a 5 per cent increase causes the minute ventilation to double. Carbon dioxide will cross the blood-brain barrier more readily than bicarbonate, and the subsequent dissociation of carbonic acid releases hydrogen ions into the cerebrospinal fluid (CSF), which is less able to buffer them than blood. The medulla possesses receptors on its ventral surface which, when bathed with acid CSF, respond by increasing first tidal volume and later respiratory rate. If the acidity of the CSF is prolonged, as may occur in respiratory acidosis due to chronic obstructive airways disease, a compensatory change occurs

in which CSF bicarbonate is increased, raising the pH again. As a result, a patient with an elevated arterial P_{CO_2} due to chronic bronchitis may have a diminished hyperventilatory response to carbon dioxide, and depends instead upon hypoxic drive. Uncontrolled oxygen therapy in such a patient may produce apnea by raising arterial P_{O_2} above the normal level, thereby leading to secondary hypoventilation and a further rise in P_{CO_2}, which raises the intracranial pressure and acts as a respiratory depressant. Depression of the respiratory center also occurs physiologically during sleep and may be deepened by hypnotic drugs or anesthetics.

The carotid body and aortic arch chemoreceptors are stimulated mainly by hypoxia and to a lesser extent by hypercarbia. The carotid bodies are also sensitive to a fall in pH. These peripheral chemoreceptors are highly active metabolically, and it has been suggested that they are stimulated by the local accumulation of products of anaerobic metabolism, occurring either as a consequence of a reduction in arterial P_{O_2} or from diminished perfusion in the presence of normoxemia as may occur in hemorrhagic shock. Their afferent signals are carried to the medulla by the glossopharyngeal and vagus nerves. The peripheral chemoreceptor response to hypoxia is not as sensitive as the medullary carbon dioxide response and the alveolar P_{O_2} is usually reduced to about 50 mm Hg before the chemoreceptors take over. Variation in the intensity of hypoxic drive among normal individuals has been reported, and it is possible that this might explain the differing clinical presentations of chronic obstructive airways disease, in which the "blue bloater" with a poor hypoxic response may be found at one end of the scale, and the "pink puffer" with a normal response at the other.

A number of vagally mediated afferent stimuli pass to the respiratory centers from the lungs and chest wall. The Hering-Breuer reflex is initiated by receptors in the bronchial and bronchiolar walls and in the diaphragm. Inhibitory signals are generated when these are stretched on inspiration. These do not affect central respiratory drive, but modify tidal volume and breathing rate during exercise and hypoxic or hypercarbic stimulation, and their role during quiet breathing is minimal. In addition to brain stem and cortical controls, the diaphragm and intercostal and abdominal muscles, which drive the "respiratory pump," are also subject to reflex influences at spinal level. Like other voluntary muscles, they contain length-sensitive spindle fibers, which when stretched produce signals that are transmitted to the spinal cord by γ-afferent fibers. Here these synapse with α-motor neurons supplying the corresponding muscle fibers. It is thought that the γ-afferent system may have a coordinative function, providing proprioceptive information about the respiratory muscles, so that motor output may be modified accordingly.

In metabolic acidosis, as occurs in renal failure or diabetic ketosis, nongaseous acid metabolites which do not cross the blood-brain barrier may stimulate respiration by acting on the peripheral carotid body chemoreceptors, leading to Kussmaul breathing. Cheyne-Stokes breathing is

characterized by a cyclical waxing and waning of tidal volume and respiratory frequency, and is commonly seen in severe cardiac failure associated with hypotension and following cerebrovascular accidents. This instability of the ventilatory control system may result from a variety of causes, such as prolonged circulation time resulting in delayed feedback signals to the respiratory centers, or from increased sensitivity of the CO_2 control system as a consequence of damage to higher centers, or paradoxically from depression of CO_2 responsiveness due to brain stem disease, enabling the less stable O_2 control system to take over.

PHYSIOLOGY OF EXERCISE

Under basal conditions a normal person requires approximately 250 ml of oxygen and produces approximately 200 ml of carbon dioxide every minute. When he starts to exercise or do strenuous work, his oxygen requirement and his carbon dioxide production increase, and the degree of change is related to the degree of increased activity. Sustained work requires adequate gas exchange. Although the body is capable of working under anaerobic conditions for short periods, this method of metabolism is inefficient and results in the build-up of toxic metabolites such as lactic acid. With an increased workload, delivery of oxygen to the tissues depends on the integrity of the three basic processes of respiration, namely, ventilation, perfusion and diffusion. Also necessary is an intact and properly functioning respiratory center, so that any increase in workload is accompanied by an appropriate increase in ventilation along with a selective redistribution of the oxygenated blood. The factors limiting working capacity are admirably discussed by Jones and Campbell in their book *Clinical Exercise Testing*.[26]

Work performance is best quantified by measuring oxygen consumption. The latter is influenced by body size, but can be standardized by expressing oxygen consumption as ml/kg of body weight or as a multiple of resting oxygen uptake (METS). During exercise the oxygen demand of the muscles involved increases. Since the oxygen saturation of arterial blood is almost complete, the additional oxygen requirements of the muscles can be met by increasing blood flow or by increasing the arterio-venous oxygen difference [(a-v)O_2] or both. Increased blood flow to the muscles is effected partly as an increase in cardiac output and partly as a consequence of a redistribution of peripheral blood so that the muscles receive a significantly greater proportion of the cardiac output. Cardiac output may be increased as a result of either an increase in heart rate or an increased stroke volume. In practice, increasing the load usually results in both of these responses.

The increased (a-v)O_2 in turn necessitates greater ventilation, with the result that the minute volume increases. The expected increases in heart rate and ventilation that occur in healthy subjects in response to

maximal exercise have been well studied, and there are numerous prediction formulae available in the literature. In contrast, during submaximal exercise, the increase in both heart rate and ventilation is variable, may be greatly influenced by anxiety and other factors, and hence cannot be predicted accurately.

In healthy subjects, maximal exercise is limited by the cardiac output and not by limitations of the respiratory reserve. During maximal exercise, minute ventilation nowhere near approaches maximal voluntary ventilation (MVV) and is usually only 65 to 75 per cent of the latter. By the same token, arterial oxygen saturation does not fall, at least under normal circumstances, although there is some evidence that in an exceptionally well-trained distance runner with extreme exertion, there may be slight reduction. Certainly there is no fall in the arterial oxygen saturation in a normal person even with maximal exercise. During maximal exercise when the cardiac output can increase no further, anaerobic metabolism takes over, and lactic acid and other metabolites are produced. The lactic acid has to be buffered by bicarbonate, so that ventilation has to increase still further to eliminate the excess CO_2 produced. The additional ventilation is "inappropriate" and the breathlessness which the subject experiences becomes intolerable. Maximal oxygen consumption reaches a peak in the late teens, remains relatively constant to around 25 to 30 years of age, and then slowly decreases. The decrease in maximal oxygen consumption occurs mainly as a consequence of the age-related decrease in heart rate (Fig. 3–20). Maximal oxygen consumption can be predicted fairly accurately from the heart rate response to submaximal exercise, provided the subject has reached a steady state.

As already mentioned, the relationship of heart rate and ventilation to exercise varies appreciably in the healthy individual. Such differences depend on many factors, including body size, hemoglobin content, physical fitness and the level of training. It is for these reasons that work done is best quantified by oxygen consumption rather than by external workload. Obese subjects utilize more energy for the same workload than do lean persons in good physical shape. Although some variations occur in the response to the same level of exercise in the same individual, such variations are relatively limited. Finally, the type of exercise performed may affect heart rate and oxygen consumption.

Thus the performance of the same amount of work on a bicycle and on a treadmill may lead to differing work outputs and oxygen consumptions. This is a consequence of the fact that certain people use one group of muscles more than another, and as a result, one particular muscle group becomes more efficient. With the decline in use of the bicycle in the United States, very few Americans are used to cycling and as a result their thigh muscles are inefficient. Hence, treadmill exercise is better tolerated by most Americans. Lack of training and physical fitness influences the body's ability to adapt to exercise. Thus inactivity leads to reduced levels of mitochondrial enzymes and energy stores, and should

oxygen delivery be inadequate, greater use is made of anaerobic metabolism. Rarely, an enzyme defect in the muscles themselves affects the ability to exercise, the classic example of which is McArdle's syndrome.

In the healthy person, the $(a-v)O_2$ becomes greater with increasing oxygen uptake. The resting value is around 50 ml/L and increases to about 130 to 150 ml/L with maximal work. Thus, the saturation of venous blood during maximal work is around 30 per cent. In a fully trained athlete, venous oxygen saturation may be appreciably lower, indicating that virtually all the oxygen that is carried to the muscles has been utilized by muscles. In subjects with heart disease, it is even more essential that the removal of oxygen from blood perfusing muscles is as great as possible. For a more detailed review of exercise physiology, the reader is referred to the paper by Wasserman and Whipp.[27]

THE RELATIONSHIP BETWEEN PULMONARY IMPAIRMENT AND DISABILITY

When the problem of industrial lung disease is viewed as a whole, it is evident that it matters little whether the physiological defect is obstructive or restrictive in nature; the presenting symptom is virtually always shortness of breath. Moreover, it is this symptom which is almost always the cause of respiratory disability and is therefore of paramount importance. Some elaboration is, therefore, necessary concerning the relationship between dyspnea and respiratory impairment.

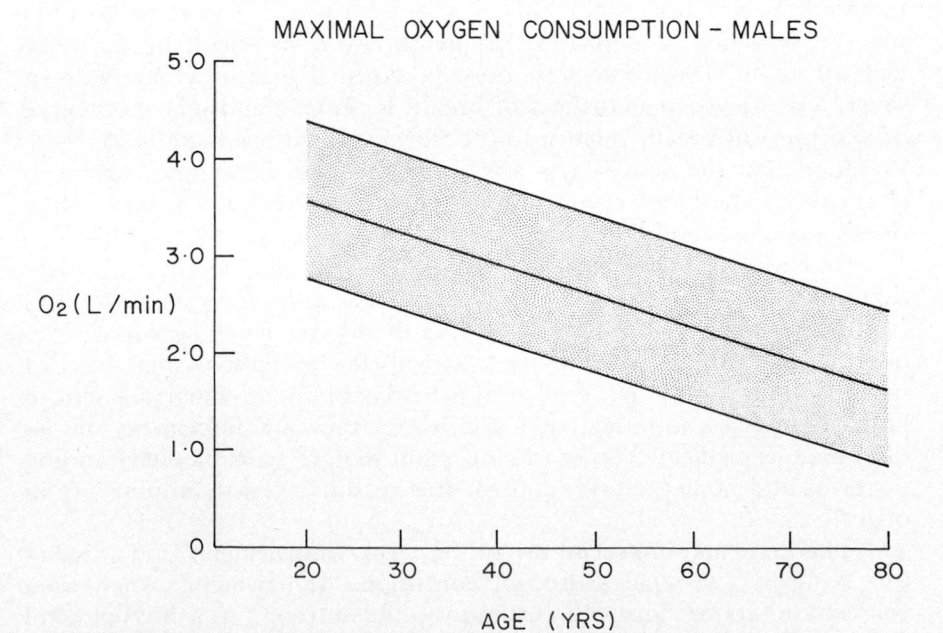

Figure 3–20. Relationship between maximal oxygen consumption and age.

Shortness of breath, like pain, is a subjective sensation and its intensity depends on both the attitude and the personality of the patient. The sensation of shortness of breath does not always correlate well with tests of pulmonary function, sometimes because the person who is affected is relatively stoical, in other instances because he or she has ulterior motives, but most often because no single test or even battery of tests has been devised that can quantify dyspnea. Not uncommonly, the severity of the symptoms is exaggerated in order to obtain financial gain, usually in the form of compensation.

In obstructive airways disease, it can be shown that there is a fairly good relationship between those tests that measure, directly or indirectly, an increased airways resistance (MVV and FEV_1) and the presence of dyspnea. This is especially true of patients who are referred to hospital for nonoccupationally related disease. In restrictive impairment this relationship is sometimes not as clear-cut. It has been suggested that the presence of dyspnea is related to the work of breathing and indeed there is appreciable evidence in favor of this contention. Nonetheless, there are certain facts which are not easily explained by this hypothesis, in particular the dyspnea experienced by a subject on a ventilator where the work of breathing is nonexistent. Campbell and Howell have suggested that length tension inappropriateness provides a better explanation for the sensation of dyspnea.[28] This theory postulates that dyspnea is experienced when there is an imbalance between the demand of the respiratory center for ventilation and the actual ventilation that takes place; in short, the ventilatory response is inappropriate and inadequate for the stimuli received. At the present time, this hypothesis provides the best explanation for the sensation of shortness of breath. Even so, much needs to be learned about this problem. It must be stressed that with moderate or severe exercise some shortness of breath is normal, and it is the degree of shortness of breath relative to the workload that needs to be assessed. Provided that the above facts are borne in mind, it becomes useful to characterize the types of respiratory impairment that are found in the pneumoconioses and other occupational lung diseases.

Nowhere is there more confusion than in the field of disability determination, and no professional group has done more to foster this confusion than lawyers. Physicians find themselves more and more frequently asked to assess disability, and with few exceptions their level of understanding and experience in this field is often an embarrassment to both themselves and the party for whom they are appearing. In no discipline in medicine is it more important to have a clear understanding of terms and nomenclature, and for this reason, a few definitions are in order.

The loose and imprecise use of the terms "impairment" and "disability" is often a seminal source of confusion. "Impairment" when used correctly in connection with respiratory disease refers to a physiological abnormality of function which persists after treatment. It is therefore best

defined as "an inability of the human respiratory apparatus to perform satisfactorily one or more of the three components of respiration, viz., ventilation, diffusion, and perfusion." Anatomical deficiencies, for example, the loss of lung, also constitute an impairment, but in the case of lung disease it is more appropriate to think in terms of physiological function. For the accurate quantification of impairment either the level of function or performance prior to the injury or illness must be known or an accurate prediction for such dysfunction in health must be available. In contrast, "disability" is best defined as "an inability to carry out a specific task or job" or, alternatively, "the development of undue distress during the performance of the job or task." What constitutes distress is, however, a subject of contention, since many perfectly normal persons may suffer some shortness of breath while performing heavy work. In this context it is vital to bear in mind that the same impairment does not necessarily lead to the same disability. Thus, were a ballet dancer to lose a leg, he or she would be completely disabled for the vocation. In contrast, the loss of a leg in a civil servant or governmental bureaucrat would interfere little with the ability to work, and indeed, since the person would be compelled to stick close to a desk, this might lead to further advancement in the bureaucracy. By the same token, because the lungs have a tremendous reserve, minimal and even moderate respiratory impairment seldom interferes with the capacity to work unless the subject earns a living as a professional athlete or in an extraordinarily physically demanding job.

While quantification of impairment is the physician's responsibility, the assessment or adjudication of disability should not be left entirely to physicians, since it requires the assessment of the role of additional factors such as educational status, job requirements, propensity for vocational training, and availability of suitable alternative work. With these provisos in mind, it is now pertinent to consider in more detail some of the factors that determine whether a particular impairment is likely to lead to disability.[29]

Educational State and Motivation

The development of shortness of breath sufficient to put a worker at a disadvantage for a particular job need not always be disabling, since in some instances the person can be moved to a less demanding job. An elderly steel worker with obstruction of the airways might be quite capable of carrying out the duties of a storekeeper or janitor, but such a simple solution is not always attainable. Thus the coal miner who is unable to continue working in the mines might have sufficient respiratory reserve to work as a bank teller or as a salesman, but may have neither the education nor the intellectual attainment for such alternative employment even should such a position be available. Should suitable alternative employment not be possible, the miner must be regarded as disabled despite his having sufficient respiratory reserve to enable him to perform a less demanding job.

In a similar context, it has been clearly established that the likelihood of a worker with a particular impairment continuing to work depends on educational and social background. The better educated the subject, the less likely he is to stop working. LeRoy-Ladurie and colleagues have shown that following a pneumonectomy about 20 per cent of laborers return to work, while 70 to 80 per cent of those with a profession return to their job.[30] In the case of children undergoing pneumonectomy, virtually all go on to obtain a job. While the loss of earnings is usually greater in the disabled professional, and this obviously provides some stimulus to return to work, it is not the only factor, and there is little doubt that if a worker finds his job interesting and stimulating, he has less desire to remain off work and claim compensation. With increasing age there is decreasing adaptability, and older persons may find it more difficult to acquire new skills. In addition, pulmonary function and reserve decline with age. These changes have an effect on working capacity and will be alluded to again.

Energy Requirements

Clearly the energy or work necessary to perform a specific task is important, since in some instances a subject's respiratory reserve may be insufficient for a particular job. As mentioned earlier, the resting requirements for oxygen in a normal person are around 250 to 300 ml/min. A face worker in the coal mine who is operating a continuous miner uses around 1.2 L/min, while farming is somewhat more arduous and demanding, and the requirement for oxygen is around 1.5 L/min and under certain circumstances appreciably higher. Heavy labor in many iron and steel foundries necessitates an oxygen consumption of around 2.1 L/min. Athletic activities require a far greater oxygen consumption, and the most arduous of all, such as cross-country skiing and running, require up to 5.0 L/min. Sustained moderate effort is tolerated less well in the subject with respiratory impairment than are short bursts of high-energy output followed by prolonged low expenditure of energy. In deciding whether a worker is capable of carrying out a task it is therefore essential to know the physical demands of the job as well as his exercise tolerance. Many jobs which were formerly regarded as arduous, e.g., coal and metal mining and construction, have become much less so with the advent of mechanization.

Pulmonary Impairment

The assessment of functional deficits in relation to disability is most often required in occupational pulmonary disease. In subjects being examined for occupationally related disability it is necessary to bear in mind that naturally occurring diseases such as asthma and emphysema may complicate the issue, since they occur concomitantly in a fair number

of subjects. It thus becomes important to separate the effects of occupation from those of naturally acquired disease. To achieve this requires a knowledge of the type and site of the impairment produced by the hazard. It is necessary therefore to know whether the particular hazard induces a response in the airways or in the lung parenchyma. Tests that enable one to diagnose and quantify the degree of impairment in a subject who is exposed to toluene diisocyanate are inappropriate for characterizing the respiratory defects in subjects with asbestosis or silicosis.

The most useful tests in the assessment of respiratory disability are those which are objective and not influenced by the behavior of the subject. This aspect of pulmonary function testing has been dealt with in detail in the chapter on Epidemiology, and the reader is referred to the appropriate section. Although it is often maintained that there is a poor relationship between pulmonary impairment and dyspnea, such a pronouncement is a quarter truth. Granted that there are some individuals in whom this is true, provided one makes allowance for personality, educational status, and whether or not the subject is claiming compensation, an acceptable correlation exists in the majority of subjects. Faute de mieux, in the determination of disability, we have to rely on the degree of impairment to indicate how short of breath a person is likely to be. The comprehensive review in which Gaensler and Wright relate symptoms to various grades and types of pulmonary impairment is still the most useful reference, despite the advent of a plethora of so-called sensitive tests for the detection of minor and insignificant degrees of pulmonary insufficiency.[31]

Turning to the grading of the severity of impairment, in general the patient's or claimant's measured value is expressed as a percentage of the predicted value for a person of the same age, height, sex, and race. That this is less than ideal and discriminates against the older worker is not apparent at first sight. Since pulmonary function declines with age, for a given percentage of the decrement to represent the same disability in an elderly man as it does in a young man would require that the ventilatory cost of performing a certain job declines with age. The reverse is true, and in reality, the young man who has an MVV which is 30 per cent of his predicted figure utilizes less of this respiratory reserve to carry out a certain task than does a 60-year-old man with the same percentage loss of MVV. The regulations devised by the United States Bureau of Disability of the Social Security Administration take this into account and award disability on the basis of a certain absolute reduction of pulmonary function, with the reduction being related only to the subject's height and sex. This appears to be a scientific approach when it is realized that considering age alone might lead to a situation in which the subject is judged disabled or prevented from doing a particular task despite the presence of normal pulmonary function.

Assessment of Shortness of Breath. Since shortness of breath is a cardinal symptom in subjects with pulmonary impairment, some attempt should be made to quantify it. Many factors render this task difficult, in

Table 3–3. ASSESSING SHORTNESS OF BREATH

Grade	Criteria
0	No shortness of breath with normal activity. Shortness of breath with exertion, comparable to a well person of the same age, height, and sex.
1	More shortness of breath than a person of the same age while walking quietly on the level or on climbing an incline or two flights of stairs.
2	More shortness of breath than, and unable to keep up with, persons of the same age and sex while walking on the level.
3	Shortness of breath while walking on the level and while performing everyday tasks at work.
4	Shortness of breath while carrying out personal activities, e.g., dressing, talking, walking from one room to another.

particular the fact that dyspnea is a subjective sensation analogous to pain and, as previously mentioned, that the symptom is often exaggerated. The criteria shown in Table 3–3 are helpful in quantifying or grading the severity of impairment.

There is a fairly good relationship between the FEV_1 and dyspnea, especially in chronic air flow obstruction, but it is remaining function rather than loss of function which governs the ability of the subject to work. Our studies in male patients who were not claiming compensation showed that the FEV_1 is closely related to exercise tolerance (Table 3–4). Other symptoms such as cough and wheeziness can seldom be regarded as disabling except under unusual circumstances.

In disability claimants the reliability of the relationship between pulmonary function and shortness of breath breaks down. This is especially true where the financial rewards exceed what the subject earns at work. Our experience with black lung claimants is shown in Figure 3–21. It is quite clear that disability claimants markedly exaggerate their symptoms, and as such, the symptom of shortness of breath can no longer be relied upon as an index of impairment.[32]

Table 3–4. RELATIONSHIP BETWEEN GRADE OF DYSPNEA AND FEV_1 IN SUBJECTS NOT SEEKING DISABILITY AWARDS

Grade of Dyspnea	Mean FEV_1
0	3.2 L
1	2.4 L
2	1.8 L
3	1.2 L
4	0.75 L

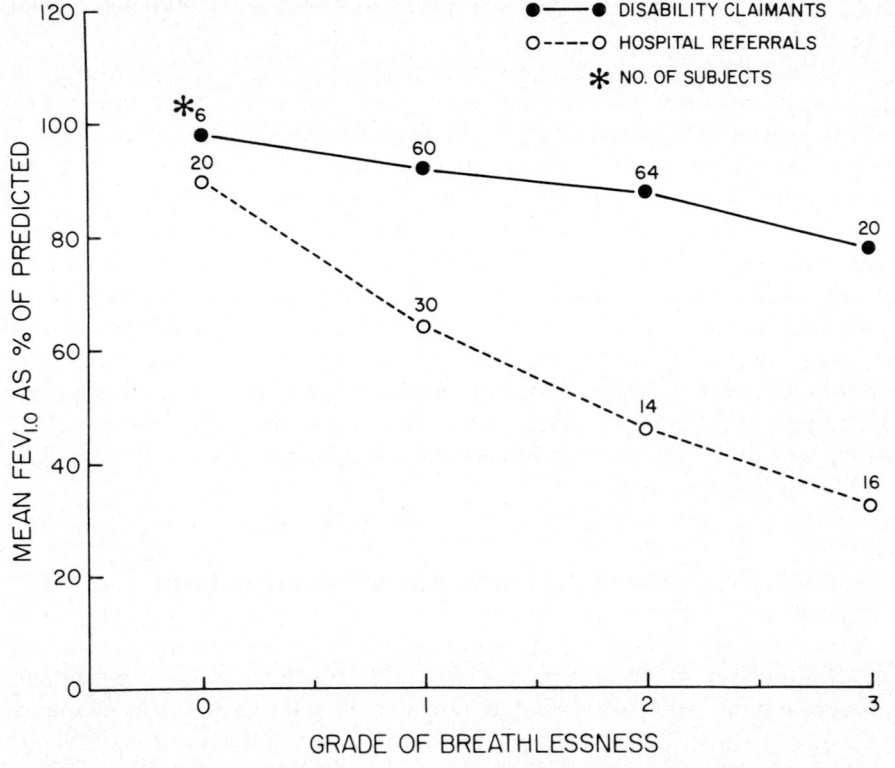

Figure 3–21. Relationship between grade of dyspnea and FEV_1 expressed as a percentage of predicted FEV_1 in black lung claimants and hospital patients. (From Morgan, W. K. C.: Disability or disinclination? Impairment or importuning? Chest, 75, 712, 1979. Used by permission.)

Physical Examination. The physical examination provides limited help in the assessment of impairment and disability. Obvious wasting and shortness of breath at rest or with minor exertion are helpful pointers. The respiratory rate is often useful in the assessment of restrictive impairment when the latter is due to pulmonary fibrosis. In many instances the subject will apparently be comfortable at rest despite the fact that he is breathing with a respiratory rate of 30 to 35 per minute. Minor exercise will often render him markedly short of breath. The presence of hyperinflation and increased resonance, the use of the accessory muscles of respiration, plus certain physical findings such as the decreased distance between the cricothyroid membrane and the suprasternal notch are all helpful indications of the severity of chronic irreversible airways obstruction. In contrast, cyanosis is an unreliable sign. Decreased breath sounds, especially at the bases, often indicate emphysema and may be helpful. Diaphragmatic excursion is difficult to assess and inaccurate.[33] The presence of wheezes indicates turbulent flow and correlates poorly with ventilatory capacity. Persistent crackles, especially medium or coarse in character, which are audible throughout mid- and late inspiration are important and suggest the presence of fibrosis. Early and persistent

inspiratory crackles at the bases indicate severe airways obstruction with overdistension.

Chest Radiograph. This is an unreliable method of diagnosing impairment and disability, and nowhere is this more true than in the field of occupationally related disease. While overdistension can be detected in the standard posteroanterior and lateral film, these changes are late and tend to be nonspecific. In the simple pneumoconioses with the exception of asbestosis, there is little or no relationship between radiographic changes and pulmonary impairment.[34] In asbestosis there is some relationship between the severity of the radiographic changes and both symptoms and pulmonary function, at least in categories 2 and 3. The relationship becomes more tenuous in the lower categories—1/0, 1/1, and 1/2.[35, 36] In conglomerate silicosis and progressive massive fibrosis of coal miners there is a relationship between shortness of breath and the size of the conglomerate opacities, and in most subjects with stages B and C there is obvious pulmonary impairment.[34]

Pulmonary Function in Determination of Impairment and Disability

Pulmonary function tests can be used in two ways to help in disability determination. First, residual function may be compared to the demands of a specified activity or a given job. Second, pulmonary function values may be related to independent indices of disability such as respiratory symptoms. Thus, the results of pulmonary function tests are often related to the degree of shortness of breath that is present when the subject is performing a certain activity. In this regard it must be remembered that a significant loss of function may be present before shortness of breath is experienced. Pulmonary function tests tend to be most useful in assessing disability in chronic conditions such as emphysema, in which the airways obstruction is irreversible. They have less application in conditions where the functional impairment tends to wax and wane or undergo exacerbations such as occur in asthma.

Spirometry. The derivation of certain indices of ventilatory capacity is the most commonly used method of assessing lung function. The various indices and the method of measurement have been described elsewhere in this chapter. Suffice it to say, the FVC, the FEV_1 and the FEV_1/FVC ratio are the most useful indices in the assessment of disabling pulmonary impairment. The tests are easily performed, simple, reproducible, sensitive, and fairly specific. Lack of effort is easily detected, and even a neophyte should have some idea that cooperation is lacking when there are disparate values. The tracings should always be inspected for reproducibility and in every instance there should be three tracings which are reproducible and within 7 per cent of the highest. The curve should be flat when the subject ceases to exhale, indicating that he has completed the maneuver. "Bumps" along the course of the curve indicate changes in

flow rates and are usually attempts by the subject to produce falsely low values. A straight line over the first 75 per cent of the forced vital capacity indicates malingering and can be produced by the subject deliberately limiting flow by pursing his lips. If reversible airways obstruction is suspected, the forced expiratory volume maneuver should be repeated following administration of a bronchodilator. Numerous prediction formulae exist. Those based on nonsmoking subjects are recommended. Nonetheless, when a claimant's value is compared to a particular predicted value, only if the claimant's value is markedly reduced is disability likely to be present, and in the context of disability determination, the choice of a particular prediction formula is not of great moment.

The MVV, although often used in disability evaluation, has certain drawbacks. First, the test requires considerable effort from the patient and is tiring and distressing, and second, it is much more difficult to assess whether the subject is making a maximal effort. Even with maximal cooperation, many nonpulmonary factors influence the MVV, including muscle coordination, heart disease, neurological function, and chest wall compliance. If the FEV_1 is multiplied by 40, this gives an accurate prediction of the MVV and enables one to see whether the subject has exerted a maximal effort during the performance of the maneuver. Because of these problems, the MVV is now used less often than previously; however, it does help in assessing the validity of the other measurements. When there is a disparity between the FEV_1 and the MVV, the latter measurement is nearly always found to be depressed, usually because of a submaximal effort.

Diffusing Capacity. This test is most useful in the determination of impairment and disability in subjects with restrictive impairment resulting from fibrotic changes in the lung. It is an overall index of gas transfer, and does not measure the diffusing capacity per se but rather the ability of the lungs to transfer gas from the alveolus to the pulmonary capillary. Though fairly reproducible, technically it is not so easily performed and is also somewhat lacking in specificity.[36] Even so, it is an essential part of the investigation of subjects with restrictive impairment in conditions such as asbestosis.[35, 36]

Arterial Blood Gases. Despite the insistence of some United States governmental agencies, blood gas analysis is not recommended, since it is nonspecific, lacking in sensitivity, invasive, and influenced by hyperventilation and the position in which the blood sample is drawn. Subjects with normal lungs may have a decrease in their PaO_2 tension, and falls of between 10 to 30 mm in the PaO_2 are common when an obese subject assumes the supine position.[37] In addition, correction factors for altitude should be applied to predicted PaO_2 values, since normal values in high-altitude cities such as Denver or Johannesburg differ markedly from the values obtained at sea level. Age likewise has a profound effect on PaO_2. While the expected PaO_2 of a 25-year-old at sea level is 95 mm, that of a 60-year-old is 76 mm, with the lower limit of normality being 70 mm (Fig. 3–22).

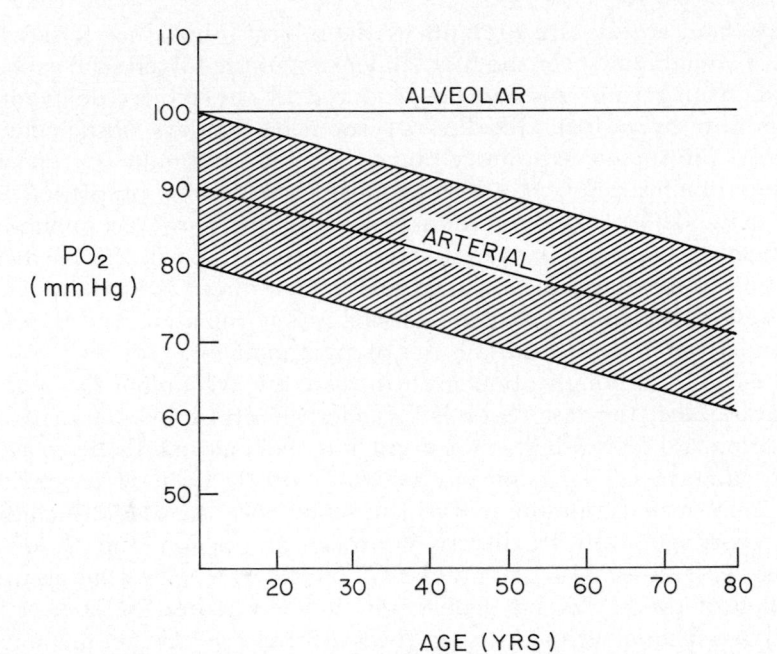

Figure 3–22. Relationship of arterial PO_2 and age. Although the standard deviation is shown as the same for young and older subjects, in practice it is greater in the older subject.

Alveolo-Arterial Oxygen Gradient [(A-a)O$_2$]. Although the (A–a)O$_2$ is a sensitive method for detecting abnormalities of gas exchange, it has little use in the assessment of disability. It is, moreover, nonspecific and affected by nonpulmonary diseases such as left ventricular failure, cirrhosis of the liver, and obesity. The size of the gradient is affected by venous admixture, ventilation perfusion mismatching, and a reduction of the diffusing capacity, with each of these factors exerting a different effect varying with the Pa_{O_2} and FI_{O_2}. Measurement of the resting (A-a)O$_2$ is unreliable as an index of impairment and often improves with exercise.[35] The average (A-a)O$_2$ at the age of 20 is around 8 mm ± 5, but by the age of 60, the mean value is 20 mm ± 8. The normal value in a 60-year-old man ranges between 15 and 28 mm (Fig. 3–23).

The (A-a)O$_2$ is affected by changes in cardiac output. As the latter changes, different fractions of the cardiac output perfuse the anatomical and physiological shunts which may be present. The coefficient of variation for the (A-a)O$_2$ is around 19 per cent, in contrast to that of the PaO_2, which is about 3.5 per cent.[38] The (A-a)O$_2$ is most useful as a means of detecting disabling impairment during exercise. Even here it is essential to ascertain that the subject has reached a steady state, and only when the (A-a)O$_2$ is over 50 mm is there any assurance that the impairment is likely to be disabling.

Lung Volumes. These show a poor correlation with shortness of breath and with respiratory disability. They are not recommended as suitable tests to be used in disability assessment.

Test of Small Airways Function. These have no place in the assessment of disability. The tests may be abnormal despite the complete absence of symptoms.

Ventilatory Equivalent (VE$_{O_2}$). In order to extract 100 ml of oxygen, a normal person has to breathe about 2.5 L of air. The number of liters of air breathed per 100 ml of oxygen uptake is usually referred to as the ventilatory equivalent (VE$_{O_2}$). This index can be measured by simple spirometry. Hyperventilation in the face of normal VE$_{O_2}$ is a normal response to exercise and is said to be metabolically justified. In contrast, when the VE$_{O_2}$ is increased, the hyperventilation is said to be metabolically unjustified and is a consequence of either cardiopulmonary disease or anxiety. The measurement of VE$_{O_2}$ at rest or at low levels of exercise is notoriously prone to inaccuracies and is of little value, but is more useful with high and sustained levels of exercise.[31] It is necessary to bear in mind that virtually every subject hyperventilates to a greater or lesser extent when first starting to breathe on a spirometer, and it is only after some time when the subject has achieved a steady state that the inappropriate hyperventilation disappears.

Dyspnea Index. A formerly popular method of trying to quantify

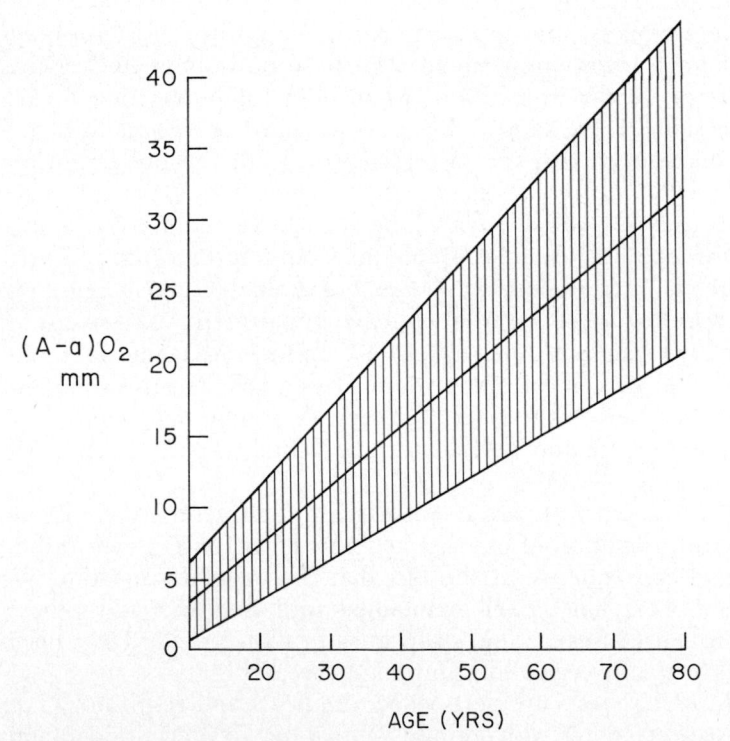

Figure 3–23. Relationship of age to the alveolo-arterial gradient for oxygen (A-a)O$_2$. The predictions are based on observations made in a selected group of older hospital patients with normal spirometry and no chest disease. Some subjects, however, were overweight and some may have had coronary artery disease in the absence of overt failure. The figure indicates that the standard deviation of the test increases with age.

impairment and shortness of breath was known as the dyspnea index. This is the percentage of the MVV required for a stated activity. The dyspnea index for walking on the flat at 2 mph is around 12 per cent ± 4. Elevation of the index can occur as a result of a reduction in the MVV or because of a pathologically increased ventilatory requirement. Any value below 35 per cent suggests that dyspnea is unlikely to be excessive, values between 35 and 50 per cent are in an intermediate zone, and all subjects with a value above 50 per cent can be assumed to be short of breath at abnormally low levels of exercise.

Exercise Testing. Although exercise testing is important physiologically, it is seldom necessary in the determination of occupationally related pulmonary disability. The main drawback to exercise testing as a means of ascertaining impairment in disability claimants is that the claimant may stop exercising before reaching the limit of his tolerance, claiming that he is short of breath, has chest pain, or is tired, when in reality he is merely disinclined. Claimants are often reluctant to undergo exercise testing, and in addition, many subjects have coincident heart disease and the risks of exercise testing in such subjects may preclude its use. For these reasons, exercise testing is best reserved for those claimants whose lung function is doubtful or borderline.

Nevertheless, this approach can be helpful in distinguishing pulmonary from cardiac impairment, and in apportioning the relative contributions to overall impairment when both pulmonary and heart disease are present in the same subject. When cardiac output fails to increase commensurately with the increased workload, the pulse rate rises inappropriately and becomes maximal at a lower than expected workload. By way of contrast, subjects with lung disease are limited by ventilation, so that with exercise their heart rate does not approach the predicted range and their limitation occurs as a result of an inability to increase ventilation to an appropriate level. In obstructive impairment, excessive shortness of breath and a high dyspnea index develop for a particular level of exercise. Impairment of gas transfer seldom plays a role because ventilation limits are reached before the arterial oxygen saturation drops to a critical level. Moreover, ventilation perfusion mismatching often lessens during exercise.

The subject with severe diffusion impairment usually demonstrates an abrupt limitation of exercise at a particular oxygen consumption level. This is a consequence of the fact that the oxygen saturation in the end pulmonary capillary is well maintained until the workload reaches a critical level, which causes a rapid drop in saturation. As the DL_{CO} declines, the critical level of oxygen consumption decreases.

If exercise tests are performed, the heart and respiratory rate should be measured along with minute ventilation, oxygen uptake, and carbon dioxide output. The subject should be monitored for arrhythmias or evidence of myocardial ischemia.

Measurement of Functional Capacity

The easiest way of estimating functional capacity is to measure oxygen consumption during maximal exercise. This can then be theoretically related to the demands of a particular job. Such an approach has disadvantages in elderly subjects in whom cardiac output is often impaired, and the stress of submaximal exercise may precipitate an infarction or arrhythmia. In the United States, up to 70 per cent of males and 55 per cent of females over the age of 50 show significant ECG changes during stress testing.

When pulmonary impairment causes a limitation of work capacity, exercise tolerance is most often determined by the maximal voluntary ventilation. An increased demand for ventilation may result from impaired gas exchange. The relationship of ventilatory capacity in gas exchange to maximal oxygen consumption was studied by Wright, who was able to derive an equation which predicted maximal O_2 consumption.[39] Armstrong and his colleagues extended Wright's study and were able to predict maximal oxygen consumption from the MVV and the ventilatory equivalent measured during submaximal exercise.[40] The predicted value corresponded closely with the measured value in both healthy and impaired subjects. This approach has been further simplified by Wehr and Johnson and can avoid the problems of maximal exercise.[41] But some doubts have been expressed as to the validity of using submaximal exercise as a means of predicting maximal O_2 consumption.

The use of submaximal exercise to predict maximal oxygen consumption has certain limitations in that heart disease may lead to a lower than normal maximal O_2 consumption. In addition, the ventilatory equivalent depends on the level of exercise, and if the measurements are made while the subject is exercising at too low a level of METS, then anxiety induced or voluntary hyperventilation can artifactually elevate the O_2 uptake. At high workloads and nearer to the anaerobic threshold, ventilation increases disproportionately to oxygen uptake, thereby increasing the ventilatory equivalent. In patients with a reduced diffusing capacity, a sudden fall in oxygen saturation often occurs at a particular oxygen consumption, and the level cannot necessarily be predicted by the ventilatory equivalent at lower workloads.

Grading of Impairment

Numerous criteria have been published for grading pulmonary impairment. These differ appreciably, and nowhere more than in the regulations promulgated by various United States governmental agencies. The criteria are listed and discussed by Epler and co-workers.[35] A rough guide to the severity of the various types of pulmonary impairment is shown in Table 3–5. These values are partly based on the work of Gaensler and Wright and partly on our own experience with coal miners

Table 3–5. CRITERIA FOR GRADING IMPAIRMENT OF PULMONARY FUNCTION

Test	Mild	Moderate	Severe
Obstructive Impairment			
MVV (% predicted)	65–80	45–60	Less than 45
VC (% predicted)	Normal	Usually normal	Slight to moderate reduction
FEV$_1$ (% predicted)	65–80	45–60	Less than 45
FEV$_1$/FVC%*	55–75	45–55	Less than 45
Blood gases† (% sat)	Normal	Usually normal	Hypoxemia
Dl$_{CO}$ (% predicted)	Normal	Normal or slight reduction	Slight to moderate reduction
Restrictive Impairment			
MVV (% predicted)	Normal	Normal	50–80
VC (% predicted)	60–80	50–60	Less than 50
FEV$_1$ (% predicted)	60–80	50–60	Less than 50
FEV$_1$/FVC%*	Normal	Normal	Normal
Blood gases % sat	Normal	Normal	Usually normal
Dl$_{CO}$ (% predicted)	Normal	50–75	Below 50
Interstitial Lung Disease			
MVV (% predicted)	Normal	Normal	60 or above
VC (% predicted)	70 or greater	50–70	Less than 50
FEV$_1$ (% predicted)	70 or greater	50–70	Less than 50
REV$_1$/FVC%*	Normal	Normal	Normal
Blood gases % sat	94–96	90–94	90 or less
(A-a)O$_2$ mm*	15–30	30–40	above 40
Dl$_{CO}$ (% predicted)	Normal	40–75	Less than 40

*Age related.
†Unreliable in obstructive impairment.

applying for black lung benefits. For full details and a lucid discussion of the application of function tests to disability determination, the reader should consult the classic paper of Gaensler and Wright.[31] Elsewhere, Richman gives an excellent description of the legal aspects and definitions of disability and discusses many of the divergent points of view that seem inevitable when physicians and lawyers are involved in lawsuits.[42]

In conclusion, the detection of impairment should be done in a simple and as noninvasive a fashion as possible, using simple and objective tests. The use of a battery of tests without regard to the likely cause of the impairment—including blood gas analysis, body plethysmography, and the determination of compliance and lung volumes such as is used in Germany—although objective, is time-consuming and puts the patient or claimant through considerable and for the most part unnecessary discomfort. Moreover, many of the more complex tests correlate poorly with symptoms. This is especially true of the use of blood gas analysis, which has been recommended by the United States Department of Labor for use in coal miners with normal or near normal ventilatory capacity.

Finally, in deciding who is disabled, what is important is not the percentage loss of function but the residual capacity or function, since this determines work capacity.

References

1. Campbell, E. J. M. et al., The Respiratory Muscles. Philadelphia, W. B. Saunders Co., 1970.
2. Barnhard, H. J., Pierce, J. A., Joyce, J. W., and Bates, J. H., Roentgenographic determinination of total lung capacity. Am. J. Med., 28, 51, 1966.
3. Reger, R. B., Young, A., and Morgan, W. K. C., An accurate and rapid radiographic method of determining total lung capacity. Thorax, 27:163, 1972.
4. Radford, E. P., Recent studies of the mechanical properties of mammalian lungs. In Remington, J. W., ed., Tissue Elasticity. Washington, D. C., American Physiological Society, 1957.
5. Pattle, R. E., Lining layer of the lung. Br. Med. Bull., 19:41, 1963.
6. Clements, J. A., Surface phenomena in relation to pulmonary function. Physiologist, 5, 11, 1962.
7. Hyatt, R. E., Schilder, D. P., and Fry, D. L., Relationship between maximum expiratory flow and degree of lung inflation. J. Appl. Physiol., 13, 331, 1960.
8. Fowler, W. S., Lung function studies, III. Uneven pulmonary ventilation in normal subjects and in subjects with pulmonary disease. J. Appl. Physiol., 2, 283, 1949.
9. First in-last out in the lung. Editorial, Br. Med. J., 3, 119, 1973.
10. Otis, A. B., McKerrow, C. B., Bartlett, R. A., et al., Mechanical factors in the distribution of pulmonary ventilation. J. Appl. Physiol., 26, 732, 1969.
11. Mackem, I. T., and Mead, J., Resistance of central and peripheral airways measured by retrograde catheter. J. Appl. Physiol., 22, 395, 1967.
12. Milic-Emili, J., Henderson, J. E. M., Dolovich, M. B., et al., Regional distribution of inspired gas in the lung. J. Appl. Physiol., 21, 749, 1966.
13. Glazier, J. B., Hughes, J. M. B., Maloney, J. E., and West, J. B., Vertical gradient of alveolar size in lungs of dogs frozen intact. J. Appl. Physiol., 23, 694, 1967.
14. Bake, B., Wood, L., Murphy, B., et al., The effect of inspiratory flow rate on the regional distribution of inspired gas. J. Appl. Physiol., 37, 8, 1974.
15. Hughes, J. M. B., Glazier, J. B., Maloney, J. E., and West, J. B., Effect of lung volume on the distribution of pulmonary blood flow in man. Resp. Phys., 4:58, 1968.

16. West, J. B., Regional differences in gas exchange in the lung of erect man. J. Appl. Physiol., *17*, 893, 1962.
17. Evans, J. W., Wagner, P. D., and West, J. B., Conditions for reduction of pulmonary gas transfer by ventilation-perfusion inequality. J. Appl. Physiol., *36*, 533, 1974.
18. Fahri, L. E., and Rahn, H., A theoretical analysis of the alveolar oxygen difference with special reference to the distribution effect. J. Appl. Physiol., *7*, 699, 1955.
19. Riley, R. L., and Cournand, A., Ideal alveolar air and the analysis of ventilation-perfusion relationships in the lungs. J. Appl. Physiol., *1*, 825, 1949.
20. Perutz, M. F., Stereochemistry of cooperative effects of haemoglobin. Nature, *228*, 726, 1970.
21. Lenfant, C., Wayes, P., Aucutt, C., and Couz, J., Effect of chronic hypoxic hypoxia on the O_2-Hb dissociation curve and respiratory gas transport in man. Resp. Physiol., *7*, 7, 1969.
22. Comroe, J. H., The Lung, 2nd ed. Chicago, Year Book Medical Publishers, 1962.
23. Ogilvie, C. M., Forster, R. E., Blakemore, W. S., and Morton, J. W., A standardized breath-holding technique for the clinical measurement of the diffusing capacity of the lungs for carbon monoxide. J. Clin. Invest., *36*, 1, 1957.
24. Filley, G. F., MacIntosh, D. J., and Wright, G., Carbon monoxide uptake and pulmonary diffusing capacity in normal subjects at rest and during exercise. J. Clin. Invest., *33*, 530, 1954.
25. Roughton, F. J. W., and Forster, R. E., Relative importance of diffusion and chemical reaction rates in determining rate of exchange of gases in the human lung, with special reference to true diffusing capacity of pulmonary membrane and volume of blood in the lung capillaries. J. Appl. Physiol., *11*, 277, 1957.
26. Jones, N. L., and Campbell, E. J. M., Exercise Testing, 2nd ed. Philadelphia, W. B. Saunders Co., 1982.
27. Wasserman, K., and Whipp, B. J., Exercise physiology in health and disease. Am. Rev. Respir. Dis., *112*, 219, 1975.
28. Campbell, E. J. M., and Howell, J. B. L., Sensation of breathlessness. Br. Med. Bull., *19*, 36, 1963.
29. Morgan, W. K. C., Disability or disinclination: impairment or importuning. Chest, *75*, 712, 1979.
30. LeRoy-Ladurie, M., Silbert, D., and Ranson-Bitker, B., Facteurs d'invalidité après pneumonectomie. Bull. Physiopathol. Respir., *11*, 182, 1975.
31. Gaensler, E., and Wright, G. W., Evaluation of respiratory impairment. Arch. Environ. Health, *12*, 146, 1966.
32. Morgan, W. K. C., Lapp, N. L., and Seaton, D., Respiratory disability in coal miners. J.A.M.A., *243*, 410, 1980.
33. Williams, T., Ahmad, D., and Morgan, W. K. C., A clinical and roentgenographic correlation of diaphragmatic movement. Arch. Intern Med., *141*, 878, 1981.
34. Morgan, W. K. C., Handelsman, L., Kibelstis, J. A., et al., Ventilatory capacity and lung volumes in U.S. coal miners. Arch. Environ. Health, *28*, 182, 1974.
35. Epler, G. R., Saber, F. A., and Gaensler, E. A., Determination of severe impairment (disability) in interstitial lung disease. Am. Rev. Respir. Dis., *121*, 647, 1980.
36. Epidemiology standardization project. Am. Rev. Respir. Dis. (Suppl.) (Part 2), *118*, 7, 1978.
37. Said, S. I., Abnormalities in pulmonary gas exchange in obesity. Ann. Intern. Med., *53*, 1121, 1960.
38. Kafer, E. R., and Donnelly, P., Reproducibility of data on spread of steady state gas exchange in indices of maldistribution of ventilation and blood flow. Chest, *71*, 758, 1977.
39. Wright, G. W., Maximum achievable oxygen uptake during physical exercise of six minutes correlated with other measurements of respiratory function in normal and pathological subjects, Fed. Proc., *12*, 160, 1953.
40. Armstrong, B. W., Workman, J. M., Hurt, H. H., and Roemich, W. R., Clinicophysiologic evaluation of physical working capacity in persons with pulmonary disease. Parts I and II. Am. Rev. Respir. Dis., 93, 90 and 223, 1966.
41. Wehr, K. L., and Johnson, R. L., Maximal oxygen consumption in patients with lung disease. J. Clin. Invest., *58*, 880, 1976.
42. Richman, S. I., Meanings of impairment and disability. The conflicting social objectives underlying the confusion. Chest (Suppl.), *78*, 367, 1980.

4

THE DEPOSITION AND CLEARANCE OF DUST FROM THE LUNGS—Their Role in the Etiology of Occupational Lung Disease

W. Keith C. Morgan

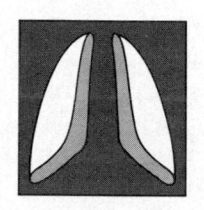

An understanding of the pathophysiology of occupational lung disease requires some knowledge of the mechanisms involved in the deposition and disposal of inhaled dust. Dust physicists have over the years studied pulmonary deposition in much detail and much is now known concerning the physical processes involved. Its subsequent transport from the sites of deposition, in particular the alveoli, to other regions is less well understood.

The basic anatomy of the lung has been known for many years and by applying this knowledge, certain outstanding workers formulated many of the theoretical concepts of dust deposition and respiratory mechanics long before appropriate fast-response electronic equipment became available to confirm their hypotheses. The advent of sophisticated and sensitive electronic measuring devices has lead to a rebirth of the study of the acute and chronic effects of inhaled particles.

DUST DEPOSITION

In 1935, Findeisen constructed a model designed to provide information on how dust particles are deposited in the lungs.[1] The model assumed that deposition depended on Newtonian mechanics and Stokes' law; the latter being the physical law which describes the fall of small particles. It has been known since the days of Lister that while inhaled air

contains numerous bacteria, viruses, and other particles, exhaled air—
apart from the early expirate which is composed of the dead space air—
is free from bacteria and particles. This was first demonstrated by Tyndall
who, by means of the Tyndalloscope, showed that expired air under
normal circumstances contained few, if any, particles and hence was
invisible in a strong light. When a person takes a breath, air is drawn
through the nares into the nasopharynx and trachea and hence into the
conducting system of the lungs. From there it reaches the alveoli by way
of the various bronchi, terminal bronchioles, respiratory bronchioles, and
atrial ducts. Most of the bronchial surface of the healthy subject is lined
by a film of mucus which is continually propelled upwards by ciliary
action. As the inspired air enters the trachea its flow rate decreases slightly.
A further reduction in velocity takes place in the main segmental bronchi.
When the third, fourth, and fifth divisions of the bronchi are reached
there is marked slowing of the air stream, so that by the time the inspired
air reaches the terminal bronchioles the flow rate is not more than 2 to 3
cm/sec.

The deposition of inhaled particles and the effects of inhaled gases
are influenced by the physical and chemical properties of the inhaled
agent, and also by sundry host factors (Table 4–1). The physical properties
of importance include particle size and density, shape and penetrability,
surface area, electrostatic charge, and hygroscopicity.[2] Among the more
important chemical properties influencing the respiratory tract's response
are the acidity or alkalinity of the inhaled agent and its ability to enter
into combination with the body's constituents. Various host factors are
also of importance and will be referred to later.

When considering particle deposition, it is useful to divide the respiratory tract into three main regions: (1) the nose and extrathoracic airways
that extend to the glottis; (2) the conducting airways, viz., dead space, or
trachea and bronchi to the terminal bronchioles; and (3) the pulmonary
parenchyma where gas exchange occurs. The nose is an exceedingly
efficient filter and most large particles are deposited in it, provided the
subject is breathing through the nares. Some small particles will, however,
reach the intrathoracic dead space, and an even smaller number will reach
the parenchyma. Those particles between 0.5 and 6.0 microns are referred
to as the respirable fraction, a term which implies their size permits their
deposition in the lung parenchyma. While this is true, not all respirable
particles are deposited in the gas-exchanging portions of the lung, and
many are deposited in the nose and dead space. The particles most likely
to be deposited in the alveoli, and of particular concern as a cause of
pneumoconiosis, are those between 0.5 and 2.5 microns.

Physical Properties

The respiratory tract's response is influenced by whether the inhaled
agent is a particulate, fume, mist, vapor, or gas, and in this connection a

few definitions are in order. An aerosol is a collection of fine particles, either liquid or solid, which is dispersed in a gas; a fume is a fine solid particulate; a mist is a fine liquid particulate; a vapor is the gaseous form of the substance which is normally a liquid; while a gas is a substance whose physical state is without fixed volume. Besides size, on occasion the shape and penetrability of a particle influence the body's reaction to it. Thus, the sharp and needle-like fibers of crocidolite asbestos are more likely to penetrate and migrate than are the serpentine fibers of chrysotile. Evidence indicates that this is an important factor in the etiology of mesothelioma and explains the increased incidence of this tumor following exposure to crocidolite. Solubility is also important, in that while insoluble particulates such as asbestos and silica produce their effects entirely or nearly entirely due to a local action, other agents, such as manganese and

Table 4–1. FACTORS INFLUENCING THE EFFECTS OF INHALED AGENTS

Physical Properties
1. Physical state—whether particle, mist, vapor, fume, or gas. SO_2 is adsorbed onto particles of carbon and hence carried into the distal airways.
2. Size and density of particles, mist, or aerosol—determines site of deposition.
3. Shape and penetrability—influences propensity for migration, chrysotile versus crocidolite.
4. Solubility.
   a. Particulates. Insoluble agents such as asbestos produce local action, whereas soluble agents such as manganese compounds have systemic effects.
   b. Gases and vapors. Insoluble agents such as oxides of nitrogen are inhaled into small air passages, while soluble agents such as ammonia and sulphur dioxide seldom pass beyond nose and nasopharynx.
5. Hygroscopicity—hygroscopic particles increase in size as they travel down respiratory tract.
6. Electric charge—influences site of deposition.

Chemical Properties
1. Acidity and alkalinity—have a toxic effect on cilia, cells, and enzyme systems.
2. Propensity to combine with substances in lung and tissues. Agents such as carbon monoxide and hydrogen cyanide have systemic effects, while fluorine compounds may have both local and systemic effects.
3. Fibrogenicity—asbestos and silica are fibrogenic; iron and carbon are nonfibrogenic.
4. Antigenicity—stimulates antibodies.

Host Factors: Genetic, Environmental, and Acquired
1. Lung defenses.
   a. Genetic determinants influence ciliary action, clearance rates, and macrophage function. Slow and rapid clearers exist, and rates of clearance are inherited characteristics.
   b. Acquired determinants, viz., drugs, cigarette smoke, temperature, and alcohol all influence ciliary and macrophage function.
2. Anatomical and physiological factors—influence of breathing patterns and airways geometry.
3. Immunological state. Response to an agent can be influenced by allergic diathesis, atopy, and tissue type.

beryllium, are soluble to a greater or lesser extent and therefore can have systemic effects on the brain, kidneys, and other organs.

The humidity and temperature of the aerosol have important influences on the site of deposition, in that hygroscopic aerosols tend to increase their size as they pass down the airways. Hence, the relative humidity of the airways becomes important. In man, inhaled air in most circumstances becomes fully saturated in the nose, partly because of diffusion and partly because of convective mixing. The large deflecting channels which are present in the anterior nares create turbulence and increase the tendency for deposition from inertial impaction. The turbinates create eddy currents and further turbulence and likewise increase deposition from inertial impaction.

Flow of air through the tracheobronchial tree may be laminar, turbulent, or transitional. In laminar flow the viscosity of the gas or mixture of gases is of prime importance, while in turbulent flow the density of the gases has a greater influence. The Reynold's number, the ratio of inertial to viscous forces, decides whether flow is turbulent or laminar. In the larger airways such as the larynx, trachea, and lobar and segmental bronchi, flow is partly turbulent and partly transitional. Increases in air flow that occur during exercise, coughing, or hyperventilation increase turbulence in the large airways. Laminar flow predominates in the small airways and their flow rates are appreciably less than are those of the larger airways. Respiratory flow rates and the size of the tidal volume affect deposition due to both inertial impaction and diffusion. Diseases which increase turbulent flow, e.g., bronchitis and asthma, increase central deposition of particles. Similarly, obstruction of the airways likewise tends to limit deposition peripherally and to increase central deposition.[2a]

Chemical Properties

The chemical properties of the inhaled agents likewise influence the effect of particles, mist, vapors, and gases. Depending on the site of deposition, the acidity or alkalinity of the agent can cause a variety of effects including paralysis of cilia, delayed particle clearance, and ciliary death, and may in addition interfere with enzyme systems which control cellular metabolism. In a like fashion, certain substances combine with the lung and tissue fluids and exert both systemic and local effects. Thus, carbon monoxide traverses the alveolocapillary membrane to form carboxyhemoglobin. Fluorine and its compounds, while having a local effect, may also be absorbed and exert systemic effects on the skeleton and other organs. The propensity of the deposited particle to induce fibrosis is likewise important, and while some particles, including asbestos, quartz, and cristobalite, are intensely fibrogenic, others, such as stannic oxide, iron, and coal, have little or no fibrogenicity. Other agents, such as *Bacillus subtilis* enzymes, when inhaled can lead to the development of antibodies

and asthma. Fungal spores and other organisms may likewise generate an immunological response.

Host Factors

Host factors may be divided into genetic, environmental, and acquired factors. The lung defenses include ciliary clearance, humoral antibody formation, and other factors which may be compromised by hereditary defects. By the same token, some persons clear particles rapidly from the ciliated airways, while others do so relatively slowly. The rate of clearing is determined to a large extent by genetic factors and is immutable in that slow and fast clearers retain their characteristics throughout life.[3, 4] Lung defenses may also be affected by environmental and occupational insults including air pollutants, cigarette smoking, drugs, and excessive cold, and by other nonspecific factors. Macrophage function, mucociliary clearance, and smooth muscle sensitivity may all be affected by such extraneous influences. The anatomy and airways geometry of individuals show marked variations. Thus the total cross-sectional area of each generation of the airways varies considerably in persons of the same age and height.[5, 6] Much the same can be said for the angles of bifurcation of the airways. Such anatomical differences affect the degree of turbulence in the airways and also the propensity for particles to settle. Breathing rates and tidal volume likewise vary appreciably, and as such may have a profound influence on the site and magnitude of particle deposition. Similarly, the immune state of the subject influences the response to inhaled agents. Thus, the presence of atopy or the allergic diathesis may predispose to the development of certain types of occupational asthma, e.g., that due to platinum salts. It has been suggested that tissue type as determined by HLA testing is also important in predicting the development of certain conditions such as asbestosis or coal workers' penumoconiosis. This is now known to be of little or no importance.[7] Smoking, on the other hand, seems to protect against the development of extrinsic allergic alveolitis, perhaps the only beneficial health fact that is known to result from this dangerous habit.[8] Whether this is due to a generalized depression of the immunological responses in smokers or occurs as a result of the fact that particles do not reach the alveoli because of an excess of mucus in the conducting airways remains conjectural.

Mechanisms of Particle Deposition

There are five physical processes involved in particle deposition (Fig. 4–1). These have been ably reviewed by Brain and Valberg[2] and are as follows:

1. Sedimentation or gravitational settling
2. Inertial impaction

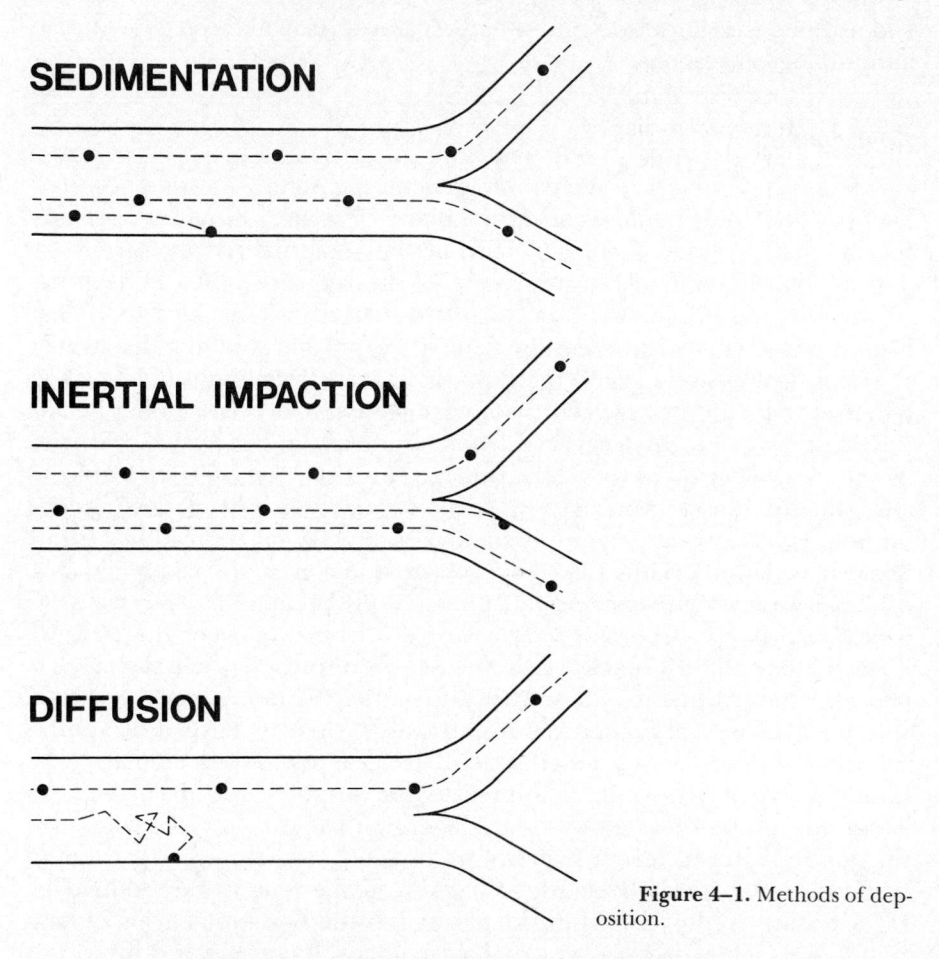

SEDIMENTATION

INERTIAL IMPACTION

DIFFUSION

Figure 4–1. Methods of deposition.

3. Diffusion or Brownian movement
4. Electrostatic precipitation
5. Interception

In man, the last two processes are of much less importance in the etiology of occupational lung disease than the others.

Sedimentation. Particles sediment under the influence of gravity, each falling at a constant speed which depends on Stokes' law. The speed at which a particle settles is known as the terminal velocity and is directly dependent on its density and the square of its diameter. Large particles settle more rapidly. Sedimentation is also affected by residence time in the alveoli, particle concentration in the various airways, the incline of the angle with respect to gravity, and the aerodynamic diameter of the particle. It must be borne in mind that in life monodispersed aerosols do not occur, and particles are not of a single size or shape. Deposition of irregular particles is usually described as a function of their aerodynamic diameter, which refers to the diameter of a unit density sphere that has

the same terminal velocity as the particle under study (see also p. 217). The distribution of aerodynamic diameters of a particular aerosol can be measured experimentally and the frequency distribution can be determined. Most heterodispersed aerosols fit a log normal distribution in which a plot of particle number density (the number of particles per given size interval, viz., 1 to 2 microns) versus the logarithm of size produces a Gaussian curve. Such an aerosol can effectively be described by two properties, namely, the count median diameter (CMD) and the geometric standard deviation (GSD). The mass median diameter (MMD) is larger than the CMD because the larger particles make a greater contribution to the total mass of the aerosol.

Inertial Impaction. When a particle is being carried along in an air current and the latter changes its direction, the momentum of the particle will carry it forward in its initial pathway. As a consequence, some particles are deposited by impaction at those regions of the bronchial tree where a bifurcation or angle is present. Deposition of the particle under such circumstances is mainly determined by its momentum, that is to say, by the product of its weight and speed. Breathing patterns characterized by increased flows tend to lead to greater inertial impaction, especially of larger particles. Turbulent impaction is more important as a cause of deposition in the larger airways and predominantly affects particles greater than 1 micron.

Diffusion or Brownian Motion. Small particles are possessed of kinetic energy as a result of being bombarded by molecules of the surrounding air. Their movement is completely random, and if a particle is in close proximity to the alveolar wall, it is likely to be deposited in this fashion. Diffusion is important in the deposition of those particles measuring up to 2 microns, and for particles below 0.5 micron is the main physical process involved.

Electrostatic Precipitation. This is a minor process in most instances. The airways are covered by a mucus layer, which is a good conductor and which precludes the development of powerful electric fields, thereby limiting the process of electrostatic precipitation.

Interception. This process involves the noninertial impaction of particles on the airway wall and is related to the physical size and in particular the length of the particle. It is of prime importance in the deposition of certain aerosols that are predominantly composed of fibers, e.g., cotton, hemp, and asbestos.

A number of theoretical models for particle deposition have been developed in which the deposition of inhaled aerosols at a given site in the respiratory tract is expressed as a percentage of the total number of inhaled particles. Most models relate particle size to the anatomical site of deposition, e.g., nose, trachea and bronchi, and lung parenchyma (Fig. 4–2).[9–11] As already mentioned, the site of deposition is influenced by the breathing rate, by tidal volume, by whether breathing is oral or nasal, and by cigarette smoking and the presence of various lung diseases. Exertion

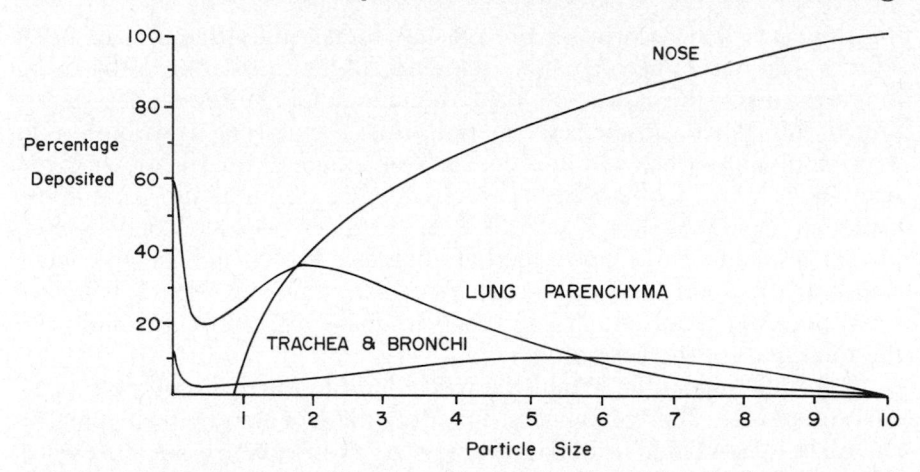

Figure 4–2. Regional deposition of particles as a function of their size in microns. This assumes a respiratory rate of 15 per minute and a tidal volume of 700 to 750 ml. (Based on data from Task Force Group on Lung Dynamics. Committee II IRCP, Deposition and retention models for internal dosimetry of the human respiratory tract. Health Phys., 12, 173, 1966.)

tends to increase oral breathing and the nose no longer acts as the efficient filter it is, with the result that a greater number of larger particles reach and are deposited in the dead space. Since there are regional differences in ventilation between the top and the bottom of the lungs, it is a reasonable assumption that there will also be regional differences in particle deposition. This has recently been confirmed.[12]

Most of the larger inhaled particles (5 microns or greater) are deposited in the nose or in the dead space long before the respiratory bronchioles are reached. In contrast, many particles below 3 microns tend to reach the gas-exchanging portions of the lung. For the most part, dust settling on the mucous film of the dead space epithelium is conveyed to the pharynx within 2 to 8 hours. Particles reaching the alveoli and gas-exchanging portions are removed by a different mechanism, which will be described later. In a normal adult subject there are three to four hundred million alveoli, each of which has a diameter of about 250 microns. Not all alveoli are in use at rest, and there is an intrapleural pressure gradient from apex to base which influences alveolar size. A normal person breathes around 5 to 6 L/min. If it is assumed that his tidal volume is 450 ml, then at a respiratory rate of 12, his minute volume will be 5.4 L. Given a dead space of 150 ml, his dead space ventilation in 1 minute will be 1.8 L and his alveolar ventilation 3.6 L. Considering that the functioning alveoli increase their volume by less than 300 ml with each breath and that the residual volume of most subjects is around 2 L, there is not much of an increase in alveolar volume in inspiration. In practice, the mean increase in the diameter of alveoli during inspiration is probably less than 5 per cent while the subject is breathing quietly. This indicates that in contrast to the gas in the conducting system and respi-

ratory bronchioles, the gas in the alveoli is turned over at a slower rate and tends to be stagnant. Because of this lower turnover and prolonged residence time, particles that reach the alveoli are likely to be retained sufficiently long to allow sedimentation to occur. Particles between 2 and 5 microns will settle in as little as 2 to 3 seconds. It is for this reason that expired air is almost free from particles of this size. With particles below 0.5 micron, sedimentation is uncommon and deposition from diffusion tends to be the major physical process involved.

Dust Deposition and Occupation

Davies has calculated the likelihood of a particle being deposited in the lungs based on the alveolar volume in different phases of respiration, the rate of breathing, and the tidal volume.[13] He has shown that an atmospheric concentration of 500,000 particles per ml is necessary to ensure that each alveolus will receive at least one particle. This dust concentration far exceeds that found in any industry. Concentrations of particles that are causally related to pneumoconiosis seldom exceed 5000/ml. Thus, under these circumstances it requires something like 1000 breaths to guarantee that a particle will first reach, and second be deposited in, an alveolus.

A coal miner working in a mine for 40 hours a week and exposed to an atmosphere containing 800 to 1000 particles/ml, all below 50 microns, for approximately 60 per cent of the time inhales between 100 and 150 gm of dust in a year. Of the dust inhaled, about 1 to 10 gm is deposited in the alveoli, but only about 0.5 gm is permanently retained. This is less than one hundredth of the total inhaled.

In some miners exposed to these conditions, radiographic changes would develop in 10 to 15 years. Since the dust levels in the United States and Britain are generally significantly below the hypothetical concentration mentioned above, the likelihood of developing category 1 simple pneumoconiosis in less than 30 years is remote. Nevertheless, it must be remembered that factors other than dust concentration influence the development of pneumoconiosis. Individual susceptibility obviously plays a role and it is apparent that certain subjects are prone to develop the disease more rapidly than others and that such differences may be related to the varying efficiency of the clearing mechanisms and possibly to differing breathing patterns (see previous discussion). It must be remembered too that the chemical properties of the deposited particles and hence their pathological effects are of prime importance. Thus at death many coal miners are found to have 20 to 30 gm of coal dust in their lungs despite the fact that during life they suffered no respiratory disability or impairment and, moreover, died of an unrelated cause. In contrast, the pulmonary deposition of 5 gm of silica would be almost certainly fatal. Although industrial hygienists use the term lifetime dust exposure in such

a way as to imply they measure accurately the dust which a worker inhales during his life, such quantifications of dust exposure are at the best approximations based on a limited number of measurements, often made at a distance from the worker's breathing zone and over a relatively short time. Even were they accurate, the relationship between the dust levels in the air and the weight of dust deposited in the lungs varies greatly from one individual to another, as does the percentage of dust cleared from the lungs.

CLEARANCE OF DUST

The mechanisms by which particulate matter is removed vary according to the site of deposition. If an insoluble particle is deposited in the dead space, it is cleared by the mucociliary escalator; however, should the particle be deposited in the lung parenchyma, it is engulfed by pulmonary macrophages, which in turn migrate either to the ciliated airways and hence to the mucociliary escalator, or to the interstitium of the lungs and from there find their way to the lymphatics.

Mucociliary Clearance

Those particles which are deposited in the anterior third of the nose are removed by blowing, wiping, sneezing, or other mechanical means. Such particles may remain at the site of deposition for 24 to 48 hours. Clearance from the posterior portion of the nose, including the turbinates, depends on the usual mucociliary mechanisms. Soluble particles when deposited in the nose are quickly absorbed. The nasal mucus layer is propelled backwards towards the nasopharynx at the rate of 4 to 6 mm per minute. There is a 4-minute half-time for particles deposited in the posterior part of the nose.

The remainder of the ciliated airways stretch from the trachea to the terminal bronchioles. The larynx is covered by mucus-secreting squamous epithelium. By way of contrast, the trachea and bronchi are covered by columnar cells, some of which are ciliated, others of which are not. Respiratory mucus is produced by submucosal mucous glands and by goblet cells. The former are situated predominantly in the large airways, while the latter occur more commonly in the smaller and more distal airways. The relative number of ciliated columnar cells progressively decreases from the trachea to the terminal bronchioles. Each columnar cell has around 200 cilia emerging from its surface, and each cilium contains longitudinal fibers which are capable of contraction. Two single fibrils form the central core. At the periphery, 9 fibrils are arranged in a concentric fashion. The peripheral fibrils converge and unite into a common structure at the top of the core.[15]

It is believed that the respiratory mucus has two layers, (1) a periciliary layer (sol) which surrounds the cilia, and (2) a mucus layer which lies on top of the cilia. It was originally thought that the mucus blanket was both continuous and contiguous, but most of the evidence suggests that this is not true and that mucus-free islands are present on the bronchial epithelium. Regeneration of destroyed ciliated epithelium usually takes between 14 and 17 days.

Cilia beat in one plane with a fast propellant stroke and a slow recovery stroke. It is theorized that one of the two subfibers in the nine peripheral filaments is shorter and that bending results from sliding between two subfibers. The gap between subfibers is bridged by dynein arms. The force of the bending filaments is transferred to the ciliary membrane by radial fibers. In the airways, the effective stroke propels the blanket of mucus towards the larynx. Ciliary motion depends on ATP as a source of energy.[16]

A normal person produces around 50 to 150 ml of mucus daily. While secretion of the mucous glands is under parasympathetic control, the goblet cells appear to respond to direct irritation. The clearance rate in man varies between 5 and 15 mm per minute, with a lower rate prevailing in older subjects and a higher rate in the young. Mucus transport rates decrease as one advances from the trachea to the peripheral airways, and the same can be said of the frequency of ciliary beating. Mucus clearance rates vary according to age and sex and are also influenced by the viscosity of the sputum and by the site of deposition of the particle. The trachea is usually cleared of particles within 10 minutes; however, the segmental and subsegmental bronchi have half-lives for particle clearance of 20 to 30 minutes. In the smaller airways, from the 10th generation and beyond, the half-life is approximately 100 to 200 minutes.

Factors Influencing Mucociliary Clearance.[16, 17] The more important physicochemical factors influencing ciliary function and clearance are cold and decreased humidity. Cold, dry air greatly depresses ciliary function and clearance, and causes many problems in patients with a tracheostomy and in those with reversible bronchospasm or asthma. The upper airways are predominantly affected. Various inorganic salts and radioactivity also depress mucociliary clearance. Acute exposure to cigarette smoke is associated in most studies with decreased mucociliary transport. Occasionally, transient increases in clearances have been observed, but these are almost certainly a consequence of the coughing that smoking engenders. Measurements of clearance rates in chronic smokers vary, and such studies tend to yield conflicting results owing to coughing and varying sites of deposition. The deposition pattern in confirmed smokers tends to be abnormal, with significantly more central deposition.[12] In chronic smokers, problems exist in regard to the confounding effects of coughing and sneezing on clearance rates. Short-term exposure to very high concentrations of air pollutants such as sulphur dioxide and the oxides of nitrogen

and ozone can be shown to impair ciliary activity transiently, but there is little evidence to suggest that air pollutants in the usual concentrations found in the ambient air of North America or Europe are likely to have a significant effect. High concentrations of oxygen, various inhalation anaesthetics, and narcotics likewise depress ciliary activity.

Particle deposition and mucociliary transport are affected in subjects with chronic bronchitis, cystic fibrosis, asthma, and other airways diseases. The removal of foreign particulates by the mucus blanket is slower in these conditions, but the decreases in ciliary activity are often compensated for by increased coughing.

Recently congenital structural defects in ciliated cells have been reported.[15] Such cells are found in the ependyma of the intracranial ventricles, the fallopian tubes, and the efferent ducts of the testes. Cilia from these different sites have the same ultrastructure as the tail of the sperm. Kartagener's syndrome is associated with a defect in the dynein arms on the outer pairs of ciliary microtubules (see above). Spermatozoa from males with Kartagener's syndrome are immotile. Additional syndromes exist in which the defects affect other parts of the dynein arms.

Alveolar Clearance

Retention of particles in the lung parenchyma is related not only to deposition but also to clearance. While animals provide a useful model for the study of alveolar clearance, most of the techniques which have been used cannot be applied to man. Even knowledge about alveolar clearance in animals is fragmentary, and we lack a detailed understanding of the basic mechanisms.

Alveolar transport depends on the alveolar epithelium, the interstitium of the septa, and the fluid and secretory pathways. The alveolar epithelium is composed of two kinds of cells, usually known as type 1 and 2 pneumocytes. The former act as a barrier between the lumen of the alveolus and the interstitium and capillary. It is assumed that their function is the transport of gases through the alveolocapillary membrane. The type 2 cell is a major secretory cell of the primary lobule and is felt by most to be responsible for the synthesis, storage, and secretion of surfactant. The latter substance is responsible for the integrity of the alveoli, which is maintained through the low surface tension of surfactant. In its absence, the alveoli collapse and the lungs become atelectatic. There seems little doubt that surfactant also plays a role in the coating and transport of deposited particles.

The other cell found in the alveoli is the alveolar macrophage. This is a mononuclear cell felt to be derived from the tissue histiocyte and which is responsible for alveolar phagocytosis. It differentiates in a unique fashion in order to adapt to the high oxygen tension that is present in the alveoli. By the same token, its activity and metabolism are seriously affected

by hypoxia. After particulate matter has been taken up by the alveolar macrophage, it may be acted upon by the cell's enzyme system or may be retained unchanged prior to being transported out of the lung.

The interstititum of the septa is made up of the basement membranes of the epithelium and capillary, and the capillary endothelium. It contains connective tissue and stroma, and is primarily affected in pulmonary edema. It may act as a pathway whereby the macrophage leaves the alveolus in order to reach the respiratory bronchiole.

As mentioned earlier, particles which may be deposited in the alveoli range from 0.01 to 8 or 9 microns, although deposition of particles above 5 microns is uncommon. Once the particle settles in the alveolus or respiratory bronchiole, subsequent clearance takes place by either absorptive or nonabsorptive processes.[18, 19] Absorptive processes involve the selective migration of the particle through the alveolar wall and hence into the bloodstream or lymph channels. Nonabsorptive mechanisms involve phagocytosis of the particle by the alveolar macrophage. Should the dust burden become excessive, clearance rates appear to reach a peak and then plateau, in which case some particles will be seen to lie free in the alveoli. It has been suggested that three phases of clearance exist, all of which have different time courses. The first involves surface transport from the proximal areas of the lobule along the respiratory surface to the respiratory bronchiole. It has been estimated that 50 per cent of the material removed by this process is cleared in 24 hours. A second and slower process has a 50 per cent clearance time of closer to 100 hours. It is suggested that the second process involves septal transport of material that has been phagocytized within the septa. The third mechanism, with a 50 per cent clearance of around 50 to 100 days, involves foreign particles that have reached dead end pathways in the perivascular and peribronchial spaces. What is becoming increasingly evident is that these generalizations cannot be applied across the board and that the clearance rate is related not only to the size of the particle but also to its density, chemical composition, and toxicity.

Deposited particles may be carried either in a free state or, in some instances, intracellularly. The mode of transport appears to depend on the physical properties and the number of particles deposited. After large challenges with particulate matter, cellular transport, as mentioned previously, is overwhelmed and many particles will be seen to be lying free on the alveolar surface and interstitial region of the septa.

The means whereby the particle is transported from its site of deposition to the nearest macrophage is unknown, and while it is possible that the macrophage itself chases particles, it has also been suggested that perhaps the particles themselves move as a result of respiratory movements and hence come into contact with the nearest macrophage.

Although it is well recognized that many macrophages migrate from the alveoli by way of the respiratory bronchioles to the terminal bronchiole and hence mount the mucociliary escalator, the exact mechanisms of

macrophage migration remain unknown. Macrophage movement entails simple amoeboid migration; however, this process is slow, especially when the cells are dust-laden. In addition, the distance from the alveoli to the terminal bronchiole is appreciable. Two pathways of macrophage migration have been suggested, one of which involves passage of the macrophage into the interstitium of the lung, the other of which is a surface route. The former hypothesis assumes that macrophages migrate into the interstitium and wend their way up to the terminal bronchiole in peribronchiolar lymph channels. The subsequent extrusion of the particle-laden macrophage onto the terminal bronchiole has been observed. This process must of necessity involve the migration of free or particle-containing macrophages through the alveolar epithelium by endocytosis. Green has suggested that particles, liquids, and cells all flow through the interstitium in the "liquid" veins of Staub.[20] He suggested that flow results from mechanical tension that acts on alveolar septa as a result of ventilatory movements, in particular the energy derived from the lung's elastic recoil and from interfacial tension. Gross, on the other hand, favors the surface route.[21] He postulates that a viscosity gradient exists within the surface fluid layer due to evaporation from the fluid surface. Thus the depth of the alveolar fluid would increase and decrease in phase with the respiratory cycle. The luminal portion of the film with the macrophages and extracellular particles resting upon it would tend to move back or retreat less easily during inspiration than the subjacent deeper portion. This would result in the macrophages and entrapped particles being propelled towards the terminal bronchioles.

No matter whether particles are transferred by the interstitial or surface routes or by both routes, the ultimate source of energy must depend on respiratory movements. Similarly, it might be inferred that these processes will be most rapid in those regions of the lung where ventilation is greatest, a factor which could explain the predilection of coal workers' pneumoconiosis and silicosis to involve the upper zones of the lungs.

Alveolar clearance seems to proceed in several temporal phases that can usually be described by a series of exponentials, with each presumably corresponding to a different type of clearance mechanism. The earliest lasts from several days or several weeks, while the terminal phase is considerably longer, and probably represents sequestration of particulate matter in the interstitial tissues. Mercer has proposed a solubility model that explains long-term clearance by a slow dissolution.[22] This theory applies to relatively insoluble particle burdens that have a log normal distribution. His theoretical results compare well with experimental data for the long-term clearance of particles that are relatively insoluble, such as uranium dioxide, but the process of alveolar clearance seems too complex to be explained by physicochemical factors alone. Part of the terminal phase of alveolar clearance probably relates to the migration of particles into the lymphatics. However, the importance of lymphatic

removal for clearing material from the lower respiratory tract has probably been exaggerated. Because particulate matter is slowly cleared from lymphatic channels and lymph nodes, the presence of particulates in these regions may be related to the pathogenesis of certain lung diseases.

In a few studies, humans have been exposed to radiotagged aerosols, with the subsequent retention being followed for several days. Morrow and his colleagues studied clearance of manganese dioxide particles and chromium-labeled ferric oxide and polystyrene particles.[23] Clearance rates for all three particles were slow, ranging from 65 to 35 days, respectively. Camner and Philipson have studied clearance in 10 healthy males using 4 microns of Teflon particles tagged with indium.[24] Half the particles were cleared during the first day, but subsequent clearance was slow. Tantalum powder has been instilled into the alveoli of man. While the trachea and bronchi are cleared within 3 to 4 days and the distal airways within 3 to 4 weeks, alveolar clearing may be incomplete after 3 to 4 years.[18] The author has a patient who still has obvious alveolar retention of tantalum 10 years after a bronchogram. It is thus evident in studies using radioactively tagged particles that there is a fast clearance phase which is usually complete within 24 to 36 hours, and a slower phase with a half-time of anything from 3 weeks to 3 months. It is important, however, to realize that other particles, for example, those of tantalum, are cleared far more slowly. Problems also exist with radioactively tagged particles in that it is sometimes difficult knowing whether measured clearance is a reflection of alveolobronchiolar transport or is a consequence of dissolution and leakage of the particulate radionucleotide.

Alveolar function and clearance are probably influenced by the same factors and agents, e.g., drugs, that affect tracheobronchial clearance. Cigarette smoke has been shown to delay alveolar clearance in man.[25]

Detoxification

Aside from the removal of particulates, normal lung defenses are dependent on the detoxification of noxious inhaled particulate matter. This latter process has as its mainstay the alveolar macrophage; however, polymorphonuclear leukocytes and histiocytes can also assume this function should the need arise. Humoral agents such as specific immunoglobulins play a dominant role against bacterial invasion, but various surface active agents, viz., enzymes such as lysozymes and lipoproteins, probably need to be present for the bactericidal properties of the phagocytes to be fully effective. These mechanisms are pre-eminent in the elimination of inhaled bacteria. The phagocytic properties of the macrophage are inhibited by hypoxia such as occurs in obstructive airways disease. This may in part explain the predisposition of subjects with chronic bronchitis and emphysema to infection.

The alveolar macrophage is thought to be derived from the bone

marrow, although in its adult form it differs significantly in structure, physiology, and metabolism from its parent cell.[26, 27] This differentiation is necessitated by the macrophage's shift to aerobic pathways for metabolic activities. By means of radioactive tagging of inhaled bacteria, it has been shown that 99 per cent of a bacterial challenge is detoxified in the first 24 hours. In contrast, only 50 per cent of the bacteria that are deposited in the lungs are removed.[26] Phagocytosis is adversely affected by the acute and chronic effects of alcohol, by steroids and immunosuppressive agents, by starvation and extreme climatic conditions, and by various air pollutants. Finally, and most deleterious of all, is the effect of cigarette smoking on the function of the alveolar macrophage.

The number of macrophages in the alveoli, as well as the exchange rate from the blood to the interstitium and alveoli, affected by the presence of inflammation and by the host's immunological response to the inhaled material. Normal macrophages have the capacity to destroy many airborne organisms, include nonpathogenic streptococci and *Escherichia coli;* however, they are unable to kill *Mycobacterium tuberculosis* and *Listeria monocytogenes.* In contrast, when activated by the mechanism of cellular immunity, they acquire the capacity to destroy pathological organisms.

Lymphocyte-mediated activation of macrophages is the chief means of defense against inhaled intracellular parasites that are deposited in the lung parenchyma. This type of acquired immunity is operative in tuberculosis and histoplasmosis and may also play a role in berylliosis. Cellular immunity has the propensity to generate a vigorous and occasionally destructive tissue response in the lung parenchyma, viz., granulomata and sometimes necrosis. The mechanisms that control and effect cell-mediated immunity and its relationship to tissue necrosis need further study.

PATHOPHYSIOLOGICAL RESPONSES TO RESPIRATORY INHALANTS

Given the chemical, physical and host factors described earlier, the ultimate response of the respiratory system still depends to a great extent on the site of deposition of the particle. The range of responses according to the site are listed in Table 4–2.

Nose

The deposition of irritants in the nose may lead to rhinitis. Chrome may cause nasal ulcerations and septal perforation, while nasal cancer in furniture workers may result from the inhalation of wood dust.[28] Hay fever results from the deposition of ragweed and other pollens in the nares and is often associated with bronchoconstriction, either reflexly[29] or because some particles bypass the nose during mouth breathing and are deposited in the airways.

Trachea and Bronchi

Several responses may occur and are listed in Table 4–2. The most important and the most frequent is bronchoconstriction. The latter may occur as a result of an immunological reaction or it can be pharmacologically induced such as probably occurs in byssinosis, in which the deposition of cotton fiber induces the liberation of mediators, for example, leukotrienes and histamine.

When inert particles are deposited in the trachea and bronchi over a prolonged period and if exposure is intense, industrial bronchitis may develop.

In this regard, most particles which are relatively insoluble, e.g., asbestos fibers and silica, and which are deposited in the airways are removed by the mucociliary escalator and hence are inert when deposited in the trachea and bronchi. This would not be the case were they deposited in the alveoli or respiratory bronchioles. When such prolonged and intense exposure occurs the mucous glands hypertrophy, the goblet cells increase, and excess mucus is produced. This leads to cough and sputum production and occasionally some evidence of a minor degree of large airways obstruction.[30] Since the particles are removed by the mucociliary escalator, they leave no radiographic traces.

Radioactive particles such as radon daughters may induce lung cancer, as can asbestos, nickel, and other agents. Finally, irritant gases and fumes may induce tracheitis.

Table 4–2. PATHOPHYSIOLOGICAL RESPONSES OF RESPIRATORY TRACT TO PARTICLES, MISTS, AND GASES

Site of Deposition	Responses
Nose	Rhinitis, hay fever Septal perforation Nasal cancer

Trachea and bronchi	Bronchoconstriction
	  1. Types I and III immunological reactions
	  2. Pharmacologically induced
	  3. Reflex; Inert particles
	Industrial bronchitis
	Lung cancer
	Acute tracheitis and bronchitis

Parenchyma	Extrinsic allergic alveolitis, types III and IV
	  immunological reactions
	Pneumoconioses
	Acute alveolitis and bronchiolitis: alveolitis,
	  pulmonary edema, and bronchiolitis obliterans
	Pulmonary alveolar proteinosis
	Emphysema

Parenchymal Responses

If the particles are organic, they may induce a hypersensitivity pneumonia or what is often referred to as extrinsic allergic alveolitis. The latter is a misnomer in that the condition is characterized not only by alveolitis but also by respiratory bronchiolitis and sometimes a terminal bronchiolitis. Many arguments exist as to the immunological origin and pathogenesis of this condition, but suffice it to say there are features of both type III and type IV immunological reactions.

If the particles are inorganic, pneumoconiosis may result. Here the term pneumoconiosis is defined as the deposition of dust in the lungs and the tissue's reaction to its presence. Nonetheless, the response differs according to the chemical and physical properties of the agent which is producing the pneumoconiosis. Four main pathological responses are seen in the pneumoconioses:

1. Interstitial Fibrosis. When this occurs the particle induces fibrosis of the alveoli and the alveolocapillary membrane becomes thickened. In addition, there may be a bronchiolitis. The gas-exchanging part of the lungs and often the respiratory and terminal bronchioles may be affected. The lungs become stiff and inelastic. The causes of this type of reaction are asbestos, beryllium, and cobalt as found in tungsten carbide (hard metal).

2. Nodular Fibrosis. The classical example of this type of fibrosis is silicosis. In this condition the silica particles are engulfed by the macrophages, which then migrate into the interstitial tissues and the lymphatic channels. There the macrophage dies and liberates toxic enzymes that induce fibrosis. The latter appears as discrete nodules separated from the alveoli, but sometimes adjacent to or situated near the respiratory bronchioles and arterioles. Most are at a considerable distance from the gas-exchanging surface. Because the nodules are separated by intervening normal lung tissue, their physiological effects are much less than those from agents which lead to the development of interstitial fibrosis. Most often in the nodular fibroses there are no detectable physiological abnormalities other than a slight increase in the stiffness of the lungs.[31] Even so, simple silicosis is a precursor of the complicated form of the disease, which is associated with both disability and premature death.

3. Interstitial and Nodular Fibrosis. This is a combined response usually only seen in exposure to diatomite, which usually contains a large amount of quartz. When the diatomite is heated and fused, some of the quartz is transformed into cristobalite and tridymite, both of which may induce interstitial fibrosis.

4. Macule Formation and Focal Emphysema. Exposure to coal, carbon, and other air pollutants may lead to the formation of macules around the second division of the respiratory bronchiole. When exposure to relatively nonfibrogenic agents is severe and prolonged, the lungs' defenses are overwhelmed and there are no longer sufficient macrophages to keep pace with dust removal. The macrophages tend to aggregate

around the respiratory bronchiole, especially in the second division, and there they die and liberate their dust burden. Since coal and carbon are only minimally fibrogenic, the fibrogenic response is limited to the production of a few reticulin fibers and occasionally scanty collagen. The pigment that is deposited appears as a mantle around the respiratory bronchiole. The smooth muscle in the latter tends to atrophy and the respiratory bronchiole subsequently dilates to form a small translucent area in the middle of the macule. This is referred to as focal emphysema and does not extend to the alveoli. Macules, usually smaller than those seen in coal miners, but occasionally with some focal emphysema, may be seen in persons who have grown up in areas with severe urban pollution. Physiologically, the presence of macules and focal emphysema leads only to a slight increase in alveolo-arterial gradient and other minimal evidence of an abnormal distribution of inspired gas.[32] Simple pneumoconiosis does, however, predispose to the development of progressive massive fibrosis.

Irritant gases such as nitrogen dioxide, chlorine, and other agents may reach the small airways and alveoli, causing severe damage to the alveolar epithelium and alveolar lining cells. Pulmonary edema may be produced, and subsequently during the recovery phase, bronchiolitis obliterans often supervenes. This is especially common following exposure to relatively insoluble gases such as the oxides of nitrogen. Massive exposure to silica may induce pulmonary alveolar proteinosis. This condition is fortunately uncommon, but in occasional instances is still seen in sandblasters. Finally, the inhalation of cadmium fumes can cause pulmonary edema and tissue destruction and lead to the development of panacinar emphysema.

It should be possible to predict the pathophysiological effects of an inhaled agent that is suspected of being a respiratory hazard by identifying its site of and propensity for deposition, along with its other properties referred to in this chapter. This same knowledge can be used as a means by which the effects of the particular hazard can be either limited or controlled completely.

References

1. Findesen, W., Über das Absetzen kleiner, in der Luft suspendierter Teilchen in der menschlichen Lunge bei der Atmung. Pfluegers Arch. Ges. Physiol., *236*, 367, 1935.
2. Brain, J. D., and Valberg, P. A., Deposition of aerosol in the respiratory tract. Am. Rev. Respir. Dis., *120*, 1325, 1979.
2a. Clague, H., Ahmad, D., and Chamberlain, M.J., et al., Histamine bronchial challenge: effect on regional ventilation and aerosal deposition. Thorax, *38*, 668, 1983.
3. Camner, P., Philipson, K., and Friberg, L., Tracheobronchial clearance in twins. Arch. Environ. Health, *24*, 82, 1972.
4. Bohning, A. E., Albert, R. E., Lippman, M., and Forster, W. H., Tracheobronchial deposition and clearance. Arch. Environ. Health, *30*, 457, 1975.
5. Lapp, N. L., Hankinson, J. L., Amandus, H., and Palmes, E. D., Variability in size of air spaces in normal human lungs as estimated by aerosols. Thorax, *30*, 293, 1975.

6. Matsuba, K., and Thurlbeck, W. M., The number and dimensions of small airways in non-emphysematous lungs. Am. Rev. Respir. Dis., *104*, 516, 1971.

7. Evans, C. C., Lewinsohn, H. C., and Evans, J. M., Frequency of HLA antigens in asbestos workers with and without pulmonary fibrosis. Br. Med. J., *1*, 603, 1976.

8. Morgan, D. C., Smyth, J. J., Lister, R. W., et al., Chest symptoms in farming communities with special reference to farmers' lung. Br. J. Ind. Med., *32*, 228, 1975.

9. Landahl, H. D., On the removal of airborne droplets by the human respiratory tract. Bull. Math. Biophysics, *12*, 43, 1950.

10. Beeckmans, J. M., The deposition of aerosols in the respiratory tract. Can. J. Appl. Physiol. and Pharm., *43*, 157, 1965.

11. Task Force Group on Lung Dynamics, Committee II IRCP, Deposition and retention models for internal dosimetry of the human respiratory tract. Health Phys., *12*, 173, 1966.

12. Chamberlain, M. J., Morgan, W. K. C., and Vinitski, S., Factors influencing the regional deposition of inhaled particles in man. Clin. Sci., *64*, 69, 1983.

13. Davies, C. N., Deposition of dust in the lungs. *In* King, E. J., and Fletcher, C. M., eds., Industrial Lung Disease. Little Brown, Boston, 1960. pp 44–58.

14. Proctor, D. F., Nasal physiology and defense of the lungs. Am. Rev. Respir. Dis., *115*, 97, 1977.

15. Afzelius, B. A., and Mossberg, B., Immotile cilia. Thorax, *35*:401, 1980.

16. Wanner, A., Clinical aspects of mucociliary transport. State of the art. Am. Rev. Respir. Dis., *116*, 73, 1977.

17. Camner, P., Clearance of particles from the human bronchial tree. Clin. Sci., *59*, 79, 1980.

18. Camner, P., Alveolar clearance. Eur. J. Resp. Dis. (Suppl.) *107*, 61, 59, 1980.

19. Lippman, M., Yeates, D. B., and Albert, R. E., Deposition, retention and clearance of inhaled particles. Br. J. Ind. Med., *37*, 337, 1980.

20. Green, G. M., Alveolo-bronchiolar transport mechanisms. Arch. Int. Med., *131*, 109, 1973.

21. Gross, P., The mechanisms of dust clearance from the lung. Am. J. Clin. Pathol., *23*, 116, 1953.

22. Mercer, T. T., On the role of particle size in the dissolution of lung burdens. Health Phys., *13*, 1211, 1967.

23. Morrow, P. E., Gibb, F. T., and Gazioglu, K. M., A study of particulate clearance from the human lungs. Am. Rev. Respir. Dis., *96*, 1209, 1967.

24. Camner, P., and Philipson, K., Human alveolar deposition of 4 μm Teflon particles. Arch. Environ. Health, *33*, 181, 1978.

25. Cohen, D., Arai, S. F., and Brain, J. D., Smoking impairs long-term clearance from the lung. Science, *204*, 514, 1979.

26. Green, G. M., The J. Burns Amberson Lecture—In Defense of the Lung. Am. Rev. Respir. Dis., *102*, 691, 1970.

27. Myrvik, Q., The role of the alveolar macrophage. J. Occup. Med., *15*, 190, 1973.

28. Acheson, E. D., Hadfield, E. H., and MacBeth, R. G.: Nasal cancer in woodworkers in furniture industry. Lancet, *1*, 311, 1967.

29. Kaufman, J., Wright, G. W., The effect of nasal and nasopharyngeal irritation on airway resistance in man. Am. Rev. Respir. Dis. *100*, 626, 1969.

30. Morgan, W. K. C., Industrial bronchitis. Br. J. Ind. Med. *35*, 285, 1978.

31. Teculescu, D., Stanescu, D. D., and Pilat, L., Pulmonary mechanics in silicosis. Arch. Environ. Health, *14*, 461, 1967.

32. Morgan, W. K. C., and Lapp, N. L., Respiratory disease in coal miners. State of the art. Am. Rev. Respir. Dis., *113*, 531, 1976.

5

EPIDEMIOLOGY AND OCCUPATIONAL LUNG DISEASE

W. Keith C. Morgan

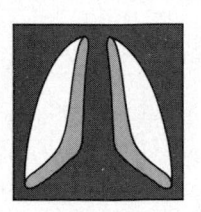

The identification, characterization, and assessment of the magnitude of both acute and chronic occupational hazards depend for the most part on the intelligent application of epidemiological methods. MacMahon has defined epidemiology as "the study of the distribution and determinants of disease in man." This definition is, however, somewhat restrictive, and much epidemiological research now takes place in normal populations, since only by delineating the range of normality can abnormality or disease be recognized. Epidemiology in more simple terms then becomes the study of normal and diseased states through the acquisition and analysis of pertinent data collected from the community.

Three methods of studying disease are commonly used:
1. Clinical observation of subjects with the disease
2. Controlled laboratory experiments using either man or animals
3. Epidemiological studies

The use of epidemiology overlaps with the first two methods and epidemiological observations are clearly important in both controlled laboratory experiments and the clinical observation of subjects with disease. In considering the epidemiological method in the study of disease, Morris described seven standard approaches:

1. *The characterization of historical patterns of disease in populations by determining the relative and absolute frequency of disease in different groups, in different areas, and at different times.* This approach is most useful when there is a single or pre-eminent factor involved in the etiology of the disease, e.g., lung cancer that develops after exposure to bischloromethyl ether or radon daughters. In the case of diseases of multifactorial origin, the problem becomes far more complex and this approach may be inadequate.

2. *The measurement of current differences in the prevalence, incidence, morbidity, and mortality of disease.* By these means it is possible to define the magnitude and effects of the problem or disease.

3. *Study of the efficacy and operation of health services.* This approach involves an assessment of the health services which are used in the prevention and control of disease.

4. *The estimation of risk of disease in individuals and selected groups.* Theoretically attractive, this method is often less than ideal, since at present identification of susceptible subjects is possible only in a few instances.

5. *The identification of disease syndromes from different patterns of disease in the population exposed.* An example of this approach would be the separation of coal workers' pneumoconiosis and industrial bronchitis in coal miners.

6. *The characterization of the range of disease from the subclinical and possibly reversible stage to the irreversible and fatal form.* This implies a full understanding of the natural history of disease and is essential when considering prevention and control of the disease.

7. *Providing an understanding of the causes of the disease through knowledge of the determinants of disease frequency in different populations.* This approach allows separation of several risk factors, e.g., the role of industrial exposure, air pollution, and cigarette smoking in the etiology of bronchitis.

Morris's methods, while neatly defining the seven approaches which can be used in the epidemiological investigation of disease, are not as precise and well defined as at first appears. Considerable overlap is present in his various defined approaches; nonetheless, they do provide a logical and helpful guide to both epidemiologists and clinicians who are concerned with the investigation and prevention of occupational disease.

Before describing the various types of studies that can be carried out on exposed populations, a few definitions of the more commonly used epidemiological terms would be in order. Prevalence means the number of subjects in a population who have a particular condition at a stated time. In occupational lung disease, the prevalence of a condition may be a reflection of recent exposure or of exposure many years previously. Thus a survey of the prevalence of coal workers' pneumoconiosis (CWP) in 1971–72 showed that about 12 per cent of working miners had radiographic evidence of the condition.[2] Most of those with CWP had developed it following prolonged exposure. The insult that was mainly responsible for the development of the condition occurred 20 to 30 years previously, when dust levels were much higher than now. A repeat survey, carried out 3 years later in 1974–75, showed the prevalence rate of CWP to have fallen to 6 per cent. Although this might conceivably be a consequence of improved dust control, this explanation appears most unlikely. The real explanations for the lower prevalence are that many of those who were originally diagnosed as having CWP in the first survey retired and claimed compensation, while those who joined the work force

and replaced them were free from disease; in addition, the reading habits of those interpreting the radiographs changed.[2]

The incidence of a condition refers to the number of persons in a particular population—in occupational lung disease it refers to exposed workers—who develop the condition over a designated time. The attack rate is somewhat similar and designates the number of subjects in a defined population who were originally normal, but subsequently developed an abnormality over a specific period of observation. Thus to define the attack rate for silicosis would require a knowledge of the number of men who initially started work with normal chest radiographs and no prior exposure, and who then went on to develop radiographic evidence of the disease over a specified time.

From data of this type attack rates may be calculated, but, here again, it is necessary to remember that the incidence or attack rate of a particular disease may be influenced by conditions prevailing much earlier. Thus were 5 out of 25 asbestos miners to develop radiographic evidence of asbestosis, one explanation would be all 25 had approximately the same work history (i.e., cumulative exposure) but that only those who were susceptible developed asbestosis. A more likely explanation would be that the 5 who contracted asbestosis had been exposed to higher concentrations than the rest, perhaps in a job in which exposure was greater and possibly at a time when dust concentrations were higher. Bearing in mind these caveats, it is useful to consider the different types of epidemiological studies or surveys which may be carried out.

TYPES OF EPIDEMIOLOGICAL STUDIES

Longitudinal Studies

A longitudinal study involves observing or measuring certain biological and medical indices over a period of time. This permits systematic observation of change with time. Such a study allows the incidence or the attack rate for a particular condition to be determined. Longitudinal studies have several drawbacks, the most important of which is the loss of participating subjects from the study. Such a loss may be due to migration, death, disability from the disease being studied, or a slackening of interest in the participants. These losses may result in the remaining subjects not necessarily being representative of the original population. Other problems include the high cost of longitudinal studies, the maintenance of standardization in measurements and tests, and the low incidence and prolonged incubation period of certain diseases. Using standard criteria is particularly important. Changing personnel may be a source of bias and may lead to different values for pulmonary function tests. Sometimes a new interviewer will cause subjects to respond differently to the administration of the same questionnaire. Technical lapses and changed equip-

ment, e.g., the type of spirometer, can invalidate several years' work by introducing substantial bias.

In any epidemiological study there must always be an initial hypothesis, and the purpose and design of the study should be to answer as simply as possible whether or not the particular hypothesis is correct. The design of the longitudinal study must take into account the end point sought. Thus some studies may be concerned with a continuing decline in pulmonary function (a continuous variable) following exposure to a certain hazard, while others seek a definite occurrence or development of a defined event such as the onset of asthma, lung cancer, or, most final of all, death. Yet other studies are concerned with the development of repeated episodes in an exposed population, for example, recurrent attacks of asthma, metal fume fever, or farmer's lung.

Historical Prospective Studies

Although these are longitudinal studies, they are carried out after the event. Thus a particular cohort identified some time previously is traced to the present and the attack rate or incidence of a particular disease or condition is then calculated. An example of such an approach would be tracing a group of asbestos miners known to have had a defined dust exposure and consequently ascertaining how many have developed lung cancer. Problems exist, in that the working population tends to be fitter than the population as a whole, since certain conditions which are prevalent in the general population automatically exclude or render a person unable to work. This effect is known as a "healthy worker effect," and much is made of it as a source of potential bias. While the healthy worker effect is important in certain industries, e.g., those involving hard physical work, it is unlikely to influence to any great extent those subjects whose work is relatively sedentary and whose physical demands are far less. Thus a survey of furnace workers in a steel plant is unlikely to turn up a large number of subjects with emphysema or asthma, since only the mildly affected could continue working. In contrast, such a survey carried out in waiters or taxi drivers would be likely to reveal that both of these occupations have a high prevalence of air flow obstruction.

Cross-sectional Studies

Cross-sectional studies, as the name implies, look at a cross section of the population on one occasion only. In the case of occupationally related lung disease, the normal practice is to examine those exposed to a particular hazard and to compare them to a nonexposed control group.

The main purpose of such studies is to estimate the prevalence of a particular condition and to characterize the type of impairment in those affected by it. In addition, the effects of various nonoccupational factors, such as cigarette smoking, air pollution, ethnic background, lifestyle, and

diet, may be assessed. Occasionally, it is possible to reconstruct past exposures from work histories and to derive a dose-response relationship. Usually, however, the dust exposure data depend on so many intangibles and assumptions that accurate inferences cannot be drawn.

A cross-sectional study has many advantages, including the fact that the study is usually finite in both time and expenditure. The main drawback involves the investigation of a survivor population in which those who have been most affected may have already retired. Missing observations on retired and impaired workers may conceal the most important part of the story, and every effort should be made to trace them so that they may be included. In cross-sectional studies, the prevalence of a particular condition may reflect environmental conditions two or three decades previously, a situation which is particularly true of the pneumoconioses. Although many statistical ploys have been devised to cope with missing or incomplete observations, they are based on a series of assumptions, the accuracy or likelihood of which cannot be vouchsafed.

Multifactorial Effects

When a condition or disease results from multiple exposures or multiple factors, some sort of statistical approach may be necessary to sort out the contribution of these various exposures or factors. Thus the development of coronary artery disease has been shown to be related to a number of risk factors, including smoking habits, obesity, lack of exercise, diet, and elevated serum cholesterol and serum triglycerides. Apportioning the relative contribution of each factor is difficult, but can be effected more or less satisfactorily using certain well-accepted statistical techniques. These include the use of matched pairs, triads, quadrads, and so on. For example, if a large population containing both exposed and nonexposed workers has been studied, it is possible to identify a series of pairs from the exposed and unexposed groups who have certain matching characteristics, e.g., age, height, sex, race, and smoking habits. Thus, when studying the prevalence of airways obstruction in textile workers exposed to cotton fibers, one could compare cardroom workers or spinners exposed to cotton with a comparable group of subjects from the same mill who worked with polyesters. If each exposed subject·can be matched with a nonexposed subject of the same age, height, sex, race, and smoking habits, then tests of ventilatory capacity such as the FVC and FEV_1 should be very similar. Provided enough pairs are available and provided results show a consistent and statistically significant difference between the exposed and nonexposed groups, it is possible to incriminate the particular agent concerned. Some authors have decried the use of matched pairs and claim the method is overused; nevertheless, with proper matching, it can be a most effective way of controlling and quantifying the confounding factors.

Other methods of controlling confounding factors include multiple

regression analyses and an analysis of covariance. The former may be unduly influenced by a few outlying points, while the latter is also subject to certain inherent influences which may introduce bias. Stratification analysis, in which all the variables are characterized so that strata are formed, thereby permitting within stratum comparisons, has recently become popular. This approach is useful when dealing with retrospective studies, but frequently the number of subjects is insufficient to allow adequate comparisons.

EPIDEMIOLOGICAL SURVEYS FOR OCCUPATIONAL LUNG DISEASE

When designing an epidemiological survey, it is essential first to pose the question or questions to be asked; second, to select the appropriate study and control population samples so as to exclude bias; and third, to use those methods which answer the questions posed as simply and as unambiguously as possible. Without a hypothesis a "fishing expedition" results, and data collection becomes an end in itself. An epidemiological study may be carried out for clinical investigative purposes, for example, to ascertain whether a new industrial process constitutes a hazard and if so to identify the factors responsible, while in other instances the main purpose of the study may be to detect or screen for a particular condition or disease so that it can be treated. Here the term "screening" is defined as "the presumptive identification of unrecognized disease by the application of tests, examinations, or other procedures which can be applied rapidly."[3] The purpose of screening is to detect disease in those who are apparently well and who are unaware that they have any disease or impairment. No matter what the purpose of the screening survey, certain methodological principles are inviolate. Before starting a screening study, those concerned need to apply the criteria shown in Table 5–1 to the condition for which they are screening. This is seldom done, and nowhere is this more true than in screening for occupational lung disease.[4] Some principles of these, e.g., the avoidance of bias in sample selection, have been touched upon already, but to date nothing has been said concerning the choice of tests and examinations which should be used. In the practice of clinical epidemiology, it needs to be borne in mind that large numbers of persons are studied and that errors in the collection of physiological or other data and in the answering of specific questions occur at random. Such errors, or perhaps variations would be a more apt description, are acceptable in epidemiology, but not in clinical practice. The one exception to this general rule is those surveys which are being conducted to screen for a specific condition such as diabetes.

All tests that are used in epidemiological surveys or, if it comes to that, in clinical practice, should be judged by the criteria shown in Table 5–2. Thus, the test must be acceptable to the patient, and in this regard

Table 5–1. PRINCIPLES FOR DECIDING IF A
SCREENING TEST IS JUSTIFIED*

1. The condition being sought should be an important health problem for the individual and the community
2. There should be an acceptable form of treatment for patients with recognizable disease
3. The natural history of the condition, including its development from latent to declared disease, should be adequately understood
4. There should be a recognizable latent or early symptomatic stage
5. There should be a suitable screening test or examination for detecting the disease at the latent or early symptomatic stage, and this test should be acceptable to the population
6. The facilities required for diagnosis and treatment of patients revealed by the screening program should be available
7. There should be an agreed policy on whom to treat as patients
8. Treatment at the presymptomatic, borderline stage of a disease should favorably influence its course and prognosis
9. The cost of case-finding (which would include the cost of diagnosis and treatment) needs to be economically balanced in relation to possible expenditure on medical care as a whole
10. Case-finding should be a continuing process, not a "once and for all" project
11. The benefits accruing to the true positive should outweigh the harm done as a result of false-positive diagnosis

*After Wilson, M. M. G., and Jungner, G.: Principles of Screening for Disease. Geneva, World Health Organization, 1968.

should neither cause pain nor be associated with risk. Invasive tests such as arterial puncture are particularly unsuited for community studies. The tests should likewise be simple, so that the patient can carry out the instructions. Closing volume can be measured reproducibly and without difficulty in a fixed laboratory using volunteer medical students and laboratory technicians; however, in a field situation in which the subjects being tested are coal miners or textile workers, reproducibility and cooperation become much more difficult to obtain. Spirometry, on the other hand, can be successfully carried out in almost 100 per cent of the population. The recommended tests should likewise be objective and uninfluenced by patient cooperation or observer bias.

Table 5–2. CRITERIA FOR TESTS

1. Acceptance by subjects: Test should not cause discomfort.

2. Simplicity: Equipment and procedure should be simple.

3. Objectivity: Results should not be influenced by whether subject cooperates fully or not.

4. Precision (reproducibility): Repetition yields the same value.

5. Accuracy: The test quantifies accurately what one needs to know.

6. Validity: sensitivity, specificity, and predictive value

Blood gas analysis and electrocardiography are uninfluenced by patient cooperation, provided that the patient consents to undergo these examinations. However, the interpretation of the electrocardiogram, in contrast to that of blood gas analysis, is greatly influenced by the interpreter. A test should be reproducible, meaning that when measured several times under the same conditions it should yield the same result. Lack of reproducibility may be a consequence of the equipment used or the person making the measurements. When an experienced pulmonary physiologist or technician measures closing volume (CV) tracings on several occasions over a period of a week, there may be considerable intraobserver variation. Such variation may affect those indices which are often assumed to be objective, e.g., CV, CC, and the other tests mentioned above. True biological variability also exists. Thus the FEV_1 is relatively reproducible and, when the test is repeated 5 to 10 times in an hour in the same subject, will vary only by about 5 per cent. In contrast, the FEF_{50}, the FEF_{75}, and the FEF_{25-75} may yield values that vary from 10 to 25 per cent when repeated under the same conditions.[5] Accuracy is even more important and must not be confused with precision or reproducibility (Fig. 5–1). Accuracy means the ability of a particular test to measure what the investigator requires to know. Accuracy and validity are really one and the same and should be assessed by considering three indices— sensitivity, specificity, and predictive value— all of which contribute to the concept of validity. The appropriate formulae for these indices are shown in Table 5–3.

Sensitivity is an index of the number of false negatives, in short, the ability of the test to give a positive result when the person being tested has the disease. Specificity is an index of the number of false positives and may be defined as the ability of the test to give a negative result in those who are truly negative. Sensitivity and specificity are competing influences and the ratio of one to the other is usually referred to by engineers as the signal to noise ratio. The predictive value of the test (ability to predict disease) is related to both specificity and sensitivity and is more useful than either of these indices alone. Furthermore, it has special application in screening studies. The predictive value of the test is largely determined by the prevalence of a particular disease in the sample being studied. Even highly specific and sensitive tests lose their predictive value when the prevalence of the condition in the population examined is low (Table 5–4).

The importance of standardization in epidemiological studies has recently received much attention from the Medical Research Council of Great Britain and from the Heart, Lung and Blood Institute of the National Institutes of Health, the American Thoracic Society, and the American College of Chest Physicians. Without adequate standardization, comparisons between different studies are impossible and bias inevitably creeps in. Nowhere is this more of a problem than in longitudinal studies, where personnel and often methods change. Measurement and hence

Table 5–3. FORMULAE FOR SENSITIVITY, SPECIFICITY, AND PREDICTIVE VALUE

$$\text{Sensitivity} = \frac{\text{True Positives}}{\text{True Positives} + \text{False Negatives}}$$

$$\text{Specificity} = \frac{\text{True Negatives}}{\text{True Negatives} + \text{False Positives}}$$

$$\text{Predictive value of a positive test} = \frac{1}{1 + \left(\dfrac{1 - y}{x}\right)\left(\dfrac{1}{z} - 1\right)}$$

Where
Sensitivity = x
Specificity = y
Prevalence = z

quantification become impossible unless the methodology has been standardized and is consistently applied. Recently, the American Thoracic Society (ATS) issued a monograph entitled *The Epidemiology Standardization Project.*[6] This monograph has as its goal the standardization of the most frequently used procedures that are applied in epidemiological surveys of lung disease. Three methods are used for the collection of medical and biological data: first, a standardized questionnaire to elicit the prevalence of respiratory symptoms, smoking habits, and other pertinent information; second, the performance of certain pulmonary function tests; and third, the radiographic examination of the chest.

The Questionnaire

An excellent questionnaire has been devised by the Medical Research Council (MRC) of Great Britain.[7] The questionnaire records the prevalence of certain symptoms including cough, sputum, wheeze, and shortness of breath. The latter is quantified as far as possible. A smoking history is obtained, and here it is important to estimate lifelong smoking habits rather than those which are current. Additional questions concerning past illnesses can be added to the questionnaire. In surveys of occupational lung disease the standard questions should be supplemented by further

Table 5–4. PREDICTIVE VALUE OF A POSITIVE TEST

Sensitivity (%)	Specificity (%)	Prevalence	Predictive Value (%)*
95	95	50/100	95
95	95	5/100	50
95	95	1/100	16
95	95	1/1000	2
60	98	1/1000	3

*Percentage of tests positive.

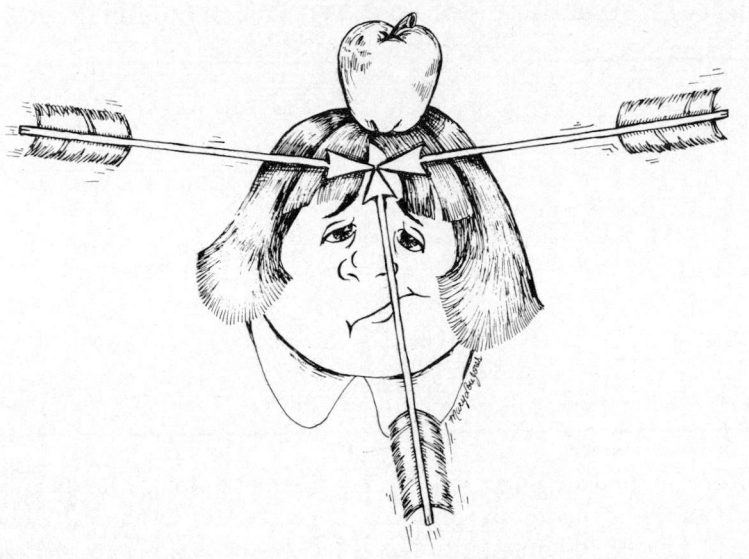

Figure 5–1. Distinction between precision (reproducibility) and accuracy.

questions which record the worker's complete occupational history from the time he started work to the present. In addition, if there are doubts as to what each job entailed, supplementary questions should be put to the worker asking for details. The MRC questionnaire has been tested in a variety of different conditions and has been shown to be a reproducible and accurate way of collecting such information. However, the questions have to be asked as written, and the subject being interviewed must not be intimidated or bullied by the tone of the interviewer. In this context it has been found that subjects who smoke will, when interviewed by a physician who is against the habit, confess more often to cough and sputum than they would have done had they been interviewed by a nurse or disinterested interviewer. For these reasons, the MRC have published a set of instructions describing how these questionnaires should be administered.[8] In addition, some form of training in the administration of the questionnaire is advisable for all interviewers prior to its use. To be an effective instrument in the accumulation of reliable data, the questionnaire should not be too long. When a questionnaire takes 30 to 60 minutes to complete, the patient becomes bored and resentful. As a result, it is often left incomplete and much of the data is useless. Self-administered questionnaires are in general less satisfactory, and their reliability is inversely proportional to their length. It must, however, be conceded that if the questionnaire is short and explicit, it can be self-administered and the data may indeed be useful and accurate.[6]

As previously mentioned, the ATS published a series of recommendations concerning the administration of standardized respiratory questionnaires. In doing so they devised their own questionnaire, which is a

modification of the original MRC version. This is known as the ATS/DLD/78 Questionnaire and has been shown to be reliable and reproducible in selected groups whether self-administered or administered by an interviewer. Additional questions can be added concerning asthma, family history, and the evaluation of pediatric disease. The ATS/DLD/78 Questionnaire has two components, an initial part designed as a bare minimum to be used in all surveys and a secondary part involving a group of supplementary questions that can be selected as appropriate by the interviewer or study designer. The questionnaire tends to be overly long, and when it is self-administered, the attention of the subject often lapses. Copies of the questionnaire can be found in a supplement to the American Review of Respiratory Disease.[6]

As with the MRC version, instructions for the use of the ATS/DLD/78 Questionnaire have been published. The instructions emphasize the need to ask the questions in an impartial fashion. It is recommended that interviewers shall be trained for a week or 10 days prior to using the questionnaire in any survey. The ATS/DLD/78 Questionnaire is recommended for use in the United States, but because of nuances in phraseology due to cultural differences and difficulties in translation, the questionnaire is somewhat less useful in Britain and other English-speaking nations, not to mention those countries where English is not the native language.

Tests of Pulmonary Function

The following are the uses of pulmonary function tests in occupational lung disease.

1. The detection of respiratory impairment and disease.
   a. Pre-employment examination.
      In many instances such tests are included as part of the pre-employment or pre-placement examination. The main aim of the tests is to detect impairment and thereby avoid employing those with compromised lung function and those who are at a greater risk of developing pulmonary impairment.
   b. Detection of occupationally related or naturally occurring disease by means of serial examinations.
      This approach represents a form of screening and the basic purpose of such examinations is to detect disease early and thereby to modify its course and prognosis. Detection in the absence of an ability to change the course of the disease is futile other than to quantify the prevalence and risk in a particular population. The World Health Organization has elaborated certain criteria which should be applied to each and every screening program (see Table 5–1).
2. For epidemiological purposes.
   a. Hazard evaluation.

If there is a suggestion that a particular job appears to be associated with the development of respiratory symptoms, then by carrying out a limited number of appropriate tests in the exposed population and in a suitable group of nonexposed controls it should be possible to determine whether such a hazard exists. The choice of the test to be used should be decided according to the type of impairment likely to be associated with the hazard. Thus, if several of the subjects are complaining of wheezing and shortness of breath, those tests measuring ventilatory capacity should be selected.

b. The derivation of standards for specific hazards.

An environmental standard has as its purpose the elimination or control of a particular hazard. In the promulgation of standards, the risk of exposure has to be weighed against the demand for and the importance of the product that is being manufactured. If it is decided that a particular product is essential, then it becomes necessary to accept a certain risk. In the process of deriving a standard, it is essential to relate biological to environmental measurements; for example, to estimate the concentration of a particular agent that produces a certain decrement in pulmonary function.

3. Disability determination.

Those pulmonary function tests that are most useful in this discipline are those which are both objective and simple. The purpose of such tests should be to determine whether significant impairment is present. Those tests that detect abnormalities not associated with symptoms, e.g., closing volume and frequency dependency of compliance, have no place in the determination of disability.

No matter what the purpose of the particular tests, the criteria already alluded to should be used to assess whether the particular choice of test is appropriate. Simplicity, accuracy, reproducibility, and reliability are the prerequisites for tests that have most use in epidemiological studies of pulmonary disease. To attain these features, some form of standardization of each test in investigation is necessary. The Appalachian Laboratory for Occupational Respiratory Disease (ALFORD) and the Division of Lung Diseases of the Heart, Lung and Blood Institute have sponsored several workshops and conferences in the hope of achieving this end. That they have been largely successful has depended on the support of a considerable number of persons and organizations, including the Environmental Health and Physiology Committees of the American College of Chest Physicians (which first published the Statement on the Assessment of Ventilatory Capacity[9]), the Division of Lung Diseases of the Heart, Lung and Blood Institute, and the American Thoracic Society.

For several years it has been apparent that not only do the techniques of performing pulmonary function tests require standardization but, in addition, many of the numerous spirometers which are on the market provide unreliable and inaccurate measurements.[10] Because of these technical problems, an effort was made by the ATS to define the appropriate

specifications for spirometer performance. A workshop was held on the standardization of spirometry at Snowbird, Utah, and the proceedings were subsequently published.[11] Specifications for pulmonary function tests were subsequently published in the Federal Register and an excellent paper by Hankinson and Gardner subsequently described the performance characteristics of a number of commonly used spirometers.[12]

As a result of much research and effort, there is now a large measure of agreement as to what tests should be done, how such tests should be done, and what equipment should be used to obtain valid results (Table 5–5).

The Epidemiology Standardization Project of the American Thoracic Society divided pulmonary function tests into essential tests and optional tests.

Essential Tests for Pulmonary Epidemiological Studies

As a minimum, all epidemiological studies involving pulmonary function should include the FVC and FEV_1. The equipment used to measure these indices of ventilatory capacity should provide a permanent record. The system used should graphically record either time versus volume or flow versus volume. Time display should be at least 2 cm/sec, volume display 1 cm/L, and flow 4 mm/L/sec. All spirometers should have a thermometer or temperature probe. In adults the tests can be performed either sitting or standing, but children should preferably be seated during the tests. A nose clip is optional but recommended, although there is little evidence to suggest that nose clips have any significant effect. If tidal volume is being recorded over a period of 30 seconds or more, nose clips are desirable. At least three acceptable forced expiratory volume maneuvers are required. Should any of these not represent a maximal effort or have other technical defects, additional maneuvers should be carried out. The two best FEV_1's and FVC's should not vary by over 5 per cent or 0.1 L, whichever is greater. Preferably, the three best results should be within 7.5 per cent. The start of the timing for the FEV_1 should be obtained by back extrapolation, and the recording of the forced expiratory volume maneuver should continue for at least 6 and preferably 10 seconds. In this connection, in subjects with severe obstruction the forced expiratory volume maneuver may be prolonged for up to 14 to 15 seconds. The largest of the three FVC's and FEV_1's should be accepted as the subject's value. All volumes should be corrected to BTPS. Calibration of the spirometer must be done regularly for both the FVC and the FEV_1.

The rationale for the number of maneuvers to be carried out is discussed elsewhere and various combinations have been tried.[13, 14] The first FVC maneuver often yields the lowest results, and it is apparent that there is a definite learning effect. This is less evident in regard to the FEV_1.

Table 5-5. RATING OF VARIOUS RESPIRATORY FUNCTION TESTS

Criteria	FVC	FEV$_1$	FEF$_{25-75}$	Peak Flow	FEF$_{50}$	FEF$_{75}$	Lung Volumes TLC and RV	CV	D$_{L-CO(b)}$	Blood Gases	(A-a)O$_2$
Acceptability	+++	+++	+++	+++	+++	+++	++	++	++	--	--
Simplicity	+++	+++	+++	++	-	-	-	±	-	-	--
Objectivity	+++	+++	++	-	++	++	+++	+	+	+++	-
Reproducibility	+++	+++	--	++	-	--	+	±	+	++	±
Accuracy	+++	+++	±	+	±	±	+	-	+	+	±
Sensitivity	+	+	++	+	++	+	-	++	++	+	+
Specificity	++	+++	-	+	-	-	-	--	±	---	-

Optional Tests for Pulmonary Epidemiological Studies

Forced Expiratory Volume Between 25 and 75 per cent of Vital Capacity (FEF_{25-75}). In certain instances the additional tests can be obtained from the standard spirometric tracing of the time versus volume maneuver or the flow volume loop. Such tests include the FEF_{25-75}, or maximal midexpiratory flow (MMF). It is often suggested that this test is more sensitive than the FEV_1 or the FEV_1/FVC ratio. The test and the method of calculation are described in Chapter 3. Calibration of the spirometer is essential, as in the case of the FEV_1 and FVC. The FEF_{25-75} is less reproducible than the FEV_1 and FVC, and although it has been suggested that it is more sensitive than the FEV_1, there is good evidence that this is not so. Thus, when the FEV_1/FVC ratio is normal—between 75 and 85 per cent—by definition the complete FEF_{25-75} is measured within the time required to complete the FEV_1 maneuver. Only if the flow rate during the first 25 per cent of the FVC were supernormal would it be possible for an abnormal FEF_{25-75} to occur.[6] The specificity of the FEF_{25-75} is low, and, moreover, the annual decrement in FEV_1 is exponential and not linear; therefore the FEF_{25-75} is less useful in longitudinal studies. Other problems include the fact that the FEF_{25-75} falls concomitantly with the FVC and with restrictive impairment. It has thus been suggested that a correction factor should be applied for lung volume when restrictive impairment is present.[15, 16] By the same token, when the FVC increases after the use of bronchodilators, the FEF_{25-75} is likewise affected, since the lung volumes often also increase.

The Flow Volume Curve (Peak Flow, FEF_{25}, FEF_{50}, FEF_{75}). The apparatus required for measurement of flow volume curves is more complex than the standard water-filled spirometer. A storage oscilloscope is desirable and a permanent record essential. Calibration for both flow and volume needs to be carried out. The various indices, e.g., FEF_{25} and FEF_{50}, should be taken off the curve in which the sum of the FVC and FEV_1 is largest. Since the equal pressure point migrates peripherally at low lung volumes, flow at these volumes (FEF_{75} and FEF_{90}) is determined by the resistance to flow in the small airways and by the elastic recoil of the lungs. In addition, flows such as the FEF_{50} and the FEF_{75} are affected by changes in lung volume.

Static Lung Volumes Other than Vital Capacity. The measurement of lung volumes, in particular total lung capacity (TLC), residual volume (RV), and functional residual capacity (FRC), in occupationally exposed populations may provide useful information under certain circumstances. In a clinical setting, a knowledge of these volumes has limited usefulness except in the performance of challenge studies, and even then dynamic lung volumes provide more useful information. Nevertheless, changes of RV and TLC often occur following exposure to toluene diisocyanate, cotton dust, and other agents, and may invalidate maximal flow measurements when the latter are expressed as a percentage of vital capacity. The

determination of lung volumes enables flow to be expressed at a percentage of TLC or at absolute lung volumes.[17] Similarly, when the body plethysmograph is being used to determine airways resistance (Raw), it is essential to express Raw at a particular lung volume. In addition, a knowledge of lung volumes enables this index of lung function to be converted to the more satisfactory measurement of specific conductance. In regard to TLC and RV, deviations from predicted values in an individual subject, even when marked, are seldom reliable as a means of assessing impairment. First, the percentage change in TLC and RV is usually less than that which occurs in the vital capacity; and second, predicted values for TLC and RV are less well established and have a larger standard error, and the effects of age and other variables are not so well documented. Moreover, many subjects have a combination of both restrictive and obstructive impairment, with the result that changes in TLC and RV are often inapparent or obscured. For these reasons it is apparent that in a clinical setting a knowledge of TLC and RV does not always help in differential diagnosis.

Other problems exist, in that TLC and RV are not easily determined and the apparatus necessary is complicated and subject to technical errors. This is especially true of the body plethysmograph, which, although the most accurate method, is also the most complex and the one in which technical errors are most difficult to detect. Furthermore, the plethysmograph is relatively immobile and cannot be used easily in the field. The helium single breath and rebreathing methods are technically more simple, but both tend to underestimate TLC, FRC, and RV when there are poorly ventilated areas of lung such as bullae present. Finally, a radiographic method of determining total lung capacity is available. This requires both a posteroanterior and lateral chest film. This method treats the lungs as a series of elliptical cylindroids and calculates the volume in this fashion.[18] If radiographs are available for other reasons, the radiographic method has considerable application, especially in epidemiological studies. It is reasonably clear that in interstitial disease, changes in TLC, RV, and FRC are insensitive and lag behind changes in VC and the diffusing capacity. In addition, they have little or no prognostic value and are unsuitable for long-term studies. In obstructive disease and diseases in which the elastic recoil of the lung decreases, a knowledge of FRC and RV is more helpful, especially as a means of relating flows to lung volume.

Diffusing Capacity ($DL_{CO_{sb}}$). There is little doubt that the $DL_{CO_{sb}}$ adds appreciably to the characterization of impairment in occupational lung disease, especially in those diseases leading to restrictive impairment, such as asbestosis, hard metal disease, and berylliosis. The steady state method is not suitable for epidemiological purposes, but can be used in diagnosis and in the assessment of impairment and disability. In surveys and field work, an automated method using a module is probably best, but here again regular calibration is vitally important. The various methods of carrying out the $DL_{CO_{sb}}$ are described in the Epidemiology Standardization

Project.[6] Duplicate values are essential and should agree within 5 per cent. The $DL_{CO_{sb}}$ is influenced by the size of the inspired volume, and if this differs by more than 10 per cent from the FVC, the value will be invalid owing to an artifactually reduced alveolar volume. The test is also affected by the duration of breath-holding and by an inadvertent Valsalva maneuver. The values obtained are also influenced by the hemoglobin level, and hence women tend to have lower values. Cigarette smoking also affects the measurement. The specificity and sensitivity in conditions such as asbestosis and interstitial lung disease have been studied in detail by Gaensler et al.[6] They found the sensitivity to be high but the specificity relatively low.

Blood Gas Analysis. Blood gas analysis at rest and with exercise is often used to help in the diagnosis of a particular condition and in the assessment of pulmonary impairment and disability. While a reduction of arterial PO_2 may be seen in occupational asthma, byssinosis, asbestosis, and several other occupational lung diseases, blood gas analysis seldom adds any additional diagnostic information and still less frequently is helpful in the assessment of occupationally related pulmonary impairment.[19] Thus the arterial PO_2 is affected by numerous nonpulmonary conditions, including cardiac disease, obesity, hepatic cirrhosis, and various neurological diseases. This lack of specificity is as great a drawback as is its relative lack of sensitivity. Moreover, there is little correlation between the arterial PO_2 and the presence of dyspnea. Thus asthmatics or byssinotic subjects may have severe ventilatory impairment and yet have a normal or near normal arterial oxygen tension. Much the same goes for a restrictive impairment, and here again the diffusing capacity is affected earlier than are the blood gases, and in addition correlates far better with the presence of dyspnea. Nonetheless, exercise studies may be helpful in assessing how much oxygen is available to the metabolic sites, and as a way of separating cardiac from pulmonary impairment.

Other Indices Derived from Blood Gas Analysis. The alveolo-arterial oxygen gradient $(A-a)O_2$, physiological dead space (VD_P), and ratio of dead space to tidal volume (VD/VT) are indices derived from blood gas analysis, and all may be abnormal in occupational lung disease. Nevertheless, for the most part they are nonspecific and relatively insensitive. The $(A-a)O_2$ has been recommended as a sensitive test for early disease, but it is now clear that its usefulness is strictly limited for a variety of reasons. First, as already mentioned, the test is nonspecific; second, the resting value may be profoundly influenced by hyperventilation and anxiety; third, the $(A-a)O_2$ increases with age; and fourth, the test is invasive. The exercise $(A-a)O_2$ is far more useful and helps to eliminate the confounding factor of hyperventilation. Despite these drawbacks, some subjects with categories 2 and 3 simple coal workers' pneumoconiosis who have an absolutely normal ventilatory capacity will show an increase in the $(A-a)O_2$. Even so, this is a late finding and is always preceded by radiographic changes.

Tests of Small Airways Function. These tests have been hailed as a means of detecting disease early in its course, thereby providing an opportunity to arrest the condition and prevent the onset of disability. Many problems exist with this approach, not least of which is the fact that the detection of abnormalities by these tests does not necessarily portend who is going to develop disabling impairment. The proportion of cigarette smokers who have an abnormal closing volume or frequency dependence of dynamic compliance is far in excess of the 12 to 15 per cent who go on to develop significant airways obstruction. Thus it is apparent that not all subjects who have these abnormalities of small airways function develop significant impairment.

Of the tests of small airways function that are available, frequency dependence of dynamic compliance has the least to recommend it. The test is difficult to carry out, and involves swallowing an esophageal balloon; the equipment used in its determination is expensive; and technical misadventures are common. In the presence of normal spirometry, a fall in dynamic compliance at high respiratory frequencies may indicate small airways obstruction or, alternatively, localized changes in the elastic recoil of the lung. Thus, while it is possible for the overall flow pressure volume curve to be normal, this would not preclude a situation in which the presence of localized areas of emphysema and fibrosis balance each other out so that the overall mechanical properties of the lung are normal.

Closing volume is less sensitive but is much simpler to carry out. Nonetheless, the test is nonspecific. While noninvasive, it is technically more difficult to perform than simple spirometry, and around 20 per cent of the general population who are tested in the field cannot follow the instructions necessary to complete the test.[20] The determination of closing volume is influenced by inspiratory and expiratory flow rates during the performance of the tests, and also by the duration of breath-holding. Compared to the FEV_1, the test is more variable, less specific, more difficult to carry out, and its performance more time-consuming. Pilot studies using the test in byssinosis and in other conditions in which there is an acute change in ventilatory capacity have shown it to be less sensitive and less reliable than the FEV_1.[20]

Flow volume curves with oxygen-helium mixtures have likewise been advocated as the ideal approach to early diagnosis. The initial enthusiasm for the test has not been vindicated, and at least in some occupationally related diseases, in particular those due to coal dust exposure, the test has been shown to be far more variable and less sensitive than the FEV_1.[21] It is doubtful whether it will prove more useful in other occupationally related disease, although controlled trials may be worthwhile.

Normal Values for Pulmonary Function Tests

Numerous prediction formulae exist for the various indices of ventilatory capacity, the FVC and FEV_1, in particular. For a variety of reasons,

it is difficult to recommend one particular set. Probably the most reliable values are those of Morris,[22] Knudson,[23] and Peterson,[24] all of which were derived from nonsmoking populations. For any given subject, age, height, sex, and race influence his or her ventilatory capacity and lung volumes. Weight and other factors make a far lesser contribution. The FVC and FEV_1 reach their maximum at about the age of 25, remain relatively unchanged to age 30 or so, and then slowly decline. The annual decrement for the FEV_1 is around 25 ml and that for the FVC around 15 to 20 ml. Although the mean annual decrement in subjects with chronic air flow obstruction tends to be linear over a period of 7 to 10 years, and may range from 30 to 200 ml, over periods of a year considerable fluctuations occur, and in some instances definite improvement takes place for no apparent reason (Fig. 5–2). Furthermore, much greater declines in both the FEV_1 and FVC occur in older subjects. In contrast, maximal expiratory flows tend to reach their maximum at an earlier age, that is to say 17 or 18, and then start to decline in the early 20s. Although it is often not realized, the FEV_1/FVC ratio likewise decreases with age, and it is inappropriate to take an arbitrary cut-off, such as 70 per cent, as the lower limit of normal. A ratio of around 65 per cent, which is definitely abnormal in a 25-year-old, may be entirely normal for a 60-year-old. The larger the subject, the greater the FVC, and the greater the tendency for the person to have a somewhat lower FEV_1/FVC ratio. Appropriate prediction formulae for this index have also been published.[25]

In a disease-free individual of any given height there is a range of values for normality, and when a large number of subjects of the same age, height, and sex are tested, the values for the FVC and FEV_1 have a Gaussian distribution. The lower limit of normality is usually defined as the value which is exceeded by 95 per cent of healthy individuals in the

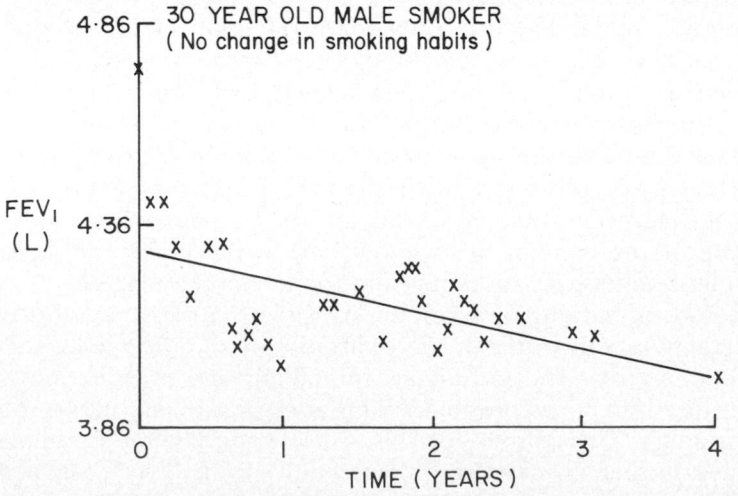

Figure 5–2. Serial measurements of FEV_1 over a period of 4 years in a heavy smoker.

population. This is approximately the mean value minus 1.64 SEE (standard error of the estimate). Black subjects have lung volumes and flow rates that are about 12 to 15 per cent less than white subjects of the same age and height.[26] Other racial differences have been reported in Eskimos, Chinese, and East Indians.[27-29]

Many laboratories report abnormal pulmonary function when the subject being tested has a value that is 80 per cent or less than the predicted figure. The use of 80 per cent as a cut-off irrespective of age and other factors is, however, incorrect. Reasons for this were discussed in a recent editorial by Sobol and Sobol.[30] A level of 80 per cent of predicted is based on the assumption that all pulmonary function tests have a variance around the predicted which is a fixed percentage of that figure. Coincidence of 80 per cent of the predicted and two standard deviations is a matter of chance and occurs at a single point only. It is apparent that small persons with normal function will deviate more readily than those who have normal function and are tall. Thus the regression line for 80 per cent of the predicted and the line for the 95 per cent confidence limit do not coincide. In older subjects the 80 per cent of the predicted line converges on the predicted, whereas the reverse is true for younger subjects. Sobol describes a method that normalizes all subjects to a single value for each function.[30] Thus, for an index whose value is represented by a simple mean and standard deviation (SD), the normalizing process requires determining the value of the mean when the mean minus 2SD represents 80 per cent of the mean.

Radiographic Examinations

The chest radiograph has for many years been one of the mainstays in the epidemiological investigation of the pneumoconioses. It remains the sole means of detecting pulmonary retention of certain dusts, e.g., silica and coal. For these and other reasons, an abnormal chest film is routinely accepted as the only legal evidence of dust exposure in workmen's compensation cases and in industrial litigation. Seldom, however, is the chest film useful in the assessment of pulmonary function, although there is some correlation between the radiographic category of asbestosis and the degree of pulmonary impairment. It nevertheless provides a measure of the amount of dust retained in the lungs and is especially useful in monitoring coal miners and those exposed to silica.

Before embarking on a respiratory disease survey that relies on chest radiography as one of the means of acquisition of epidemiological data, it is imperative that the techniques for taking and interpreting films be standardized as far as possible.[31] This is especially important in longitudinal studies. The reasons for this are several. The chest radiograph is used as a means of quantifying the amount of dust that is retained in the lungs. The retention of dust leads to the development of certain shadows

or opacities in the chest film, and in general, the more opacities, the more retained dust.[32-34] While the radiographic opacities may not always be produced by the dust itself—rather, they may originate as a fibrogenic response to the retained dust—it is reasonable to assume that the more fibrosis present, the more retained dust. Thus it is evident that there is a continuum from no dust in the lungs to maximal dust, whatever the latter might happen to be. In an attempt to quantify the amount of dust in the lungs, various radiological classifications of the pneumoconioses have been introduced. Since 1950, the International Labor Organization (ILO) has published a series of classifications that have been widely accepted. The latest and most comprehensive is the ILO 1980 classification, which provides the means of classifying not only the pneumoconioses but also pleural thickening and pleural calcification.[31] Classifications rely on the partly arbitrary selection of certain films as being typical of the various stages of the disease. The films used in the 1980 ILO classification have been reproduced and are available from the ILO as standard sets.

The pneumoconioses were originally divided into simple and complicated forms of the disease. The simple form was diagnosed by the presence of either regular or irregular opacities less than 1 cm in diameter, plus a significant exposure history. When one of the opacities were larger than 1 cm in diameter, complicated pneumoconiosis was said to be present. Simple pneumoconiosis was subdivided into categories 1, 2, and 3, according to the extent and profusion of the opacities. Similarly, complicated pneumoconiosis was divided into stages A, B, and C, according to the size of the large opacity or opacities. A group of experts selected a series of chest films that in their opinion could be used as standards for the various stages and categories. It was, moreover, suggested that any unknown, unclassified film that was being categorized should be compared to the standards. While such an exercise is essential when approximating the unknown to the standard, it must be realized that no other radiograph exactly matches any of the standards. The amount of dust retained in the lungs of the subject whose film is being interpreted is bound to be either slightly more or less than that retained in the lungs of the subject from whom the standard film was made. In addition the volume of the lungs and soft tissue shadows will influence the radiographic appearances.

It subsequently became apparent that a classification that relies on major categories alone, viz., 1, 2, and 3, lacked sufficient sensitivity for longitudinal epidemiological studies. It also became evident that those studies in which an attempt was made to relate environmental measurements to radiographic progression needed a more sensitive indicator. This led to the introduction, by Liddell and May, of the 12-point scale.[35] This modification subdivides each major category of simple pneumoconiosis into three subcategories (Fig. 5–3). Category 0 is divided into subcategory 0/−, in which the film was absolutely normal and under no conceivable circumstances could anyone consider it otherwise (in British parlance, a "barndoor" normal); 0/0, in which the film was normal; 0/1, in which the

CATEGORY
&
SUB-CATEGORY

0			1			2			3		
0/-	0/0	0/1	1/0	1/1	1/2	2/1	2/2	2/3	3/2	3/3	3/+

Figure 5–3. ILO elaboration of the classification of simple pneumoconiosis.

interpreter decided that it was category 0, but considered category 1 as well. Category 1 is made up of subcategories 1/0, 1/1, and 1/2. In the case of subcategory 1/0, it was decided that the film should be placed in category 1 but category 0 was also seriously considered; 1/1 represents a typical category 1, and closely resembles the standard film. In the case of category 1/1, neither category 0 nor category 2 was considered. The classification goes up to category 3/+, in which there are more opacities present in the film than in the midcategory 3/3 standard radiograph. Thus, the numerator represents the category in which the radiograph was placed, while the denominator describes any other category that was considered.

The Liddell classification divides the continuum from no dust to maximal dust into a 12-point scale. Most persons assume that the scale is made up of equal intervals, and that the weight of additional dust retained for each increase in category is the same, i.e., it takes the same amount of dust to change a 0/1 to a 1/0 as it does to change a 2/2 to a 2/3. This assumption may not be valid, but has much to recommend it in practical terms, especially when it comes to the assessment of progression in pneumoconiosis. Moreover, studies have been carried out which have related radiographic subcategories to the coal content of the lungs, and these have shown that for the most part there is a straight line relationship.[32-34]

Extent

The lungs are divided into three zones on each side: upper, middle, and lower. This division is made by projecting horizontal lines drawn at 1/3 and 2/3 of the vertical distance between the lung apices and the domes of the diaphragm. Profusion of small opacities is determined as mentioned earlier by considering all the affected zones of the lungs, and by comparing the unknown film with the standard radiographs. When there is a marked difference in profusion of different zones of the lungs, the zone or zones showing the lesser involvement or profusion are ignored when classifying the film.

Small Opacities

Those opacities that are present in the lungs and that are found in various pneumoconioses can be classified as either rounded (regular) or irregular.

Small Rounded Opacities. These opacities have a fairly rounded and regular margin, at least when viewed without magnification. They are classified according to their size into p, q, and r; p being up to 1.5 mm, q varying between 1.5 and 3 mm, and r between 3 and 10 mm. While there is usually only one type of opacity present, occasionally mixtures occur. The reading of the film should be based on the predominant type of opacity noted. Provision is made for recording different types of opacity, e.g., p and q or p and r in the same film, and reference to this will be made later. Progression from category 1 to 2 and further up the scale is seldom if ever associated with a change in the type of opacity. When the chest x-ray changes from normal to abnormal and p-type opacities appear, these usually persist should the film progress further to category 2 or 3. While p-type opacities occur for the most part in coal workers' pneumoconiosis (CWP), q-type opacities are seen in both CWP and silicosis, though r-type opacities are more commonly found in silicosis. Progression may occur in silicosis with or without further exposure, while in simple CWP the progression and development of more small opacities is seen only with further exposure. Regression rarely if ever occurs in silicosis, and while regression or clearing is not thought to occur in CWP, the possibility cannot be categorically denied. Regression has been observed in welders' siderosis.

Irregular Opacities. These are classified as s, t, or u and were previously designated without measurements as fine, medium, or coarse opacities; however, in the 1980 ILO classification, dimensions have been given to irregular opacities. Thus s opacities have a width up to 1.5 mm, t opacities vary between 1.5 and 3 mm, and u opacities between 3 and 10 mm. Irregular opacities are characteristically seen in asbestosis; however, scanty irregular opacities may also be present in cigarette smokers and in those with airways obstruction.[36, 37] Nevertheless, in the absence of dust exposure seldom does the film of a smoker rank higher than 1/0 and more usually it is 0/1.

Rounded and irregular opacities may occur in the same film, but one or the other usually predominates. The 1980 ILO classification makes provision for recording both regular and irregular opacities when both are present in the same radiograph. Thus the designation q/t means that the predominant small opacity is of the q type, but that there are a significant number of small irregular opacities of the t type. In this way, all combinations of opacities may be recorded. Repetition of the same letter, for example p/p, t/t, indicates that the opacities are all predominantly one shape and size. A word of caution should be added in regard

to the designation of size of the irregular opacities: it must be remembered that the s, t, and u dimensions are approximations.

Large Pneumoconiotic Opacities

A large opacity is defined as any opacity greater than 1 cm that is present in a film in which there is sufficient evidence to indicate a diagnosis of pneumoconiosis. This definition therefore excludes large opacities due to other causes such as cancer of the lung. Category or stage A is defined as a large opacity between 1 and 5 cm in diameter or several opacities each greater than 1 cm in diameter but whose combined diameter is less than 5 cm. Category or stage B is present when an opacity or opacities whose combined width is greater than 5 cm or whose area does not exceed the equivalent of the right upper zone. Category or stage C is present when there are one or more opacities whose combined area exceeds the equivalent of the right upper zone or a third of one lung field.

Pleural Thickening

The site—the chest wall, diaphragm, or costophrenic angle—and the width and the extent of pleural thickening should be recorded separately.

Chest Wall. Chest wall pleural thickening may be circumscribed (plaques) or diffuse. Both plaques and diffuse thickening can occur in the same subject. Thickening should be recorded separately for the right and left pleural surfaces, and when seen along the lateral chest wall, the maximal width should be recorded. Width is measured from the inner aspect of the chest wall to the inner margin of the shadow cast by the pleural thickening at the border of the lung and pleura. It is subdivided into stages A, B, and C, with A representing a maximal width of 5 mm; B, a maximal width of between 5 and 10 mm; and C, a maximal width of over 10 mm. When pleural thickening is seen en face, it should be recorded, although it may also be seen in profile. When viewed en face alone, width usually cannot be determined. The extent of pleural thickening is defined in terms of the degree of involvement of the lateral chest wall and is quantified into three grades. Grade 1 indicates involvement of up to a quarter of the lateral projection of the chest wall; grade 2 indicates involvement of between one-quarter and one-half, and grade 3 more than one-half of the lateral projection of the chest wall.

Diaphragm. A plaque involving the diaphragmatic pleura should likewise be recorded as present. Here again, the right or left side should be indicated, and this is as illustrated in the example in the standard radiographs.

Costophrenic Angle. Obliteration of the costophrenic angle should be recorded. If the thickening extends up the chest wall, the findings should be recorded as both costophrenic angle obliteration and pleural thickening, provided the latter is of grade 1 or greater. The site involved

should be specified. The scalloping or leafing of the diaphragm that is sometimes seen in severe airways obstruction and that creates an artificial appearance of costophrenic angle obliteration should not be recorded.

Pleural Calcification. One or both sides may be involved but should be recorded separately. Here again, the site and extent must be documented. In regard to the site, provision is made for recording involvement of the chest wall, diaphragm, and other structures including the pericardium and mediastinum. The extent of pleural calcification is subdivided into grades 1, 2, and 3, with 1 being an area of calcified pleura with the greatest diameter up to 20 mm, or a number of such areas whose combined diameter does not exceed 20 mm. Grade 2 includes calcification in an area or areas whose greatest diameter exceeds 20 mm but not 100 mm. Grade 3 includes pleural calcification in one or more areas where the greatest diameter exceeds 100 mm.

Equipment and Technique

The new ILO classification and guidelines for its use contain a number of recommendations as to the x-ray equipment to be used and the most suitable technique for taking chest radiographs.[31] In regard to certain of the recommendations, unanimity was not forthcoming. The criteria for obtaining a quality film are included in the booklet that accompanies the standard radiographs. Film quality should be assessed and recorded. Four grades are recognized: 1, good quality; 2, acceptable with no technical defect likely to impair the classification of the radiograph for pneumoconiosis; 3, poor with some technical defect, but still acceptable for classification purposes; and 4, unreadable. When a film is unacceptable or of poor quality, some mention should be made as to why it is unsatisfactory, i.e., whether it is overpenetrative or underpenetrative, fogged, or grey.

Classifying Unknown Films

It is recommended that when a reader who is interpreting a series of unknown films sees a film that obviously demonstrates the features of pneumoconiosis, rather than arbitrarily awarding a category to the film, he or she should compare it to the appropriate standard films, trying to match the profusion and type of opacities in the unknown with the appropriate standard. Only in this fashion will the interpretation of films become an objective exercise. Many readers feel that the standard films are so fixed in their minds that they have no need to refer to them when interpreting unknowns. The refusal to use standard films has been shown by Morgan and Reger to lead to what they refer to as the middling tendency.[38] Thus when certain readers are faced with interpreting an unknown radiograph that shows pneumoconiosis, instead of comparing it to the standards, they immediately attach a category to it. In doing so, they virtually always use a midcategory (1/1, 2/2, or 3/3). Had they

compared it to the standards, an element of uncertainty might have entered their mind. As it is, their mental processes leave them never in doubt but often wrong. Thus in one study involving several interpreters, all of whom were consultants to the U.S. Public Health Service, all but one showed a pronounced middling tendency.[38] The one exception was the sole reader who regularly used the standards while interpreting unknowns.

Nevertheless, it must be remembered that there is no guarantee that the 12-point scale is made up of equal intervals, and indeed its originators felt that the intervals were probably unequal.[39] If the scale were of equal intervals, the weight of additional dust obtained for each increase in subcategory would be the same. When independent randomized reading is used to determine radiographic progression, should several readers be afflicted with the middling tendency, the bias would tend to eliminate or decrease progression, especially when change is small (1/1 to 1/2). Further references to the problems of reading progression will be found later in the chapter. In the few instances in which progression is marked, viz., two subcategories, the middling tendency would tend to exaggerate it even further.

Observer Variation

Despite the standardization of techniques for taking and interpreting films, the radiographic interpretation of pneumoconiosis still remains a subjective exercise. Marked interobserver and intraobserver variations occur,[40–42] as they also do in the interpretation of chest films for tuberculosis, barium enemata for colitis, and electrocardiograms for myocardial infarction. Interobserver variation is usually greater than intraobserver variation, and it is essential in an epidemiological survey to compare and standardize the radiographic interpretations of various readers. Marked differences between British and North American readers have been shown to exist—while the British appear to have been disciplined into conformity with their most experienced reader, the North Americans show too much individuality.[41] Those readers who differ greatly from their colleagues should be excluded. Multiple readings are to be preferred to single readings, but even then the panel of readers should be tested at regular intervals to ensure that their reading habits have not changed. This can be done by having them re-read several series of films at regular intervals. Such a series should range over all categories and should have at least 100 films in it. During the interpretation of the series of unclassified films, all x-rays thought to be positive for pneumoconiosis should be matched with the appropriate standard. When reading an unclassified series of films, the introduction of "marker films" at fairly regular intervals, that is to say, good quality x-rays that several readers have read independently and classified in an agreed category, helps keep the readers' "thermostat" in line with the consensus. Thus when a marker film is interpreted, the reader should agree fairly closely with the prior consensus category (within

1 subcategory). Should the reader deviate by more than one subcategory, the error should be pointed out to him. The reader is then aware that his readings are out of line with the consensus and can make a conscious effort to adjust his reading scale up or down.

The interpretation of films for pneumoconiosis is greatly influenced by technique, and therefore techniques should be standardized as far as possible prior to starting the survey. Individual radiologists can no more agree on an optimal technique than they can on the degree of pneumoconiosis present in individual films. For these reasons a uniform technique should be adopted, since were each radiologist allowed to use his own preference, the range would be infinite. Such recommendations for standardization of techniques have been published and, while certainly not ideal, can with intelligent application help reduce interobserver variation.[31, 43] Nonetheless, there have been film trials comparing various radiographic techniques using high versus low kilovoltage, and the results have shown that the interpretation is little affected by using high as opposed to low kilovoltage techniques.[44]

The depth of inspiration, the duration of exposure, and the method of developing the film all may influence interpretation. It has been shown that overpenetrative films are likely to decrease the category awarded, whereas if the film is unduly soft or underpenetrative, a higher category is likely to be awarded.[45] The effect of such changes may be profound and may change prevalence and progression rates by as much as 50 per cent.

The Chest Radiograph and Dust Exposure

Serial chest radiographs have been used in numerous epidemiological studies of occupational lung disease as a means of monitoring dust exposure in exposed populations. When conducting studies in which chest radiographs have been made on dust-exposed populations it is customary to consider several indices, including the prevalence of the condition, the attack rate, and the progression rate. The prevalence rate may not reflect present conditions, and hence is one of the less useful measurements. The attack rate is better as a rule, but in silicosis and CWP, diseases that seldom develop without prolonged exposure, the disease may appear at a time when exposure is decreasing. In certain instances, the main insult may have occurred several years previously, and the onset of abnormalities is related in the main to prior exposure. The best way of relating environmental exposure to the radiographic response is to measure the progression rate, that is to say, the change in category over a period of time during which dust exposure was measured and is known. This is best achieved by comparing diads, triads, or quadrads of films from exposed workers.

Serial films can be used to improve clinical diagnosis and also to determine progression. Thus when a tentative diagnosis is based on a solitary film which shows only equivocal changes, the diagnosis may

subsequently be established when a radiograph is taken at a later date and shows that the characteristic features have appeared. The assessment of radiographic progression and regression needs further description.

Methods of Assessing Progression and Regression

Two kinds of change may be detected through comparison of serial films: first, the appearance of disease or abnormality in previously normal films; and second, progression or regression in a film already interpreted as abnormal.[46] In the first instance the frequency of abnormalities appearing in a series of previously normal films allows one to calculate an attack rate, while in the second instance a progression index can be derived. The films may be presented for comparison to the reader in two ways.

Independent Method. This involves presentation to the interpreter of a series of films so that he cannot remember when the other radiograph(s) from the same subject was presented to him. The independent method permits several modes of presentation of the films, namely, immediately, that is to say as soon as the films are available for comparison; serially, with all the first films on one occasion and all the second films on another occasion; and independently randomized, with the films of the first and the second series mixed. Since it is known that the reading habits of an interpreter are subject to change, it is obviously desirable to read all the films of the randomized series within a relatively short time.

Side by Side Method. When two or more films of the same subject are available, they may be presented in the correct chronological sequence or the order may be disguised. However, attempts at disguising the order are often unsuccessful, and the technical qualities of the films usually permit recognition of the temporal sequence. When three or more films are available, possible sequences become many and the only useful approach is to completely reverse the order. Two or more films may be interpreted as a simple series (triad, tetrad, pentad) or as separate diads, e.g., as the first and fourth films of a series. The latter involves comparing the first film with the second, then with the third, etc. The logistics of such complex comparisons become enormous.

The main arguments concerning the reading of progression in pneumoconiosis center around which method is preferred, the side by side or the independent. Implicit in the use of the side by side method is the bias introduced by a knowledge of chronological sequence of the films. However, it must not be forgotten that bias exists with the independent method. In any two chest radiographs of the same subject taken at an interval, there are several differences between the films of the diads, for example, the age of the patient examined, his weight in certain circumstances, and also technical factors affecting film quality. Experienced readers make allowance for age and technique, but only if these compensatory mechanisms are entirely consistent, which they are obviously not, can it be said that the independent method is without bias. Advocates of the side by side method claim it allows readers to compensate for differing

techniques, and in addition reduces the variation that is inherent in independent reading.

The problem of bias introduced by knowledge of chronological sequence was investigated by Reger and his colleagues.[47] The results of their studies indicated that the side by side method is prone to bias, and the assumed chronological sequence of the diad greatly influenced the progression score. The design of their study was somewhat contrived in that the readers, believing they knew the temporal sequence, were presented with a pair of films showing up to eight steps of regression. This was effected by reversing the order of the films without the interpreter's knowledge. In addition, it was shown that a progression score was often recorded in two copies of the same film when the reader believed that they were taken at different intervals. It is thus apparent that the assumed chronological sequence greatly influences the reading of progression when the side by side method is used. Although this trial may be criticized in that it was somewhat foreign to the experience of most readers, a similar investigation utilizing serial radiographs from subjects with tuberculosis and sarcoidosis showed exactly the same findings. In this case it cannot be claimed that regression is unknown, since the interpreters should have known that both tuberculosis and sarcoidosis are prone not only to improve but to regress.[48]

Liddell and Morgan compared side by side with independent reading according to standard scientific criteria and they also reviewed several published series.[46] They did this by comparing the methods in terms of differentiability, consistency, validity, and simplicity. Since there is a continuum from no dust to maximal dust with no exact end point to indicate the presence of disease, the definition of sensitivity has to be modified. The authors concluded that at the present time, side by side reading is the method of choice, since independent randomized reading tends to lack specificity and the signal-noise ratio is likewise less satisfactory. In general there is more variability with the independent method of reading, and regression may be recorded in a proportion of the paired films. Comparison of independent and side by side reading usually shows that the independent method yields about half as much progression as the side by side method.[49] Only when it becomes possible to guarantee exactly the same technique when taking films over a period of several years will it be possible to limit the problem of bias in the independent method.

The few comparative trials that have been carried out in which progression has been read by interpreters from different nations have shown some startling differences. This is especially true of one trial in which British and North American readers were compared. The cause of such variability was not immediately apparent, but clearly much needs to be done in order to obtain more uniform and less variable readings of progression.

It is often assumed that the interpretation of the films for pneumo-

coniosis requires profound knowledge and perspicacity, and that the ideal interpreter is a god-like blend of Sherlock Holmes, Albrecht Dürer, and Socrates. In reality, the interpretation of a film for pneumoconiosis is a glorified guess or estimate of the number of dots present on it. The more educated the observer, the more likely he is to be rigid in his interpretation. If the observer happens to have an opinion that coincides with an accepted consensus, this is ideal, but if he does not, it is most unlikely that he will change his reading habits. If the latter state of affairs is the case—and this is a frequent occurrence among eminent radiologists and to lesser extent in chest physicians—then that observer must be excluded from epidemiological studies. The distinction between epidemiology and clinical diagnosis is often difficult to explain to radiologists and clinicians, but its importance cannot be overestimated. We have shown that lay readers can be trained to read films for pneumoconiosis.[50] Since they have no preconceived ideas and hence tend to be more open to suggestion, they are more likely to record than to interpret and in many ways are to be preferred.

A report of a workshop sponsored by the National Heart and Lung Institute offers much useful advice for those who are involved in the use of the chest x-ray in epidemiology.[51] The main recommendations are that in epidemiological studies involving radiographic examinations of the chest, at least three readers, whose comparability has been assessed prior to the study, should be used. All readings should be carried out independently, and consensus or collaborative reading sessions should be avoided, since the consensus frequently represents the opinion of the most forceful and biased reader. A mean reading is the best measure of the prevalence of the condition. In addition, standard films should be used in order to achieve comparability and chest films of unexposed workers should be included in the series for control purposes. A percentage of the films should be recycled to ensure reproducibility.

References

1. Morris, J. N., Uses of Epidemiology. New York, Churchill Livingstone, 1975, pp. 318–320.
2. Attfield, M., and Hudak, J., Prevalence of coal workers' pneumoconiosis: comparison of first and second rounds. In Rom, W. N., and Archer, V. E. eds., Health Implications of New Energy Technologies. Ann Arbor, Mich., Ann Arbor Science, 1980.
3. Whitby, L. G., Screening for disease: definitions and criteria. Lancet, 2, 819, 1974.
4. Morgan, W. K. C., Screening for occupational lung cancer. Chest, 74, 239, 1978.
5. McCarthy, D. S., Craig, D. B., and Cherniack, R. M., Intraindividual variability in the maximal expiratory flow volume and closing volume in asymptomatic subjects. Am. Rev. Respir. Dis., 112, 407, 1975.
6. Epidemiology Standardization Project. Am. Rev. Respir. Dis., 118 (Suppl II), 1–88, 1978.
7. Research Council Committee on the Aetiology of Chronic Bronchitis, Standardized questionnaires on respiratory symptoms. Br. Med. J., 1960, 2, 1965.
8. Medical Research Council Committee on the Aetiology of Chronic Bronchitis, Instructions for the Use of the Questionnaire on Respiratory Symptoms. Dawlish, England, W. J. Holman, Ltd., 1966.

9. Morgan, W. K. C., and Schmidt, C. D., Joint statement of the Committees of Environmental Health and Physiology: The assessment of ventilatory capacity. Chest, 67, 95, 1975.
10. Fitzgerald, M. X., Smith, A. A., and Gaensler, E. A., Evaluation of electronic spirometers. N. Engl. J. Med., 289, 1283, 1973.
11. ATS Statement, Snowbird workshop on standardization of spirometry. Am. Rev. Respir. Dis., 119, 831, 1979.
12. Gardner, R. M., Hankinson, J. L., and West, B. J., Evaluating commercially available spirometers. Am. Rev. Respir. Dis., 121, 73, 1980.
13. Tager, I., Speizer, F. E., Rosner, B., and Prang, G., A comparison between the three largest and the last of five forced expiratory maneuvers in a population study. Am. Rev. Respir. Dis., 114, 871, 1976.
14. Ferris, B. G., Speizer, F. E., Bishop, Y., and Prang, G., Spirometry for an epidemiologic study. Bull. Eur. Physiopath. Respir., 14, 175, 1978.
15. Sherter, C. B., Connolly, J. J., and Schilder, D. P., The significance of volume adjusting the maximal midexpiratory flow in assessing response to a bronchodilator drug. Chest, 73, 568, 1978.
16. Cockcroft, D. W., and Berscheid, B. A., Volume adjustment of maximal midexpiratory flow. Chest, 78, 595, 1980.
17. Hankinson, J. L., Reger, R. B., and Morgan, W. K. C., Maximal expiratory flows in coal miners. Am. Rev. Respir. Dis., 116, 175, 1977.
18. Reger, R. B., Young, A., and Morgan, W. K. C., An accurate and rapid radiographic method of determining total lung capacity. Thorax, 27, 163, 1972.
19. Morgan, W. K. C., Lapp, N. L., and Seaton, D., Respiratory disability in coal miners. J.A.M.A., 243, 2401, 1980.
20. Fairman, R. P., Hankinson, J. L., Lapp, N. L., and Morgan, W. K. C., Pilot study of closing volume in byssinosis. Br. J. Ind. Med., 32, 235, 1975.
21. Boehlecke, B., Piccirillo, R. E., and Hankinson, J. L., Use of helium oxygen spirometry in the detection of small airways disease in coal miners. Paper presented at the International Conference on Occupational Lung Disease, sponsored by the American College of Chest Physicians, San Francisco, 1979.
22. Morris, J. F., Koski, A., and Johnson, L. C., Spirometric standards for healthy nonsmoking adults. Am. Rev. Respir. Dis., 103, 57, 1971.
23. Knudson, R. J., Slatin, R. C., and Lebowitz, N. J., The maximal expiratory flow volume curve: normal standards, variability and effects of age. Am. Rev. Respir. Dis., 113, 587, 1976.
24. Petersen, M. R., Amandus, H., Reger, R. B., et al., Ventilatory capacity in normal coal miners: Prediction formulae for the FEV_1 and FVC. J. Occup. Med., 15, 899, 1973.
25. Morris, J. F., Temple, W. P., and Koski, A., Normal values for the ratio of one second forced expiratory volume to fast vital capacity. Am. Rev. Respir. Dis., 108, 1000, 1973.
26. Lapp, N. L., Amandus, H., Hall, R., and Morgan, W. K. C., Lung volumes and flow rates in black and white subjects. Thorax, 29, 185, 1974.
27. Rode, A., and Shephard, R. J., Pulmonary function of Canadian eskimos. Scand. J. Respir. Dis., 54, 4, 1973.
28. DeCosta, J. L., Pulmonary function studies in healthy Chinese adults in Singapore. Am. Rev. Respir. Dis., 104, 128, 1971.
29. Corey, P. N., Ashley, M. J., and Chan-Yeung, M., Racial differences in lung function: search for proportional relationship. J. Occup. Med., 21, 395, 1979.
30. Sobol, E. J., and Sobol, P. G., Percent of predicted as the limit of normal in pulmonary function testing: a statistically valid approach. Thorax, 34, 1, 1979.
31. Guidelines for the use of the ILO international classification of radiographs of pneumoconiosis. No. 22 (Rev.), Occupational Safety and Health series. Geneva, International Labour Office, 1980.
32. Rivers, D. E., Wise, M. E., King, E. J., and Nagelschmidt, G., Dust content, radiology and pathology of simple pneumoconiosis of coal workers. Br. J. Ind. Med., 17, 87, 1960.
33. Rossiter, C. E., Relation of lung dust content to radiological changes in coal workers. Ann. N.Y. Acad. Sci., 200, 465, 1972.
34. Caplan, H., Correlation of radiological category with lung pathology in coal workers' pneumoconiosis. Br. J. Ind. Med., 19, 171, 1962.

35. Liddell, F. D. K., and May, J. D., Assessing the Radiological Progression of Simple Pneumoconiosis. London, National Coal Board (Medical Service), 1966.
36. Carilli, A. D., Kotzen, L. M., and Fischer, M. L., The chest roentgenogram in smoking females. Am. Rev. Respir. Dis., *107*, 133, 1973.
37. Amandus, H. E., Lapp. N. L., Jacobson, G., and Reger, R. B., Significance of irregular small opacities in the radiographs of coal miners in the U.S.A. Br. J. Ind. Med., *33*, 13, 1976.
38. Morgan, W. K. C., Petersen, M. R., and Reger, R. B., The "middling" tendency. Arch. Environ. Health., *29*, 334, 1974.
39. Liddell, F. D. K., An experiment in film reading. Br. J. Ind. Med., *20*, 300, 1963.
40. Reger, R. B., and Morgan, W. K. C., On the factors influencing consistency in the radiologic diagnosis of pneumoconiosis. Am. Rev. Respir. Dis., *102*, 905, 1970.
41. Reger, R. B., Amandus, H. E., and Morgan, W. K. C., On the diagnosis of coal workers' pneumoconiosis: Anglo-American disharmony. Am. Rev. Respir. Dis., *108*, 1186, 1973.
42. Amandus, H. E., Pendergrass, E. P., Dennis, J. N., and Morgan, W. K. C., Pneumoconiosis: inter-reader variability in the classification of the type of small opacities in the chest roentgenograms. Am. J. Roent., *122*, 740, 1974.
43. Jacobson, G., Bohlig, H., and Kiviluoto, R., Essentials of chest radiology. Radiology, *95*, 445, 1970.
44. Washington, J. S., Dick, J. A., Jacobsen, J., and Prentice, W. M., A comparison of conventional and grid techniques for chest radiography in field surveys. Br. J. Ind. Med., *30*, 365, 1973.
45. Reger, R. B., Smith, C. A., Kibelstis, J. A., and Morgan, W. K. C., The effect of film quality and other factors on the roentgenographic categorization of coal workers' pneumoconiosis. Am. J. Roent., *55*, 462, 1972.
46. Liddell, F. D. K., and Morgan, W. K. C., Methods of assessing serial films of the pneumoconioses: a review. J. Soc. Occup. Med., *28*, 6, 1978.
47. Reger, R. B., Butcher, D. F., and Morgan, W. K. C., Assessing change in the pneumoconioses using serial radiographs. Am. J. Epidemiol., *98*, 243, 1973.
48. Reger, R. B., Petersen, M. R., and Morgan, W. K. C., Variation in the interpretation of radiographic change in pulmonary disease. Lancet, *1*, 111, 1974.
49. Amandus, H. E., Reger, R. B., Pendergrass, E. P., et al., The pneumoconioses: methods of measuring progression. Chest, *63*, 736, 1973.
50. Peters, W. L., Reger, R. B., and Morgan, W. K. C., The radiographic categorization of coal workers' pneumoconiosis by lay readers. Environ. Res., *6*, 60, 1973.
51. Weill, H., and Jones, R., The chest roentgenogram as an epidemiologic tool. Arch. Environ. Health, *31*, 435, 1975.

6

PATHOLOGICAL REACTIONS OF THE LUNG TO DUST

A. R. Gibbs, R. M. E. Seal,
and J. C. Wagner

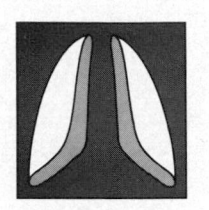

The changes resulting from the inhalation of foreign material should be considered from the viewpoint of the various ways in which the lung may react. It becomes apparent that inhalation of vapors and dusts encountered occupationally may produce almost the full range of possible pulmonary responses other than those due to invasion by multiplying microorganisms and certain systemic diseases.[1] The inhaled material can behave as an acute irritant evoking an acute nonspecific inflammatory reaction, or as a low-grade irritant evoking a low-grade, nonspecific response, or when combined with or containing protein it may become antigenic and elicit a variety of hypersensitivity lung reactions.

Phylogenetically, the mammalian lung has developed efficient defense mechanisms to deal with the majority of inhaled materials; overloading of this mechanism allows retention of particles leading to diverse disease patterns, the effect on the lung being largely dependent on the biological activity of the material encountered.

Host factors clearly form a variable that will modify the consequences of exposure; the intervention of chronic inflammation and ill-understood background states such as the rheumatoid diathesis and the atopic state are examples. Anatomical variations, for example, of lymphatic drainage, may also alter the site of dust retention in different individuals. The response to a dust may be modified by exposure to another. It is not surprising therefore that the clinicopathological entities encountered are varied and complex, particularly since exposure in an industrial society is seldom as pure as that in a designed laboratory experiment.

Anatomically, the response and damage will occur to a varying degree in the large or small conducting airways, the respiratory parenchyma, the

pulmonary vascular bed, the pleura, and the reticuloendothelial system. The varied biological responses to retained inhaled material and the nature of the body's attempts at healing by fibrosis and cellular proliferation lead to a wide range of chronic destructive lung diseases and also in some instances to the development of neoplasms.

DIFFUSE ALVEOLAR DAMAGE

The term diffuse alveolar damage describes the pathological picture encountered when a noxious agent damages the bronchioalveolar lining cells and endothelial cells of the lung. Although a wide variety of agents, e.g., viruses, irradiation, drugs, collagen diseases, and oxygen, may cause this reaction, the pathological appearances are similar.[2] The outcome of the reaction is dependent on the intensity and duration of exposure, and varies from death in the acute phase to resolution or interstitial fibrosis and/or obliterative bronchiolitis. Industrial agents which may cause the reaction include fumes of nitrogen, cadmium, beryllium, nitrogen dioxide, and ammonia.

Macroscopic Appearance

The lungs are heavy, edematous, and hemorrhagic, with varying degrees of induration. Similar changes occur in the larynx, trachea, and bronchi. The more soluble the inhaled substance, the more proximal the area of damage.

Microscopic Appearance

The microscopic features can be divided into early changes (1 to 7 days after exposure) and late changes (more than 7 days after exposure). These changes are often complicated by secondary infection.

Early changes:
  1. Intra-alveolar and interstitial edema
  2. Intra-alveolar hemorrhage
  3. Hyaline membranes (2 to 7 days)
  4. Focal alveolar lining cell hyperplasia (3 to 7 days)
  5. Necrosis of bronchiolar epithelium
  6. Fibrin thrombi within capillaries or small arteries
  7. Interstitial mononuclear infiltrate (after 5 days)

Late changes:
  1. Interstitial and intra-alveolar fibrosis
  2. Proliferation of smooth muscle fibers
  3. Vascular changes—subintimal fibrosis of veins and arteries, muscular hypertrophy of pulmonary arterial walls
  4. Conspicuous alveolar lining cell hyperplasia.

Figure 6–1 illustrates the early changes of diffuse alveolar damage in a patient dying two days after exposure to oxides of nitrogen. Figure 6–2 illustrates a slightly later phase in a patient dying after exposure to cadmium fumes. After survival for 6 to 7 days, alveolar lining cell hyperplasia and metaplasia become conspicuous (Fig. 6–3), although focal changes may be seen after 3 days. Similar histological changes may result from noxious agents arising by inhalation or via the blood stream. The pointer to an intraluminal route is that in the least involved lobules, the inflammatory damage is more intense in the center and in smaller conducting airways.

Some of the late sequelae described may be found on lung biopsy of patients presenting with chronic lung changes without a history of a dramatic illness following acute exposure. Exposure may be minimal over a long period, the lung lesions developing insidiously until the patient presents with the late changes described.

The total clinical picture may not be that of a pure respiratory problem, since many substances have effects on other organs; for example, cadmium has nephrotoxic effects and fluoride has skeletal effects.

Desquamative Interstitial Pneumonia

Desquamative interstitial pneumonia (DIP) is characterized by a uniform filling of alveolar spaces by plump rounded or polygonal, deeply

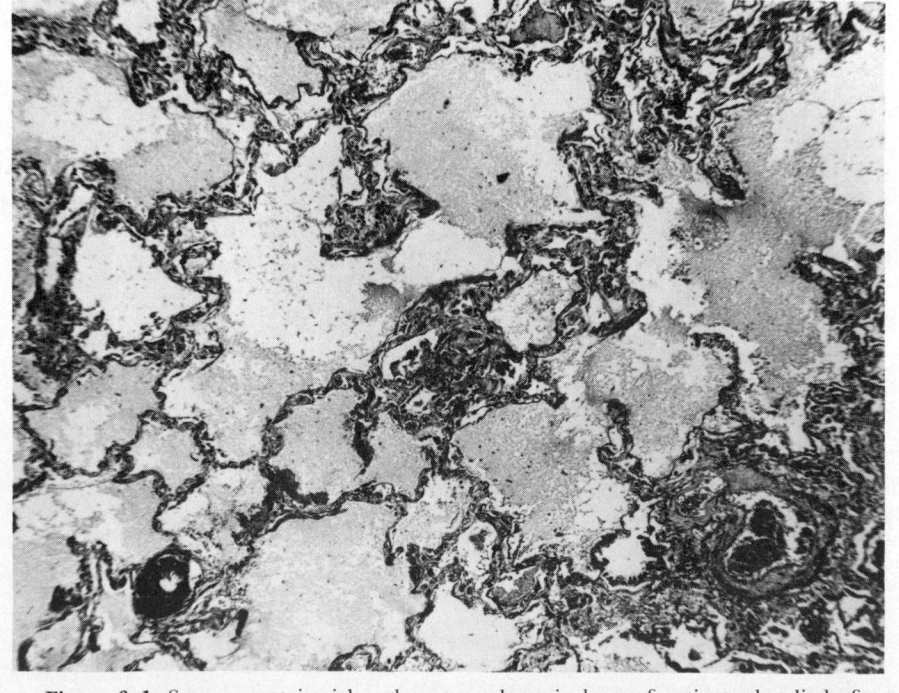

Figure 6–1. Severe, protein-rich pulmonary edema in lung of patient who died after acute exposure to nitrous fumes.

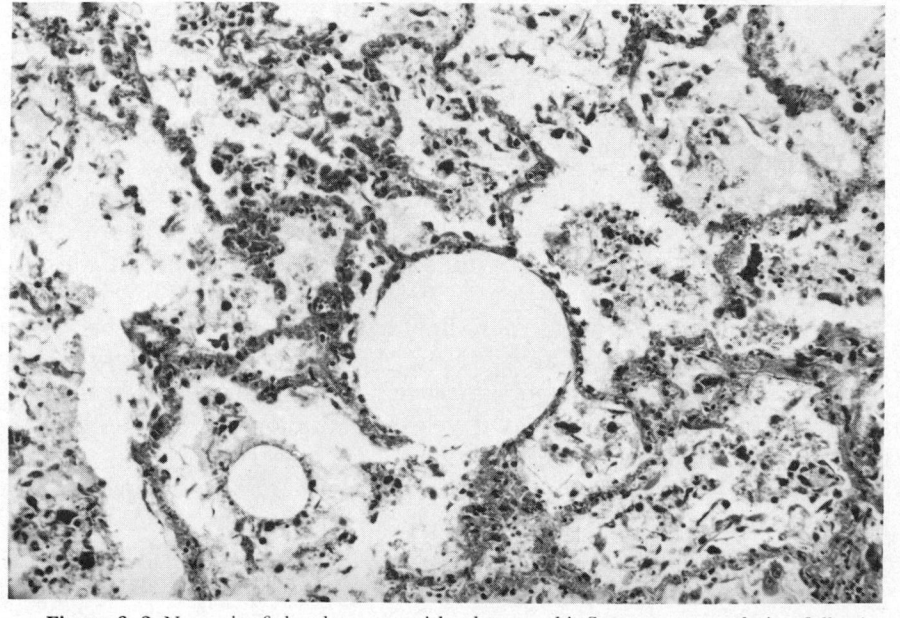

Figure 6–2. Necrosis of alveolar septa with edema and inflammatory exudation following cadmium fume exposure (H and E).

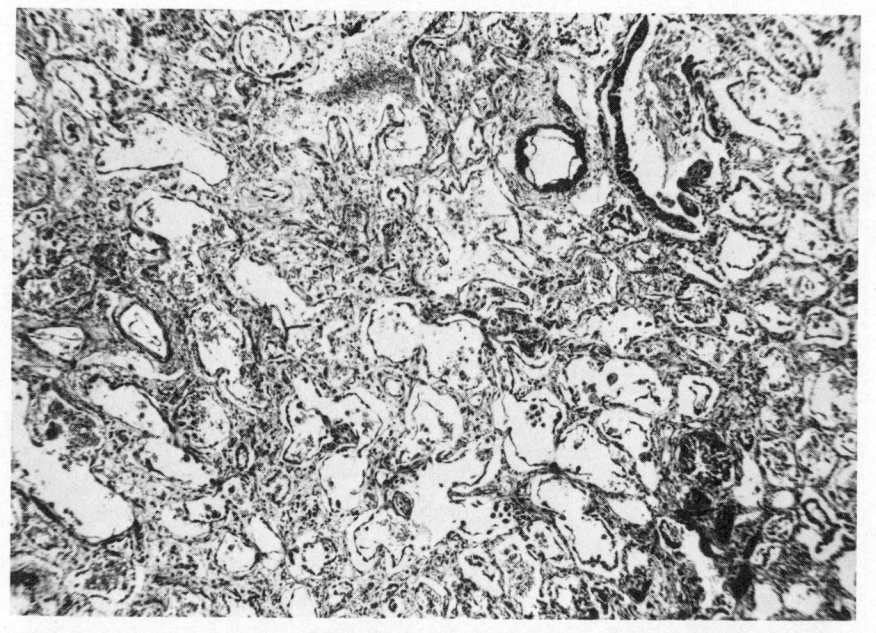

Figure 6–3. Lung of patient who died a week after acute exposure to cadmium fumes, showing detachment of alveolar epithelial cells and a few desquamated cells in alveolar sacs. Interalveolar septa are thickened from edema and cellular infiltration. Hyperplasia of bronchiolar epithelium is seen (top right) (H and E).

eosinophilic mononuclear cells.[3] Although many cases are idiopathic, it is now recognized that an identical morphological picture can be produced by drugs and occupational agents. The latter include asbestos, silica, talc, tungsten carbide, aluminum, and a variety of silicates.[4-6] Whenever this pathological reaction is encountered it is very important to obtain a detailed occupational history and, if possible, to utilize sophisticated methods of analysis, e.g., energy dispersive x-ray analysis with scanning or transmission electron microscopy, in order to establish or eliminate an occupational cause.

In DIP there is little interstitial fibrosis, an absence of hyaline membranes and necrosis, and uniform filling of alveolar spaces by mononuclear cells. These cells are very eosinophilic and may contain cytoplasmic vacuoles and yellow-brown granules that are periodic acid-Schiff (PAS) positive but negative to iron staining. Electron microscopy has demonstrated these cells to be mainly macrophages with a smaller proportion of type II pneumocytes.[5]

Giant Cell Interstitial Pneumonia

Giant cell interstitial pneumonia is a very rare type of interstitial pneumonia characterized by numerous bizarre, large, giant cells within the alveolar spaces superimposed upon either the desquamative form of interstitial pneumonia or chronic interstitial fibrosis. Recently it has been recognized that several of these cases may be due to hard metal (tungsten carbide) exposure.[7]

Pulmonary Alveolar Proteinosis

In pulmonary alveolar proteinosis there is filling of the alveoli by eosinophilic, amorphous exudate that is PAS positive. There is a variable amount of interstitial inflammation and fibrosis. It has been proposed that excessive surfactant and associated lipids are discharged by the type II pneumocytes due to damage from a variety of agents and inadequately removed.[8] Inhalation of large amounts of finely particulate silica may cause this reaction.[9] Other inorganic particles have been implicated in this reaction.[10]

HYPERSENSITIVITY OCCUPATIONAL DISEASE

Although it is probably an oversimplification to regard hypersensitivity reactions as falling into four distinct and separate types, it is nevertheless a useful way of separating the mechanisms for an initial understanding.

Immediate, anaphylactic, Type I hypersensitivity reactions occur when IgE (or IgG_4) molecules on the surface of mast cells (or basophils) bind

with their corresponding antigen. The reaction initiates the release of pharmacologically active substances, e.g., histamine, 5-hydroxytryptamine, bradykinin, and slow-reacting substance of anaphylaxis from these cells. The resulting tissue response is seen within minutes of introduction of the antigen—in the skin, by the production of a wheal; in the lung, by bronchoconstriction. Eosinophilia is often associated with Type I reactions to fungi and other parasites, but this may represent a link with other hypersensitivity states to the infection. Certain individuals appear to be genetically predisposed to Type I reactions; these are the so-called atopic people, who tend to have higher levels of specific IgE.

Type II response is a cytotoxic or cytolytic tissue–damaging reaction mediated by antibody directed against components of cell surfaces. Damage is caused by interference with membrane function due to antibody combination. When complement-fixing antibodies are present cell lysis can occur, e.g., transfusion mismatch. Sometimes certain drugs complex with protein on cell surfaces, with stimulation of antibody production giving rise to purpura. This type of hypersensitivity reaction is not usually thought to be concerned in pulmonary hypersensitivity disease, yet features consistent with Type II reactions may be seen.

Arthus or Type III hypersensitivity occurs when precipitating antibody (usually IgG) combines with antigen. Complement is fixed and polymorphonuclear leukocytes are attracted. The microprecipitate-complement complex is phagocytosed and enzymatically digested. It is considered, however, that the incomplete fusion of the exterior cell membrane around the precipitate during phagocytosis allows enzymes to "leak" out, and it is the action of these enzymes that causes the tissue damage seen in Type III reactions. When the immune precipitate is "nonphagocytosable," polymorphonuclear leukocytes secrete their lysozymal granules onto the precipitate, and adjacent tissue damage is subsequently greater. Recent work has shown macrophages to be capable of releasing hydrolases after ingestion of immune precipitate. The response is seen largely around smaller blood vessels and polymorphonuclear leukocytes are abundant. In classical Type III reactions, hemorrhage, thrombus formation, and necrosis occur, being maximal at 6 hours. Later, mononuclear cells are seen, but are not considered to be part of the typical Type III response. While Arthus-type hypersensitivity classically involves immune precipitates, complement, and polymorphonuclear leukocytes, there are substances capable of acting on complement independent of antibody. Thus, activation of the alternative pathway of complement may lead to an Arthus reaction, as has been shown in tick bite injury. Many dusts including moldy hay dust can activate the alternative pathway.[11]

Delayed, tuberculin, Type IV hypersensitivity is mediated by sensitized lymphocytes interacting with appropriate antigen, resulting in the release of biologically active materials. These so-called lymphokines include transfer factor, cytotoxic factor, macrophage inhibitory factor (MIF), and interferon.

The tissue damage due to a Type IV response is maximal at 48 to 72 hours, with edema, necrosis, mononuclear infiltration of the tissues, and formation of epithelioid tubercles considered to be derived from blood monocytes held in situ by MIF from sensitized lymphocytes.

However, even in a designed Type IV reaction using BCG-sensitized experimental animals and introducing tuberculoprotein into the tissues, a mild Arthus component with neutrophil exudation can be seen contributing to the total histological picture.

While this thumbnail sketch is an oversimplification, it suffices as a background to examine the pulmonary pathology of several occupational diseases operating largely through hypersensitivity mechanisms. The response to organic dusts is determined by a number of factors including dose of inhaled material, particle size, physiochemical properties, biological properties, prior exposure, and genetic predisposition.

Asthma

Asthma occurring as an occupational disease results from inhaled substances combining with protein and becoming antigenic. A wide variety of such substances, including complex salts of platinum and toluene diisocyanate, may cause industrial asthma.

The contribution of the histopathologist to the understanding of asthma is to remind clinicians that asthma is not a disease characterized by bronchospasm alone and that an intraluminal obstructive exudate is certainly not confined to a small group of severe cases in status asthmaticus. The inflammatory exudate is a universal component, and if the sputum is fixed in alcohol and processed as a paraffin section, a characteristic appearance will be found in the majority of asthmatics. The diagnostic features are, in the acute stage, a proteinaceous and mucus-containing matrix in which clumps of respiratory epithelial cells (sometimes in spherical masses called "Creola bodies") and linear accumulations of eosinophils are seen. At a later stage, a characteristic exudate containing linear necrotic eosinophils, eosinophilic spirals, and Charcot-Leyden crystals may be observed. It is presumably in the prevention of this intraluminal obstructing infiltrate that steroid therapy is mainly effective. In the wall of the bronchus there is thickening of the basement membrane, eosinophilic infiltration, hyperplasia of smooth muscle, presumably reflecting repeated stimulation, and also, as in nonallergic chronic bronchitis, hyperplasia of the mucus-secreting apparatus. That asthma is regarded as a hypersensitivity reaction is justified by the presence of the eosinophil as the inflammatory cell, the immediate wheal produced in the skin when the appropriate antigen is used, and the rapid development of airways obstruction on inhalation of appropriate extracts.

Nevertheless, a Type III reaction or predominantly pharmacological events may operate in these individuals with prolonged asthma or who

develop late bronchoconstriction (4 to 10 hours) after inhalation provocation tests.[12] Industrial agents may result in immediate, delayed, or mixed types of asthma; specific antibodies have been demonstrated in a few instances.

Extrinsic Allergic Alveolitis

The concept inherent in the generic term applied to this group of diseases is that they all have in common the inhalation of antigenic material, resulting in an allergic inflammation affecting the alveolar wall. While this concept is in large part true, the condition is best understood if this concept is examined further. The pathological change is certainly not confined to an infiltration of the interalveolar septa, as there is also a bronchiolitis and the inflammatory damage is more severe in the center of the lung lobule than at its periphery; an additional and prominent feature in the acute stage is the presence of "sarcoid-like" noncaseating epithelioid granulomata. An early account of farmer's lung was more accurate in describing the histopathological feature as "an acute granulomatous interstitial pneumonitis."[13] The pulmonary arterioles are also involved in the acute stage. Extrinsic allergic bronchiolar alveolitis would now be a preferable term.

The tissue response in most members of this group includes the presence of foreign body–type giant cells, and a "nonallergic" foreign body reactive component may well contribute materially to the total lung damage.

Extrinsic allergic alveolitis in the acute stage differs from pulmonary sarcoidosis in that the granulomata are accompanied by the additional inflammatory features and by the centrilobular accentuation of the pathological change, suggesting an explanation of why the patient with allergic alveolitis may be dyspneic with minimal radiographic mottling, while the sarcoid patient is minimally disabled despite extensive radiographic changes.

Evidence that these diseases are of an allergic nature, mainly of Type III (Arthus) but possibly with contributions from Type II and Type IV hypersensitivity, is derived from inhalational challenges in susceptible individuals, serology (precipitins), and animal models. The clinician must nevertheless accept that the condition occasionally has to be diagnosed in spite of failure to demonstrate the appropriate antigen, and must remember that heavy exposure to foreign material such as moldy hay may induce a high titer of antibody in the absence of any tissue lesion.

Extrinsic allergic alveolitis creates problems as, on the one hand, complete resolution may occur with or without steroid administration in patients with extensive interstitial infiltration and with numerous granulomata, and, on the other, the inflammatory process may be more insidious, with interstitial fibrosis and architectural derangement found on the initial lung biopsy, after an apparently short clinical history.

Occasionally, after a single severe acute episode, the disease will be seen to progress to fine interstitial fibrosis and finally to extensive contractural fibrosis with honeycomb change more marked in the upper lobes, though the chronic stage of the disease is usually reached only after repeated acute episodes or after prolonged insidious exposures. In the chronic stage granulomata are absent, though a variable degree of interstitial mononuclear infiltration is present, suggesting the possibility of a continuing antigenic presence. The reasons for a continuous smoldering activity leading to chronic disease are not fully understood. It is possible that this is explained by differences in ability to handle inhaled particles and to process antigen and immune complexes. Thus a slowly continuing hypersensitivity inflammation may persist and this may be of Types II, III, or IV.

The pattern of fibrosis in chronic extrinsic alveolitis is variable, with a fine, interstitial process (mural fibrosis of interalveolar septa) and a more coarse pattern of intercommunicating bands of peribronchial and bronchiolar fibrosis. The enlargement of related air spaces also is variable, ranging from coarse cystic honeycombed areas to distorted, thin-walled emphysematous alveolar sacs around small focal areas of fibrosis. Some patients after an acute attack proceed to a prominent emphysematous appearance with a fine fibrosis that could well be overlooked on cursory examination. Such patients have an obstructive profile on lung function testing; many are nonsmokers. In the chronic stage of farmer's lung some patients have an increase in goblet cells. Goblet cell hyperplasia is certainly not confined to cigarette smokers, and exposure of experimental animals to *Micropolyspora faeni* is associated with goblet cell hyperplasia as a later feature in the pathological course.

There is still much to be learned about the mechanisms of progression to the permanent fibrosis and associated parenchymal changes of the chronic stage of extrinsic alveolitis.

Other Occupational Granulomatous Interstitial Diseases

Beryllium exposure causing diffuse alveolar damage has already been discussed. Beryllium exposure more frequently causes chronic interstitial fibrosis with many "sarcoid-like" granulomata. That this disease evokes a delayed (Type IV) response is suggested by the 48- to 72-hour period before the beryllium patch test lesions appear, and the prominence of "tubercles" in the pathological picture. It has also been shown that *in vitro* lymphocyte transformation by beryllium is positive in chronic beryllium disease.[14] However, it is not yet known whether the beryllium acts directly on stimulated lymphocytes or whether it is combined with tissue or serum proteins before eliciting a Type IV response. Occasional cases of spread of the disease along lymphatic pathways after cutaneous implantations and of possible systemic spread have been reported. However, in such

cases it is difficult to exclude the possibility of inhalational exposure, as apparently only minute amounts of beryllium are necessary to initiate disease.

In practice, the differential diagnosis of chronic beryllium lung from sarcoid is difficult, though extensive interstitial fibrosis with lymphocytic infiltration favors the former. In many cases the pathologist and clinician must depend on the results of microanalysis by sophisticated means available only in a few laboratories throughout the world. In the authors' experience such analyses have yielded negative results in the lesions of patients with known industrial exposure.

PULMONARY RESPONSES TO INHALED INORGANIC DUST

The reactions of the lungs to inorganic dust is dependent upon the nature, dosage, and duration of exposure of the dust inhaled. The reaction may be modified by the presence of another dust, immunological factors, and the coexistence of other pulmonary diseases. The dusts to be considered are those particles which have dimensions of suitable size to penetrate to and be retained in the respiratory portions of the lungs, that is, beyond the terminal bronchioles. The size of round or irregular particles to meet these requirements would be less than 10 microns in diameter and of fibrous particles less than 3 microns in diameter, a fibrous particle being defined as one having a greater than 3:1 length-diameter ratio. All dusts smaller than these dimensions may penetrate to the respiratory airways, but the lower limit of retention is more difficult to define; dust particles of standard density less than 1 micron in diameter have an extremely low settling speed, and the smaller the particle the less likely it is to be deposited on the walls of the airways.

The majority of the dust particles that have penetrated below the level of the ciliated epithelium are taken up by macrophages, which migrate up to the terminal bronchioles, and are then removed via the mucociliary apparatus. If the amounts of dust encountered are too great, this mechanism becomes overloaded, and a small proportion of the dust will enter the type I pneumocytes and interstitium.[15] Some of this will be cleared via the lymphatics which have been shown to be present in respiratory bronchioles in proximity to the alveoli.[16] It should be remembered that cigarette smoke and other pollutants will modify the clearance of inhaled particles. If the dust inhaled is nontoxic (e.g., tin, iron, and pure carbon), the only reaction is accumulation of dust within macrophages in those alveoli arising from the respiratory bronchioles. Eventually, a few fibroblasts are attached to the site and the macrophages are held in situ by a thin net of reticulin fibers. This is of particular interest in the case of tin smelters, where the presence of the radiopaque dust gives the impression of severe disease, in contrast to the relatively normal lung parenchyma containing centrilobular collections of dust-laden mac-

rophages without any emphysema or fibrosis. This is certainly the picture seen in post-mortem material in young adult smelters dying of other conditions.

Fiber Exposure and Parenchymal Disease

Interest has mainly focused on the asbestos groups of fibrous hydrated silicates, but recently knowledge has accrued on asbestos substitutes such as man-made mineral fibers, noncommercial forms of asbestos, fibrous zeolites (erionites), and fibrous clays. Clinical and experimental studies have indicated that fiber dimensions are of great importance in determining whether a particular fiber produces or does not produce pulmonary disease. For instance, tremolite, an amphibole mineral, occurs in several physical forms: flake-like, fine, and coarse fibered. Clinical and experimental studies have shown that the flake-like form is unassociated with pulmonary disease, the coarse fibered form is associated with pleural plaques and not mesothelioma, and the fine fibered form is associated with the development of mesothelioma.[17]

Fiber diameter determines penetration to peripheral airways. Fibers possessing diameters below 3 microns deposit in peripheral airways, whereas fibers with diameters greater than 3 microns in diameter are intercepted in airways higher up. Fiber diameter is also important in determining neoplastic potential; the ability to cause mesothelioma requires a fiber diameter of less than 0.5 micron.[18]

Fibrogenic activity and neoplastic potential are also dependent on fiber length; fibers greater than 8 microns in length appear to be the important ones.[19–22] The majority of fibers deposit in the alveolus and at the alveolar ducts nearest to the respiratory bronchioles and may be taken up by macrophages and type I pneumocytes soon after exposure.[23] Experimental work has demonstrated that short fibers (less than 5 microns) are cleared more efficiently than larger fibers via the conducting airways.[24] Long fibers have a greater propensity for bridging the alveolar ducts and alveoli and penetrating the type I pneumocytes. They may then be transported to the interstitium, lymphatics, or capillary endothelial cells. Some are carried to the regional lymph nodes. Fibers which are not cleared (greater than 8 microns in length), macrophages, and cell debris become enmeshed in a fibronectin/reticulin network which coarsens with time and becomes replaced by collagen fibers.[25] The adjacent alveolar epithelium undergoes metaplasia from type I to type II pneumocytes. In some alveoli, epithelium is shed into the lumen but in others there is walling off of the alveoli by these cells. This occurs usually at the bifurcation where groups of alveoli are closed off from the lumina of the respiratory bronchioles, giving the so-called pseudo-acinar appearance. Initially, lesions are confined to occasional discrete respiratory bronchioles scattered throughout the pulmonary parenchyma. After further exposure greater numbers of respi-

ratory bronchioles become involved; all respiratory bronchioles arising from individual terminal bronchioles become thickened as the fibrous tissue network extends into the wall of the respiratory bronchiole. This interstitial process extends centrifugally to involve all acinar structures. With progression, individual lesions tend to coalesce, resulting in the development of a diffuse interstitial fibrosis. The density of the fibrous tissue may gradually increase, ultimately resulting in the replacement of the pulmonary parenchyma by a dense collagenous network surrounding distal air spaces. In cases due to asbestos exposure, large clumps of asbestos bodies and fibers may be observed.

In asbestosis the lesions commence subpleurally at the base of the lower lobes and gradually extend upward as the disease progresses. Once sufficient asbestos dust has been retained, the lesions will progress even if no further exposure occurs. In a minority of cases the air spaces become completely sclerosed and massive fibrotic areas are observed.

The observance of ferruginous bodies within the lung is utilized by pathologists as a marker of asbestos exposure, although ferruginous bodies can be formed on other fibers such as of talc and glass. However, using routine autopsy studies Pooley[26] and later Churg and Warnock[27] have shown that 98 per cent of ferruginous bodies have an asbestos core. All types of asbestos fibers may become coated with complexes of hemosiderin and glycoproteins to form bodies, but long fibers have a greater propensity to do so than short fibers.[26] Therefore, counts of coated fibers by light microscopy more accurately reflect amphibole load than chrysotile. A further factor impairing pathological interpretation of fiber loads is that chrysotile fibers are removed from the lung parenchyma more quickly by dissolution and preferential lymphatic clearance.

In cases of severe asbestosis, fiber counts reasonably accurately reflect pulmonary disease. In patients who have had severe respiratory disability, the lungs show severe interstitial fibrosis both macroscopically and microscopically, many ferruginous bodies are seen in sections, and the fiber count exceeds 10^6 per gram of lung tissue. However, with less severe degrees of asbestosis, correlation of fiber counts with pulmonary fibrosis is more problematic. This is of particular importance whenever a patient dies with a pulmonary carcinoma, since if death can be shown to be consequent to asbestosis, industrial compensation may be paid, whereas lung carcinoma in the absence of asbestosis is usually not compensatable. There are two major problems: (1) quantifying the amount of pulmonary fibrosis, and (2) attributing the pulmonary fibrosis to asbestos exposure. Several schemes for grading pulmonary fibrosis in asbestosis have been proposed but none is wholly satisfactory because there are difficulties in allowing for both macroscopic and microscopic degrees of fibrosis. The following is a reproducible and useful method for assessing the degree of fibrosis in these cases. Careful macroscopic examination of the cut surface of a well-inflated lung is performed, perhaps with barium sulfate impregnation, and the area of interstitial fibrosis expressed as a percentage of

the total lung surface. Representative sections are then taken and examined microscopically and graded as follows:[28]

Grade 0—None

Grade 1—Slight focal fibrosis around respiratory bronchioles.

Grade 2—Lesions confined to respiratory bronchioles of scattered acini, but fibrosis extends into alveolar ducts, atria, and the walls of adjacent air spaces.

Grade 3—Further increase and condensation of the peribronchiolar fibrosis, with early widespread interstitial fibrosis.

Grade 4—Widespread diffuse fibrosis with few recognizable alveoli; honeycombing may or may not be present.

In attributing the fibrosis to asbestos exposure, quantification of asbestos fibers, although problematic, is very useful. There are a number of technical difficulties in obtaining accurate counts of fibers and bodies within lung tissue. These include (1) loss of fibers by adherence to glass surfaces of the apparatus used, (2) maceration, which may damage and cause the break-up of fibers, leading to artificially high counts, and (3) variations in counts from one area of a lung to another. These problems can be overcome to a large extent by carefully following a standardized procedure, but it makes the comparison of results from one laboratory to another extremely difficult. It is better to become familiar with the range of results from a particular laboratory. In our laboratory, utilizing the method of Ashcroft and Heppleston,[29] we usually obtain fiber counts of approximately 60,000/gm of lung tissue in mesothelioma cases and counts between 20,000 and 50,000/gm of lung tissue in cases with pleural plaques. Electron microscopical counts are perhaps even more useful, since the exact fiber types can be identified and quantified and fibers not resolved by the light microscope may be revealed. Electron microscopical counts are between 10^2 and 10^4 higher than light microscopical counts. Table 6–1 shows some examples of light and electron microscopical counts. By utilizing a combination of macroscopical and microscopical evaluation of lung specimens together with fiber counts, we subdivide asbestosis into minimal, slight, moderate, and severe degrees (Table 6–2).[28]

Fibrous dusts have an unexplained tendency to drift toward the pleura. If this drift is contained by the elastic lamina of the visceral pleura, it leads to extensive pleural fibrosis, the whole lung becoming encased in a dense layer of fibrous tissue up to 1.0 cm in thickness. In other cases, the fibers escape through the visceral pleura, penetrate the parietal layer, and are obstructed by the dense subpleural fibrous tissue. This most commonly occurs in the lower region of the thorax. The fibers elicit a widespread fibroblast response and become surrounded by dense collagen with a regular woven appearance. The centers of these lesions undergo ischemic necrosis with gradual deposition of calcium phosphate, leading after many years to the typical large calcified pleural plaques.[30] They are most common on the dome of the diaphragm and are seen bilaterally on

Table 6–1. COMPARATIVE LIGHT AND ELECTRON MICROSCOPICAL COUNTS OF FIBERS (BODIES) IN LUNG PARENCHYMA IN PATIENTS EXPOSED TO ASBESTOS*

Case	L.M. Count† Bodies	Fibers	Total E.M. Count	Ratio of E.M. to L.M.	Chrysotile (%)	Crocidolite (%)	Amosite (%)	Tremolite (%)	Mullite (%)
1	45,360	10,640	4,800,000	85:1	8.8	—	10.8	—	76
2	300	2,700	23,480,000	7820:1	12.2	9.6	1.3	0.6	76.2
3	1,045,000	9,955,000	157,500,000	14:1	4.6	65.4	30	—	—
4	1,608,500	5,431,500	238,600,000	21:1	5.4	4.5	90.1	—	—
5	90,432	663,258	95,200,000	126:1	2.4	80.6	9.7	—	—

*L.M. = light microscopy; E.M. = electron microscopy.
†Data from Ashcroft and Heppleston.[29]

Table 6–2. GENERAL GUIDELINES FOR THE DIAGNOSIS AND GRADING OF ASBESTOSIS

Asbestosis Grade	Macroscopic Appearance	L. M. Appearance*	Usual L.M. Count of Fibers†	Clinical and Radiological Features
Minimal	No fibrosis visible.	Grade 1 lesions. Prolonged search reveals an occasional asbestos body.	> 50,000	None
Slight	Careful inspection of inflated lung reveals fine interstitial fibrosis occupying less than 25% of the total area.	Grade 1 to 3 lesions. An occasional asbestos body is seen.	> 100,000	None
Moderate	A combination of induration with fine to moderate fibrosis involving 25–50% of the total lung area.	Grade 2 to 4 lesions. Moderate numbers of asbestos bodies are seen.	> 250,000	Mild clinical symptoms and slight radiological changes.
Severe	Interstitial fibrosis involving more than 50% of the lung with or without honeycombing.	Grade 3 to 4 lesions. Numberous bodies usually observed.	> 1,000,000	Severely dyspnoeic. Interstitial changes observed radiologically.

*L.M. = light microscopy.
†Per gram of dried lung tissue.

the lower chest wall, frequently following the line of the ribs. Pleural plaques are usually associated with parenchymal fiber counts of 20,000 to 50,000/gm of dried lung tissue counted by phase microscopy and consisting mainly of lung amphibole fibers seen by electron microscopy.[31] This is surprising, since it has been shown by Sebastien et al.[32] that when the pleura itself is examined short chrysotile fibers greatly outnumber long amphibole fibers. These workers also found no correlation between the pleural fiber content and the parenchymal fiber content.

Silica Exposure

The interstitial reticuloendothelial reaction to quartz dust is seen when the quartz dust particles are in the 2 to 5 micron range. Initially, when deposited in the lung parenchyma these quartz particles are ingested by the macrophages and held in phagosomes. As demonstrated by Harrington and Allison,[33] the quartz has the ability to attract numerous lysosomes from the cytoplasm of the macrophage into the phagosome and disrupt them. The quartz crystals then become attached to the lipoprotein membrane surrounding the phagosome and separate the segments to which they adhere. This allows the contents of the phagosome, which now contains numerous active enzymes, to escape into the cytoplasm and destroy the organelles. This kills the cells, releasing the enzyme-rich fluid and the quartz crystals into the alveoli. Either the quartz crystals are then taken up by additional macrophages and the process is repeated or, if no more macrophages are available (or if there are insufficient macrophages to deal with the number of quartz crystals present), the crystals are taken up by the type II alveolar epithelial cells (granular pneumocytes). This causes these cells to discharge the lamellar bodies and the associated lipids into the air spaces, leading to a localized alveolar lipoproteinosis. If numerous type II cells are destroyed as a consequence of very high silica exposure, a subsequent generalized alveolar proteinosis will develop.

Most of the fluid containing the active enzymes, lipids, and silica crystals is taken up by the lymphatics which start at the junction of the alveolar ducts and the atria; there are usually four lymphatic channels accompanying the arterioles at the level of the respiratory bronchioles. At irregular intervals along these lymphatics are small clumps of reticuloendothelial cells consisting of lymphocytes, macrophages, and reticulin cells with occasional fibroblasts. The arrival of the debris from the origins at these sites elicits a marked reaction, the silica crystals being engulfed by the connective tissue histiocytes, which are destroyed in a similar manner to the alveolar macrophages. The lipid and enzymes initiate a proliferative response by the reticulum cells, and more fibroblasts and macrophages are attracted to the area. As a result of this, the arteriole at this point is surrounded by a mass of tissue consisting of proliferating mononuclear cells, dead and dying macrophages, and fibroblasts producing reticulin

and collagen fibers in which all the cells are becoming enmeshed. Meanwhile, some quartz crystals and the other materials have continued up the lymphatics toward the hilum of the lung, causing similar lesions in subsequent aggregations of reticuloendothelial cells and, finally, nodules in the sinuses of the lymph glands. Others track along the lymphatics leading to the visceral pleura, resulting eventually in the development of fibrotic nodules in the subpleural lymph nodes. While this process spreads through the interstitium of the lung, the perivascular reaction around the arteriole supplying the respiratory bronchiole is progressing with an overwhelming production of concentric collagen fibers that have destroyed the perivascular lymphatics and are steadily reducing the lumen of the arteriole. If this process is gradual, the lumen will become completely constricted and all that will remain will be the elastic tissue in a mass of concentric collagen fibers. However, if the process is accelerated, ischemic necrosis will intervene and the center of the nodule will consist of a focus of gray necrotic tissue. Previously these foci were thought to be due to tuberculous infection and these nodules were known as tuberculosilicotic islets. This is not correct, the appearance being due to ischemic necrosis. As the collagen proliferation increases, the cellular elements are prevented from reaching the center of the nodule and tend to collect on the periphery, taking the quartz crystals with them. Thus in a fully developed silicotic nodule no quartz crystals can be seen in the center but are actively destroying the macrophages around the edge of the nodule.

In certain situations, the amount of crystalline quartz deposited in the lung parenchyma can be so great that the periarteriolar lymphatics are completely blocked and the quartz is taken along the perivenous lymphatics in the interlobular septa leading to a perilobular interstitial fibrosis; in addition to this, numerous type II alveolar epithelial cells are destroyed, resulting in a generalized alveolar lipoproteinosis. These are the features of acute silicosis.

Following moderate but prolonged exposure to quartz dust, the silicotic islets continue to proliferate in both the lung parenchyma and the lymph glands. The involvement of the lymph glands extends beyond the hilum of the lungs, and silicotic nodules may be found in the cervical glands and along the aortic chain down to the inguinal glands.

In the lungs the silicotic islets initially are discrete and most common at the apices of the upper and lower lobes. These islets are about 0.5 mm in diameter but can increase up to more than 50 mm, many of the larger examples having necrotic centers. As the disease progresses (and the fibrosis associated with quartz, like that with asbestos, continues after exposure to the dust has ceased), individual lesions coalesce leading to conglomerate lesions, which in turn may become massive and occupy large areas of the lung. Ischemic necrosis can intervene, causing large ragged cavities without the presence of tubercle bacilli. However, infection with mycobacteria in association with the response to quartz is still a major complication.

Coal Dust Exposure

In coal workers' pneumoconiosis, the miners are exposed to a dust that is a mixture of coal, kaolin, mica, and silica. Particles less than 10 microns in diameter may enter beyond the terminal bronchioles. The amount deposited is determined by the concentration and physiocochemical nature of the dust, and host factors such as breathing pattern of the individual. At first there is an increase in the number of macrophages which phagocytose the particles and carry them up again to the mucociliary escalator which commences in the terminal bronchioles; most of the dust is cleared in this way. If there is an excessive amount of coal dust present or if the mucociliary appartus is interfered with, e.g., by cigarette smoke, this route for clearance is overwhelmed, and phagocytes begin to accumulate in the alveoli which arise directly from the respiratory bronchioles. These phagocytes may be held up for an excessive time. This is a signal for fibroblasts to be sent to the alveolus, where they begin to secrete a thin network of fibronectin along which reticulin fibers are developed. This then entraps macrophages, some of these lyse and more fibroblasts arrive to produce more reticulin fibers. This constitutes the usual central dust focus which is almost noncollagenous. If the dust contains a small amount of crystalline silica (quartz), the macrophages may be killed more rapidly and collagen fibers coarsen the network. In this manner the alveoli that arise directly from the respiratory bronchioles are gradually plastered up with a mesh containing coal dust, dying macrophages, and fibroblasts. If the quartz content of the dust is ten per cent or more, the pathogenesis is closer to that seen in silicosis. The macrophages are rapidly destroyed by the quartz particles, and their cytoplasmic and dust contents are taken up in clumps by the lymphatics, which drain from a sump at the level of the atria. These lymphatics, in groups of four, accompany the blood vessels to the hila of the lungs. At intervals, the small lymphatics enter aggregations of reticuloendothelial cells or, later, lymph nodes. The first of the collections of cells seems to be around the arteriole at the level of the second order of respiratory bronchioles, in the center of the primary lobule. The arrival of the cell debris and dust at this point elicits a fibroblastic response and the arteriole is rapidly surrounded by a network of reticulin fibers enmeshing fibroblasts, disintegrating macrophages, reticuloendothelial cells, and a large amount of dust. Gradually, the cellular component decreases and the fibers become more prominent, with collagen taking over from reticulin. This fibrous tissue mass surrounds the arteriole, gradually encroaching on its lumen until eventually the vessel is "strangled," leaving behind its elastic tissue outline and a center of ischemic necrosis. Such collagenous lesions are palpable and may be gray in color and circumscribed when mainly silicotic, but blacker, still palpable, and often stellate when coal dust predominates—the lesion in anthracosilicosis.

The lesions of simple coal workers' pneumoconiosis can be categorized

into three distinct types: central, numerous, widely distributed peribronchiolar irregular nonpalpable lesions that form the background in simple pneumoconiosis—primary coal dust foci *(a)*, and larger, less numerous, nodular lesions that are termed secondary dust foci and are divided into *(b)* stellate and *(c)* circumscribed according to configuration. When examining a lung in coal workers' pneumoconiosis we assess the primary lesions on a 0 to 3 scale both for size (0, 0/1, 1, 1/2, etc.) and profusion (1 = up to 33 per cent, 2 = 33 to 66 per cent, and 3 = more than 66 per cent). Secondary dust foci are measured with a graticule and the lesion recorded in the ranges of less than 5 mm, between 5 and 10 mm, and over 20 mm. Other features such as emphysema, interstitial fibrosis, dust impregnated septa, and pleural thickening can be scored in a similar fashion.

We believe that the secondary dust foci are produced by some additional factors such as tubercle bacilli, the rheumatoid diathesis, or increased quartz in the respired dust, when, as previously described, this occurs *in situ.* Depending upon factors that are not understood these nodules may remain small and discrete or enlarge and conglomerate with neighboring nodules, and these conglomerates can eventually aggregate with other nodules and produce massive fibrosis. In all these changes, there is always a perivascular element, and ischemic necrosis may occur either in small foci or in large areas. Four factors have been implicated in the production of massive fibrosis: (1) total lung dust, (2) composition (quartz), (3) tubercle bacilli, and (4) immunological status.

Radiological and pathological studies have shown that progressive massive fibrosis (PMF) usually occurs on a background of high categories of simple pneumoconiosis. However, exceptions occur. Mineralogic analysis of the dust from miners' lungs has shown that the mean levels of total lung dust tend to be greater in those with PMF than in those with simple pneumoconiosis.[34] Nevertheless, there is considerable overlap between the two categories. In addition, the total lung dust within the PMF group varies with coal rank, being greater in the highest rank group. Davis et al.[34] found no significant differences in the percentage of coal or mineral composition of lung dust between differing levels of pathology in the high-rank coal mines. However, in low-rank groups, the percentage of coal was smaller and non-coal mineral (quartz, kaolin, mica) greater in lungs with massive fibrosis compared to simple pneumoconiosis. Thus there appears to be considerable variation in quantity and composition of lung dust in lungs with similar pneumoconiotic lesions. Davis et al.[34] have suggested that the composition of dust within a lung may alter during the progress of the disease.

Mycobacterium tuberculosis has also been implicated in the development of secondary lesions and progression to massive fibrosis. Several studies have reported finding tubercle bacilli, by direct microscopic examination or bacteriological culture, in the massive fibrotic lesions of coal miners.[35–37] Experimental studies have demonstrated that the tubercle bacilli result in dust fibrosis indistinguishable from PMF.[38] Treatment of miners with early

massive fibrosis with antituberculous drugs has failed, however, to arrest the progression of the lesions.[38] In coal miners with massive fibrosis we have been impressed by the consistent finding of enlarged hilar lymph nodes which show breach of their capsule by coal dust and macrophages which extend through the wall and into the lumen of the adjacent branch of the pulmonary artery or appropriate bronchus (Fig. 6–4). Even in the occasional case of massive fibrosis with minimal background lesions we have found the supplying bronchus or branch of the pulmonary artery invaded by coal dust and macrophages from the adjacent enlarged hilar node. It is tempting to surmise that an event such as a primary tuberculous infection may have resulted in the breach of the lymph node by the coal dust and macrophages and set up a local immune response which led to the production of massive fibrosis. The initial evidence of previous tuberculous infection may then have disappeared. Other immunological factors such as the rheumatoid diathesis have also been implicated in its causation.

As far as the nonmineral content of these massive lesions, Wagner et al.[40] examined a small number of cases, studying biochemical, pathological, ultrastructural, and immunological features of the same material. The preliminary results suggest that collagen is present in the capsule of these lesions but that at the center it is replaced by another insoluble protein (or proteins), which is probably stabilized by some form of cross linking. This protein complex accounts for about one third, consisting of approximately equal amounts of mineral dusts and calcium phosphate. Serum proteins were also observed, but their association with the lesions has yet to be determined. Recently, it has been confirmed that these lesions contain a large amount of fibronectin.[25]

On occasion coal miners may evince irregular opacities radiologically; this is caused by a combination of emphysema and interstitial fibrosis.[41] This interstitial fibrosis may be pigmented or unpigmented. The cause of this interstitial fibrosis is unknown.

All the forms of progression may well depend upon immunological factors. This could occur with *Mycobacterium tuberculosis* acting as an adjuvant or in the rheumatoid diathesis. In the remaining subjects there may be subtler changes which can be detected only by the immunological monitoring of populations at risk.

Emphysema and Coal Workers' Pneumoconiosis

The three forms of emphysema considered in relation to coal dust exposure are "focal emphysema," centrilobular emphysema, and irregular emphysema. This terminology of the original CIBA classification of emphysema is followed, though recently alternatives have been used by some workers in the field.[42] For example, Heppleston[43] dropped the use of his own term focal emphysema and used proximal acinar emphysema attributable to dust as distinct from proximal acinar emphysema attribut-

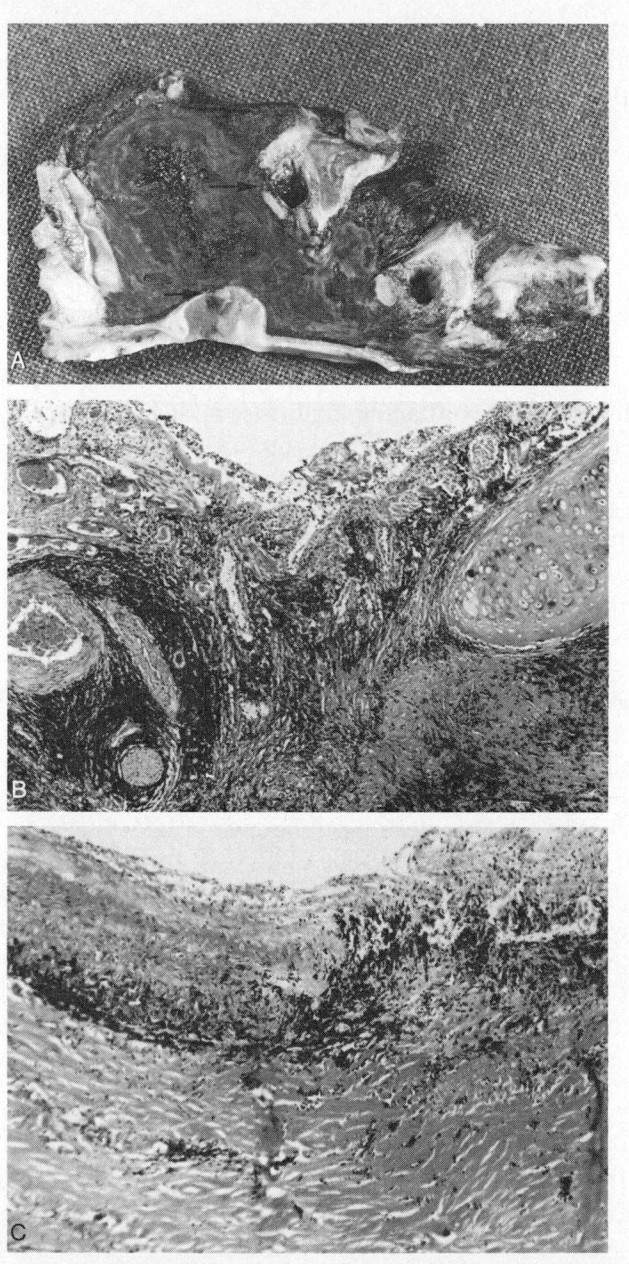

Figure 6–4. A, Photograph of hilum from a patient with massive fibrosis, showing hilar lymph node impregnated with coal dust which extends beyond the capsule into the related bronchial wall and lumen (upper arrow) and pulmonary artery (lower arrow). B, Section from capsule of lymph node and related bronchus in same patient showing spread of dust-laden macrophages through the bronchial wall into its lumen (original × 54). C, Section from branch of pulmonary artery showing spread of dust-laden macrophages through the vessel wall into its lumen (original × 80).

able to inflammation (centrilobular emphysema of Leopold and Gough[44]). Reid[45] prefers centriacinar to centrilobular emphysema. Destructive panacinar emphysema diffusely involves alveolar sacs throughout the acinus and, since in our experience a rim of peripheral normal alveoli is found, even in severe emphysema of coal workers, this variety has not been included.To add to the confusion of terminology, panacinar is sometimes referred to as panlobular emphysema. Irregular emphysema related to pulmonary scarring has a potentially wide application if the destructive enlargement of air spaces related to diffuse fibrosis from many causes is included in addition to small focal lung scars.

Focal Emphysema. This is a distention of the respiratory bronchiole which has been daubed on its luminal surface by a plaster consisting of the reticulin network containing coal dust and distintegrating cells. It is presumed that the plaster has a splinting effect against the tractive forces of respiration. This is distention and not a destructive emphysema, and the lesions, small in size, may be widespread but not considered to significantly impair lung function. It is generally agreed that these nondestructive enlargements of respiratory bronchioles are attributable to the dust. Whether these lesions progress to destruction owing to the disruptive effect of the dusts alone, and therefore by definition become centrilobular emphysema, is controversial.

Centrilobular Emphysema. When lungs of older miners with simple pneumoconiosis are examined most will have some degree of the destructive centrilobular emphysema. In a coal miner such lesions will also naturally be anatomically related to the coal focus, also situated in the center of the lobule. It will be readily appreciated that a wide range of combinations are therefore possible. The dust focus may be insignificant, moderate in size, or large, occupying much of the lobule, and similarly, the anatomically related emphysema may be minimal in extent, may be moderate, or may occupy almost all of the lobule as judged by careful naked eye inspection of appropriate large lung preparations. That the latter are examples of centrilobular emphysema, however, becomes apparent on examination of histological preparations when the peripheral "rim" of normal alveolar sacs are seen. Figures 6–5 to 6–11, all of which are taken from Gough whole-lung sections, illustrate the range of combinations. Figure 6–12 shows extensive centrilobular disease.

A further variable in assessing the pathological changes is that there is often a great difference between the most severely and the least affected lobule (Fig. 6–13). A mean must somehow be found, whether by the use of somewhat subjective assessment using standards or by more sophisticated quantitative techniques. A problem often encountered is the interpretation of extensive enlargement of air spaces involving the whole lobule where there is also widespread thickening of the interstitial tissue. Here one has to decide whether the lesion is either basically extensive centrilobular or panacinar emphysema with resolving superadded inflammatory change or an example of interstitial fibrotic disease. Two examples of this

Text continued on page 154

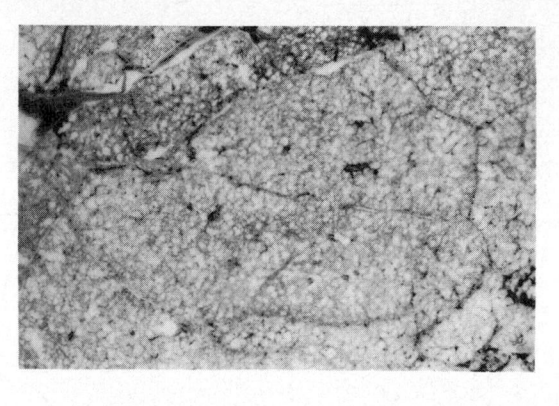

Figure 6–5. Lobules of a normal urban dweller.

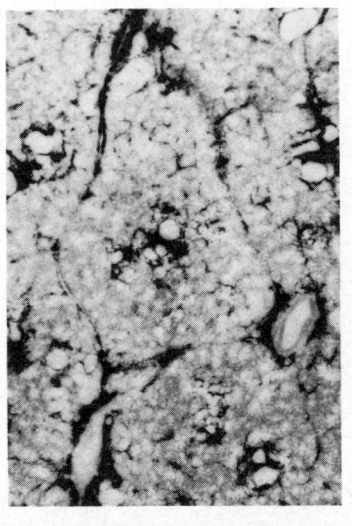

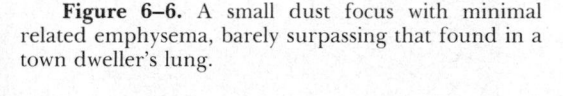

Figure 6–6. A small dust focus with minimal related emphysema, barely surpassing that found in a town dweller's lung.

Figure 6–7. Several lobules with moderate central coal dust and minimal related emphysema.

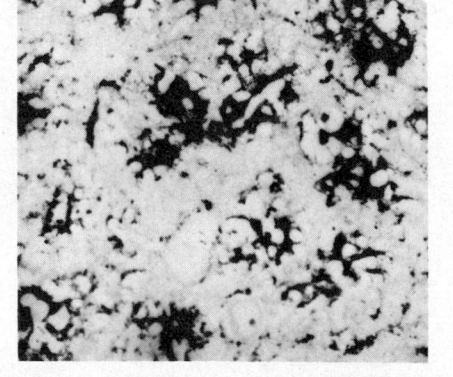

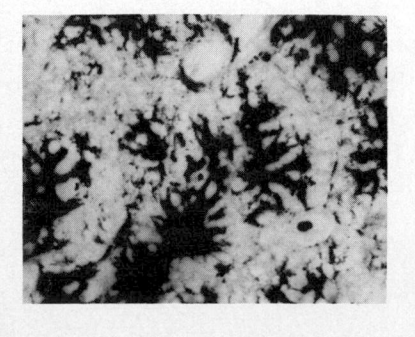

Figure 6–8. Coal foci occupying much of the lobule, but without significant related emphysema.

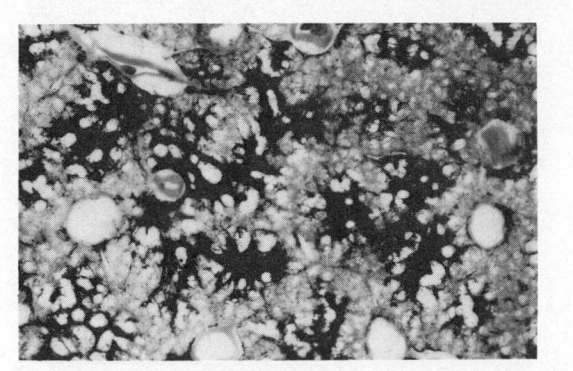

Figure 6–9. Minimal emphysema around a moderate central coal dust focus.

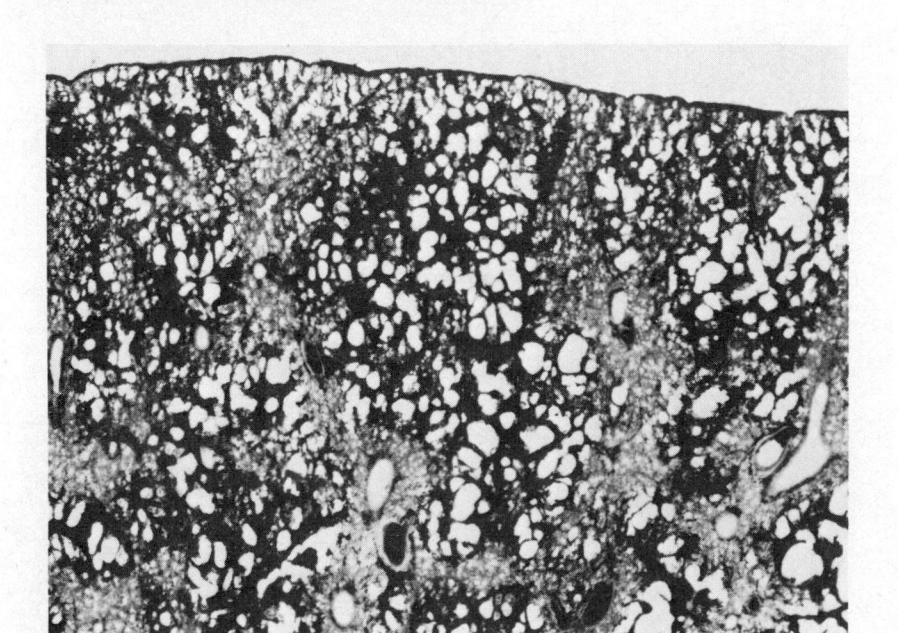

Figure 6–10. Moderate emphysema in lobules associated with extensive focal dust deposition.

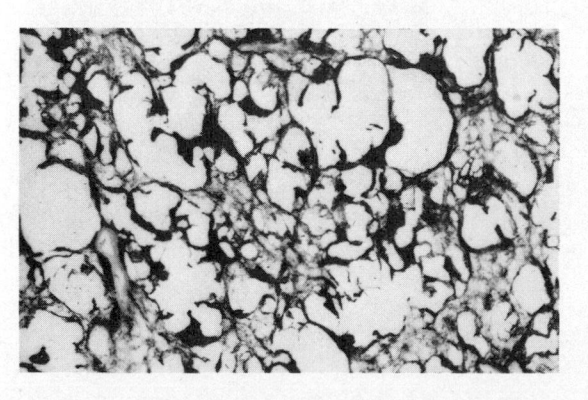

Figure 6–11. Extensive centrilobular emphysema around coal dust foci.

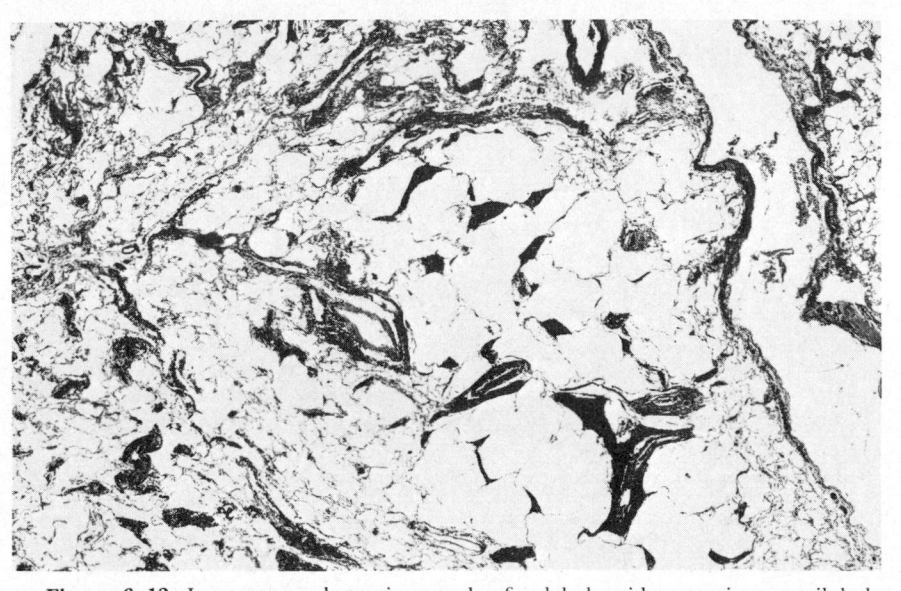

Figure 6–12. Low power photomicrograph of a lobule with extensive centrilobular emphysema. The rim of normal alveoli can be clearly seen.

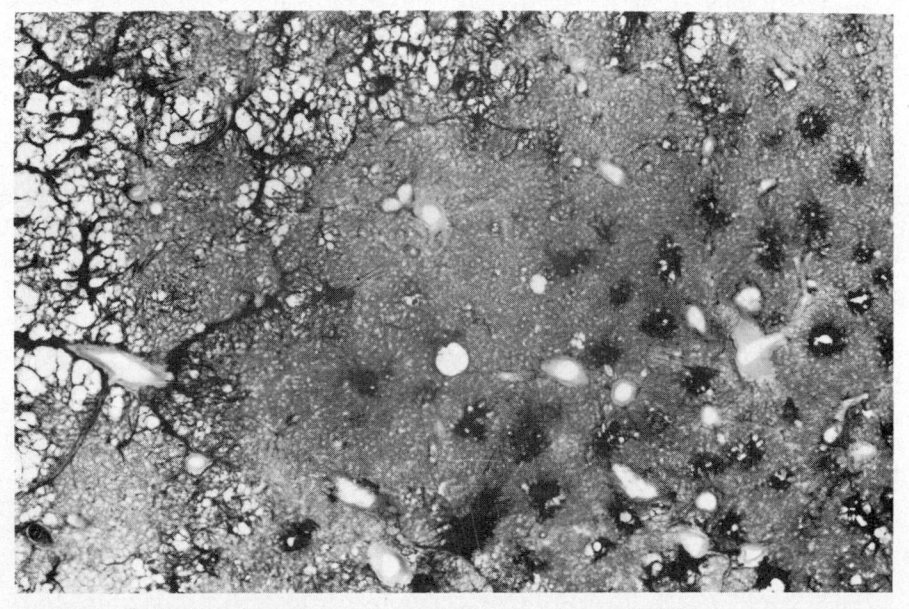

Figure 6–13. Gough paper section of coal miner's lung. Portion of lower lobe ($\times$2), showing dust foci without emphysema on right while on left several severely emphysematous lobules are seen.

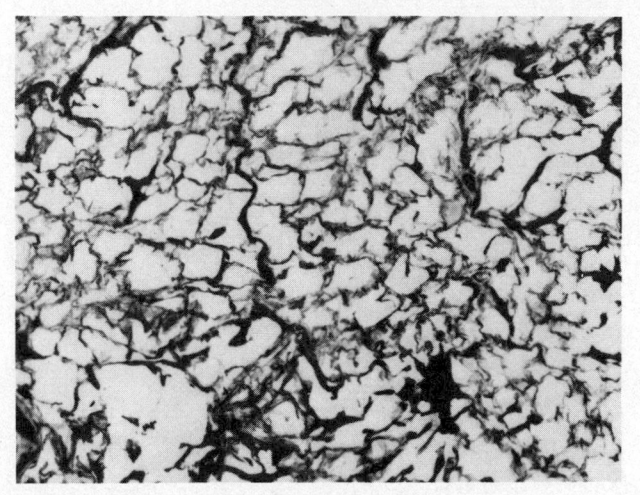

Figure 6–14. Gough paper section showing extensive "emphysema" and thickening of all septa.

problem are shown in Figures 6–14 and 6–15, where well-marked emphysema is present in association with definite interstitial fibrosis and cellular infiltration. To what extent this association is cause and effect is not clear.

The majority of clinicians and pathologists in the pneumoconiosis field appear to accept that the size of the dust nodule is related to exposure and has little influence on lung function in the absence of progressive massive fibrosis. Furthermore, most consider any disabling emphysema to be unrelated to the presence of the dust and to be attributable to nonindustrial factors.

While smoking is a major factor in airways obstruction and disability, in some miners it is not the only factor. The occurrence of moderate to severe centrilobular emphysema with disability in a group of lifelong nonsmoking miners throws suspicion onto the dust itself.[34, 46] It would not be surprising if the continued presence of foci of macrophages and neutrophils in simple coal workers' pneumoconiosis eventually led to their "stimulation" and consequent release of destructive proteolytic enzymes.[47] The release of fibroblastic stimulating factors has been postulated. All the cellular components are seen in the centrilobular location in coal workers' pneumoconiosis, together with varying degrees of extension by the macrophages peripherally, collagenization of interalveolar septa, and destructive emphysema.

Irregular Emphysema. This occurs as a result of traction in relation to scars and bears no consistent relationship to acinar anatomy. Such emphysema may also occur around large coal lesions and, for reasons that are not clear, is uncommon if the dust has a high quartz content or if rheumatoid factor is present (Fig. 6–16). The enlargement of air spaces in a diffusely fibrotic area of lung can be regarded as irregular emphysema,

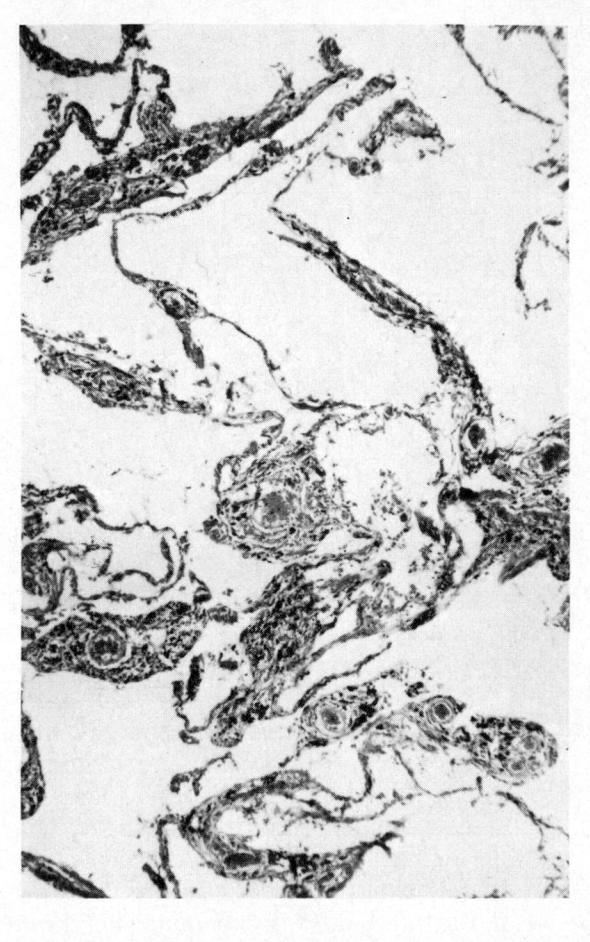

Figure 6–15. Van Gieson stained section showing the periphery of a lobe in a coal miner in whom chronic bronchitis and emphysema were diagnosed during life. The alveolar septa show thickening and there is perivascular cellular infiltration.

in which case the borderland between irregular emphysema and "honeycomb" or cystic lung is blurred.

CORRELATION OF RADIOGRAPHIC APPEARANCES AND PATHOLOGY IN PNEUMOCONIOSIS

When the inhaled dust is both radiodense and does not damage or "stimulate" macrophages, i.e., is nonfibrogenic, extensive radiographic mottling may be seen, as, for example, when the only lesion is a harmless centrilobular accumulation of macrophages containing tin oxide.

In extrinsic allergic alveolitis with centrilobular granulomata, bronchiolitis, and a diffuse interstitial pneumonitis, the patient may be severely dyspneic with a radiograph that is often passed as normal. In this situation the radiograph is a crude index of pathological change. More extensive involvement in the acute stage is represented by a fine miliary "spotting" radiologically. In those patients whose disease progresses to the chronic

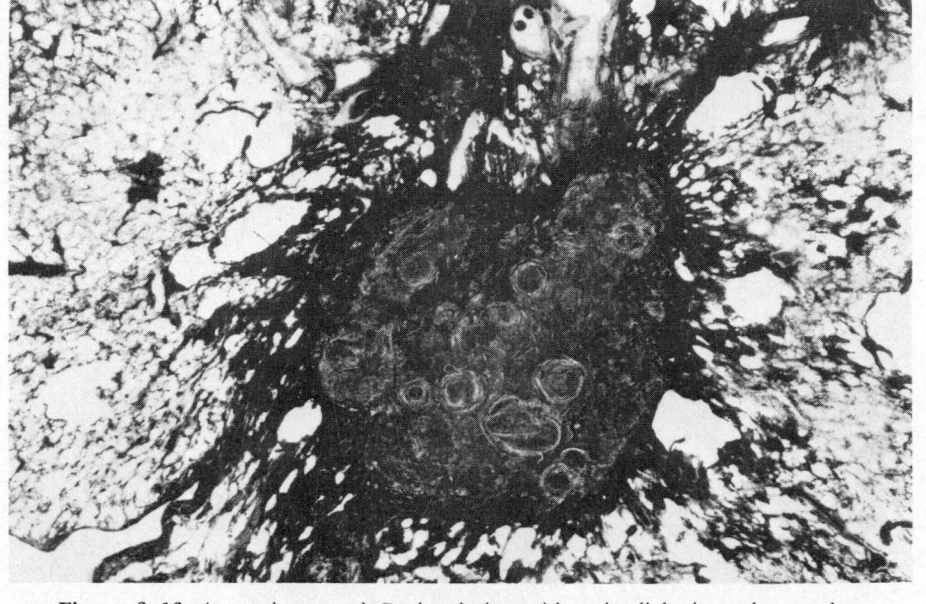

Figure 6–16. A conglomerated Caplan lesion with only slight irregular emphysema around the edge.

stage, the granulomata resolve, but the chronic stage radiographically is evidenced by a persistence of the mottling. The classical radiographic features of pulmonary fibrosis follow later.

Some patients with chronic disease may have a relatively normal radiograph, when a "balance" between fibrosis and honeycomb or cystic change or related irregular emphysema is present.

In the inorganic dust pneumoconioses other than asbestosis, the extent and degree of the nodular opacification evident in a radiograph are usually thought to relate well to the amount of dust entrapped in the centrilobular area. Though the correlation is reasonable it must be remembered that radiology is a relatively insensitive method of demonstrating the earlier nodular and fibrotic lesions. In correlated studies on men exposed to quartz and asbestos dusts, it was shown that when the earliest evidence of the disease could be detected radiologically, the subject had a moderate degree of pneumoconiosis as assessed by pathological examination[48, 49]

When emphysema is superadded to the pathological picture, the "category" (grading of severity) of the radiograph may regress as the patient's disability increases. Although somewhat heretical, it can be said that in simple coal workers' pneumoconiosis the severity of disabling pathological change may vary inversely with the nodular opacification and directly with the degree of emphysema, the latter being difficult to assess radiologically. In inorganic dust pneumoconiosis causing interstitial fibrosis, the radiograph may be pinpoint nodular or have fine irregular

opacities, and even in this situation, the radiological appearances may be minimized by related cystic or emphysematous change.

The importance of assessing irregular opacities has recently been stressed, for they may well indicate the change from simple centrilobular macrophage collection to diffusion of the process peripherally in the lobule, with development of emphysema and sometimes fibrosis.

DUST EXPOSURE AND CANCER

The association of exposure to various types of dust and fumes and cancers of the respiratory tract is largely concealed by the relative frequency of bronchial carcinoma in the urban population and the overwhelming importance of cigarette smoking as shown by epidemiological studies. Nevertheless, there is also a relationship between lung cancer and the work environment, and it is probable that the etiology of this disease is multifactorial. Pollutants, infections, and individual susceptibilities—as, for example, the integrity of the mononuclear macrophage system— should also be considered in investigating the etiology of lung cancer; to forget these other factors may hinder further research. It is important to realize that while epidemiological evidence has shown that there is a multiplicative effect between asbestos exposure and smoking in the development of lung cancer, experimentally it is relatively simple to produce these tumors by exposure to asbestos but extremely difficult to do so with cigarette smoke.

As a result of these difficulties and the high incidence of bronchogenic carcinoma in the general population, it is not easy to obtain definite pathological evidence of an association between dust exposure and cancer unless there is an unusual histological appearance or site of tumor origin, for example, the presence of carcinoma of the nasal sinuses and of the bronchi in men exposed to chromate fumes or to fumes from the processing of nickel, the adenocarcinoma of the nasal sinuses in woodworkers and shoemakers and the histological picture of carcinoma developing around areas of silicotic fibrosis which is practically pathognonomic of exposure to radon in the St. David's Mine at Schneeberg, Saxony.

The relationship of asbestos to malignant disease is complex. Diffuse mesotheliomata of the pleura and peritoneum have been shown to be associated with exposure to crocidolite asbestos dust from fiber mined in the Cape Province in South Africa and the Wittenoon area of Western Australia; evidence of an association with other types of asbestos fiber is not conclusive. However, recent animal experiments suggest that other mineral fibers of less than 0.5 micron in diameter injected into the pleural cavity may be capable of producing a mesothelioma. The majority of the commercially used types of asbestos fiber do not fall into this category.

It is generally accepted that carcinoma of the lung is causally related to the presence of moderately severe fibrosis of asbestosis and originates

peripherally in the areas of fibrosis in a similar manner to the "scar cancer" described by Raeburn and Spencer.[50] The carcinomata described in the 1930s were mainly squamous and multicentric in origin, but recently these peripheral tumors have been mainly adenocarcinomata. In addition, endobronchial carcinomata of all the usual types are now seen in men with asbestosis. This is probably a result of the same factors that initiate these tumors in the general population. As in both New York and London, epidemiological studies have confirmed the multiplicative effects of cigarette smoking and asbestos exposure, and examinations of the lungs from the general population throughout the world indicate the everyone living in an industrial community has some asbestos in the lungs, it becomes increasingly difficult to state how much asbestos exposure is required to be considered a contributing factor in the development of carcinoma of the lung.

The current state of knowledge can be summarized as follows:

1. All types of asbestos produce pulmonary fibrosis if there has been excessive exposure to the dust, providing the length of the fiber exceeds 8 microns and the diameter is less than 3 microns.

2. Cancer of the lung occurs among workers who have pulmonary fibrosis due to excessive exposure to asbestos dust and tends to parallel the degree of fibrosis.

3. Cancer of the lung is far more common among workers who are cigarette smokers. (The two carcinogens asbestos and cigarette smoke appear to combine multiplicatively in the production of lung cancer.)

4. Mesotheliomata of the pleura and peritoneum occur with fibers greater than 8 microns in length and less than 0.5 micron in diameter. These occur with exposure to asbestos, tremolite, and erionite.

5. Mesotheliomata have occurred in people who have had neighborhood exposure to asbestos dust either from living in close vicinity to mills and factories before the dust was controlled or from cleaning the protective clothing of relatives who brought their work clothes home before this practice was forbidden.

6. There is no evidence that exposure of the general population to the small amounts of asbestos fiber in beverages, drinking water, food, or pharmaceutical preparations increases the risk of cancer.

It will therefore be necessary to continue careful monitoring of exposed populations. Accurate pathological and mineralogical studies also need to be continued to establish a dose-response relationship between exposure to specific types and dimensions of fibers and the development of lung cancer.

EXAMINATION OF LUNGS IN INDUSTRIAL DISEASE

Even today the majority of lungs are assessed by naked eye inspection of the cut surface of the uninflated organ in the postmortem room, much

as any other organ is evaluated macroscopically; blocks for histological examination are also usually taken at this time. It has become evident since the work of Professor Jethro Gough that more careful attention to the preparation of the lung for assessment of the distribution of dust and its effect on pulmonary structure is mandatory for a full evaluation of the degree and distribution of lesions. For lungs to be submitted for further examination by authorities who are responsible for awarding compensation, after fixation and gross section in an uniflated state, is demanding too much of interpretative skills.

A Suggested Routine for Proper Evaluation of Pulmonary Disease

1. At least one lung should be fixed by formol saline inflation, if possible within 12 hours of death.

2. A representative coronal section of the lung should ideally be used to produce a thick whole-lung paper-mounted section, according to the Gough-Wentworth technique.[51] This technique is certainly of great value in assessing the extent and severity of emphysema (Figs. 6–5 to 6–11); see also Fig. 13–7).

3. Many departments may not possess facilities for preparing the whole-lung paper sections, but the simple barium sulfate impregnation technique of Heard[52] is within the scope of any department with photo-

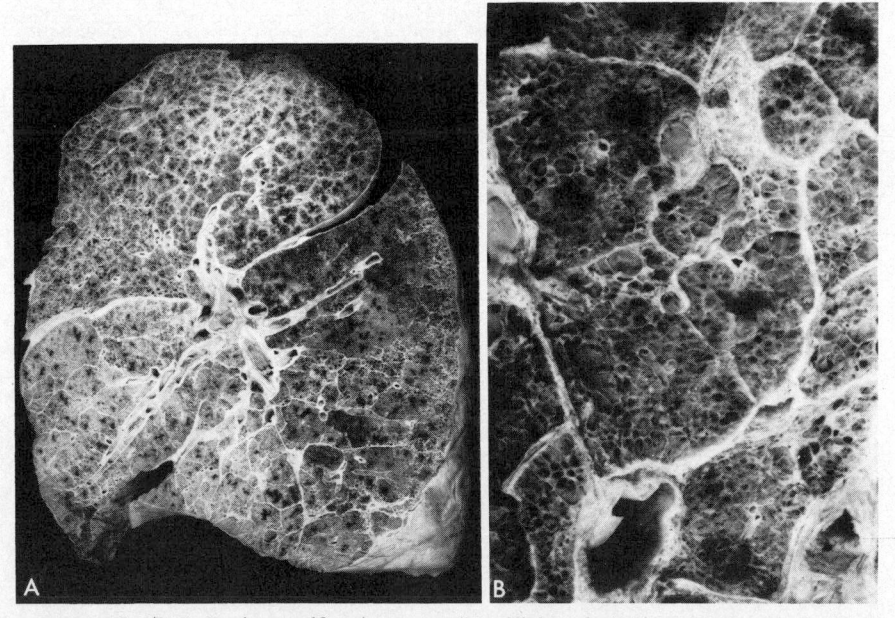

Figure 6–17. *A*, Barium sulfate impregnation. Slight asbestosis seen posteriorly in the lower lobe. The large paper section in this case was relatively uninformative. *B*, Enlargement (×4) of a part of lower lobe in *A* showing more detail of the interstitial fibrosis.

graphic facilities. This technique has deficiencies in portraying centrilobular dust lesions but has a definite advantage in demonstrating the degree of interstitial fibrosis (Fig. 6–17). The method can be utilized to produce known magnifications of portions of upper lobe and lower lobe. We employ a ×4 enlargement as a routine.

4. We find that an additional highly informative simple procedure is the preparation of 5 cm by 5 cm blocks with 20 micron sections mounted on 5 cm by 5 cm projection slides and covered by an appropriate coverslip. Such slides stained by hematoxylin and eosin or Van Gieson's stain can be projected in a 35-mm projector, and detailed viewing of much of the lung parenchyma can be undertaken by pathologists, radiologists, and clinicians. Such a preparation may be placed in an enlarger and a low-power photograph of high quality prepared by projection onto process film. This negative may be used to produce further enlargements.

5. Special examinations that may be undertaken include injection of pulmonary vasculature by radiopaque material and the production of radiographs, quantification and identification of inorganic material, the assessment of birefringent material before and after incineration, and bacteriological and immunological studies.

6. Examination of the lung is incomplete without careful examination of bronchi and their walls, and of the hilar nodes.

References

1. Gibbs, A. R., and Seal, R. M. E., Atlas of Pulmonary Pathology. Current Histopathology, Vol. 3. Lancaster, England, M. T. P. Press Ltd., 1982, p. 83.
2. Katzenstein, A. L. A., Bloor, C. M., and Liebow, A. A., Diffuse alveolar damage—the role of oxygen, shock and related factors. Am. J. Pathol., *85*, 210, 1976.
3. Liebow, A. A., Steer, A., and Billingsley, J. E., Desquamative interstitial pneumonia. Am. J. Med., *39*, 369, 1965.
4. Abraham, J. L., and Hertzberg, M. A., Inorganic particles associated with desquamative interstitial pneumonia. Chest, *805*, 67, 1981.
5. Corrin, B., and Price, A. B., Electron microscopic studies in desquamative interstitial pneumonia associated with asbestos. Thorax, *27*, 324, 1972.
6. Herbert, A., Sterling, E., Abraham, J., and Corrin, B., Desquamative interstitial pneumonia in an aluminum welder. Human Pathol., *13*, 694, 1982.
7. Abraham, J. L., and Spragg, R. G., Documentation of environmental exposure using open biopsy, transbronchial biopsy and bronchopulmonary lavage in giant cell interstitial pneumonia (GIP). Am. Rev. Respir. Dis., *119*(Suppl.), 197, 1979.
8. Corrin, B., and King, E., Pathogenesis of experimental pulmonary alveolar proteinosis. Thorax, *25*, 230, 1970.
9. Suratt, P. M., Winn, W. C., Brady, A. R., et al.: Acute silicosis in tombstone sandblasters. Am. Rev. Respir. Dis., *115*, 521, 1977.
10. Abraham, J. L., and McEuen, D. D., Inorganic particles associated with pulmonary alveolar proteinosis. Am. Rev. Respir. Dis., *119*(Suppl), 196, 1979.
11. Edwards, J. H., Wagner, J. C., and Seal, R. M. E., Pulmonary responses to particulate materials capable of activating the alternative pathway of complement. Clin. Allergy, *6*, 155, 1976.
12. Turner-Warwick, M., Immunology of Occupational Disease of the Lung. London, Edward Arnold, 1978, p. 191.
13. Dickie, H. A., and Rankin, J., Farmer's lung: an acute granulomatous interstitial pneumonitis occurring in agricultural workers. J.A.M.A., *167*, 1069, 1958.

14. Williams, W. R., and Jones Williams, W., Comparison of lymphocyte transformation and macrophage migration inhibition tests in the detection of beryllium hypersensitivity. J. Clin. Pathol., *35*, 684, 1982.
15. Leak, L. V., Pulmonary lymphatics and their role in the removal of interstitial fluids and particulate matter. *In* Brain, J. D., Proctor, D. F., and Reid, L. M., eds., Respiratory Defense Mechanisms. New York, Marcel Dekker, 1977, p. 631.
16. Lauweryns, J. D., and Baert, J. H., The role of the pulmonary lymphatics in the defenses of the diseased lung: morphological and experimental studies of the transport mechanisms of intratracheally instilled particles. Ann. N.Y. Acad. Sci., *221*, 244, 1974.
17. Wagner, J. C., Chamberlain, M., Brown, R. C., et al., Biological effects of tremolite. Br. J. Cancer, *45*, 352, 1982.
18. Stanton, M. F., Layard, M., Tegeris, A., et al., Carcinogenicity of fibrous glass: pleural response in the rats in relation to fibre dimensions. J. Natl. Cancer Inst., *58*, 587, 1977.
19. Stanton, M. F., and Wrench, C. J., Mechanisms of mesothelioma induction with asbestos and fibrous glass. J. Natl. Cancer Inst., *48*, 797, 1972.
20. Wright, G. W., and Kuschner, M., The influence of varying length of glass and asbestos fibres on tissue response in guinea pigs. *In* Walton, W. H., ed., Inhaled Particles, Pergamon Press, Oxford, 1977, pp. 455.
21. Wagner, J. C., Berry, G., Skidmore, J. W., and Pooley, F. D., The comparative effects of three chrysotiles by injection and inhalation in rats. *In* Wagner, J. C., ed., The Biological Effects of Mineral Fibres, Vol. 1. Lyon, France, IARC, 1980, p. 363.
22. Stanton, M. F., Layard, M., and Tegeris, A., Relation of particle dimension to carcinogenicity in amphibole asbestosis and other fibrous minerals. J. Natl. Cancer Inst., *67*, 965, 1981.
23. Brady, A. R., Hill, L. H., Adkins, J. B., and O'Connor, R. W., Chrysotile asbestos inhalation in rats: deposition pattern and reaction of alveolar epithelium and pulmonary macrophages. Am. Rev. Respir. Dis., *123*, 670, 1981.
24. Morgan, A., Talbot, R. J., and Holmes, A., Significance of fibre length in the clearance of asbestos fibres from the lung. Br. J. Ind. Med., *35*, 146, 1978.
25. Wagner, J. C., Burns, J., Munday, D. E., and McGee, J. O. D., Presence of fibronectin in pneumoconiotic lesions. Thorax, *37*, 54, 1982.
26. Pooley, F. D., Asbestos bodies, their formation, composition and character. Environ. Res., *5*, 363, 1972.
27. Churg, A. A., and Warnock, M. C., Asbestos and other ferruginous bodies, their formation and clinical significance. Am. J. Pathol., *102*, 447, 1980.
28. Gibbs, A. R., and Seal, R. M. E., Occupational lung disorders, II. Silicate Pneumoconioses. *In* Atlas of Pulmonary Pathology. Lancaster, England, M. T. P. Press, 1982, p. 91.
29. Ashcroft, T., and Heppleston, A. G., The optical and electron microscopic determination of pulmonary asbestos fibre concentration and its relation to the human pathological reaction. J. Clin. Pathol., *26*, 224, 1973.
30. Meurman, L., Asbestos bodies and pleural plaques in a Finnish series of autopsy cases. Acta Pathol. Microbiol. Scand. Suppl., *181*, 1, 1966.
31. Churg, A., Fibre counting and analysis in the diagnosis of asbestos-related disease. Human Pathol., *13*, 381, 1982.
32. Sebastien, P., Janson, X., Gaudichet, A., and Bignon, J., Asbestos retention in human respiratory tissues: comparative measurements in lung parenchyma and in parietal pleura. *In* Wagner, J. C., ed., The Biological Effects of Mineral Fibers, Vol. 1. Lyons, France, IARC Scientific Pub. No. 30, 1980, p. 237.
33. Harrington, J. S., and Allison, A. C., Lysosomal enzymes in relation to the toxicity of silica. Med. Lavora, *56*, 471, 1965.
34. Davis, J. M. G., Chapman, J., Collings, P., et al., Autopsy studies of coal miners' lungs. Report No. TM/79/9. Edinburgh, Institute of Occupational Medicine, 1979.
35. James, W. R. L., The relationship of tuberculosis to the development of massive pneumoconiosis in coal workers. Br. J. Tuber. *48*, 89, 1954.
36. Rivers, D., James, W. R. L., Davies, D. G., and Thomson, S., The prevalence of tuberculosis at necropsy in progressive massive fibrosis of coal workers. Br. J. Ind. Med. *14*, 39, 1957.
37. Naeye, R. L., Mahou, J. K., and Dellinger, W. S., Rank of coal and coal workers' pneumoconiosis. Am. Rev. Respir. Dis., *103*, 350, 1971.

38. Byers, P. D., and King, E. J., Experimental and infective pneumoconiosis with coal, kaolin and mycobacteria. Lab. Invest., *8*, 647, 1959.

39. Ball, J. D., Berry, G., and Clarke, W. G., A controlled trial of anti-tuberculosis chemotherapy in the early complicated pneumoconiosis of coal workers. Thorax, *24*, 399, 1969.

40. Wagner, J. C., Wustermann, F. S., Edwards, J. H., and Hill, R. J., The composition of massive lesions in coal miners. Thorax, *30*, 382, 1975.

41. Cockcroft, A. E., Wagner, J. C., Seal, R. M. E., et al., Irregular opacities in coal workers' pneumoconiosis—correlation with pulmonary function and pathology. Ann. Occup. Hyg. *26*, 767, 1982.

42. Report of the conclusions of a CIBA guest symposium. Terminology, definitions and classifications of chronic pulmonary emphysema and related condition. Thorax, *14*, 286, 1959.

43. Heppleston, A. G., The pathological recognition and pathogenesis of emphysema and fibrocystic disease of the lung with special reference to coal workers. Ann. N.Y. Acad. Sci., *200*, 347, 1972.

44. Leopold, J. G., and Gough, J., The centrilobular form of hypertrophic emphysema and its relation to chronic bronchitis. Thorax, *12*, 219, 1957.

45. Reid, L., Pathology of Emphysema. London, Lloyd Luke, 1967.

46. Lyons, J. P., Ryder, R. C., Seal, R. M. E., and Wagner, J. C., Emphysema in smoking and non-smoking coal workers with pneumoconiosis. Bull. Europ. Physiopath. Resp., *17*, 75, 1981.

47. Werb, Z., and Gordon, S., Secretion of a specific collagenase by stimulated macrophages. J. Exp. Med., *142*, 346, 1975.

48. Hurwitz, M., and Wagner, J. C., Correlation of radiological and necropsy findings in silicosis. *In* Orenstein, A. J., ed., Proceedings of the Pneumoconiosis Conference in Johannesburg, 1959. London, J. & A. Churchill, 1960, p. 242.

49. Caplan, A., Gibson, J. C., Hinson, K. F. W., et al., A preliminary study of observer variation in the classification of radiographs of asbestos exposed workers and the relationship of pathology and x-ray appearance. Ann. N.Y. Acad. Sci, *132*, 379, 1965.

50. Raeburn, C., and Spencer, H., Lung scar cancers. Br. J. Tuberc. *51*, 237, 1957.

51. Gough, J., and Wentworth, J. E., The use of thin sections of entire organs in morbid anatomical studies. J. Roy. Microsc. Soc., *69*, 231, 1949.

52. Heard, B. E., A pathological study of emphysema of the lungs with chronic bronchitis. Thorax, *13*, 136, 1958.

7

CELLULAR AND MATRIX MECHANISMS IN OCCUPATIONAL LUNG DISEASE

J. Bernard L. Gee
and Jamson Lwebuga-Mukasa

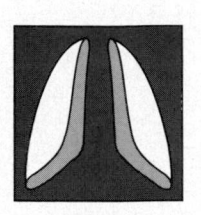

This chapter will focus on the terminal units of gas exchange, the alveolocapillary units. Airways disorders will not be considered, even though it is recognized that disorders affecting these terminal units also involve alveolar ducts and terminal bronchioles. It is axiomatic that occupational lung hazards will cause disease by interference with normal lung biology; our continual reference to better studied nonoccupational disorders is therefore appropriate.

The past two decades have witnessed a radical change in the approach to lung disease. First came the ability to obtain two alveolar capillary unit cells for morphological and functional study. A notable achievement was Myrvik's use of pulmonary lavage to obtain rabbit alveolar macrophages (AM) and later the isolation from whole lungs of type II cells by Kikkawa,[1] Mason,[2] and other workers.[3] The second development was the understanding of phagocytic cell function in terms of both antimicrobial defenses and tissue injury mechanisms. About this time the subclasses and functions of lymphocytes were being elucidated. Bienenstock simultaneously emphasized that the lung can mount a distinctive local immune response particularly through the bronchus-associated lymphoid system. More recently, connective tissue biochemistry advances have been applied to the lung by Crystal and others.[4] The interaction between cells and connective tissue matrix proteins has become apparent in the past five years. Finally, while classical anatomical pathology defined many characteristics of occupational and other lung disorders, the recent advances have come from direct studies of the effects of specific occupational hazards on cellular and matrix behavior. These studies employ both *in vitro* techniques and

163

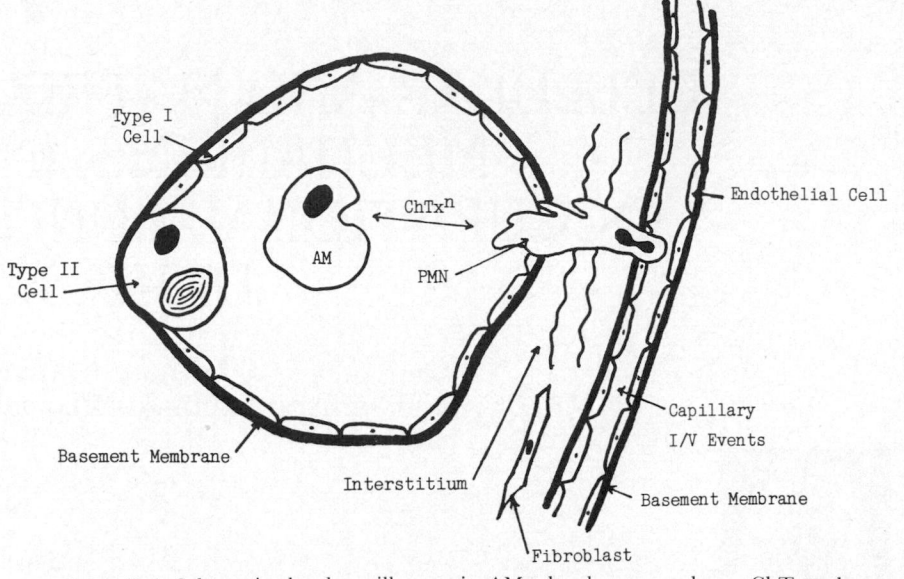

Figure 7–1. Schematic alveolocapillary unit. AM, alveolar macrophage; ChTx^n, chemotaxin. Neutrophil migration (PMN) is rare in normal lungs.

the isolation of cells and soluble products from healthy and diseased lungs by bronchoalveolar lavage (BAL), a technique applied to man by Reynolds,[5] and Hunninghake and Crystal,[6] and briefly reviewed elsewhere.[7, 8]

ALVEOLOCAPILLARY UNIT: STRUCTURAL CELLS

Figures 7–1 and 7–2 depict the structure of the alveolocapillary units. Figure 7–1 is diagrammatic and indicates the distribution of blood vessels, alveolar spaces, and cellular populations. Detailed morphology of these is more apparent in the electron microscopical picture (Fig. 7–2). The alveolar surface is lined by type I epithelial cells, which are flattened and have a large surface area, thus providing a suitable framework for gas exchange. Nothing is really known about the biochemistry of these epithelial cells, which do not undergo mitosis. Tight junctions between neighboring type I cells and also with a subjacent second lung cell type (type II) occur. Review of the nature of these junctions and their role in water solute exchange may be found elsewhere. The junctions between type I and type II cells are a common location for the migration from capillary to lung air spaces of polymorphonuclear neutrophils (PMN) following intra-alveolar inflammatory states.

The second cell type mentioned, the type II cell, tends to occur in the alveolar corners. When mature, they are characterized by the presence of lamellar bodies (Fig. 7–3). Type II cells derive from a primitive cuboidal epithelium which invades the mesenchyma at an early embryological stage.

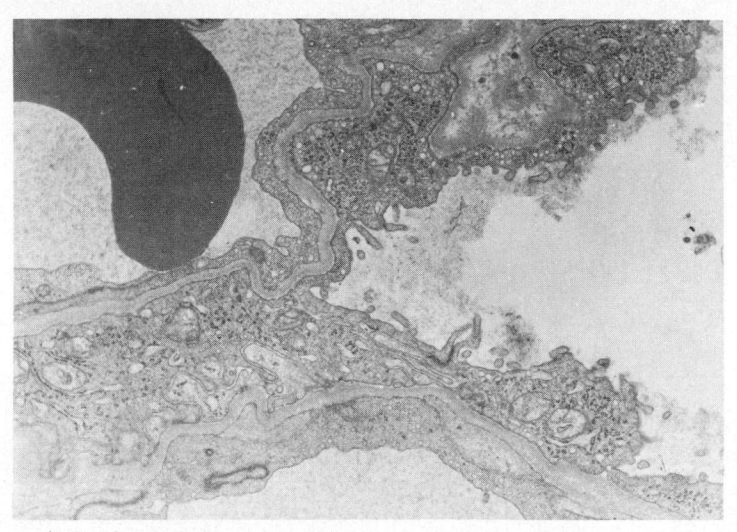

Figure 7–2. Alveolocapillary unit. Alveolar capillaries are seen at top left and bottom. Alveolar surface is lined by attenuated cytoplasm of differentiating type I pneumocytes.

Near term, the type II cells both mature and differentiate. The maturation is characterized by the appearance of lamellar bodies and the secretion of surfactant. The maturation is under hormonal control (corticosteroids, thyroxine, etc.), and the secretion depends on the usual microfilament, microtubule, and hormonal factors. These type II cells also differentiate into type I cells. Both maturation and differentiation are partly controlled by a fibroblast-derived peptide.[9] These later embryological developments form the basis for the function of type II cells in the adult lung, where

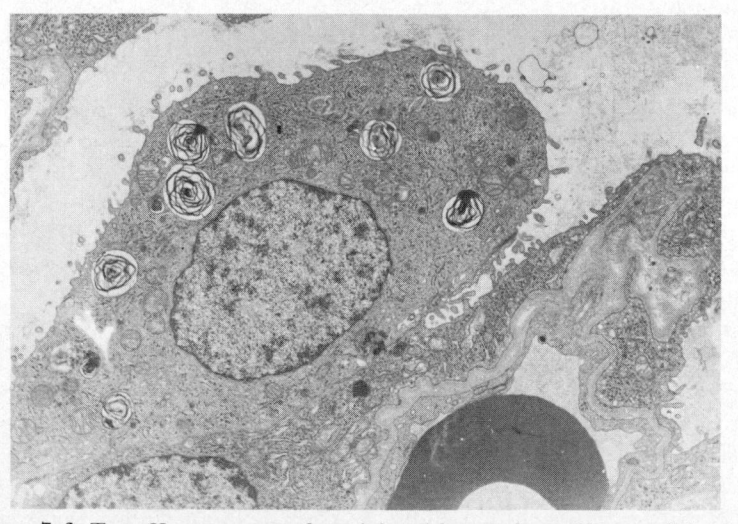

Figure 7–3. Type II pneumocyte from injured human lung. Characteristic structures include surface microvilli and lamellar bodies.

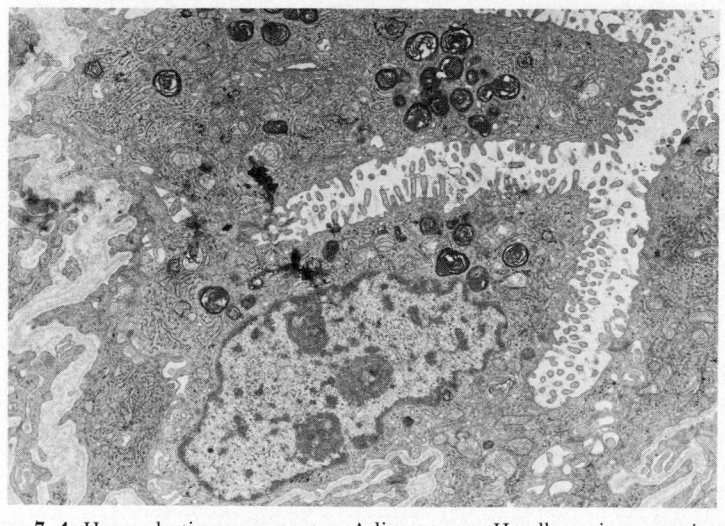

Figure 7–4. Hyperplastic pneumocytes. Adjacent type II cells project prominently into alveolar spaces. Lambellar bodies are numerous and microvilli elongated and club-shaped.

they also serve to regenerate type I cells. This process is relatively slow in normal lungs but provides a rapid repair mechanism following alveolar injury. Studies employing low levels of toxic gases such as nitrogen dioxide or hyperoxia[10] have shown that injury to type I cells following inhalation of oxidants leads to hyperplasia (Fig. 7–4) and proliferation of type II cells with their subsequent differentiation into type I cells. These studies have employed tritiated thymidine as a tracer to show that differentiation and complete type II cell turnover occurs within 2 to 4 days following acute airspace injury.

Some recent *in vitro* studies have demonstrated that type II cells only retain normal morphology when grown upon basement membranes and do not function well when grown on a collagenous stroma lacking a basement membrane. Among the affected functions are the production of surfactant, organization into a monolayer, and probably the production by type II cells of basement membrane.[10a] Much remains to be done to define the surface characteristics that best serve these type II cell functions, but it is already clear that repair following injury critically depends on this cell–basement membrane surface relationship.

Endothelial cells form the equivalent in the capillaries of the air surface type I cells. They constitute 40 per cent of all pulmonary cells. In healthy lungs, about 1 per cent of endothelial cells turn over each day. Following injury, these cells rapidly proliferate and can readily repopulate the basement membrane. Pure lines of such cells are available from a number of larger blood vessels, including pulmonary vasculature and umbilical cords. Thus, much more is known about them; for instance, they synthesize clotting factor VIII.[11] While these cells share with type I

cells an extensive surface area with flattened cytoplasm, they additionally increase their surface area by the presence of small almost spherical indentations termed caveolae on the blood surface of the cell. Studies by Ryan and Ryan[12] have demonstrated these caveolae to be the site of many surface ectoenzymes such as those responsible for the degradation of serotonin, prostaglandins, and adrenergic compounds. Additionally, angiotensin converting enzyme (ACE) is also localized at this site and degrades both angiotensin I to angiotensin II, and bradykinin. Both actions involve the removal of two C-terminal amino acids from oligopeptides, and hence this enzyme is a generalized dipeptidylpeptidase. The large surface area and cell surface enzymes enhance not only alveolocapillary gas exchange but also enhance vascular clearance of chemical mediators of inflammation. Defects in endothelial cell function can be detected early in lung disease by measurements of the clearance of such compounds,[13] e.g., serotonin.

The alveolocapillary interstitium contains such mesenchymal cells as fibroblasts and smooth muscle cells. The cells are part of the connective tissue system and are a source of matrix materials described later. The fibroblast is paradoxically capable of generating both collagen and a specific collagenase[14] which attacks collagen types I and III. Fibroblasts are phagocytic cells. Uptake of particles, e.g., latex, promotes the release of collagenase and other proteases. Both cell types proliferate in interstitial pulmonary fibrosis. Additionally, myofibroblasts, cells with contractile properties and probably related to smooth muscle cells, also proliferate in idiopathic pulmonary fibrosis (IPF).

These cells and their response to injury have been recently succinctly reviewed.[15] In certain acute onset occupational lung diseases, both type I epithelial cells and endothelial cells are injured. For instance, they are damaged by oxidant gases (NO_2, O_3), paraquat, chlorine, phosgene, acid mists, and such materials as sublimates of cadmium and mercury. This damage is manifest as a capillary leak pulmonary edema. When not fatal, the repair processes often lead to complete recovery, but an obliterative fibrosing terminal bronchiolitis and alveolitis can also result.

Recent studies have also emphasized that the alveolocapillary units also leak in the early phases of such chronic diseases as asbestosis.[16] In a sheep model, intratracheal asbestos installation causes transudation of albumin and transferrin from blood to air spaces. This can readily be demonstrated with intravenous radioactive gallium scanning. Gallium largely binds to transferrin. Following its appearance in the air space, the gallium is sequestered in the AM; a similar phenomenon occurs in both idiopathic and asbestos-induced pulmonary fibrosis.

Type II cells are more resistant to injury; their role in tissue repair is discussed in detail below. In some patients with silicosis, BAL has shown many type II cells to be present. The significance of this observation is unclear, but there are reports of a proliferative type II cell response and alveolar proteinosis in acute experimental silicosis.

ALVEOLOCAPILLARY UNIT: MATRIX

The extracellular matrix of the lung parenchyma consists of a basement membrane on which alveolar epithelial cells rest, a second basement membrane on which endothelial cells reside, and a collagenous interstitium separating these two membranes. In certain regions, known as the thin segments of the capillary loop, these two membranes fuse. These structural components form a scaffold on which normal cell function is maintained and an architectural framework for normal repair after injury.

The extracellular matrix of the alveolar wall consists of four broad classes of structural macromolecules: (1) collagen types I, III, IV, and V, (2) noncollagenous adhesive glycoproteins laminin and fibronectin, (3) elastin, and (4) glycosaminoglycans. The purification of these macromolecules and the preparation of specific antibodies thereto by Furthmayr, Madri and others[17] permit histochemical localization in human lung.

Collagens

There are several genetically distinct varieties of collagen, all of which contain hydroxyproline. Types I and III collagens form triple helix fibrils and are located in the interstitium of the lung. Types IV and V do not form fibrils and contain helical collagenous, as well as noncollagenous, globular domains. The fibrillar character of collagen, in general, requires the preservation of a glycine occurring as every third amino acid in the collagen molecule sequence. In type IV collagen the glycine content comprises less than one-third of the amino acids, and there are interruptions in the tertiary repetition of glycine. Type IV collagen is exclusively found in the basement membrane. Type V has both a basement membrane and interstitial localization. Type II collagen is found only in cartilagenous tissues and therefore is not a component of the alveolar wall.

Collagen comprises about 65 per cent of the normal lung connective tissue. Recent work by Madri and Furthmayr[18] has demonstrated a 2.5-fold increase in the collagen content of fibrotic lungs when compared to normal ones. In IPF, there are profound changes in the distribution of the various collagens. There is an increase in type I collagen in thickened alveolar septa and a concomitant disappearance of type III collagen from that location. Type V collagen content is increased and found around smooth muscle cell clusters. Only type IV collagen in the basement membrane appears unchanged in both location and extractable amounts. No measurements of collagen composition are available in such occupational lung fibroses as asbestosis.

While the exact significance of the above changes in the distribution of collagen types for lung function is unclear, the role of collagen in modifying cell and other matrix protein behavior is becoming increasingly apparent.[19] Such studies have, so far, focused largely on other organs than

the lung and perhaps are best exemplified by the behavior of myoblasts, which mature into myotubes only when the former are grown on collagen. In the developing murine lung, epithelial branching can be prevented by using an analogue of proline, an important cross-linking amino acid present in collagen.[20] This suggests tissue differentiation requires a normal collagen matrix. For a wide range of cells, it is now becoming clear that collagen directly influences cell proliferation, cellular differentiation and migration, and more importantly the orientation of epithelial cells in a particular polar direction. Furthermore certain cells match preferentially to specific collagen types. For instance, platelet aggregation is most stimulated by type III collagen, whereas epidermal and smooth muscle cells adhere more readily to types IV and V, respectively.

Noncollagenous Proteins: Laminin and Fibronectin

These two proteins are important in that they can interact with both collagens and cell surfaces, and thereby function as adhesive agents. Laminin, a large protein of molecular weight 1 million daltons, spontaneously forms aggregations.[21] The molecule has a cruciate shape with irregular arms, and some of its amino acid structure is now becoming apparent. These arms serve as cross-linking agents to other proteins and cell surfaces. Laminin has an exclusive basement location where it has been demonstrated to play a role in the attachments of such cells as liver epithelial cells. Recent studies by Couchman and co-workers[22] have demonstrated that fibroblasts also have laminin receptors in addition to fibronectin receptors. The precise role of laminin in the lung is presently unclear.

Fibronectin is a somewhat smaller molecule than laminin. Structural and functional aspects of this molecule have recently been reviewed.[23, 24] In its dimeric, near linear form, it has a molecular weight of 450,000 daltons. Fibronectin has been found in both the interstitium and the basement membrane, as well as in plasma. Several molecular domains exist within this linear molecule with separate binding sites for collagen, heparin, fibrin, and other fibronectin molecules, and for cell surfaces. Fibronectin is produced by endothelial cells, platelets, fibroblasts, and macrophage lines. While fibronectins from various sources may exist in several minor molecular variations, a number of general functions are becoming clear. For instance, fibronectin in plasma serves as a general opsonin for phagocytosis by promoting nonspecific "sticking" of particulates to phagocyte cell surfaces. It thus differs from such immunospecific opsonic immunoglobulins as those produced in response to specific bacterial materials. Additionally, fibronectin has been shown to play a role in cell attachment, cellular shape, and differentiation of many mesenchymal cell lines. One important function of fibronectin is that it provides a surface upon which fibroblasts can migrate. This can be shown under *in*

vitro conditions with chemotactic chambers. Additionally, fibronectin is itself a true chemoattractant for fibroblasts which will migrate towards increasing fibronectin concentrations. Employing various proteolytic enzymes, one may separate fibronectin-fibroblast binding sites from those responsible for collagen-fibronectin interactions. Thus, as the name suggests, fibronectin can serve as a nexus relating cells to structural proteins.

Enhanced production of fibronectin by rodent AM occurs following the ingestion of certain forms of asbestos. The fibronectin content of BAL fluid is increased in IPF but does not appear to correlate with clinical progression in that disorder.[25] A recent important observation is that fibronectin is quantitatively important in the "fibrous" material of the lungs of patients with progressive massive fibrosis.[26] Fibronectin stimulates proliferation of fibroblasts by rendering them competent to respond to other proliferative factors such as those secreted by AM.

Elastin

Electron microscopical observation of mature elastin fibers reveals two distinct components.[27] There is a microfibrillar tubular structure some 1100 nm in diameter with a 400-nm central core.[28] The second component is amorphous under electron microscopy and appears to fill the spaces between the microfibrils. Elastin is difficult to solubilize owing to its unusually high content of nonpolar amino acids and particularly to the presence of certain cross-linking amino acids, desmosine and isodesmosine. This cross-linking depends on the activity of a Cu^{++}-containing enzyme, lysyl oxidase. The cellular origin and factors determining the architectural arrangement of lung elastin are poorly understood. Presumably, as in other tissues, lung elastin is generated by fibroblasts and smooth muscle cells. Elastin is found in the noncapillary blood vessel linings and also in the basement membrane and lung interstitium. Elastinolysis and loss of elastic recoil are usually regarded as hallmarks of emphysema. The individual contributions of elastin and other matrix proteins to stress-strain lung mechanics are poorly understood, but it appears likely that elastin confers high extensibility and excellent recoil but low tensile strength. Fibrillar collagens probably confer limits to lung distensibility.

Glycosaminoglycans

These macromolecules comprise complex polysaccharide moieties (alternating uronic acid and hexosamine) and are usually covalently linked to a protein core to form a proteoglycan. Glycosaminoglycans can interact with collagen, fibronectin, laminin, and cell surfaces. They too have been demonstrated to play a role in the differentiation of a number of structures in embryonic development. In basement membranes, they may act as

charge-dependent filtration mechanisms. Their precise function in the lung is, at present, unclear, but the lung is a rich source of many glycosaminoglycans—for instance, heparin. Furthermore, other glycosaminoglycans, such as hyaluronic acid, are readily oxidized by such inflammatory compounds as superoxide anion (v.i.), with a resulting sharp increase in its viscosity. In at least one connective tissue matrix—that secreted by smooth muscle cells—digestion of glycosaminoglycans appears to be a prerequisite for the action of enzymes on subjacent fibrillar proteins such as elastin. The glycosaminoglycan content of lungs from patients with progressive massive fibrosis is increased.

LUNG DEFENSES: POTENTIAL FOR INJURY

The sterility of the normal human lung requires many mechanisms, which include airway ciliary clearance, local humoral immune mechanisms (e.g., secretory IgA), and the native ability of AM to kill microorganisms in the lung air spaces. Additional factors maintaining lung sterility are the immunological responsiveness to previously encountered microorganisms as mediated by local lymphocyte populations, AM activation, and also the recruitment of polymononuclear neutrophils (PMNs) into air spaces under acute inflammatory reactions associated with bacterial invasion. Detailed considerations of these defense mechanisms may be found elsewhere. This discussion will emphasize the inherent ability of the "normal" activities of these three cell types (PMN, AM, and lymphocytes) to cause lung injury. This potential is readily apparent in many lung diseases and is relevant to certain occupational disorders. The pathogenetic potential of the normal physiology of each of these three cell types will be described and the role of the mast cell will be discussed.

Neutrophils

Polymorphonuclear leukocytes (PMN) are professional phagocytes.[29] They are normally absent from the lung parenchyma, are uncommon in normal airways, and are infrequently found in BAL fluid from normal nonsmoking subjects. In human BAL fluid, PMN constitute about 1 per cent and from 3 to 5 per cent of nucleated cells in normal nonsmoking and smoking subjects, respectively. However, neutrophils are sequestered in the pulmonary microcirculation where they form a large pool adherent to the vascular surface of endothelial cells, a phenomenon known as margination. Following a number of inflammatory responses in the lung, they are readily mobilized and cross into air spaces by the process known as diapedesis (Fig. 7–5A and B). PMN have a relatively short circulating half-life of 2 to 3 days and a tissue life of a few hours. They provide a powerful antibacterial defense mechanism. Three physiological and path-

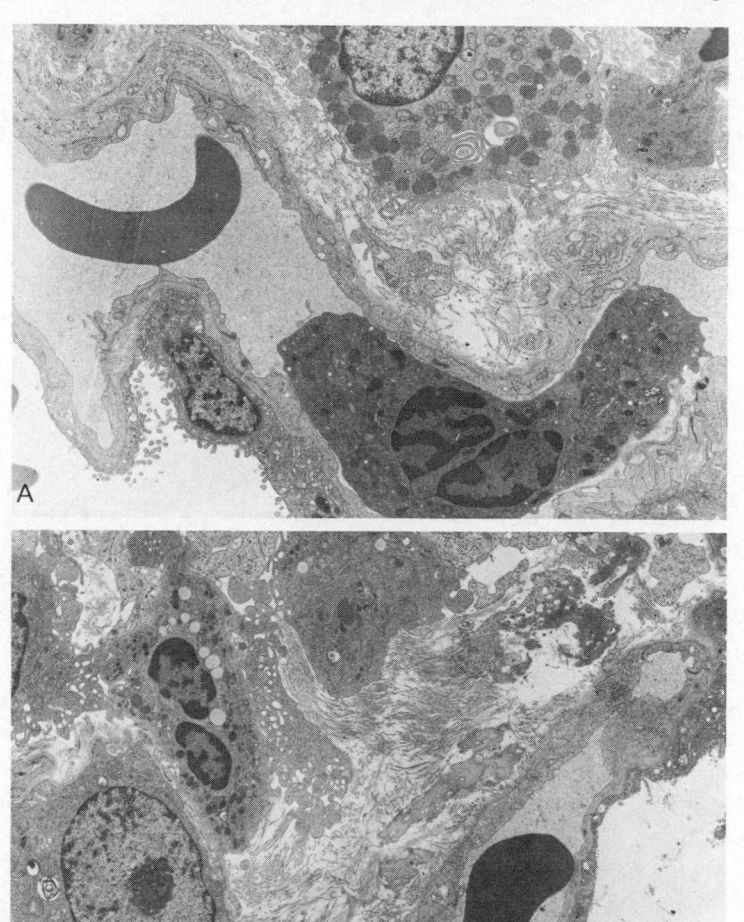

Figure 7–5. *A*, Lung inflammation. A mature polymorphonuclear leukocyte appears to conform to the endothelial surface lining the thick portion of the alveolocapillary unit. Note edema of adjacent interstitial space. *B*, At top left a polymorphonuclear leukocyte migrates in the interstitium along the basement membrane of a type II pneumocyte. Interstitium is edematous.

ogenetic features of these cells are the release of oxidants, the release of degradative enzymes and chemotactic responsiveness.

   Oxidants. PMN contain few mitochondria and their resting respiration is relatively low. However, there is a brisk rise in oxygen consumption following either phagocytosis of particles or the exposure of the cells *in vitro* to stimulants such as complement factors (C5a), AM-derived chemotactic factors, and certain other low-molecular-weight peptides associated with bacteria. This brisk rise in oxygen consumption depends upon a cyanide-insensitive flavoprotein NADPH oxidoreductase found on the external surface of the PMN membrane. During phagocytosis, this external

surface of the cell membrane necessarily becomes internalized with the invagination of the fully enclosed phagocytic vacuole. However, the oxidant products of this enzyme are released extracellularly both following nonparticulate stimulation and during the process of internal vacuole formation during phagocytosis. The major biological products of this enzyme are highly reactive oxidants, which are listed in Table 7–1. Of these, the immediate and most important product is superoxide anion, which can undergo spontaneous or enzymatic dismutation (by superoxide dismutase) to form hydrogen peroxide. Additionally, in the presence of halides present in normal extracellular fluid, a hypohalide ion may be formed (e.g., $HOCl^-$). One particular enzyme, myeloperoxidase, which constitutes 5 per cent of the dry weight of the PMN, is important in the production of hypohalide ions and also in subserving oxidation of many substrates.

There is ample evidence that such oxidant materials are powerful microbicidal agents, but the mechanisms for this are unclear. However, for our purposes, such oxidants are highly injurious to the lung. For instance, in a number of experimental models of inflammatory lung disease[30] in which PMN mobilization and activation is produced by such agents as C5a, protection occurs when antioxidants such as superoxide dismutase are employed. Fibroblasts and umbilical vessel endothelial cells are damaged by activated PMN by an oxidation-dependent mechanism. Likewise, matrix materials such as hyaluronic acid can be oxidized by superoxide anion.[31]

An important effect of oxidants is on alpha-1-antiprotease.[32] This specific protein, normally present in the circulating blood and in BAL fluid, is an important constituent of the antiprotease screen. It combines in a molar ratio with a number of important proteases discussed below. At its active site is a methionine molecule containing a reduced sulfhydryl group. This group may be oxidized by superoxide anion, hydrogen peroxide, and a number of other oxidizing materials, probably including cigarette smoke, rendering the alpha-1-antiprotease incapable of inhibiting certain proteases. Oxidation of alpha-1-antiprotease is greatly enhanced by myeloperoxidase, which is liberated by PMN degranulation. This effect

Table 7–1. OXIDANTS PRODUCED BY PHAGOCYTES

Superoxide anion	$O_2^{\cdot}$
Hydrogen peroxide	H_2O_2
Hydroxyl free radical	$OH \cdot$
Hypochlorite ion	$HOCl^-$
Singlet O_2	$1_{O_2^*}$
$O_2^{\cdot}$ generation	$2O_2 + NADPH \rightarrow 2O_2^{\cdot}$ $+ NADP^+ + H^+$
H_2O_2 generation* (dismutation of $O_2^{\cdot}$)	$O_2^{\cdot} + O_2^{\cdot} + 2H^+ \rightarrow$ $H_2O_2 + O_2$
Haber Weiss reaction	$O_2^{\cdot} + H_2O_2 \rightarrow OH \cdot +$ $OH^- + 1_{O_2^*}$

*Some oxidases convert O_2 to H_2O_2 directly without an $O_2^{\cdot}$ dismutation step.

is preventable by catalase. Such oxidation does not affect the basic structure of the molecule, which can still be detected by specific antibodies, but does severely impair the antiprotease activity as measured, particularly with PMN elastase. Direct oxidant damage to endothelial cells, direct injury of matrix proteoglycans, and indirect damage to matrix proteins resulting from impairment of antiproteolytic mechanisms all combine to injure the alveolocapillary unit. Such injury may be manifest on an acute basis as a capillary leak and subsequent pulmonary edema or as more chronic tissue injury.

The release of oxidants has been demonstrated *in vitro* employing asbestos fibers and PMN.

Degradative Enzymes: Proteases. PMN contain a wide range of enzymes capable of degrading lipid, proteinaceous, and carbohydrate-containing molecules. Many such enzymes are localized within the two types of neutrophil granules that may properly be termed lysosomes. Aside from the substrate specificity, there are two distinct groups of degradative enzymes characterized by the relative pH optima. Those with acid pH optima tend to be more strictly granule associated and probably operate when the lysosomal granuole fuses with a phagocytic vacuole to produce a phagolysosome in which the pH is about 6.0. The second group is more important with respect to matrix injury, and includes certain neutral proteases whose pH optima is in the range of 7.4 to 8.0. These enzymes are released from PMN into the extracellular fluid and can attack native, insoluble, cross-linked structural matrix materials in the extracellular environment whose pH is presumed to be approximately 7.4. Two of the best studied of these enzymes are elastase and collagenase,[33] both of which are stored pre-formed in the PMN granules. These enzymes are released by the same factors that promote oxidant activity by PMN. Proteolytic tissue injury depends on an initial attack on insoluble matrix materials in the extracellular environment, followed by partial degradation of such molecules which are subsequently either further degraded by other proteases or ingested and exposed to intralysosomal acid proteases.

There is an important distinction, however, between the release of oxidants and proteases. The latter require functioning cytoplasmic microtubular structures for granule movement and hence protease exteriorization. Oxidant release, however, is a surface phenomenon and does not require such microtubule-directed crytoplasmic granule migration. Thus, colchicine, an inhibitor of microtubule reassembly, will diminish lysosomal degranulation and protease release, but has little or no effect on oxidant responses by PMN.

Two key PMN enzymes in matrix digestion are collagenase and elastase. These enzymes are biochemically well characterized, and their molecular actions are relatively well defined.[33, 34] PMN elastase attacks elastin, type IV collagen,[35] laminin, fibronectin, and blood clotting factors. As such, it is a more general protease than its name suggests. PMN elastase activity against elastin is enhanced by a platelet product (PF_4), thus indirectly involving platelets in tissue injury,[36] PMN elastase reacts on a

molar basis with alpha-1-antiprotease in its reduced form and also with alpha-2-macroglobulin to form protease-antiprotease complexes. Such complexes with alpha-1-antiprotease are inactive against native elastin. Those with alpha-2-macroglobulin have been reported to be active against elastin[37] and certainly attack certain low-molecular-weight elastin residues and oligopeptides. Once these complexes are formed, they can be subsequently ingested by macrophages. There is also a low-molecular-weight bronchial protease inhibitor of neutrophil elastase. Thus, there are natural inhibitor systems for this enzyme.

Neutrophil collagenase is a more specific enzyme for collagen[38] and fibronectin.[35] It has no effects on elastin. It attacks native insoluble collagen fibrils (type I but not type III), cleaving collagen molecules at a single point. Such cleavage permits unfolding of the collagen helical structure and its subsequent attack by other less specific proteolytic enzymes active both at neutral and acid pH. Collagenase also differs from elastase in that it does not have a serine group at its active site, is a zinc-containing metalloproteinase, and is not inhibited by alpha-1-antiprotease.

Both of these enzymes are implicated in the pathogenesis of a number of nonoccupational lung diseases. The currently accepted theory of the pathogenesis of emphysema states that this disorder largely results from the digestion of structural proteins including elastin as a result of an imbalance between proteases and antiproteases. The digestion of elastin and other matrix proteins leads to a loss of elastic recoil. Elastase may also play an important role in more acute diseases such as the adult respiratory distress syndromes (ARDS), in which large numbers of PMNs, high concentrations of free elastase, and significant oxidation of alpha-1-antiprotease have all been demonstrated in BAL fluid.[39] While there are no known occupational diseases that parallel generalized emphysema, local emphysema-like changes and cavitation are features of certain pneumoconioses, e.g., silicosis and coal workers' pneumoconiosis. Some occupational disorders resemble ARDS. Among these are paraquat inhalation, polyethylene fume fever, and perhaps exposure to sublimates of metals. Certainly PMN mobilization to the lung has been demonstrated in paraquat exposure, and paraquat itself is a powerful oxidizing substance. There are no direct studies of this mechanism in other acute occupational diseases.

There are two diseases in which both BAL leukocytosis and free collagenase in BAL fluid occur, idiopathic pulmonary fibrosis (IPF)[40] and asbestosis.[41, 42] Collagenase may be responsible for disordered collagen metabolism, but precisely how this leads to fibrosis is presently unclear.

Mononuclear Phagocytes

Mononuclear phagocytes derived from maturation of bone-marrow stem cells differentiate first into circulating blood monocytes and subsequently into tissue macrophages which in the lung are termed alveolar

macrophages (AM). AM are easily recovered from human lungs by BAL and their biochemistry and other functions can be readily examined. In the normal nonsmoking person, BAL cellular yield is around 10 million cells, of which approximately 80 per cent are AM. Lavage of otherwise healthy smokers' lungs yields 5 to 10 times more cells, of which 95 per cent are AM. When studied in tissue culture, the cells from smokers are more adherent to tissue culture vessels and show enhanced secretory activity, particularly of such enzymes as lysozyme (muramidase). Classically, following Metchnikoff, macrophages were largely regarded as scavenger cells. While this is an important function, there are other very important functions of mononuclear phagocytes which will be detailed in the following discussion.[43-45]

Adaptive and Biosynthetic Activity. The differentiation of circulating monocytes into tissue phagocytes varies with local organ conditions. For instance, macrophages found within the peritoneum are characteristically anaerobic in their energy metabolism, whereas AM, which reside at the relatively high oxygen tension in the lung, preferentially use aerobic metabolism as a source of ATP generation. Both animal and human AM are relatively rich in mitochondria and show brisk oxidative phosphorylation. In addition to adaptations specific for the tissue in which the macrophage resides, other adaptations to local perturbations of the chemical environment in the lung occur. Such specific intrapulmonary adaptations include the production of aryl hydrocarbon hydroxylase by human AM derived from cigarette smokers, who have necessarily been exposed to such polycyclic hydrocarbons as benzpyrene. Additionally, tissue-cultured rabbit AM grown in the presence of red cells develop a heme-oxidase which is not present in the normal cell.

Biosynthetic Products. Table 7–2 lists a number of the more important of the some 50 known products of AM.

Chemotactic Factor for PMN. The AM can regulate the migration of PMN from circulation to lung tissue and air spaces by factors produced by macrophages in many species including man. These factors have been recently reviewed by Reynolds[46] and include protein- and lipid-containing factors released by AM following phagocytosis of many materials including bacteria, antigen-antibody complexes, asbestos fibers, and certain forms of silica. Chemotactic factor not only mobilizes PMN, but also stimulates PMN to release oxidants and proteases. The combination of mobilization and secretogogue functions of the chemotactic factors is an interesting economy of nature's signaling system. In this manner, therefore, the AM can serve as a regulator of acute inflammatory responses within the lung. These responses may be appropriate where bacteria invade the lung, since they induce a PMN antimicrobial response. However, persistent PMN mobilization occurring with nonbiodegradable factors such as asbestos fibers may be injurious. These factors are readily released by relatively minimal stimuli. For instance, in primates, repeated BAL alone results in their release, and accumulation of PMN within the air spaces rises from a

normal of 1 per cent to about 10 per cent with repeated lavages. Thus, it is likely that many occupationally inhaled stimuli may trigger chemotactic factor release.

In patients with IPF, AM recovered by BAL when placed in tissue culture rapidly release supernormal amounts of PMN chemoattractants in those patients with high PMN counts in their lavage fluid. In IPF, the factor is a low-molecular-weight lipid component. There are suggestions that in this disease, the excessive release is associated with immune complex deposition. It has been suggested that asbestos may form a nidus upon which complexes may be deposited or alternatively act as an adjuvant in promoting immune responses, thus enhancing local antibody-antigen complexing.

There are two groups of inflammatory mediators generated by AM (Table 7–2). The first group are products of arachidonic acid. Of these,

Table 7–2. SECRETORY PRODUCTS OF MONONUCLEAR
PHAGOCYTES*

Enzymes	*Bioactive Lipids*
Lysozyme	Arachidonate metabolites
Neutral proteases	Prostaglandin E$_2$
Plasminogen activator	6-keto-Prostaglandin F$_{2a}$ (from
Collagenase	prostacyclin)
Elastase	Thromboxane
Angiotensin convertase	Leukotriene (including slow-
Acid hydrolases	reacting substance of
Proteases	anaphylaxis)
Lipases	Hydroxy-eicosatetraeneoic acids
(deoxy)Ribonucleases	Platelet-activating factor
Phosphatases	
Glycosidases	*Neutrophil Chemotactic Factor*
Sulfatases	
Arginases	*Factors Promoting Replication of:*
	Interleukin I (endogenous
Complement Components	pyrogen)
C1	Myeloid precursors (colony-
C4	stimulating factors)
C2	Erythroid precursors
C3	Fibroblasts
C5	Microvasculature
Factor B	
Factor D	*Factors Inhibiting Replication of:*
Properdin	Lymphocytes
C3b inactivator	Tumor cells
Enzyme Inhibitors	*Nucleosides and Metabolites*
Plasmin inhibitors	Thymidine
Alpha-2-macroglobulin	Uracil
	Uric acid
Binding Proteins	
Transferrin	
Transcobalamin II	
Fibronectin	

*Modified from Nathan, C. F., Murray, H. W., Cohn, Z. A., et al.: The macrophage as an effector cell. N. Engl. J. Med., *303*:622, 1980.

some products (for instance, prostaglandin E_2) are antichemotactic. However, other arachidonic acid products by the lipoxygenase pathway (certain leukotrienes) are extremely potent PMN chemoattractants. The second group are complement-derived factors, some of which are synthesized in vitro by human AM (C3 and C5). It is likely that both groups are produced in response to particulate challenge. In addition, free complement factors are present in BAL fluid from normal subjects, for which AM may be one source. Parenthetically, many solid phase materials (asbestos fibers, insoluble antigen-antibody complexes) activate the complement system, producing, among other materials, the powerful secretogogue and chemoattractant C5a.

To summarize, there is ample evidence that the AM exerts an important influence on the PMN responses in the lung so regulating inflammation.

Other Cell Interaction Factors. Human AM are a source of interleukin 1, a compound responsible for the activation of lymphocytes. This compound is now known to be identical with endogenous pyrogen. Another important compound is platelet-activating factor, whose chemistry is now well known.[47] This factor may play a role in asthma, mediating bronchoconstriction and also changes in capillary permeability. Human AM also release a fibroblast proliferating factor of importance in fibrosing occupational lung disorders.

Oxidant Responses. As previously indicated, PMN generate highly toxic free radicals. Monocytes and tissue macrophages, including human AM, also generate oxidants[48] that are probably important intracellular antimicrobial factors, e.g., against mycobacteria. However, they release smaller amounts of such materials into the tissue culture medium and presumably into the extracellular fluid *in vivo*. During the differentiation of monocytes into tissue macrophages, there is an increase in the activity of a number of systems that detoxify these oxidants within the cell, thereby limiting their extracellular oxidant release. These systems include catalase, present in high concentrations in rabbit and human AM, which causes the oxidoreduction of hydrogen peroxide to water and molecular oxygen. Additionally, AM contain superoxide dismutase, which generates hydrogen peroxide from superoxide anion. More importantly, a cytoplasmic glutathione system similar to that present in the red cells exists in AM. The pathways involved in glutathione system are indicated in Fig. 7–6. The pathway is quantitatively the single most important antioxidant defense system of the cell. Regeneration of NADPH by the pentose shunt and glutathione reductase are responsible for maintenance of high levels of reduced glutathione, which in turn maintains normal microtubular function. This same glutathione system is important in detoxificaiton of lipid hydroperoxides generated by the oxidation of unsaturated fatty acids. Lipid hydroperoxides initiate self-perpetuating chain reactions that irreversibly impair cell membrane function and structures. Both glutathione and vitamin E (alpha-tocopherol) are important defense mechanisms against oxidant injury by biologically generated oxidizing free radicals and

those present in cigarette smoke and by environmental exposure to oxidants. All three of these antioxidants are largely intracellular, though catalase release follows phagocytosis by PMN and AM. There is one other important circulating antioxidant, an acute phase-reactant copper containing protein ceruloplasmin, whose role in lung diseases is largely univestigated.

Degradative Enzymes. AM contain a wide range of lysosomal enzymes. Some of these, including such proteolytic enzymes as the cathepsins, are stored in pre-formed lysosomes. In addition, beta-glucuronidase, beta-galactosidase, and a number of lipid-splitting enzymes are also present. One important enzyme, lysozyme (muramidase), which is partially stored in the cytoplasm, requires relatively continuous synthesis for its secretion into the external medium. Lysozyme is weakly microbicidal and exerts an interesting antichemotactic effect on PMN.

In mononuclear phagocytes, there is considerable species variation in the presence of the two important neutral proteases described by PMN, collagenase and elastase. Collagenase is certainly present in rabbit AM, where it is in turn activated by another neutral protease. Neither of the latter enzymes is stored in the cell and both require continuous protein synthesis. Rat AM produce an elastase with similar properties to the mouse peritoneal macrophage, a metalloproteinase capable of attacking native elastin. Human monocytes contain a nonsecreted serine protease elastase.[49] Activation of peritoneal macrophages evokes the secretion of a metalloproteinase elastase, which attacks native elastin and also degrades alpha-1-antiprotease.[50] In human AM there is considerable debate concerning the presence of such an elastase but collagenase has not been detected in human AM. As regards elastase, there are three reports claiming the presence of a metalloenzyme based on assays employing three substrates: a chromophore-like elastin peptide (succinyl-trialanine-paranitrophenylphosphate), solubilized elastin, and tritium-labeled native elastin. Conclusive proof that this is true extracellular elastase is lacking.[51] However, human AM can ingest complexes of PMN elastase with either alpha-1-antiprotease or alpha-2-macroglobulin. In addition, human PMN elastase

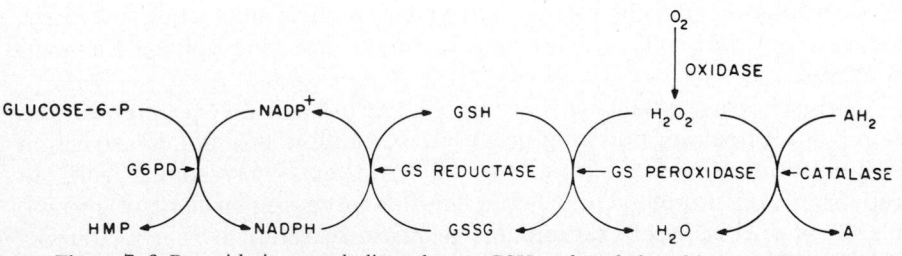

Figure 7–6. Peroxidative metabolic pathways. GSH, reduced glutathione; GSSG, oxidized glutathione; G6PD, glucose-6-phosphate dehydrogenase; HMP, hexose monophosphate shunt; AH$_2$ represents unknown hydrogen donors for catalase. GS reductase and GS peroxidase refer to glutathione enzymes.

Table 7–3. THE ROLE OF ALVEOLAR MACROPHAGES (AM) IN
PROTEOLYSIS

*Increased Proteolysis:**
1. Mobilizes PMN (chemotaxins)
2. Provokes PMN elastase relase
3. Secretes neutral proteases, collagenase, and elastase
4. Contains lysosomal acid proteases, cathepsins
5. Other lysosomal hydrolases
6. Oxidant damage to protease inhibitors

Decreased Proteolysis:
1. Binds and ingests PMN elastase
2. Contains alpha-1-antitrypsin
3. Contains cytosol antiprotease
4. Alpha-2-macroglobulin synthesis
5. Ingests protease:antiprotease complexes

*Numbers 1 through 5 depend on AM activation.

can bind to human AM cell membranes and be subsequently ingested without precomplexing with either of the antiproteases. Some of this PMN elastase can be released as an active elastase. Thus, the role of AM in regulation of elastinolysis is a complex one (Table 7–3) and exhibits much species variation.[52]

The distinction between the two types of elastase has been shown by studies employing inhibitors. The macrophage enzyme, a metalloproteinase, is inhibited by chelating agents, whereas the PMN enzyme (serine protease) is inhibited by a group of relatively specific oligopeptide chloromethylketone inhibitors and also by alpha-1-antiprotease.

Mouse peritoneal macrophages and human monocytes also secrete another neutral protease, plasminogen activator,[53] which catalyzes the formation of plasmin from plasminogen (a circulating enzyme). Plasmin, in turn, lyses fibrin and activates complement factors (C_1 and C_3) and Hageman factor, thus releasing several inflammatory mediators. Plasmin also acts on tissue matrices, possibly on glycosaminoglycans. This action may be important in exposing fibrillar proteins to the action of collagenases and elastases. These actions are potentiated by direct surface contact between macrophages and the matrix.[54] Additionally, there is a positive feedback loop inherent in these enzyme activities, since their products, complement and collagen cleavage fragments, are macrophage chemoattractants.

Mononuclear phagocytes are important in such diverse processes as skin wound healing, postpartum uterine involution, and bone destruction in periodontal disease. Monocytes and AM may play similar roles in repairing and inducing lung injury by the foregoing proteolytic mechanisms. Suppression of macrophage protease secretion by corticosteroids and lymphocyte-activated protease secretion have been demonstrated to date only in animal studies; determination of the factors affecting human AM function requires further study.

Response to Inhaled Materials. Macrophage activity in occupational lung disease focus partly on its scavenger function (Fig. 7–7). The ultimate response of the macrophage depends on the nature of the particle scavenged.[55] For instance, in occupational infectious diseases the macrophage plays an antimicrobial role and can kill and digest bacteria. For nonbiodegradable particles, the AM sequester and transport such materials as coal dust, hematite, and a number of other minerals. Neither of the first two particles causes any long-term change in macrophage function. A third type of particle, silica, is readily ingested by phagocytes but produces major cellular dysfunction.[56] Morphological and biochemical evidence of mcarophage lysosomal membrane injury is well documented, but the precise mechanism for this remains uncertain. Two mechanisms are generally proposed, (1) hydrogen bonding of silica to lysosomal membranes with subsequent fragility of that membrane, and (2) activation of a lysosomal membrane phospholipase, thus degrading the lipids of the membrane. However, silica ultimately causes cell autolysis by lysosomal digestion of the cytoplasm. Thus, silica particles can be recycled through a series of macrophages. Silica (quartz) causes *in vitro* lipid peroxidation in guinea pig macrophages.[57] Vitamin E has been reported to prevent lung fibrosis following quartz exposure *in vivo*. These impaired macrophages exhibit deficient antimycobacterial activity.

Asbestos fibers produce different effects.[56] In general, asbestos fibers are relatively nontoxic for macrophages. Fibers longer than 10 to 20 micrometers are not completely ingested by macrophages, which presumably transport them poorly. Fibers of these or greater lengths, when deposited in the lung, are thought to be more fibrogenic than smaller

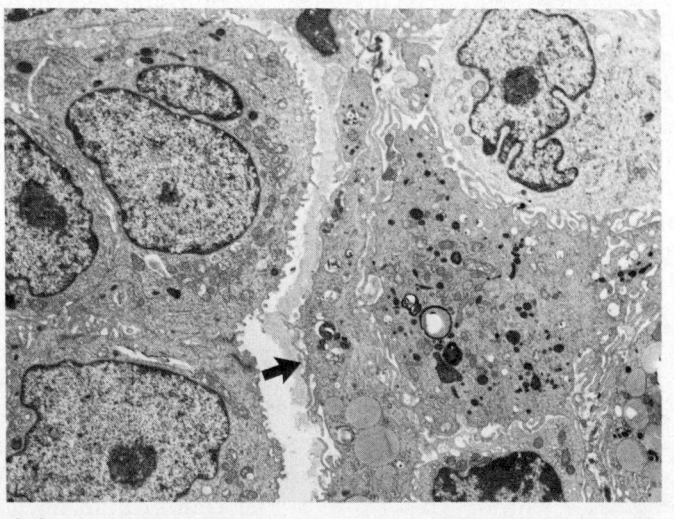

Figure 7–7. Macrophage response. Patient is an industrial worker with pulmonary fibrosis. An AM (arrow) with ruffled cell surface and many inclusions is seen adjacent to the two undifferentiated pneumocytes at left.

ones. The action of asbestos fibers may depend on sialic acid groups in cell membrane glycoproteins and be mediated by the surface charge of the fiber.[58] Asbestos fibers release lysosomal enzymes, cause variable changes in the secretion of neutral proteases, and activate a cell membrane phospholipase, with resulting release of arachidonic acid, the precursor of both prostaglandins and such lipoxygenase products as the leukotrienes. However, there is little or no cell autolysis seen morphologically or suggested biochemically by the release of cytosol LDH into tissue culture media. Asbestos also stimulates macrophages to release fibronectin. Ingestion of crocidolite by AM increases the number of surface receptors for complement (C3) and the Fc component of IgG. This and other observations on AM are of uncertain significance but could imply a heightened immune responsiveness.[59]

Finally, in immunological occupational lung diseases such as farmer's lung, pigeon breeder's lung, and beryllium disease, the presentation of antigens to lymphocytes requires processing by macrophages. In sarcoidosis, experimental studies show enhanced processing of an exogenous antigen, tetanus toxoid, by human AM. Whether similar enhancement occurs in occupational hypersensitivity diseases needs examination.

Lymphocytes

The recognition of a well-organized lymphoid system in the lung dates back to the 1880s. Bienenstock has emphasized the ability of the bronchus-associated lymphoid tissue to mount a specifically local immune response within the lung itself. In addition to their role in immune defenses, lymphocytes have recently been heavily implicated in the control of such mesenchymal cells as fibroblasts. BAL has permitted detailed studies of cell-mediated immunity in many and detailed observations on the nature of lymphocytes present within lavage fluid.

Lymphoid Organization. Lymphoid structures contain four anatomical groups: (1) the classical hilar, paraductal, paratracheal, and subcarinal lymph nodes, (2) the bronchus-associated lymphoid tissue, (3) lymphoid clusters and free lymphocytes within the alveolocapillary parenchyma, and (4) free lymphocytes within the peripheral air spaces available to study by BAL. The bronchus-associated lymphoid tissue has a lymphoepithelial junction permitting the direct exposure of airways antigens to superficial lymphocytes within the organized lymphoid tissue. Likewise, free luminal lymphocytes are presumably capable of responding immediately to antigens presented to them. Some 10 to 20 per cent of the total nucleated cells in normal BAL fluid are lymphocytes. In certain stages of immunologically mediated diseases (sarcoidosis, berylliosis), there is a sharp rise in the percentage of lymphocytes, up to 80 per cent of total nucleated cells in BAL fluid.

Cell Types. Lymphocytes are of three general types, whose charac-

Table 7–4. GENERAL LYMPHOCYTE TYPES IN NORMAL HUMAN BRONCHOALVEOLAR LAVAGE (BAL)

Type	Total % Lymphocytes	Source	Some Functions
T cells	18–47	Thymus	Antigen Recognition Lymphokine Formation
B cells*	4–19	Bone Marrow	Antibody Production
Null cells†	Balance	?	?

*B cells show surface immunoglobulins of IgG, IgA, IgM, and IgD classes, the latter two being more prevalent. The quantities of IgG, IgA, and IgM classes of antibodies secreted are similar in normal lavage cells but will presumably change with the stage of B-cell proliferation and antibody secretion in disease.

B cells are responsible for the production of specific antibody in antigen-specific diseases, e.g., farmer's lung. They can also produce many different antibodies, present in low serum concentrations in such disorders as asbestosis and silicosis, a feature termed polyclonal B-cell activation.

†Null cells may be undifferentiated T or B cells.

teristics are summarized in Table 7–4. In addition to the recognition of these general types, there has been a recent explosion of information on the subsets of the T-cell population.[60] Aside from specific immunological responses, these cells control inflammation, repair, and lung defense and injury. The three T-cell subsets can be recognized functionally and can be identified with variable precision in different species by the use of monoclonal antibodies directed specifically against distinctive surface antigenic proteins present on the cellular subsets.

Helper T Cells (T_H). Some features of this subset of T cells are indicated in Table 7–5. T_H cells play roles in both humoral and cell-mediated immunity. For instance, the first two functions listed in Table 7–5 are important in the creation of a granulomatous response. After processing of an antigen by a combined macrophage-lymphocyte interaction, lymphocytes release a monocyte chemotactic factor which attracts monocytes to the site of antigen deposition. During this migration, monocytes mature into macrophages, which, together with the resident tissue macrophages, are immobilized in the granuloma by macrophage inhibition factor. The latter, together with a number of other materials elaborated by lymphocytes, appears to lead to activation of macrophages. Activation includes increased oxidant metabolism, lysosomal enzyme content, and

Table 7–5. FEATURES OF HELPER T CELLS (T_H)

1. Monocyte chemotactic factor release.
2. Macrophage immobilizing and activating factors.
3. Promotion of antibody production by B cells. For haptene-protein complexes (e.g., beryllium-protein complexes), B cells are antibody specific, with T_H is carrier specific.
4. Activation of cytotoxic T cells that attack "foreign" and tumor cells.
5. Reaction with macrophages. Macrophages present antigen to T cells and activate T-cell populations via interleukin I.

probably protease release. Subsequent maturation of macrophages into epithelioid giant cells occurs. These phenomena are readily seen in sarcoid and in certain stages of such immunological occupational disorders as farmer's lung and berylliosis.

The third and fourth items (Table 7–5) also serve host defense functions operating against microbes and tumors. The third feature is antibody production against specific microorganisms or other antigenic materials. Thus, aided by T_H, B cells are responsible for the precipitating antibodies in a variety of immune responses. In patients with pigeon breeder's disease, antibodies against pigeon serum exist in BAL fluid.[61] Whether they are formed by local lung B-cell transformation is uncertain. However, in a sensitized host, reinhalation of the antigen will lead to antigen-antibody complex formation within both peripheral air spaces and lung tissue. Depending on the particular ratio of antigen to antibodies and the physical form of the complexes, secondary alveolar inflammatory responses will result. These responses include activation of complement and of macrophages to release oxidants and PMN chemotactic factor, PMN mobilization, and further phagocyte-related tissue injury. The extent of this phenomenon in the lung may depend on local antibody formation and therefore not directly relate to serum antibody levels which reflect more systemic lymphocyte activation. This phenomenon is an example of normal lung antimicrobial defense mechanisms being subverted into a tissue injury mechanism in which the lung becomes secondarily injured, much as an innocent bystander at a crime.

The final feature, namely macrophage-active processing of antigen for presentation to T cells, is an important initiating event in many immune reactions.*

Elegant studies by BAL of pulmonary sarcoidosis by Hunninghake[63] and colleagues have demonstrated an alveolitis characterized by activated macrophages and a sharp increase in T-lymphocytes, largely T_H cells. To our knowledge, there are so far no such studies of this phase of such hypersensitivity lung diseases as those associated with thermophilic *Actinomycetes*. However, following lymphocyte transfer from one animal sensitized to pigeon serum to a second animal, the second animal develops disease following aerosol challenge with pigeon serum. This depends on a memory function, served by a subset of T cells.[61] A similar alveolitis has been described by Daniele and his colleagues in beryllium lung disease.[62]

Suppressor T Cells (T_S). The recognition of suppressor T cells by Gershon and colleagues affords a new dimension in immunoregulation. While much is known of the basic aspects of their lymphocyte biology

---

*For at least some of these reactions to occur, particularly foreign antigen recognition, both T cells and macrophages must recognize not only that the antigen is foreign to the host, but also that the two cell types themselves derive from the same host. This latter self-recognition is mediated by various components of the major histocompatibility complex. This latter phenomenon is termed "genetic restriction" and also affects reactions between certain lymphocyte subsets.

(including the presence on T_S of type 2 histamine receptors), their relevance to granulomatous disease is only beginning to emerge. It has been suggested that in the later stages of sarcoidosis, in which there is relative steroid resistance, the lung lavage lymphocyte population shifts from largely T_H to largely T_S cells.[63] The interplay between T_H and T_S cells probably also operates in pigeon breeder's disease. This interplay is suggested by studies of the disease in man[64] and in monkeys. Among pigeon breeders, only some become diseased. Both healthy and diseased breeders show somewhat similar levels of antibody to pigeon serum in serum and in BAL fluid. Similarly, the proliferative responses of both circulating and BAL lymphocytes to the predominantly T cell mitogen, phytohemagglutinin, differ little in health and disease. The difference specifically associated with disease seems to reside in the presence in diseased subjects of BAL lymphocytes which react with pigeon serum. The specific activation of lung lymphocytes could reflect either enhanced T_H cell activity in disease or enhanced T_S cell activity in healthy subjects. There are two lines of evidence that T_S activity may be very important. The first derives from studies on a small group of monkeys exposed to pigeon serum. All developed antibodies but only some acquired the disease. Low-dose irradiation, which mainly impairs T_S cell function, leads to disease in the healthy monkeys. Thus, the absence of disease is not a passive failure, but appears to be actively maintained by T_S cell function. The second evidence comes from preliminary studies by Moritz,[65] who showed increased numbers of T_S cells in the lung lavage of patients with pigeon breeder's disease in an inactive phase some months after recovery from the acute disease.

The notion that T_S cells play a role in terminating not only antibody production[60] but also both granulomata formation and lymphocytic alveolitis in postexposure hypersensitivity lung diseases is an appealing one. The suggestion also derives largely from analogies with schistosomiasis, another more fully studied granulomatous disorder that also affects the lung. Granulomata in this disorder undergo spontaneous "modulation" some 10 weeks after infestation. At this time T_S cells predominate among the T-cell populations within the granuloma around the schistosome egg. Further, granuloma size in this disorder can be manipulated by agents affecting either the number or the degree of activity of T_S cells. Enhanced T_S cell activity diminishes granuloma size.

Aside from the interplay between T_H and T_S cells in tissue injury and disease, evidence is now emerging that lymphocytes can modulate the behavior of mesenchymal cells involved in repair. For instance, prostaglandin E_2 produced by "lymphocytes" inhibits fibroblast proliferation. T-lymphocytes, stimulated by mitogens, promote fibroblast growth.[66-68] The factor responsible differs from phagocyte-derived factors. Likewise, in one granulomatous disorder, that due to Schistosoma mansoni, fibroblast stimulation factors also occur.[69] Asbestos also produces effects on lymphocytes, but their relevance to disease is unclear.[69, 70]

Mast Cells

The involvement of mast cells in asthma is recognized widely. Their role in immunoregulation, their control by lymphocytes, and their relation to mesenchymal cell function and IPF are now becoming evident.

Most of these cells are normally found in the lung parenchyma, below the basement membrane of the epithelial cells of the airway lumen, but a small number of these cells may also be found in the airways. Their granules are sources of a number of inflammatory mediators and smooth muscle constrictive agents, including histamine, serotonin (5-hydroxytryptamine [5HT]), eosinophil chemotactic factors, heparin, a number of proteases, and slow reacting substances (leukotrienes).

The involvement of 5HT in delayed hypersensitivity reactions,[71] at least in mice, has been established by a number of pharmacological studies, notably those by Askenase and Gershon. For instance, reserpine, a 5HT-depleting agent, diminishes these reactions. The effect of reserpine can be abrogated by preventing the oxidation of monoamines such as 5HT with a monoamine oxidase inhibitor (pargyline). Cyproheptadine, a competitive antagonist of both 5HT and histamine, also modifies these reactions. Morphological and autoradiographical (with tritiated 5HT) studies of mast cell degranulation confirm this effect. In contrast with anaphylaxis, massive degranulation of mast cells does not occur in delayed hypersensitivity reactions. However, in delayed reactions, pseudopodial movement, fusion of some granules with the cell membrane, and accompanying release of 5HT all occur during the evolution of murine-delayed skin hypersensitivity reactions. The release of 5HT causes gaps to be formed between vascular endothelial cells. Colloidal carbon and PMN move from the circulation to tissue spaces through these gaps. In this manner, tissue mast cells regulate both vascular integrity and the inflammatory effects of PMN on tissues.

Pharmacological and immunological manipulations in this system demonstrate that the function of mast cells is regulated by T-lymphocytes, as opposed to the IgE-mediated antigen-antibody complexes seen in allergic asthma. Whether histamine, another major mediator produced by mast cells, terminates the immune responses by reacting with the type 2 histamine receptor on T_s cells needs further study.

The relation between mast cells, T-lymphocytes, PMN, and vascular endothelial cells provides an integrated feedback circuit between inflammatory, immunological, and structural cells. Another example of this type of cellular cooperation between inflammatory and structural cells involves fibroblasts and mast cells.[72] In tissue culture, a single fibroblast can phagocytose many extruded mast cell granules, a phenomenon also microscopically observable in skin biopsies. Thereby, the proteolytic actions of such granule-associated materials as chymotrypsin are terminated. In turn, these granules influence fibroblast behavior. Depending on the number of granules ingested, the enzymes beta-hexosaminidase and col-

lagenase are released by the fibroblasts. Such collagenase is capable of injuring matrix proteins.

In idiopathic pulmonary fibrosis (IPF), lung biopsies show excess numbers of mast cells, some of which are partially degranulated.[73] Haslam showed an average twofold rise in the histamine content of BAL fluid from patients with IPF.[74] Histamine levels correlated with the neutrophil and eosinophil counts from the BAL fluid in these patients. While there was no statistical correlation with the biopsy mast cell counts, both the BAL leukocytosis and histamine levels appeared to be related to a measurement of fibrosis in these biopsies. These clinical studies, although suggestive, do not define a pathogenetic sequence which is implied by the foregoing cell biology studies. A role for mast cells in occupational lung disease is therefore suggested in asbestosis and delayed hypersensitivity disorders.

REPAIR AND INJURY: PULMONARY FIBROSIS

Pulmonary fibrosis is an all too common chronic disabling disorder resulting either spontaneously or from several industrial diseases, including asbestosis and silicosis. Occupational causes also include repeated acute or chronic exposure to substances known to cause hypersensitivity lung disease. In IPF, the involvement of the immunological system in the production of pulmonary fibrosis is evident from the association of this disorder with a variety of diseases of an autoimmune type (rheumatoid arthritis, scleroderma, etc). Likewise, pulmonary fibrosis of industrial origin is frequently associated with extrapulmonary manifestations of an immune type, e.g., Caplan's syndrome or scleroderma in silicosis.

It is not currently possible to give a comprehensive account of the mechanisms of pulmonary fibrosis; however, three general conceptual points can be made. First, during the growing period and throughout life, lung cells and lung matrix are continually recycled, with renewal producing either expansion or preservation of normal architecture and function. Second, following injury, under many circumstances the lung is capable of reconstituting a relatively normal architectural and functional framework with little evidence of fibrosis. Thus, an important conceptual question concerning pulmonary fibrosis is, why do certain acute or chronic inflammatory states so disrupt this repair function as to lead to fibrosis?

Third, as classical anatomical pathologists have for many years insisted, pulmonary fibrosis is seen only in disorders in which there is significant damage to the basement membranes upon which endothelial and type I cells reside. They have thus emphasized that cellular renewal following injury requires a preservation at least of this component of the normal lung architecture. For the lung, the first experimental support for this view was provided by Vracho,[75] who employed oleic acid to produce an ARDS model. Where the basement membrane was preserved, type II

cells regenerated a normal lung architecture. Destruction of the basement membrane resulted in fibrosis. This view is consistent with the evidence presented earlier, which suggested the critical importance of the matrix cellular interactions in the differentiation and normal function of lung cells. However, the matrix itself is synthesized by epidermal and mesenchymal cells including type II cells, fibroblasts, and smooth muscle cells. Thus there is a complex interplay between the effects of matrix upon the cell function and the effects of cell function on matrix formation. The intimate details of this regulation are currently the subject of much investigation, the results of which will provide a more firm basis upon which to develop a comprehensive view of pulmonary fibrosis and ultimately ameliorate it by therapeutic maneuvers.

The following bear upon the hypothesis that impaired cell matrix repair leads to disorderly fibrosis.

1. We have already reviewed the evidence, summarized in Table 7–6, that matrix materials can be degraded by secretion products of phagocytes such as oxidants, proteases, and other degradative enzymes. Both asbestosis and IPF are associated with free uninhibited collagenase in the air spaces, and it has been suggested that the prognosis in IPF directly relates to the number of PMN obtained by BAL. The matrix proteins generally attacked by AM (in some species) and PMN products include collagen, elastin, proteoglycans, and fibronectin. These comprise the major components not only of basement membranes but also of lung interstitium, and inflammatory damage to them clearly can occur. Such damage specifically extends to the basement membrane.

2. The interrelation between the injury cell, e.g., PMN or AM, and the matrix is important. For instance, the products and movements of these cells may vary with the nature of the surface on which they reside. Certainly, enhanced matrix injury occurs at points of contact between macrophages and the matrix surface.[54] Campbell et al.[76] examined the relative importance of cell-surface contact and oxidative inactivation of protease inhibitors. They employed PMN layered to provide direct contact with ^{125}I-labeled fibronectin surfaces. They showed that PMN-derived oxidants did not protect secreted elastase from inhibition by alpha-1-antiprotease. Additionally, they demonstrated that under these conditions, both alpha-1-antiprotease and alpha-2-macroglobulin did not inhibit PMN elastase as effectively as they could inhibit PMN elastase in solution. This observation suggests that cell-surface contact zones may exclude various soluble phase materials such as antiproteases and antioxidants as ceruloplasmin. Matrix injury is even more complicated than the degradation of a single material such as elastin and involves several enzymes in sequence, e.g., plasmin and elastase. Finally, the matrix has profound effects on platelets, which can release powerful mediators. For instance, exposed "collagen" activates platelets. Exposure of collagen can readily occur following basement membrane injury, thus amplifying an already injurious cascade.

Table 7–6. MATRIX INJURY MECHANISMS

Injury Mechanisms		AM	PMN	Protective Mechanisms	Target Extracellular Macromolecules
O$_2^-$, etc.		+ +	+ + +	SOD* Catalase CP*	Hyaluronic acid
Elastase	S/M*	±	+ + +	Alpha-1-antiprotease	Elastin Collagen IV Fibronectin Glycosaminoglycans
Collagenase	M	0	+ + +		Collagen I–IV Fibronectin
Trypsin†	S	ND*	+ + +	Alpha-1-antiprotease	Collagen III
Chymotrypsin†	S	ND	+ + +	Alpha-1-antiprotease	Fibronectin

*S = serine; M = metallo; CP = ceruloplasmin; SOD = superoxide dismutase; ND = not done.

†Trypsin and chymotrypsin are acid proteases and are relatively tightly bound to PMN granules. While they certainly act on the indicated substrates, the physical or contact conditions for this action need elucidation.

3. The cell-to-cell sorting and cell-to-matrix adhesion for fibroblasts, macrophages, endothelial cells, and smooth muscle cells has already been stressed. These cells not only adhere to the matrix, but can generate many of the proteins contained in the matrix. There are suggestions that type II cells can produce basement membrane proteins. Collagen is not the sole component of the acellular material present in lung fibrosis; probably all matrix components are present in a "disorganized" manner. Fibronectin is the major component present in the progressive massive fibrosis in coal workers' lungs.[26]

4. Fibroblasts, a source of many matrix proteins, respond to beta-agonists and a number of factors produced by other cells, including macrophages and lymphocytes, and also to other chemoattractants such as fibronectin and species of prostaglandins. Macrophages from patients with IPF produce larger quantities of fibronectin.[25] Silica has long been known to stimulate macrophages to produce filterable compounds capable of activating fibroblasts.[77] Initially, much of the research suggested enhanced collagen production by a given number of fibroblasts; however, some of the early methods employed to measure collagen production were invalid. More recent evidence suggests the effects are largely chemoattractant and proliferative but in some instances cause an increase in the production rates of matrix proteins. However, the evidence clearly indicates that fibroblasts will be recruited to areas of active inflammation by macrophage and lymphocyte activation at those inflammatory sites.

In addition to cell-derived factors affecting fibroblast functions, hu-

man type I, II, and III collagens and certain collagen degradation products are also skin fibroblast chemoattractants under *in vitro* conditions.[78] Synthetic tri- and dipeptides present in collagen molecules, notably those containing hydroxyproline, are also chemotactic. Postlethwaite and colleagues have proposed the following sequence, whereby tissue injury leads to fibroblast mobilization. In normal matrices, collagen is shielded by interfibril glycosaminoglycans. Degradation of the latter by inflammatory processes exposes the collagens to cleavage and further degradation. These degradation products in turn evoke fibroblast migration. As a result, tissue injury evokes tissue repair mechanisms.

There is room for more research on questions concerning lung fibroblasts. Do fibroblast clones with widely differing production rates for different collagens exist? What regulates the relative amounts of collagen and collagenase secretion? Fibroblasts are phagocytic cells; what does this imply for repair processes? Fibroblasts in tissue culture show "contact inhibition" of their replication. Does this phenomenon operate *in vivo*?

5. The replacement of injured type I cells by proliferation and differentiation of type II cells has already been mentioned. Thus, even in the presence of a normal basement membrane, following some inflammatory or toxic destruction of type I cells, the factors affecting the differentiation of type II cells assume considerable importance. These factors are poorly understood, and the need for more research on them is clearly emphasized by some important experiments by Witschi and colleagues.[79] This group employed a number of injury mechanisms, including hyperoxia, chemical compounds, and radiation, to investigate the effects of a second injury applied some three days after an initial injury—for example, the application of hyperoxia following radiation. They showed, under certain circumstances, that type II cell proliferation can be prevented by such second injuries at that time. Where a second injury was employed, there was a somewhat greater general inflammatory response, and, more importantly, the failure of type II cell proliferation was associated with subsequent fibrosis. Under these circumstances, fibroblast proliferation replaces the normal type II cell differentiation. This may lead to a disorderly excessive deposition of matrix proteins, rather than an organized re-epithelialization by type II–derived type I cells. Alternatively, the cuboidal epithelium, often seen lining the air spaces in IPF, may arise from type II cell failure. These cuboidal cells morphologically resemble those present in the early embryonic stage of lung development and may redevelop in the face of type II cell failure.

Bleomycin, an antimitotic cancer chemotherapy drug, affects DNA synthesis and causes pulmonary fibrosis. Bleomycin is believed to affect type II cell division, and leads to the formation of abnormal giant cells.

In hard metal lung disease, nongranulomatous, intra-alveolar, interstitial inflammatory and mildly fibrosing responses occur. Transmission electron microscopy shows the presence of bizarre giant forms of AM in BAL fluid and of type II cells in biopsy specimens obtained from the

lungs of tool grinders who work with tungsten carbide–cobalt high-speed steels.[80] While the mechanisms responsible for this disease remain poorly defined, it is clear that in addition to the predictable uptake of metal dust by AM, type II cells are also affected.

6. A unifying theory for fibrosis, therefore, focuses on matrix injury and impaired type II cell function, together with the proliferative and secretory activities of mesenchymal cells. Nonbiodegradable particulates and repeated exposure will produce persistent inflammatory responses, thus perpetuating injury to both matrix and type II cells. This hypothesis has implications for both prevention and therapy. In accord with clinical observations, established fibrosis is irreversible, since slow turnover matrix proteins are already laid down. Blocking collagen synthesis in the lung alone is probably unachievable. Thus, therapy must focus on modifying the inflammatory response and protecting and enhancing the differentiation of type II cells. Aside from the removal of causal agents from the workplace, modification of the inflammatory potential of the agents may be important and can be examined *in vitro* with AM and PMN, and also with type II cells. Protection against the inflammatory compounds will require the development of either administerable antioxidants or antiproteases or the modulation of their release by steroid and nonsteroid antiinflammatory drugs and perhaps microtubule poisons like colchicine.

A novel approach to granulomatous disease therapy is based on the association of angiotensin converting enzyme (ACE) with certain granulomata and both macrophages and T-lymphocytes therefrom.[81, 82] Captopril, an inhibitor of ACE, diminishes the size of two granuloma types, those due to *S. mansoni*[83] and *M. tuberculosis*[84]; whether it diminishes postgranulomatous fibrosis is not known.

A further novel approach might employ analogues of vitamin A. These agents are cancer chemotherapeutic drugs that facilitate epithelial cell differentiation and diminish bronchial metaplasia in experimental animals exposed to asbestos,[85] and are also potential anti-inflammatory agents. One agent, retinoic acid, has an interesting anti-inflammatory effect on rheumatoid synovial cells.[86] Many joint diseases are, like lung diseases, due to oxidant and proteolytic tissue matrix injury. The latter depends on a collagenase and is influenced by prostaglandin E_2. Both these materials are produced by synovial cells under the control of a monocyte-derived factor. This bicellular system resembles the mononuclear phagocyte fibroblast relationship described earlier for lung disease. Collagenase production and PGE_2 formation, respectively, were completely and partially inhibited *in vitro* by two forms of retinoic acid at noncytotoxic concentrations that are probably safely achievable in man. While the biological actions of vitamin A analogues are complex, they offer a potentially fruitful therapeutic approach to lung disease.

Theoretically, drugs affecting basophil function and products might also be useful.

CONCLUSION

The foregoing account has been based on normal cellular and matrix biology, together with studies of lung disease in man. It is clear that the interplay between structural, phagocytic, and lymphocytic cells and basophils determines the inflammatory response and the repair mechanisms. Examples of these mechanisms in other tissues are instructive, particularly where they illuminate chronic tissue injury mechanisms. With these newer basic mechanisms as a background, much earlier work on occupational lung disease deserves re-study. One fruitful area of study is the role of lymphocyte and epithelial growth factors in the regulation of repair, cell differentiation, and fibrogenesis.

References

1. Kikkawa, Y., and Yoneda, K., The type II cell of the lung. I. Method of isolation. Lab. Invest., *30*, 76, 1974.
2. Mason, R. J., Williams, M. C., Greenleaf, R. D., et al., Isolation and properties of type II alveolar cells from rat lung. Am. Rev. Respir. Dis., *115*, 1015, 1977.
3. Dobbs, L. G., Geppert, E. F., Williams, M. C., et al., Metabolic properties of ultrastructure of alveolar type II cells isolated with elastase. Biochim. Biophys. Acta, *618*, 510, 1980.
4. Hance, A. J., and Crystal, R. G., Collagen. *In* Crystal, R. G., ed., The Biochemical Basis of Pulmonary Function. New York, Marcel Dekker, 1976, p. 215.
5. Reynolds, H. Y., Fulmer, J. D., Kazmiorowski, W. C., et al., Analysis of cellular and protein content of bronchoalveolar lavage fluid from patients with idiopathic pulmonary fibrosis and chronic hypersensitivity pneumonitis. J. Clin. Invest., *59*, 165, 1977.
6. Hunninghake, G. W., Gadek, J. E., Kawanami, O., et al., Inflammatory and immune processes in the human lung in health and disease: evaluation by bronchoalveolar lavage. Am. J. Pathol., *97*, 149, 1979.
7. Gee, J. B. L., and Fick, R. B., Jr., Bronchoalveolar lavage. Thorax, *35*:1, 1980.
8. Keogh, B. A., and Crystal R. G., Alveolitis: the key to the interstitial lung disorders. Thorax, *37*, 1, 1982.
9. Smith, B. T., Lung maturation in the fetal rat: acceleration by injection of fibroblast-pneumocyte factor. Science, *204*, 1094, 1979.
10. Adamson, I. Y. R., and Bowden, D. H., Type 2 cell as a progenitor of alveolar epithelial regeneration. A cytodynamic study in mice after exposure to oxygen. Lab. Invest. *30*, 35, 1974.
10a. Lwebuga-Mukasa, J., Unpublished observations, 1983.
11. Carvalho, A. C. A., Bellman, S., Saullo, J., et al., Altered plasma factor VIII antigen: a sensitive indicator of endothelial damage. Am. Rev. Respir. Dis., *123*, 98, 1981.
12. Ryan, U. S., and Ryan, J. W., Correlations between the fine structure of the alveolar-capillary unit and its metabolic activities. *In* Bakhle, Y. S., and Vane, J. R., eds., Metabolic Functions of the Lung. New York, Marcel Dekker, 1977, p. 197.
13. Gillis, N., and Greene, N. M.: Possible clinical implications of metabolism of blood borne substrates by the human lung. *In* Bakhle, Y. S., and Vane, J. R., eds., Metabolic Functions of the Lung. New York, Marcel Dekker, 1977, p. 173.
14. Kelman, J., Brin, S., Horwitz, A., et al., Collagen synthesis and collagenase production by human lung fibroblasts. Am. Rev. Respir. Dis., *115*, 343, 1977.
15. Bowden, D. H., Alveolar response to injury. Thorax, *36*, 801, 1981.
16. Begin, R., Rola-Pleszczynski, M., Sirois, P., et al., Early lung events following low-dose asbestos exposure. Environ. Res., *26*, 535, 1981.
17. Furthmayr, H., Immunization procedures, isolation by affinity chromatography and serological and immunochemical characterization of collagen-specific antibodies. *In*

Furthmayr, H., ed., Immunochemistry of the Extracellular Matrix, Vol I. Boca Raton, Fla., CRC Press Inc., 1982.

18. Madri, J. A., and Furthmayr, H., Collagen polymorphism in the lung: an immunochemical study of pulmonary fibrosis. Human Pathol., *11*, 353, 1980.

19. Kleinman, H. K., Rohrbach, D. H., Terranova, V. P., et al., Collagenous matrices as determinants of cell function. *In* Furthmayr, H., ed., Immunochemistry of the Extracellular Matrix, Vol II. Boca Raton, Fla., CRC Press Inc., 1982, p. 151.

20. Alescio, T., Effect of a proline analogue, azetidine-2-carboxylic acid, on the morphogenesis in vitro of mouse embryonic lung. J. Embryol. Exp. Morphol., *29*, 439, 1973.

21. Timpl, R., Rohde, H., Robey, P. G., et al., Laminin—a glycoprotein from basement membranes. J. Biol. Chem., *254*, 9933, 1979.

22. Couchman, J. R., Hook, M., Rees, D. A., et al., Adhesion growth and matrix production by fibroblasts on laminin substrates. J. Cell Biol., *96*, 177, 1983.

23. Mosesson, M. W., and Armani, D. L., The structure and biological activities of plasma fibronectin. Blood, *56*, 145, 1980.

24. Pearlstein, E. L., Gold, I., and Garcia-Pado, A., Fibronectin: a review of its structure and biological activity. Mol. Cell. Biochem., *29*, 103, 1980.

25. Rennard, S. I., and Crystal, R. G., Fibronectin in human bronchoalveolar lavage fluid. J. Clin. Invest., *69*, 113, 1981.

26. Wagner, J. C., Burns, J., Munday, D. E., et al., Presence of fibronectin in pneumoconiotic lesions. Thorax, *37*, 54, 1982.

27. Ross, R., The elastic fiber. J. Histochem. Cytochem., *21*, 199, 1973.

28. Sear, C. H. J., Grant, M. E., and Jackson, D. S., The nature of the microfibrillar glycoproteins of elastic fibres. Biochem. J., *194*, 587, 1981.

29. Klebanoff, S. J., and Clark, R. H., The Neutrophil: Function and Clinical Disorders. New York, North-Holland Publ. Co., 1978.

30. Fantone, J. C., and Ward, P. A., Role of oxygen-derived free radicals and metabolites in leukocyte-dependent inflammatory reaction. Am. J. Pathol., *107*, 396, 1982.

31. DelMaestro, R. F., An approach to free radicals in medicine and biology. Acta Physiol. Scand., *492*(Suppl), 153, 1980.

32. Janoff, A., Carp, H., Laurent, P., et al., The role of oxidative processes in emphysema. Am. Rev. Respir. Dis., *127*, S31, 1983.

33. Havemann, K., and Janoff, A., Neutral Proteases of Human Polymorphonuclear Leukocytes. Baltimore, Urban & Schwarzenberg, 1978.

34. Barrett, A. J., Proteinases in Mammalian Cells and Tissues. New York, North-Holland Publ. Co., 1977.

35. Crystal, R. G., and Rennard, S. I., Pulmonary connective tissue and environmental lung disease. Chest, *80*, 33S, 1981.

36. Lonky, S. A., and McCarren, J., Neutrophil enzymes in the lung: regulation of neutrophil elastase. Am. Rev. Respir. Dis., *127*, S9, 1983.

37. Stone, P. J., Calore, J. D., Snider, G. L., et al., Role of alpha-2-macroglobulin-elastase complexes in the pathogenesis of elastase-induced emphysema in hamsters. J. Clin. Invest., *69*, 920, 1982.

38. Horwitz, A. L., Hance, A. J., and Crystal, R. G., Granulocyte collagenase: selective digestion of type I over type III collagen. Proc. Natl. Acad. Sci. U.S.A., *74*, 897, 1977.

39. Cochrane, C. G., Spragg, R. G., Revak, S. D., et al., The presence of neutrophil elastase and evidence of oxidation activity in bronchoalveolar lavage fluid of patients with adult respiratory distress syndrome. Am. Rev. Respir. Dis., *127*, S25, 1983.

40. Gadek, J. E., Kelman, J. A., Fells, G. A., et al., Collagenase in the lower respiratory tract of patients with idiopathic pulmonary fibrosis. N. Engl. J. Med., *301*, 737, 1980.

41. Jaurand, M. C., Gaudichet, A., Atassi, K., et al., Relationship between the number of asbestos fibres and the cellular and enzymatic content of bronchoalveolar fluid in asbestos exposed subjects. Bull. Europ. Physiopath. Resp., *16*, 595, 1980.

42. Gadek, J., Hunninghake, G., Schoenberger, C., et al., Pulmonary asbestosis and idiopathic pulmonary fibrosis: pathogenetic parallels. Chest, *80*, 63S, 1981.

43. Gee, J. B. L., and Fick, R. B., Jr., Alveolar macrophage and nonrespiratory functions of the lung. *In* Altura, B. M., and Saba, T. M., ed., Pathophysiology of the Reticuloendothelial System. New York, Raven Press, 1981.

44. Nathan, C. F., Murray, H. W., and Cohn, Z. A., The macrophage as an effector cell. N. Engl. J. Med., *303*, 622, 1980.

45. Van Furth, R., Mononuclear Phagocytes in Immunity, Infection, and Pathology. Oxford, Blackwell Scientific Publications, 1975.
46. Reynolds, H. Y., Lung inflammation: role of endogenous chemotactic factors in attracting polymorphonuclear granulocytes. Am. Rev. Respir. Dis., 127, S16, 1983.
47. Arnoux, B., Duval, D., and Benveniste, J., Release of platelet-activating factor (PAF-acether) from alveolar macrophages by the calcium ionophore A23187 and phago-cytosis. Europ. J. Clin. Invest., 10, 437, 1980.
48. Gee, J. B. L., and Khandwala, A. S., Motility, transport and endocytosis in lung defense cells. In Brain, J. D., Proctor, D. F., and Reid, L. M., eds., Respiratory Defense Mechanisms. New York, Marcel Dekker, 1977, p. 927.
49. Senior, R. M., Campbell, E. J., Landis, J. A., et al., Elastase of U-937 monocyte-like cells: comparisons with elastases derived from human monocytes and murine macro-phage-like cells. J. Clin. Invest., 69, 384, 1982.
50. Banda, M. J., Clark, E. J., and Werb, Z., Limited proteolysis by macrophage elastase inactivates human alpha-1-proteinase inhibitor. J. Exp. Med., 152, 1563, 1980.
51. Hinman, L. M., Stevens, C. A., Matthay, R. A., et al., Elastase and lysozyme activities in human alveolar macrophages. Am. Rev. Respir. Dis., 121, 263, 1980.
52. Cohen, A. B., Chenoweth, D. E., and Hugli, T. E., The release of elastase, myeloperox-idase, and lysoyme from human alveolar macrophages. Am. Rev. Respir. Dis., 126, 241, 1982.
53. Gordon, S., The secretion of lysozyme and a plasminogen activator by mononuclear phagocytes. In Van Furth, R., ed., Mononuclear Phagocytes in Immunity, Infection, and Pathology. Oxford, Blackwell Scientific Publications, 1975.
54. Werb, Z., Vainton, D. F., and Jones, P. A., Degradation of connective tissue matrices by macrophages. J. Exp. Med., 152, 1537, 1980.
55. Allison, A. C., Mechanisms of macrophage damage in relation to the pathogenesis of some lung diseases. In Brain, J. D., Proctor, D. F., and Reid, L. M., eds., Respiratory Defense Mechanisms. New York, Marcel Dekker, 1977.
56. deShazo, R. D., Current concepts about the pathogenesis of silicosis and asbestosis. J. Allergy Clin. Immunol., 70, 41, 1982.
57. Gabor, S. Z., Anca, Z., Sugravu, E., et al., In vitro and in vivo quartz-induced lipid peroxidation. In Brown, R. C., Chamberlain, M., Davies, R., and Gormley, I. P., eds., The In Vitro Effects of Mineral Dusts. London, Academic Press, 1980, p. 131.
58. Light, W. G., and Wei, E. T., Surface charge and asbestos toxicity. Nature, 265, 537, 1977.
59. Kagan, E., The alveolar macrophage: immune derangement and asbestos-related malig-nancy. Semin. Oncol., 8, 258, 1981.
60. Golub, E. S., The Cellular Basis of the Immune Response, 2nd ed. Sunderland, Mass., Sinauer Associates, Inc., 1981.
61. Schlueter, D. P., Infiltrative lung disease hypersensitivity pneumonitis. J. Allergy Clin. Immunol., 70, 50, 1982.
62. Epstein, P. E., Dauber, J. H., Rossman, M. D., et al., Bronchoalveolar lavage in a patient with chronic berylliosis: evidence for hypersensitivity pneumonitis. Ann. Intern. Med., 97, 213, 1982.
63. Hunninghake, G. W., and Crystal, R. G., Pulmonary sarcoidosis. A disorder mediated by excess helper T-lymphocyte activity at sites of disease activity. N. Engl. J. Med., 305, 429, 1981.
64. Moore, V. L., Pedersen, G. M., Hauser, W. C., et al., A study of lung lavage materials in patients with hypersensitivity pneumonitis: in vitro response to mitogen and antigen in pigeon breeders' disease. J. Allergy Clin. Immunol., 65, 365, 1980.
65. Moritz, E. D., Smiejan, J. M., Keogh, B. A., et al., Non-fibrotic pigeon-breeder's syndrome: a disorder characterized by a chronic suppressor cell alveolitis. Clin. Res., 30, 435a, 1982.
66. Postlethwaite, A. E., Snyderman, E. R., and Kang, A. H., The chemotactic attraction of human fibroblasts to a lymphocyte-derived factor. J. Exp. Med., 144, 1188, 1976.
67. Wahl, S. M., Wahl, L. M., and MacCarthy, W. Y., Lymphocyte-mediated activation of fibroblast proliferation and collagen production. J. Immunol., 121, 942, 1978.
68. Wahl, S. M., and Gately, C. L., Modulation of fibroblast growth by a lymphokine of human T cell and continuous T cell line origin. J. Immunol., 130, 1226, 1983.
69. Wyler, D. J., and Postlethwaite, A. E., Fibroblast stimulation in schistosomiasis. IV. Isolated egg granulomas elaborate a fibroblast chemoattractant in vitro. J. Immunol., 130, 1371, 1983.

70. Rola-Pleszczynski, M., Masse, S., Sirois, P., et al., Early effects of low-dose exposure to asbestos on local cellular immune responses in the lung. J. Immunol., *127*, 2535, 1981.
71. Askenase, P. W., Bursztajn, S., Gershon, M. D., et al., T cell–dependent mast cell degranulation and release of serotonin in murine delayed-type hypersensitivity. J. Exp. Med., *152*, 1358, 1980.
72. Rao, P. V. S., Friedman, M. M., Atkins, F. M., et al., Phagocytosis of mast cell granules by cultured fibroblasts. J. Immunol., *130*, 341, 1983.
73. Kawanami, O., Ferrans, V. J., Fulmer, J. D., et al., Ultrastructure of pulmonary mast cells in patients with fibrotic lung disorders. Lab. Invest., *40*, 717, 1979.
74. Haslam, P. L., Cromwell, O., Dewar, A., et al., Evidence of increased histamine levels in lung lavage fluids from patients with cryptogenic fibrosing alveolitis. Clin. Exp. Immunol., *44*, 587, 1981.
75. Vracko, R, Significance of basal lamina for regeneration of injured lung. Virchows Arch. (Path. Anat.), *355*, 264, 1972.
76. Campbell, E. J., Senior, R. M., McDonald, J. A., et al., Proteolysis by neutrophils. Relative importance of cell-substrate contact and oxidative inactivation of proteinase inhibition in vitro. J. Clin. Invest., *70*, 845, 1982.
77. Heppleston, A. G., The mechanism of macrophage recruitment in lungs occupied by siliceous dust. *In* Brown, R. C., Gormley, I. P., Chamberlain, M., and Davies, R., eds., The In Vitro Effects of Mineral Dusts. New York, Academic Press, 1980, p. 275.
78. Postlethwaite, A. E., Seyer, J. M., and Kang, A. H., Chemotactic attraction of human fibroblasts to type I, II, and III collagens and collagen-derived peptides. Proc. Natl. Acad. Sci. U.S.A., *75*, 871, 1978.
79. Witschi, H. R., Haschek, W. M., Klein-Szanto, A. J. P., et al., Potentiation of diffuse lung damage by oxygen: determining variables. Am. Rev. Respir. Dis., *123*, 98, 1981.
80. Davison, A. G., Haslum, P. L., Corrin, B., et al., Interstitial lung disease and asthma in hard-metal workers: bronchoalveolar lavage, ultrastructural, and analytical findings and results of bronchial provocation tests. Thorax, *38*, 119, 1983.
81. Hinman, L. M., Stevens, C., Matthay, R. A., et al., Angiotensin convertase activities in human alveolar macrophages: effects of cigarette smoking and sarcoidosis. Science, *205*, 202, 1979.
82. Silverstein, E., Friedland, J., Shanek, A. E., et al., Pathogenesis of sarcoidosis. Mechanism of angiotensin converting enzyme (ACE) elevation: T-lymphocyte modulation of enzyme induction in mononuclear phagocytes: enzyme proterties. *In* Proceedings of the 9th International Conference on Sarcoidosis and Other Granulomatous Disorders. Paris, 1981.
83. Weinstock, J. V., Ehrinpreis, M. N., Boros, D. L., et al., Effect of SQ 14225, an inhibitor of angiotensin I–converting enzyme, on the granulomatous response to *Schistosoma mansoni* eggs in mice. J. Clin. Invest., *67*, 931, 1981.
84. Schrier, D. J., Ripani, L. M., Katzenstein, A. L., et al., Role of angiotensin-converting enzyme in bacille Calmette-Guérin–induced granulomatous inflammation. J. Clin. Invest., *69*, 651, 1982.
85. Mossman, B. T., Craighead, J. E., and MacPherson, B. V.: Asbestos-induced epithelial changes in organ cultures of hamster trachea: inhibition by retinyl methyl ether. Science, *207*, 311, 1980.
86. Brinckerhoff, C. E., McMillan, R. M., Dayer, J. M., et al., Inhibition by retinoic acid of collagenase production in rheumatoid synovial cells. N. Engl. J. Med., *303*, 432, 1980.

8

IMMUNOLOGY OF OCCUPATIONAL LUNG DISEASES

Robert Burrell

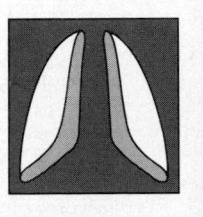

Owing partly to their function and partly to their anatomical location, the lungs and skin are the organ systems most in contact with the external environment. Both the gas-exchanging regions of the lung and the airways are constantly bathed in large volumes of air containing great varieties of suspended mineral and organic dusts. Such particulates either may be antigenic in themselves, may interfere with immune functions of the lung, or may, as a result of an immunological reaction, lead to pulmonary damage. Although most immunological reactions are beneficial, there is a growing realization that they can be two-edged swords and may occasionally be accompanied by harmful side effects. Pulmonary immune injury is seen most often in subjects exposed to dusts as a result of either their occupation or their hobby.

Although the lung is usually thought of as an organ of respiration, it also has important immunological functions. The lung clears itself of inhaled foreign particles by means of cells lining the airways. It also cleanses the internal pulmonary environment of harmful agents that are carried to the lungs by the pulmonary circulation. This it does through a series of aggregates of lymphoid tissue. Since with many antigens phagocytosis is a necessary prelude to antibody production, the immunological importance of the pulmonary macrophage specifically and the lungs in general should be apparent.

Of first order of importance in the defense of the lungs are the immunological effectors known to be present in the pulmonary tissue. Of the five major classes of immunoglobulins, two, IgA and IgE, are characteristically produced in lymphoid tissues associated with external secretions such as those found lining the lamina propria of the bronchial mucosa. Secretory IgA, unlike its humoral counterpart, possesses an extra chain or secretory piece which is acquired as the molecule passes from the site

196

of its synthesis in a plasma cell through the epithelial cells into the mucosa. Such antibody appears to be stimulated locally by antigenic contact and is not necessarily reflected in the antibody content of the peripheral circulation. Molecules of the IgE class are synthesized in plasma cells of bronchial lymph nodes and respiratory mucosa, but do not have a secretory piece. Other classes of immunoglobulins may also be found in respiratory secretions,[1] particularly if the individual is IgA-deficient.[2]

Such secretory antibody is therefore the body's first line of specific humoral defense against respiratory pathogens, and protection against respiratory infection depends more on these antibodies than it does on the antibodies found in the serum. All immunoglobulins may be stimulated by antigenic contact with respiratory tissues, particularly if the stimulus is accompanied by irritation. This type of immunity is dependent on cells whose origin is the stem cells of the bone marrow, and is sometimes referred to as B cell–dependent.

Another form of immunity is associated with the presence of mature lymphocytes, the maturation of which is controlled by the thymus. This type of immunity is referred to as T cell–dependent and is responsible for resistance to many intracellular infections, delayed hypersensitivity, graft rejection, and certain other immunological responses. Such cellular immunity has been recognized to be of great importance in regard to the lymph nodes of respiratory tissue, but its protective role in regard to the air passages and alveoli is just beginning to be appreciated.

Both B- and T-cell systems of the lung are capable of being stimulated by direct antigenic contact with the respiratory tissues, but this is not necessarily so if antigenic contact is made via extrapulmonary routes.[3, 4] Pulmonary T- and B-cell responses may occur with such extrapulmonary contact with antigen if the latter is accompanied by nonspecific pulmonary stimulation.[3]

TYPES OF IMMUNE INJURY

A practical system has been formulated for classifying the different modalities of immune injury.[5] The classification has formerly proved useful not only to the experimentalist but also to the clinician who must take etiological pathophysiology into consideration for diagnostic and therapeutic purposes. Four distinct immunological responses were originally described, all of which can play a role in the etiology of pulmonary disease (Fig. 8–1), but knowledge of modern immunopathology dictates that other important mechanisms also be considered.

IgE–Dependent Allergy

Type I reactions are those dependent upon reagin or antibody of the IgE class. Clinically such reactions are seen in the atopic patient with the

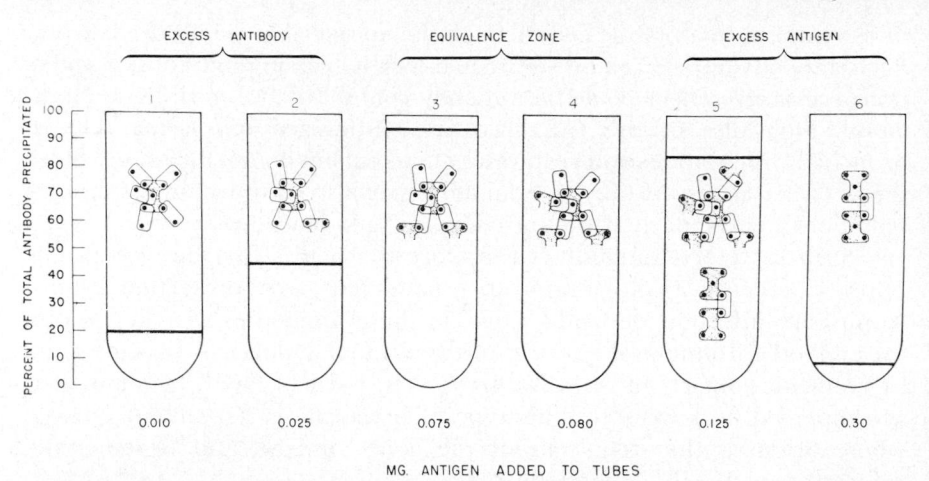

Figure 8–1. Schematic representation of a precipitin curve showing the composition of soluble immune complexes in ratios of antigen excess (Tube 6). Not enough antibody is available to build a lattice among the complexes, but such complexes are still capable of fixing complement. (From Raffel, S.: Immunity, 2nd ed., 1953. Courtesy of Appleton-Century-Crofts, Publishing Division of Prentice-Hall, Inc., Englewood Cliffs, N.J.)

classical forms of immediate hypersensitivity or allergy. IgE antibodies become fixed to certain receptor sites on mast cells by means of the nonantigen-reactive ends of the heavy chains of the globulin when specific antigen reacts with such cell-bound antibody. When two or more IgE molecules react with one molecule of antigen, it is postulated that the heavy chains are stressed in such a fashion that damage results to the attached cell, causing it to release various pharmacologically active mediators that result in the clinical manifestations.[6] Histamine, acetylcholine, heparin, 5-hydroxytryptamine, slow-reacting substance of anaphylaxis (SRS–A), and various plasma kinins are among those substances known to be released in Type I reactions.[7]

These mediators physiologically activate secondary target organs, e.g., smooth muscle and vascular tissue. If the inhaled particles are large (between 20 and 60 microns), the site of IgE activation is usually in the nasal turbinates, resulting in the allergic rhinitis–hay fever diathesis. When smaller (6 to 20 microns) antigenic particles are inhaled, they lodge in the bronchi and bronchioles and if they react with specific IgE, bronchial asthma may result. Chronic stimulation of this kind may result in certain forms of cellular hyperplasia leading to the development of nasal polyps and bronchial smooth muscle hypertrophy as seen in hay fever and chronic bronchial asthma, respectively. Mucous metaplasia in which the ciliated cells are often replaced by goblet cells also occurs. The basement membrane may be often thickened or even ruptured, possibly owing to antigen-antibody complexes, but IgE may not be the only immunoglobulin involved in such basement membrane damage.[8, 9]

The immunological methods for incriminating a Type I response rely

on demonstrating the physiological effect of specific IgE present in the patient. This is more easily effected either by skin testing or by measuring the subject's ventilatory capacity following an aerosol challenge. Positive immediate skin tests (Type I) are characterized by the sudden appearance (within 1 to 2 minutes after challenge) of an edematous wheal and an erythematous flare. In subjects in whom extreme hypersensitivity is suspected or in whom there are contraindications to direct testing, specific laboratory tests should be used.

If interpreted with care, inhalation challenge tests are an excellent means of diagnosing immediate allergies and distinguishing them from other forms of immune injury.[10] Although care is required for their performance, the response correlates well with clinical pulmonary disease. In such tests, the patient's forced expired volume in 1 second (FEV_1) is measured before and shortly after an aerosol challenge. If the subject is sensitive, the FEV_1 falls significantly within an hour, and slowly reverts to normal, usually in 2 to 4 hours. The fall likewise may be reversed by adrenergic drugs. After the initial reaction in some subjects, an additional decline in FEV_1 may occur after 3 to 4 hours; such a latent fall is currently not understood, but could be an indication of another mechanism of response.

Two excellent laboratory means of diagnosis of immediate hypersensitivity are radioallergosorbent (RAST) testing[11] and *in vitro* histamine release.[12] RAST testing involves reacting the patient's serum with specific antigen coupled to an insoluble matrix. After washing to remove unreacted protein, radiolabeled anti-Ig is added to the antigen matrix and the results observed in a scintillation counter. *In vitro* histamine release testing involves incubating the patient's leukocytes with specific antigen and then measuring histamine release either fluorometrically or enzymatically.

Cytotoxic Reactions

Type II reactions are those that result from antibody reacting with either an intrinsic antigenic constituent of the cell, an intrinsic antigen that is adherent to the cell, or an intrinsic antigenic specificity coincidentally similar to an extrinsic antigen. Several such antibodies have been associated with various forms of occupational respiratory disease.

Chief among the antibodies to intrinsic antigenic constituents of lung tissue are the humoral antibodies to an insoluble lung connective tissue component.[13] This antigen is collagen or reticulin and is also present in WI-38 human embryonic lung fibroblast cell cultures.[14] Circulating antibodies to this antigen are spontaneously produced in a variety of chronic pulmonary diseases,[13] are of the IgA class,[15] and are demonstrable by the antiglobulin consumption test.[13] The role of these antibodies in the pathogenesis of pulmonary disease has been well studied. They are cytotoxic for lung fibroblast cell cultures,[16] induce increased production

of serum LDH_2 and LDH_3, localize in focal patches of certain alveolar septa,[17] cause increased localization in the lung of bacteria cleared from the blood stream,[17] induce an increase of interstitial alveolar connective tissue leading to a distention of the terminal airways,[17] and predispose the host to a more invasive form of tuberculous infection.[18-20] They seem to arise as a result of any chronic lung disease in which there is appreciable tissue damage and may in turn contribute to further injury.

Another important lung antigen is a glycoprotein associated with capillary basement membranes.[14, 21] It is found in these membranes in kidney, lung, placenta, and other organs. Caution is necessary in working with this antigen prepared with glomerular basement membrane preparations, since such preparations are often contaminated with collagen fibrils with similar antigenicity to the antigen described above.[14] True capillary membrane glycoprotein antigen induces complement-fixing antibodies (IgG or IgM), thereby distinguishing it from the connective tissue antigen. The former antigen seems to be the target for antibodies and is associated with the injury seen in Goodpasture's syndrome.[22] How these antibodies arise is unknown, but they may well be due to coincidental specificity with an extrinsic antigen.

Another antigen reported from lung tissue in association with disease states includes a material which is probably reticulin, but no information is available about the nature of its antibody or its relation to pathological changes.[23]

Rheumatoid factor (RF) and antinuclear factor (ANF), primarily IgM and IgA antibodies, respectively, have been reported to occur in association with a variety of chronic occupational respiratory diseases. RF is found in both human[24] and experimental silicosis,[25] asbestosis,[26] and coal workers' pneumoconiosis (CWP)[27, 28] significantly more often than in the normal population. The antibody may develop owing to the adjuvant effect of materials such as silica[29] and be a reflection of chronic tissue damage, but some experimental evidence indicates that RF also contributes to the development of the lesion. Passively administered RF was found to result in more intensive vasculitis when granulomata were induced with Freund's adjuvant.[30]

ANF seems to be a better indicator of the prevalence and severity of disease in CWP[27] and asbestosis,[26, 31] in that its presence correlates well with the extent of radiographic abnormality and its prevalence in subjects with these diseases is greater than that of RF. Little is known about the function, if any, of ANF in vivo. The suggestion has been made that the cytotoxic antibody may form immune complexes with nucleoproteins and lead to interstitial pulmonary fibrosis, idiopathic forms of which are associated with an increased prevalence of ANF.[32] Should this hypothesis prove correct, the reaction more closely resembles an immune complex-mediated injury response (see below). Finally, evidence has been obtained that passively administered human ANF increased the polymorphonuclear counts and mean volume of pleural effusion in artificially induced pleurisy

in experimental animals.[33] None of these antibodies appears to be primarily pathogenic, but rather intensify pre-existing pulmonary insults from other causes.

Little evidence is available to incriminate antibodies to extrinsic antigens adsorbed to normal lung tissue, although the suggestion has been made that fungal antigens associated with farmer's lung may do so and that subsequent antibody reaction with these leads to injury.[34]

Immune Complex–Mediated Inflammation

An explanation of Type III or soluble immune complex reactions requires an understanding of some of the fundamentals of antigen-antibody reactions. Serum antibodies to many soluble antigens may be demonstrated by the precipitin reaction, but visible reactions will be seen only if certain conditions are met. The formation of a visible precipitate depends on the development of a lattice structure between bivalent IgG antibodies and multivalent antigens. Since the ratio of valence between antigen and antibody is so great, the two reactants are able to combine in different proportions depending on the relative concentrations of each. A range of such reactions through various concentrations is depicted in Figure 8–1.[35]

In regions of antigen excess, the number of antigen valences so outnumbers antibody valences that there are not enough antibody molecules to act as bridges between the antigen-antibody complexes (represented by the tube on the right in the figure); hence, no lattice of visible precipitate develops even though an antigen-antibody reaction has taken place. These complexes remain soluble and are capable of fixing complement.

Once the complement cascade has been activated through the C3 component, small peptide cleavage products become chemotactic for neutrophils. These cells are drawn to the area of immune complex deposition and may release their lysosomal enzymes which injure the adjacent tissue. Whether exposure to an antigen develops into such an injury reaction depends on many factors. The concentration of antigen is very critical; if it is too high, apparently the complexes are too small or possess only one antibody molecule per complex so that complement is not fixed. If the complexes form at equivalence, i.e., relatively lower concentrations of antigen, they are precipitated and phagocytized in the circulation without incident.

Type III reactions are responsible for the dermal Arthus reaction, part of the serum sickness syndrome, and the most common form of glomerulonephritis.[36] These conditions differ mainly in the site of deposition of the soluble complexes. Immune complex–mediated injury in pulmonary disease has been considered in two areas. It has been suggested that immune complexes which form intravascularly may deposit in the

lung and possibly result in interstitial pneumonitis and fibrosis. Antibodies such as RF and ANA, discussed above, may act in this fashion.[37] There is also a large body of literature suggesting that immune complexes resulting from serum antibody reacting with inhaled, soluble antigens may lead to hypersensitivity pneumonitis.[38] There is very little immunological, pathological, physiological, or even epidemiological evidence, however, to support this hypothesis.[39] Patients with clinical hypersensitivity pneumonitis often, but not universally, possess precipitins to the responsible environmental agents that initiated the disease,[40] but far too many people without evidence of active disease or without history of past disease also demonstrate these antibodies yet are clinically unaffected following occupational exposure to the antigens. The demonstration of precipitins merely identifies inhalational agents from environments to which an individual has been exposed.

The presence of precipitins against extracts of appropriate fungi is often demonstrated by the Ouchterlony method of immunodiffusion.[41, 42] Better and quicker results may be obtained by electrophoretically forcing the antigen to migrate to the anode against the cathodally migrating globulins of the patient's serum (Fig. 8–2).[43] With *Aspergillus* antigens, the presence of more than two lines is usually indicative of aspergilloma or invasive aspergillosis.[42]

Provocation tests by means of aerosol challenge are useful in differentiating early and late reactions,[10] but immunological evidence is unavailable to explain the late response. A parenchymal response is indicated when there are significant falls in both FEV_1 and forced vital capacity (FVC) about 4 to 6 hours after challenge. The ratio of FEV_1/FVC remains unchanged in such a response, but the decline in lung volumes may be accompanied by a reduction of the carbon monoxide–diffusing capacity. An obstructive response is also seen in which only the FEV_1 decreases, thereby leading to a change in the $FEV_1:FVC$ ratio. Late responses are more prolonged than Type I responses, are often accompanied by fever, and can be reversed by the administration of steroids. Often a patient will show a dual response (Fig. 8–3), indicating the coexistence of Type I and late reactions. In such instances, the time of appearance and resolution of such changes is important in differentiating them.

Cell-Mediated Immunity

Type IV reactions differ from the previous three in that humoral immunoglobulins are not involved. Rather, this form of reaction is due to cell-mediated immunity or delayed-type hypersensitivity. The prototype of this kind of reaction is the delayed skin reaction to tuberculin seen in persons who have been exposed to tubercle bacilli.

The principal cells responsible for this type of reaction are the thymus-dependent lymphocytes, although it is becoming apparent that bone marrow-dependent lymphocytes may also be involved. When antigen

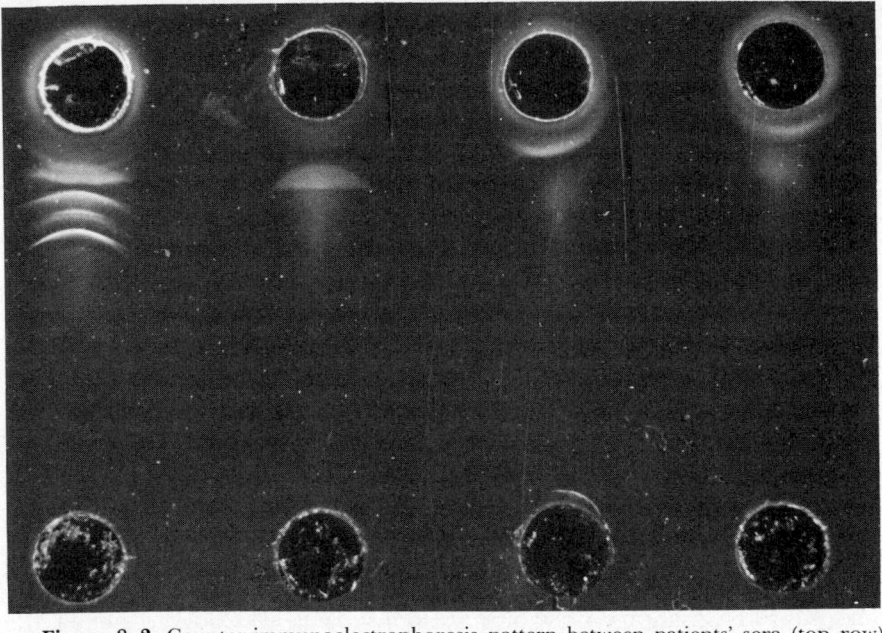

Figure 8–2. Counter-immunoelectrophoresis pattern between patients' sera (top row) and Aspergillus antigens (bottom row). Electrophoretically, the anode is at the top and the cathode is at the bottom. The patient on the left demonstrates a pattern indicating intimate antigenic contact with the fungus. Precipitation shown by the other sera is regarded as nonspecific.

reacts with specifically sensitized lymphocytes, a variety of effectors are released that account for such manifestations as migration inhibition of macrophages, target cell cytotoxicity, mitogenesis, chemotaxis, and transfer of specific sensitivity.[44] These factors all participate *in vivo* in producing the gross and histological appearances of the lesions of delayed hypersensitivity. As with humoral mechanisms of defense, such a line of immunity is ordinarily beneficial, but may also be injurious.

Figure 8–3. FEV$_1$ results obtained from two patients after aerosol challenge with fungal antigen. The dotted line was obtained from a patient who exhibited only a Type I atopic response. The solid line was from a patient who exhibited a dual response: an initial Type I reaction which resolved by 2 hours was followed by an additional late reaction between 4 and 6 hours. (Redrawn from Pepys, J.: Hypersensitivity diseases of the lungs due to fungi and organic dusts. Monogr. Allergy *4*, 1, 1969.)

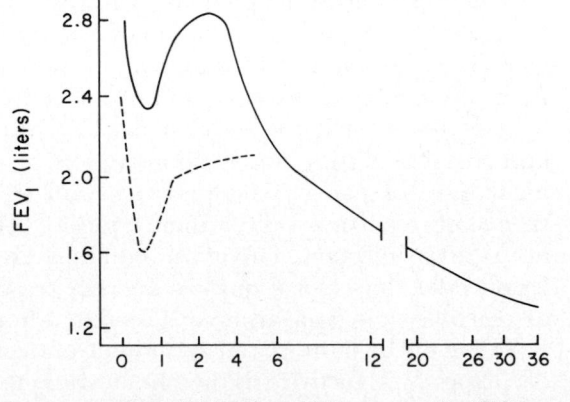

TIME (HOURS) AFTER Ag INHALATION

Cell-mediated immune reactions in the lung may be directed against either extrinsic or intrinsic antigens. One of the most important extrinsic antigens that may lead to such injury in the lung is beryllium.[45] Several soluble mediators are demonstrable *in vitro* following incubation of patient's lymphocytes with beryllium salts and in turn correlate well with skin reactivity. However, skin or patch testing with beryllium salts is contraindicated because such testing may indeed induce primary sensitization or cause an exacerbation of pre-existing lesions in diseased subjects.[46]

Experimental evidence suggests that in animals exhibiting Type IV skin sensitivity, severe pulmonary changes are produced if the animals are challenged with aerosolized antigen.[47-50] These changes consist of peribronchial and perivascular infiltrates of lymphocytes, some interstitial infiltrates, interalveolar septal thickening, dilatation of capillaries, and increased respiratory frequency with no change in airways resistance.

There are reports of Type IV responses to certain extrinsic antigens, notably bagasse, *Micropolyspora faeni*, and pigeon excreta, all of which antigens are usually associated with Type III reactions.[51, 52] The varied clinical picture seen in hypersensitivity pneumonitis appears to depend not only on variation in the host response, but also on the site of the antigen-antibody reaction.[53]

Just as there is a humoral aggressive response against lung antigens in certain forms of chronic pulmonary disease, so there is also a cell-mediated counterpart. Such a mechanism has been described that reacts against a soluble connective tissue antigen of lungs.[54] Evidence of Type IV reactivity to this antigen has been found in a variety of experimental pulmonary diseases, e.g., experimental berylliosis and coal workers' pneumoconiosis, but also in a limited number of patients with chronic respiratory disease.[55] Under these circumstances, the pathological change initiated by an extrinsic agent apparently leads to a Type IV reaction against an intrinsic antigen. Additional information that cell-mediated immunity to intrinsic antigen exists has been obtained from studies on patients with idiopathic pulmonary fibrosis (IPF), where it was shown that the lymphocytes of 94 per cent of such patients were reactive against collagen as compared to only 17 per cent of those from patients with nonfibrotic disease and none in normal controls.[56]

Methods for detection of Type IV sensitivity are limited to intracutaneous skin testing and demonstration of mediators following *in vitro* incubation of patient's lymphocytes with test antigen. Positive delayed-type skin tests consist of erythema and 10 mm or more of induration 48 hours after injection. The induration may proceed to necrosis; hence, the lesion does not resolve quickly. In very sensitive individuals, initial signs of reactivity may appear as early as 6 to 8 hours following injection.

One of the more popular methods of demonstrating *in vitro* correlates of Type IV reactivity is by the technique of macrophage migration inhibition. If macrophages and sensitized lymphocytes are incubated in

tissue culture media within a capillary tube, the macrophages will begin
to migrate out of the tube within 24 hours. If the cells are incubated with
specific antigen, this migration pattern is greatly inhibited. The difference
between normal migration and specific inhibition due to beryllium in a
berylliotic patient's lymphocytes may be seen in Figure 8–4.[57] Another
Type IV mediator commonly sought following incubation of lymphocytes
with test antigen is lymphocytotoxin. In this procedure, the supernatant
fluid from the lymphocyte-antigen mixture is placed on selected target
cell cultures, e.g., fibroblasts. Either the cultures are examined directly for
cytopathogenic effects or, if the cells have been labeled with a radiochem-
ical, release of the label into the medium is detected instrumentally.[58] One
final method involves stimulating blast formation in a patient's lymphocytes
with antigen.[58] Sensitized cells will begin to divide, as evidenced by uptake
of radioactively labeled thymidine following antigenic stimulation. It has
been suggested that immunological analysis of pulmonary lavage fluids
may become more important in the future.[59] In one such study of lavage
fluids from patients with IPF and chronic hypersensitivity pneumonitis,

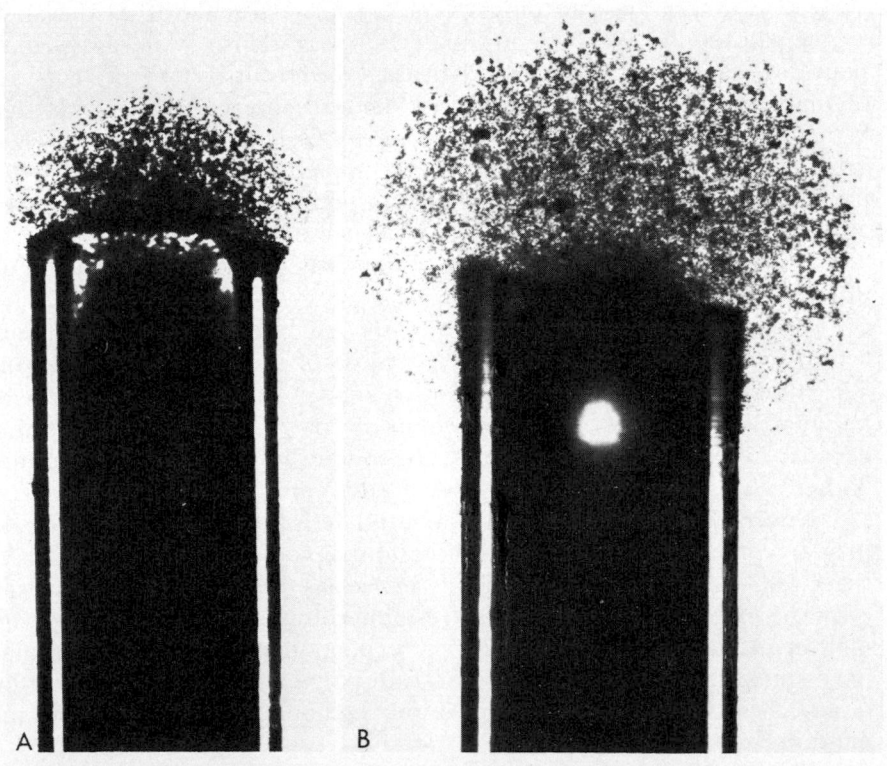

A   B

Figure 8–4. Enlarged views of macrophage migration inhibition using beryllium fluoride
as antigen. *A* shows the macrophage migration from a patient with clinical berylliosis; *B* was
obtained from a normal control. The beryllium salt markedly inhibited the normal migration
of macrophages from the capillary tube only when the patient's cells were used. (Reproduced
through the courtesy of Dr. J. J. Marx.)

elevated IgG levels were found in lavages from both kinds of patients, but only the lavages from patients with the latter disease showed the presence of high numbers of T lymphocytes.

OTHER TYPES OF IMMUNE AND IMMUNE-LIKE INJURY

The original Coombs and Gell[5] classification of immune injury into four basic types is subject to two limitations. First, a given disease rarely is due to only one type, but usually consists of a mixture of types. More importantly, modern studies of immunopathology and inflammation have revealed additional immunological mechanisms of injury or mechanisms either which involve immunological accessory cells and molecules or in which the timing is sufficiently close to known immunological reactions so as to resemble them. The following is a brief listing of some possible causes of immunological disturbances and their relation to lung disease.

Nonspecific Complement Activation. It is now well known that certain biochemical substances may nonspecifically activate (i.e., in the absence of antibody) the complement cascade, particularly via the alternative pathway, to produce an inflammatory response. Materials such as peptidoglycans[60] and lipopolysaccharides,[61] the essential cell wall structures of many microorganisms, are two well-known materials that can do this. When microorganisms such as *Micropolyspora faeni* or *Aspergillus terreus* are inhaled in large quantities, their known complement-activating activity[62, 63] takes place *in vivo*, resulting in changes in peripheral complement activity and pulmonary function even in the absence of prior immunization.[64, 65] The possibility also exists that inhaled bacterial endotoxins may trigger an inflammatory reaction.[66]

Hyperplasia. The continuous presence of humoral antibody in subcytotoxic amounts may result in hyperplasia of the target cells or tissue. The lung connective tissue antibodies known to occur in the sera of patients with chronic pneumonoconiosis[13] may act in such a fashion because in experimental situations, the long-term presence of such antibodies results in appreciable interseptal thickening of the alveolar walls.[17]

Nonspecific Reaction with Globulin. It is well known that certain protein components of staphylococci and streptococci may nonspecifically react with the Fc portion of antibody molecules (the antigen reactivity site is on the Fab portion) and possibly result in complement-mediated inflammation. At least one inhalant in an occupationally related disease may have this property. A tetrahydroxyflavan polymer associated with cotton bracts is capable of reacting with immunoglobulins in a pseudoimmune manner.[67]

Nonspecific Mediator Release. Inflammatory mediators such as histamine are usually thought to be released by antigen-IgE reactions, but there is a growing realization that such mediators may be released in the absence of specific IgE. A substance called methyl piperonylate, also found

in cotton bracts, may directly cause histamine release,[68] while substances like *Aspergillus* spores can effect such release through nonspecific complement activation.[65]

β-Adrenergic Blockage. β-Adrenergic activators of adenylate cyclase result in accumulation of cylic AMP in cells which modulate the action of histamine. If these activators are inhibited (β-blockage), the result would be unopposed cholinergic stimulation of smooth muscle constriction, and if applied to bronchial smooth muscle, an asthmatic-like reaction results. The inhalation of toluene diisocyanate (TDI), a common industrial material, leads to asthmatic reactions, and although IgE may also be produced for TDI, much evidence indicates that this material exerts its main effects through a β-blockage.[69, 70]

Potentiation by Other Environmental Agents. The simultaneous contact of additional agents in the environment may modify the response to a second agent. The potentiating effect of silica on tuberculous infection is well known,[71] but the coincidental temporal contact of an individual with either the same or a different agent is just being realized. Inhalation of something as common and innocuous as *Escherichia coli* may be quite harmful in experimental situations if followed in a certain period of time by a septicemia of the same microorganisms such as might occur during dental or surgical manipulation.[72] Streptococcal exotoxin is known to enhance the effect of gram-negative endotoxin,[73] but the effect of a streptococcal infection on a worker exposed to a gram-negative aerosol has not been explored.

Inhalant Interference of Immune Function. There are a number of occupational inhalants that can cause various immunological disturbances. Chief among these is silica, a profound macrophage toxin, which also produces in silicotic patients a high incidence of antinuclear and rheumatoid factors and elevated IgA levels, as well as connective tissue antibodies capable of localizing in silicotic nodules. A number of these processes, e.g., those that result in macrophage activation or death, in immune complex formation, or in globulin deposition, may lead to fibrosis.[74] Coal workers' pneumoconiosis is another disease in which similar immunological abnormalities may occur.[75] In both of these diseases, infective components play a significant but as yet unexplained role in lesion production. The possibility that coal mine dust has lymphocytic depression functions aside from that exerted on macrophages must be considered because such effects could lead to inhibition of immune responsiveness.[76, 77]

The inhalation of asbestos dust has also received considerable attention. In addition to the increased prevalence of antinuclear and rheumatoid factors in patients with inhalation disease due to asbestos,[75] certain forms of this material also cause interference with interferon induction,[79] altered lymphocyte function,[80] and elevated immunoglobulin levels.[81] Of great interest has been the discovery that the prolonged inhalation of asbestos causes changes in the macrophage membrane, which results in prolonged binding of these cells to macrophages.[82] This alteration of the

macrophage could possibly be antigenically related to crocidolite and would explain some of the immunological abnormalities associated with asbestosis.[82]

All of the above inhalants are related to occupational exposure, but there are many other environmental inhalants that can depress pulmonary immune function, including cigarette and marijuana smoking, air pollutants such as sulfur and nitrous oxides, and even halothane anesthesia. If a worker exposed to inhalation of industrial materials is also exposed to these other materials, e.g., cigarette smoking in a coal miner, the combined effects could be more serious than from either agent alone. Similary, the depressive effect of prolonged secondary pulmonary infection could possibly be enhanced by simultaneous inhalation of an industrial aerosol.

References

1. Ford, R. J., Jr., and Kuhn, C., Immunologic competence of alveolar cells. II. Modification of the plaque-forming response by inhibitors, tolerance, and chronic stimulation. Am. Rev. Resp. Dis., *107*, 771, 1973.
2. Tomasi, T. B., Jr., Secretory immunoglobulins. N. Engl. J. Med., *287*, 500, 1972.
3. Nash, D. R., and Holle, B., Local and systemic cellular immune responses in guinea pigs given antigen parenterally or directly into the lower respiratory tract. Clin. Exp. Immunol., *13*, 573, 1973.
4. Kaltreider, H. B., and Salmon, S. E., Immunology of the lower respiratory tract. J. Clin. Invest., *52*, 2211, 1973.
5. Coombs, R. R. A., and Gell, P. G. H., The classification of allergic reactions underlying disease. *In* Gell, P. G. H. and Coombs, R. R. A., eds., Clinical Aspects of Immunology. Philadelphia, F. A. Davis Co., 1964, p. 317.
6. Ishizaka, K., Human reaginic antibodies. Ann. Rev. Med., *21*, 187, 1971.
7. Austen, K. F., Histamine and other mediators of allergic reactions. *In* Samter, M., ed., Immunological Diseases, 2nd ed. Boston, Little, Brown, 1971, p. 332.
8. McCarter, J. H., and Vazquez, J. J., The bronchial basement membrane in asthma. Arch. Path., *82*, 328, 1966.
9. Callerame, M. L., Condemi, J. J., Bohrod, M. G., and Vaughn, J. H., Immunologic reactions of bronchial tissues in asthma. N. Engl. J. Med., *284*, 459, 1971.
10. Fink, J. N., The use of bronchoprovocation in the diagnosis of hypersensitivity pneumonitis, J. Allergy Clin. Immunol., *64*, 590, 1979.
11. Berg, T. L. O., and Johannson, S. G. O., Allergy diagnosis with the radioallergosorbent test (RAST). J. Allergy Clin. Immunol., *54*, 209, 1974.
12. Osler, A. G., Lichtenstein, L. M., and Levy, D. A., *In vitro* studies of human reaginic allergy. Adv. Immunol., *8*, 183, 1968.
13. Burrell, R., Wallace, J. P., and Andrews, C. E., Lung antibodies in patients with pulmonary disease. Am. Rev. Resp. Dis., *89*, 697, 1964.
14. Burrell, R., Esber, H. J., Hagadorn, J. E., and Andrews, C. E., Specificity of lung reactive antibodies in human serum. Am. Rev. Resp. Dis., *94*, 743, 1966.
15. Hagadorn, J. E., and Burrell, R., Lung-reactive antibodies in IgA fractions of sera from patients with pneumoconisis. Clin. Exp. Immunol., *3*, 263, 1968.
16. Esber, H. J., and Burrell, R., Further characterization of the specificity of lung-reactive antibodies in human serum. Arch. Environ. Health, *21*, 502, 1970.
17. Burrell, R., Flaherty, D. K., DeNee, P. B., et al., The effect of lung antibody on normal lung structure and function. Am. Rev. Resp. Dis., *109*, 106, 1974.
18. Rheins, M. S., and Burrell, R., Further studies on auto-tissue substances in tuberculous rabbits. Am. Rev. Resp. Dis., *81*, 213, 1960.
19. Burrell, R., and Cate, C. C., The effect of lung reactive antibodies on the pathogenesis of tuberculosis. Clin. Exp. Immunol., *9*, 809, 1971.

20. Burrell, R., and Lewis, D. M., Further studies on the effect of lung antibodies on the pathogenesis of tuberculosis. J. Lab. Clin. Med., *86*, 741, 1975.
21. Krakower, C. A., and Greenspon, S. A., The localization the "nephrotoxic" antigen(s) in extraglomerular tissues. Arch. Pathol., *66*, 364, 1958.
22. Hagadorn, J. E., Vazquez, J. J., and Kinney, T. R., Immunopathologic studies of an experimental model resembling Goodpasture's syndrome. Am. J. Pathol., *57*, 17, 1969.
23. Hennes, A. R., Moore, M. Z., Carpenter, R. L., and Hammarsten, J. R., Antibodies to human lung in patients with obstructive emphysema and pulmonary tuberculosis. Am. Rev. Resp. Dis., *83*, 354, 1961.
24. Schroeder, W., Franklin, E. C., and McEwen, C., Rheumatoid factors in patients with silicosis with round nodular fibrosis of the lung in the absence of rheumatoid arthritis. Arth. Rheum., *5*, 10, 1962.
25. Esber, H. J., and Burrell, R., An immunologic study of experimental silicosis. Environ. Res., *1*, 171, 1967.
26. Turner-Warwick, M., and Parkes, W. R., Circulating rheumatoid and antinuclear factors in asbestos workers. Br. Med. J., *3*, 492, 1970.
27. Lippman, M., Eckert, H. L., Hahon, N., and Morgan, W. K. C., The prevalence of circulating antinuclear and rheumatoid factors in United States coal miners. Ann. Intern. Med., *79*, 807, 1973.
28. Wagner, J. C., and McCormick, J. N., Immunological investigations of coal-worker's disease. J. Roy. Coll. Physicians Lond., *2*, 49, 1967.
29. Pernis, B., and Paronetto, F., Adjuvant effect of silica (tridymite) on antibody production. Proc. Soc. Exp. Biol. Med., *110*, 390, 1962.
30. DeHoratius, R. J., and Williams, R. B., Rheumatoid factor accentuation of pulmonary lesions associated with experimental diffuse proliferative lung disease. Arth. Rheum., *15*, 293, 1972.
31. Turner-Warwick, M., Immunology and asbestosis. Proc. Roy. Soc. Med., *66*, 927, 1973.
32. Nagaya, H., Elmore, M., and Ford, C. C., Idiopathic interstitial pulmonary fibrosis. An immune complex disease. Am. Rev. Resp. Dis., *107*, 826, 1973.
33. Hughes, P., and Rowell, N. R., Aggravation of turpentine-induced pleurisy in rats by "homogenous" and "speckled" antinuclear antibodies, J. Pathol., *101*, 141, 1970.
34. Wenzel, F. J., Emanuel, D. A., and Gray, R. L., Immunofluorescent studies in patients with farmer's lung. J. Allergy Clin. Immunol., *48*, 224, 1971.
35. Raffel, S., Immunity, 2nd ed. New York, Appleton-Century-Crofts, 1961, p. 137.
36. Roy, L. P., Fish, A. J., Michael, A. F., and Vernier, R. L., Etiologic agents of immune-deposit disease. *In* Schwartz, R. S., ed., Progress in Clinical Immunology, Vol. 1. New York, Grune and Stratton, 1972, p. 1.
37, Haslam, P. L., Thompson, B., Mohammed, I., et al., Circulating immune complexes in patients with cryptogenic fibrosing alveolitis. Clin. Exp. Immunol., *37*, 381, 1979.
38. Roberts, R. C., and Moore, V. L., Immunopathogenesis of Hypersensitivity Pneumonitis. Am. Rev. Respir. Dis., *116*, 1075, 1977.
39. Burrell, R., and Rylander, R., The role of precipitins in hypersensitivity pneumonitis. Eur. J. Resp. Dis., *62*, 332, 1981.
40. Marx, J. J., Jr., Emanuel, D. A., Dovenbarger, W. V., et al., Farmer's lung disease among farmers with precipitating antibodies to the thermophilic actinomycetes: a clinical and immunological study. J. Allergy Clin. Immunol., *62*, 185, 1978.
41. Senzel, F. J., Emanuel, D. A., and Zygowica, P. M., Simplified serologic test for farmer's lung. Am. J. Clin. Pathol., *49*, 1983, 1968.
42. Coleman, R. M., and Kaufman, L., Use of the immunodiffusion test in the serodiagnosis of aspergillosis. Appl. Microbiol., *23*, 301, 1972.
43. Gordon, M. A., Almy, R. E., Greene, C. H., and Fenton, J. W., II, Diagnostic mycoserology by immunoelectrophoresis: a general, rapid, and sensitive microtechnic. J. Clin. Pathol., *56*, 471, 1971.
44. Lawrence, H. S., and Landy, M., eds., Mediators of Cellular Immunity. New York, Academic Press, 1969.
45. Marx, J. J., Jr., and Burrell, R., Delayed hypersensitivity to beryllium compounds. J. Immunol., *111*, 590, 1973.
46. Shelley, W. B., and Hurley, H. J., The immune granuloma: late delayed hypersensitivity to zirconium and beryllium. *In* Samter, M., ed., Immunological Diseases, 2nd ed. Boston, Little, Brown, 1971, p. 728.

47. Pernis, B., Role of lymphocytes in infiltrative lung diseases. Arch. Environ. Health, *10*, 289, 1965.
48. Miyamoto, T., Kabe, J., Noda, M., et al., Physiologic and pathologic respiratory changes in delayed type hypersensitivity reaction in guinea pigs. Am. Rev. Resp. Dis., *103*, 509, 1971.
49. Richerson, H. B., Acute experimental hypersensitivity pneumonitis. J. Lab. Clin. Med., *79*, 745, 1972.
50. Kabe, J., Aoki, Y., and Miyamoto, T., Antigenicity of fractions from extracts of *Candida albicans*. J. Allergy, *47*, 59, 1971.
51. Kawai, T., Salvaggio, J., Lake, W., and Harris, J. O., Experimental production of hypersensitivity pneumonitis with bagasse and thermophilic actinomycete antigen, J. Allergy Clin. Immunol., *50*, 267, 1972.
52. Caldwell, J. R., Pearce, D. E., Spencer C., et al., Immunologic mechanisms in hypersensitivity pneumonitis. J. Allergy Clin. Immunol., *52*, 225, 1973.
53. Katz, R. M., and Kniker, W. T., Infantile hypersensitivity pneumonitis as a reaction to organic antigens. N. Engl. J. Med., *288*, 233, 1973.
54. Cate, C. C., and Burrell, R., Lung antigen induced cell mediated immune injury in chronic respiratory disease. Am. Rev. Resp. Dis., *109*, 114, 1974.
55. Dill, J., Fox, R., Landrigan, P., Macsween, M., et al., A study of lung-specific, cell-mediated immunity in chronic pulmonary diseases. Clin. Allergy, *7*, 539, 1977.
56. Kravis, T. C., Ahmed, A., Brown, T. E., et al., Pathogenic mechanisms in pulmonary fibrosis. J. Clin. Invest., *58*, 1223, 1976.
57. Marx, J. J., Delayed hypersensitivity to beryllium compounds. Ph.D. Dissertation, West Virginia University, 1972, p. 60.
58. Bloom, B. R., and Glade, P. R., eds., Conference on In Vitro Methods in Cell-Mediated Immunity, New York University Medical Center, 1970. New York, Academic Press, 1971.
59. Reynolds, H. Y., Fulmer, J. D., Kasmierowski, J. A., et al., Analysis of cellular and protein content of broncho-alveolar lavage fluid from patients with idiopathic pulmonary fibrosis and chronic hypersensitivity pneumonitis. J. Clin. Invest., *59*, 165, 1977.
60. Smith, S. M., Burrell, R., and Snyder, I. S., Complement activation by cell wall fractions of *Micropolyspora faeni*. Infect. Immun., *22*, 568, 1978.
61. Ulevitch, R. J., and Cochrane, C. G., Role of complement in lethal bacterial lipopolysaccharide-induced hypotensive and coagulative changes. Infect. Immun., *19*, 204, 1978.
62. Marx, J. J., Jr., and Flaherty, D. K., Alternative pathway activation of complement by antigens associated with hypersensitivity pneumonitis. J. Allergy Clin. Immunol., *55*, 70, 1975.
63. Edwards, J. H., A quantitative study of the alternative pathway of complement by mouldy hay dust and thermophilic actinomycetes. Clin. Allergy, *6*, 19, 1976.
64. Olenchock, S. A., and Burrell, R., The role of precipitins and complement activation in the etiology of allergic lung disease. J. Allergy Clin. Immunol., *58*, 76, 1976.
65. Burrell, R., and Pokorney, D., Mediators of experimental hypersensitivity pneumonitis. Int. Arch. Allergy Appl. Immunol., *55*, 161, 1977.
66. Rylander, R., Haglind, P., Lundholm, M., et al., Humidifier fever and endotoxin exposure. Clin. Allergy, *8*, 511, 1978.
67. Edwards, J. H., and Jones, B. M., A pseudoimmune precipitation by the isolated byssinosis "antigen." J. Immunol., *110*, 498, 1973.
68. Hitchcock, M., Piscitelli, D. M., and Bouhuys, A., Histamine release from human lung by a component of cotton bracts. Arch. Environ. Health, *26*, 177, 1973.
69. VanErt, M., and Battigelli, M. C., Mechanism of respiratory injury by TDI (toluene diisocyanate). Ann. Allergy, *35*, 142, 1975.
70. Butcher, B. T., O'Neill, C. W., Reed, M. A., and Salvaggio, J. E., Radioallergosorbent testing of toluene diisocyanate–reactive individuals using *p*-tolyl isocyanate antigen. J. Allergy Clin. Immunol., *66*, 213, 1980.
71. Policard, A., Sur la pathogénie de la silicose pulmonaire; mode de formation du nodule silicotique. Presse Med., *41*, 89, 1933.
72. DeMaria, T. F., and Burrell, R., Effects of inhaled endotoxin-containing bacteria. Environ. Res. *23*, 87, 1980.

73. Schlievert, P. M., and Watson, D. W., Group A streptococcal pyrogenic exotoxin: pyrogenicity and enhancement of lethal endotoxin shock. Infect. Immun., *21*, 753, 1978.
74. Burrell, R., Immunological aspects of silica. *In* Dunnom, D. D., ed., Health Effects of Synthetic Silica Particulates. Philadelphia, ASTM, 1980.
75. Burrell, R., Immunological aspects of coal workers' pneumoconiosis. Ann. N. Y. Acad. Sci., *200*, 94, 1972.
76. Miller, S. D., and Zarkower, A., Effects of carbon dust inhalation on the cell-mediated immune response in mice. Infect. Immun., *9*, 534, 1974.
77. Zarkower, A., and Morges, W., Alteration in antibody response induced by carbon inhalation: a model system. Infect. Immun., *5*, 915, 1972.
78. Turner-Warwick, M., Immunology and asbestosis. Proc. Roy. Soc. Med., *66*, 927, 1973.
79. Hahon, N., and Eckert, H. L., Depression of viral interferon induction in cell monolayers by asbestos fibers. Environ. Res., *11*, 52, 1976.
80. Haslam, P. L., Lukoszek, J. A., Merchant, J. A., and Turner-Warwick, M., Lymphocyte responses to phytohemagglutinin in patients with asbestosis and pleural mesothelioma. Clin. Exp. Immunol., *31*, 178, 1978.
81. Kagan, E., Solomon, A., Cochrane, J. C., et al., Immunological studies of patients with asbestosis. II. Studies of circulating lymphoid cell numbers and humoral immunity. Clin. Exp. Immunol., *28*, 268, 1977.
82. Miller, K., Weintraub, Z., and Kagan, E., Manifestations of cellular immunity in the rat after prolonged asbestos inhalation., J. Immunol., *123*, 1029, 1979.

9

THE MEASUREMENT OF DUSTS AND FUMES

Jim Dodgson

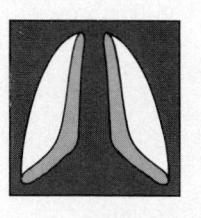

Dusts are present in the air we breathe at home, at work, in town, and in the country. This is not surprising when one considers the wide-ranging opportunities for solid particles to become dispersed in air. Windborne particles, including spores, pollens, bacteria, and viruses, as well as naturally occurring minerals, are dispersed naturally. In industry, airborne dusts arise when solid materials are crushed, ground, drilled, cut, blasted, and machined in various ways or when powdered material is disturbed by air movement or vibration during transport or packing. Spraying operations (e.g., paint, cement), emissions from combustion processes, farming operations, personal clothing, and furnishings are illustrative of other possible dust sources. Aerosols of small, submicron solid particles (fumes) are also formed by condensation of supersaturated vapors from gas phase reactions (e.g., metal and welding fumes) and from the products of combustion. These are usually much finer in particle size than airborne dusts formed by dispersion.

Airborne dusts may constitute a whole spectrum of inorganic and organic solid particles, both naturally occurring and manmade. Mixtures of different types of dust particles commonly occur in air. Fortunately, most dusts are relatively harmless and body defense systems have developed to cope with normal exposures. Nevertheless, some dusts may cause nasal cancer (wood dust), upper respiratory disorders (spores, pollens), chronic lung diseases (quartz, asbestos), lung carcinoma or mesothelioma (asbestos), or systemic poisoning (heavy metals, lead, cadmium) when inhaled or ingested to a sufficient extent. Contact with the skin may cause dermatitis or skin cancer (resins, chromates).

Many methods of dust measurement have evolved over the last 50 or more years. The available methods characterize airborne dusts in terms of their mass and particle number concentration, particle size distribution, and chemical, mineralogical, or microbiological composition. The sampling

212

and analysis methods selected in a given situation must be relevant to the potential health risk, and the sampling strategy adopted should be compatible with the purpose for sampling. Sampling may be carried out for a variety of reasons:

1. To identify environmental contaminants and sources
2. To assess the exposure of individuals in relation to national control limits or other safety standards
3. To monitor the effectiveness of environmental control equipment
4. For epidemiological research purposes

This chapter outlines the physical principles underlying current sampling practices and the main measurement methods. Information is provided on the more important practical aspects, including the selection of sampling filters and pumps. The importance of relating the sampling procedures to the subsequent analytical requirements is also discussed.

PHYSICAL PRINCIPLES OF DUST SAMPLING

Particle Size

Airborne dusts seldom consist of particles of the same size but are usually polydisperse. Similarly, particles of solid materials can vary enormously in shape from being flat and platelike (e.g., clay minerals, mica) to long, thin fibers (asbestos, glass, and rockwool fibers). Spherical particles are uncommon but can occur, for example, in the case of plant spores or from solidification from the liquid state (e.g., metal fumes, fly ash from pulverized fuel in power plants). More common are the crystalline or quasicrystalline asymmetric particles such as quartz, feldspars, carbonates, or most coals. These particles may be considered to approximate to spheres. Typical microscope images of particles of different shape are illustrated in Figure 9–1. The projected area of particles of approximate spherical shape can be equated to the diameter of a sphere of equivalent area, the diameter (referred to as the projected diameter) of which defines the particle size in microns. In the case of fibrous dusts, particle size must be expressed in terms of both fiber diameter and length. On the other hand, if the diameters of thin, flat, platelike particles are determined in this way, their physical size in relation to spheres in terms of mass or volume will be overestimated. A summary of typical particle diameters for a range of airborne dusts is shown in Figure 9–2.

Deposition of Particles in the Respiratory Tract

It is evident from Figure 9–2 that airborne dusts often contain coarse particles with diameters ranging up to 100 microns or more. While dusts that contact the face or eyes can cause discomfort or skin disorders, only those particles inhaled through the nose and mouth can be involved with

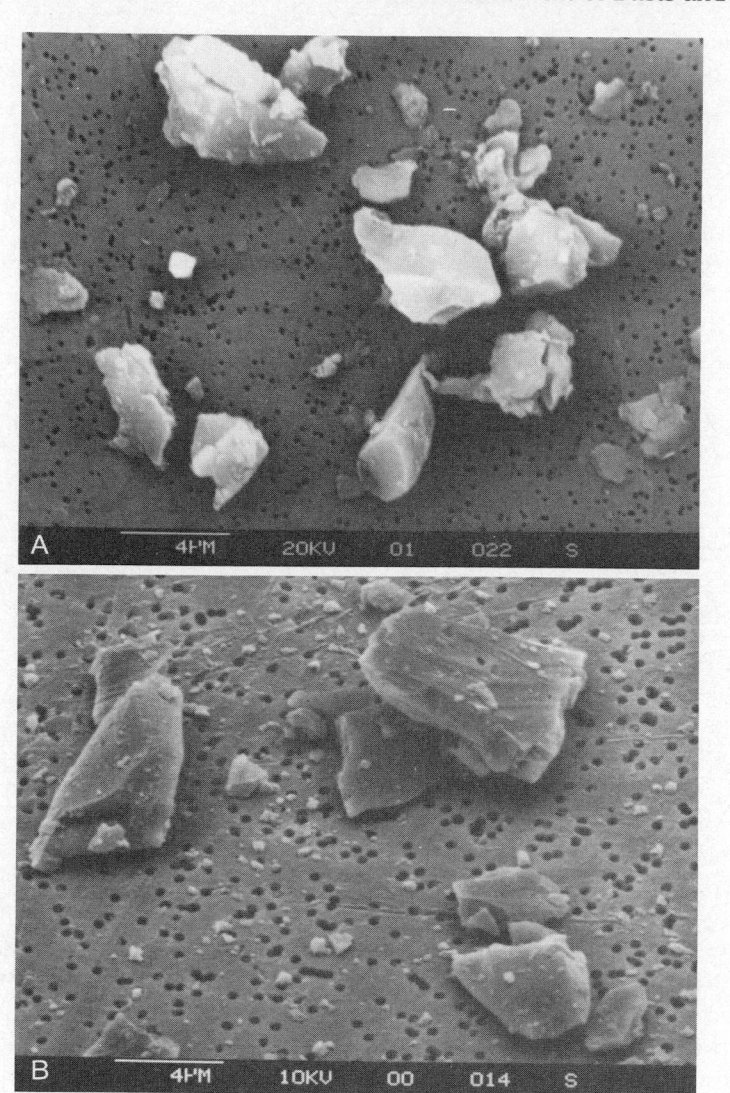

Figure 9–1. Typical photomicrographs of *(A)* coal, *(B)* quartz.

respiratory disease. It has long been known from autopsy studies on South African gold miners that the lung dusts consisted mainly of quartz particles, less than 5 microns in diameter, the mass of particles present being associated with the degree of silicosis. Subsequent research on many diseases involving epidemiological, autopsy, animal inhalation, and clinical studies have confirmed that dust-related diseases of the lung, such as silicosis, asbestosis, and coal workers' pneumoconiosis, are caused by the mass of fine, respirable particles that penetrate to the alveolar region of the lung. In the case of rapidly soluble and/or strongly reactive dusts, biological responses can occur wherever the particles are deposited in the

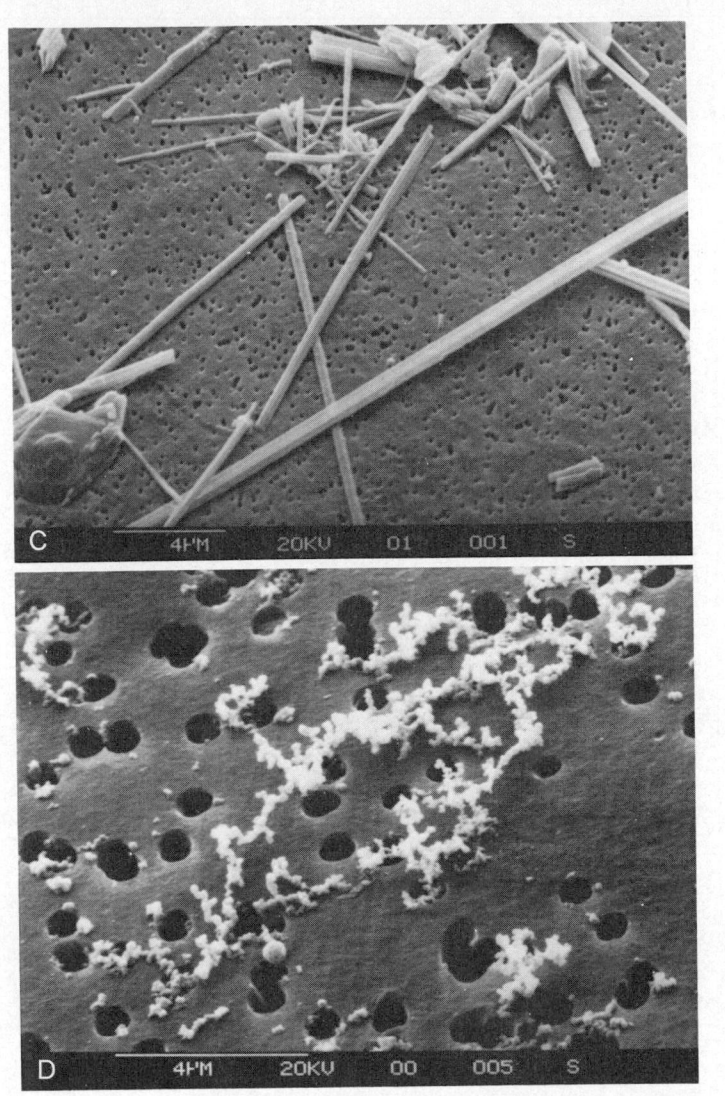

Figure 9–1 *(Continued)*. *(C)* Amosite asbestos, and *(D)* welding fume particles taken by scanning electron microscopy at magnifications indicated by the line marker. All samples mounted on Nuclepore filters and gold coated.

respiratory system or by swallowing. Some dusts when they deposit in the nonalveolated part of the lower respiratory tract may promote the development of bronchitis. Thus, the potential hazard from inhaled particles has been shown to depend on the:

1. Dust exposure (dust concentration × time at risk)
2. Site of dust deposition in the respiratory tract
3. Rate of dust clearance by cilia, macrophages, or body fluids
4. Biological toxicity and solubility of the dust

Studies of the regional deposition of inhaled particles in the respira-

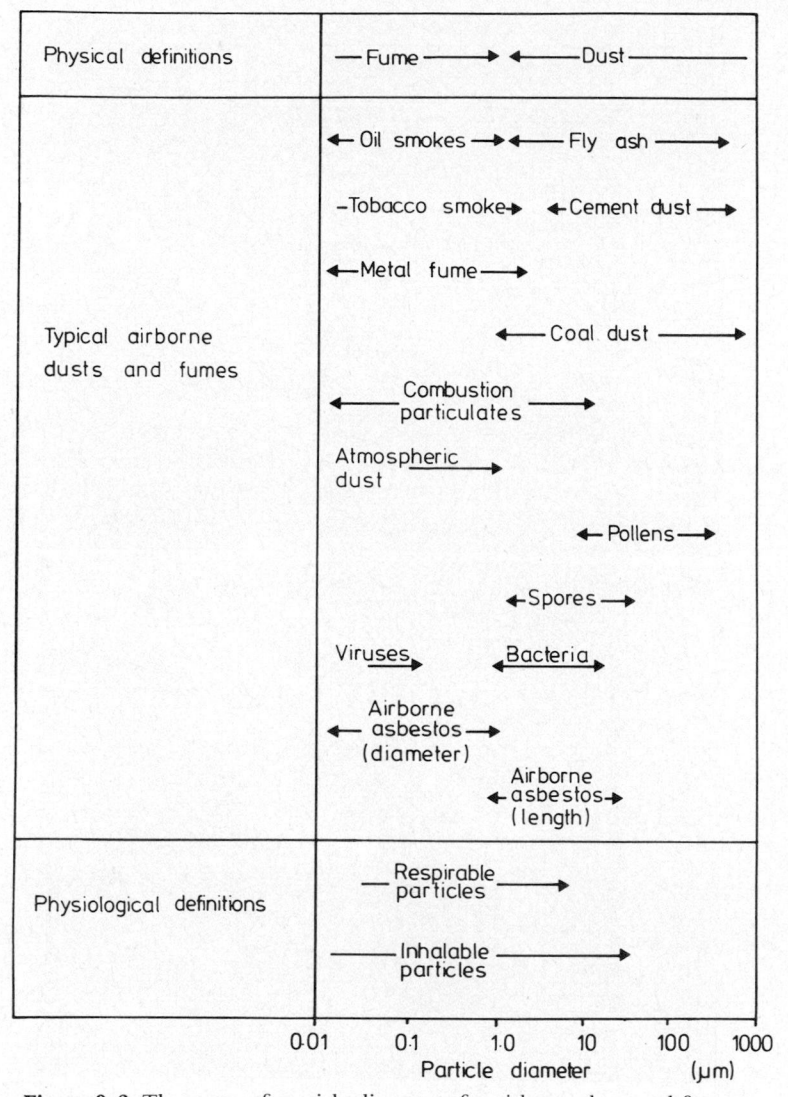

Figure 9–2. The range of particle diameters for airborne dusts and fumes.

tory tract of humans under varying breathing conditions have indicated that the amount deposited in the various regions is determined effectively by the *falling speed* of the particles in air. The *aerodynamic diameter* of a particle is used to describe the way in which particles settle or fall in still air. This is defined as the diameter (microns) of a spherical particle of unit density (1 gm/ml) that settles at the same speed as the particle in question.

The relationship between falling speed and aerodynamic diameter is well known. A freely falling particle within the size range found in dust and fumes rapidly attains a constant or terminal velocity when the

aerodynamic drag on the particle is equal to the weight of the particle. In most cases the terminal velocity, v, for spherical particles of diameter, d, may be calculated from Stokes' law:

$$v = \frac{gd^2 (p - p^1)}{18\eta}$$

where g = gravitational acceleration, η = viscosity, p = density of particle, and p^1 = density of air. Special corrections to the equation need to be applied for very small particles of a size (less than 0.01 microns) comparable with the mean free path of the air molecules and for large particles (greater than 77 microns) in which inertial effects arise due to the displacement of the air by the particle.

It should be noted that the aerodynamic diameter of a particle will usually differ from its projected diameter as measured under the microscope. The diameters will only be equal for spherical particles of unit density. Large differences occur between these parameters for particles that differ substantially from spherical shape or from unit density. For example, the terminal settling velocity (and hence aerodynamic diameter) of a long fiber or a platelike mineral is much less than that of a sphere of equivalent projected diameter or mass. This may be easily demonstrated by taking two equal size pieces of paper, crumpling one piece into a small ball, and comparing the falling speed with that of the other piece, which is held flat on the palm of a hand and dropped from the same height. Typical relationships between settling speeds and diameters of spherical particles of unit density are shown in Table 9–1. For example, all particles with a falling speed of 3.06×10^{-1} cm/s have an aerodynamic diameter of 10 microns, while those settling at 1.19×10^{-2} cm/s have an aerodynamic diameter of 2 microns, and so on.

In 1966 the Task Group on Lung Dynamics[1] considered the results of research on the deposition of particles in the respiratory tract and

Table 9–1. RELATIONSHIPS BETWEEN TERMINAL VELOCITIES AND AERODYNAMIC DIAMETERS OF SPHERICAL PARTICLES OF UNIT DENSITY*

Terminal Velocity (cm/s)	Aerodynamic Diameter (microns)
8.71×10^{-5}	0.1
2.27×10^{-4}	0.2
6.85×10^{-4}	0.4
3.49×10^{-3}	1.0
1.19×10^{-2}	2
5.00×10^{-2}	4
3.06×10^{-1}	10
1.2	20
5	40
25	100

*In air at 760 mm Hg and 20°C.

proposed a working classification to aid further studies. They divided the respiratory tract into three regions: nasopharyngeal (the head down to and including the larynx), tracheobronchial (the trachea and the bronchial tree down to the terminal bronchioles), and alveolated (the respirable region where the gas exchange takes place). Conventionally, the fractions of dust deposited in the three regions are expressed as functions of particle aerodynamic diameter for given breathing conditions. It should be noted that these are all expressed as subfractions of the dust that is actually inhaled through the nose and mouth during breathing, that is, the inhaled fraction of dust present in the ambient air. The inhaled fraction may be defined as the ratio of the dust concentration for particles of a given size in the air entering the body to that in the ambient air.

Results of research in this field may be combined in various ways to help frame quantitative definitions of dust subfractions that should be sampled selectively to aid investigations or control of different dust related diseases. A typical set of examples, illustrated in Figure 9–3, derives from recently published data[2] for mouth or nose breathing, selected to give the worst case for each region. The respirable and tracheobronchial deposition curves are taken from Stahlhoffen et al.[3] for "normal work" at a nominal minute volume of 20 L. The deposition curve for nasopharyngeal deposition was derived from Mercer[4] for similar conditions. These examples show that while particles of all sizes may be deposited in the nasopharyngeal region, only particles with aerodynamic diameter up to about 15 microns may be deposited in the tracheobronchial region, and only

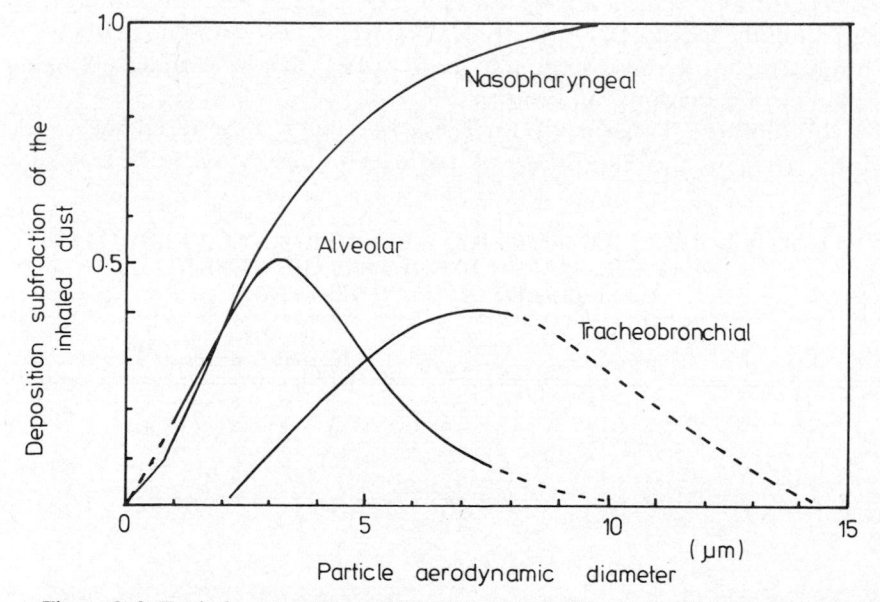

Figure 9–3. Typical curves of the regional deposition subfractions of the inhaled fraction of ambient airborne dust for human subjects.

particles with aerodynamic diameter up to about 10 microns may be deposited in the alveolar region.

In designing samplers broadly simulating the mechanism of deposition in the respiratory tract, it is necessary to make various approximations and assumptions if a practical system of sampling is to be achieved. At the suggestion of the World Health Organization, an Ad Hoc Working Group of the International Standards Organization (ISO) Committee on Air Quality[5] recently considered the available evidence and proposed a formal set of quantitative definitions for the sampling of subfractions of inhalable dust. In this context the term "inspired dust," favored by the ISO group, is synonymous with "inhaled dust," used by British and German workers in this field.

While considerable agreement has been reached on the working criteria for sampling subfractions of inhaled dust to assess health effects, the practical achievement of suitable devices—except for that for the measurement of respirable subfraction—remains to be accomplished.

SAMPLING METHODS

Dust-sampling methods have changed considerably since the early part of this century. Different physical principles have been used in the collection of dust particles, and methods of evaluation have also changed. Data obtained using measurement techniques different from those in current practice frequently form the basis of current control limits, and any earlier measurements that are available need to be taken into account during epidemiological research. Results from different methods are not usually directly comparable, and the reliability of the data needs to be assessed. In this context it is helpful to consider the changes in dust-sampling practice and the physical principles involved before discussing current procedures.

Many methods have been developed for collecting dust samples for weighing, counting, or analysis in terms of particle shape, size, and mineralogical, chemical, or biological composition. The earliest methods were developed in South Africa during the years 1902 to 1911 in the fight against silicosis among gold miners.[6] At first a known volume of dusty air was aspirated through a cotton filter and the weight of "total" dust determined after incineration of the filter. Subsequently, a "sugar tube"[7] was used, in which the dust was trapped by impaction on sugar granules, which were then dissolved and the dust filtered and weighed. These mass measuring methods did not separate the aerodynamically fine particles, and the weights obtained were dominated by the presence of small numbers of large particles. This, together with the recognition of the importance of the fine particles in silicosis, led to the development of dust-sampling techniques that enabled the number of fine particles to be counted by optical microscopy. These methods, giving results in terms of

particle counts as opposed to mass measurements, were used internationally until the development of gravimetric samplers for respirable dust during the 1960s. The latter were fitted with aerodynamic size-selectors to exclude the aerodynamically large particles. Microscopical dust-counting methods continue to be used for fibrous dusts, especially asbestos, in which it is necessary to distinguish the fiber count from the other particles present. Similarly, so called "total mass" measurements continue to be used for lead and other dusts in which measurements of the total respiratory exposure are relevant. It is anticipated that methods for measuring the total inhalable fraction of dust will become available shortly and will gradually replace the "total dust" methods.

Other developments in sampling methods include the increasing availability of direct reading instruments for both number count and mass concentrations. Increased emphasis is now placed on the use of small, personal samplers that can be located in the breathing zone of a worker for a more accurate determination of personal exposures. Large differences can occur between samples taken by instruments mounted on the worker in this way and static samples taken at fixed points near the individual. Recently reported studies in the asbestos industry have illustrated the difficulties in relating personal and static measurements.[8]

Exposures of individuals carrying out similar work may vary according to differences in personal working procedures or location relative to a source of dust. Variations in dust level may also occur during a day or over longer periods. For these reasons a reasonably reliable assessment of the conditions necessitates an appropriate sampling strategy involving both the selection of a relevant sampling method and a sufficient number of repetitive measurements. Ideally, the frequency of sampling should be based on a statistical evaluation of the variability in relation to the purpose of the measurements, whether these be for research or to test compliance with health and safety standards.

Measurement of Particle Number Concentrations

Until 20 years ago, the most widely used dust-count instruments were konimeters, impingers, and Owen's jet impaction devices, together with thermal precipitators.[6] The Kotze konimeter[9] was first developed in South Africa, and various versions have been used throughout the world, including Germany, Britain, and the United States; the small size, portability, and short sampling time have probably contributed to its popularity. It employed the principle of inertial impaction of particles from a high-speed air jet directed against a glass plate coated with petroleum or glycerine jelly as an adhesive. The Kotze konimeter utilized a spring-loaded pump to draw a 5-ml sample of air through a 0.5-mm orifice to deposit a small spot of dust on the plate for subsequent counting. Samples were taken in a fraction of a second, and successive samples could be taken on the same slide. Later versions of the device also included a built-in microscope.[10]

Since the early 1920s, impingers[11] and midget impingers[12] have been extensively used in the United States and Canada, where they became the standard dust-sampling instruments. In this case the airborne particles were drawn through a small orifice under water or other liquid and trapped by an impingement process. The suspensions could be diluted if necessary to give an optimum density for counting, thus giving flexibility in terms of sampling time and dust concentration.

The Owen's jet dust counter[13] also relied on the impingement principle. In this case the sampled air was first humidified by passage through a chamber lined with wetted blotting paper and then passed through a slit, where adiabatic expansion caused condensation of water on the dust particles. This increased the deposition efficiency onto glass slides and no adhesive was necessary. The Owen's jet was widely used in Britain during the 1920s and 30s, until the development of the thermal precipitator. It remained until very recently the standard dust-sampling instrument in Australia.

Impaction and impingement devices suffer from serious limitations that affect particle collection. Large particles are not collected efficiently— they may bounce off the slide or shatter and increase the count of small particles. Clumps may break up in the air jet or in the liquid of the impinger. Thermal precipitators[14, 15] are highly efficient for the collection of small particles below 5 microns in size, but incomplete thermal precipitation occurs at larger sizes and gravitational fall-in can occur. In these instruments air is drawn past an electrically heated wire situated between two adjacent glass coverslips on each of which a "strip" of dust is deposited. Air flow rates were low, 7 ml/min in the case of the Standard Thermal Precipitator; successive sets of short-period samples were required to cover a working shift. A modified thermal precipitator was developed for use in South Africa,[16] which provided a single dust deposit for counting. A long-running thermal precipitator[17] was developed for use in British coal mines. This instrument incorporated an aerodynamic size-selector that allowed the respirable dust to pass to settlement and thermal precipitation zones, where the deposited dusts were collected on one slide over periods of up to 8 hours.

The number count instruments were all used as static samplers located at fixed points either in the ventilating air stream near the worker or at a point close to potential sources of contaminant emission. The quantities of dust collected were small, and the composition of the dust could only be investigated by microscopical methods or by specialized microanalytical techniques.

Measurement of Respirable Dust

During the last 20 years, dust-sampling instruments have been developed that simulate the deposition of particles in the alveolar region of the respiratory tract. These instruments use aerodynamic preselectors to

remove the faster falling particles of large aerodynamic diameter that would deposit in the upper airways and allow the slower falling, fine, respirable particles to penetrate to a filter where they are collected for weighing. Sufficient respirable dust can be sampled with these devices over a working shift to permit direct measurements of the mass concentration and dust composition. Long-term investigations in the British coal-mining industry[18] have shown that the mass concentration of respirable dust measured in this way provides a much better index of the pneumoconiosis hazard than number counts of small (<5 micron) particles.

The most widely used aerodynamic preselectors are those based on horizontal elutriators or cyclones. Figure 9–4 schematically illustrates the MRE gravimetric sampler, Type 113A, which incorporates a horizontal elutriator.[19] Both the British and United States federal dust regulations for coal mines are based on this instrument. It operates at a flow rate of 2.5 L/min using a built-in pump and can collect 1 to 20 mg of respirable dust in a work shift. The horizontal elutriators give a parabolic selection curve, as illustrated in Figure 9–5, and have the advantage that their performance in practice agrees closely with that predicted theoretically.[20] They have been designed to select the respirable fraction of dust recommended by the British Medical Research Council (BMRC)[21] and the 1959 Pneumoconiosis Conference in Johannesburg.[22]

All particles with an aerodynamic diameter greater than 7.1 microns settle in the channels of the elutriator, while 50 per cent of the particles of 5 microns aerodynamic diameter and 100 per cent of very small sizes penetrate to the filter. The selection curve differs from the alveolar deposition curve, with which it is compared in Figure 9–5, particularly above 7.1 microns and in the very fine size ranges. Nevertheless, the advantages of having a physically well-defined and practically robust "standard" device were considered to be more important. The MRE gravimetric sampler is illustrated in Figure 9–6.

The United States Atomic Energy Commission[23] has proposed an alternative selection curve that more closely matches alveolar deposition (see Figure 9–5). Cyclones have been produced that can approximate to this selection curve, though a complete theoretical understanding of their performance is lacking. Nevertheless, their performance can be matched empirically to the required selection curve at a specified flow rate. In the typical cyclone shown in Figure 9–7 dust-laden air enters the cylindrical chamber B via the tangential inlet A and takes a spiral path downwards, inwards, and then finally upwards towards outlet E. The dimensions of the cyclone may be chosen so that the unwanted particles of large aerodynamic diameter are thrown outwards by inertial forces to the walls of cone C and then swept downwards in the rotating air stream to dust hopper D. The particles of small aerodynamic size remain airborne and are swept through outlet E, where they are collected on a filter. A major advantage of the cyclone system of preselection is that small cyclones can be manufactured that can be worn by the worker together with a small

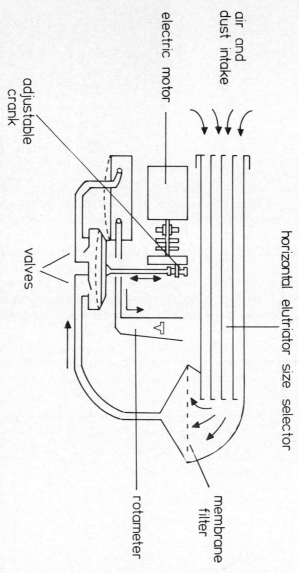

air and
dust intake

electric motor

horizontal elutriator size selector

adjustable
crank

valves

membrane
filter

rotameter

Figure 9–4. A schematic drawing of the MRE gravimetric sampler, Type 113A, illustrating the horizontal elutriator size-selector for respirable dust.

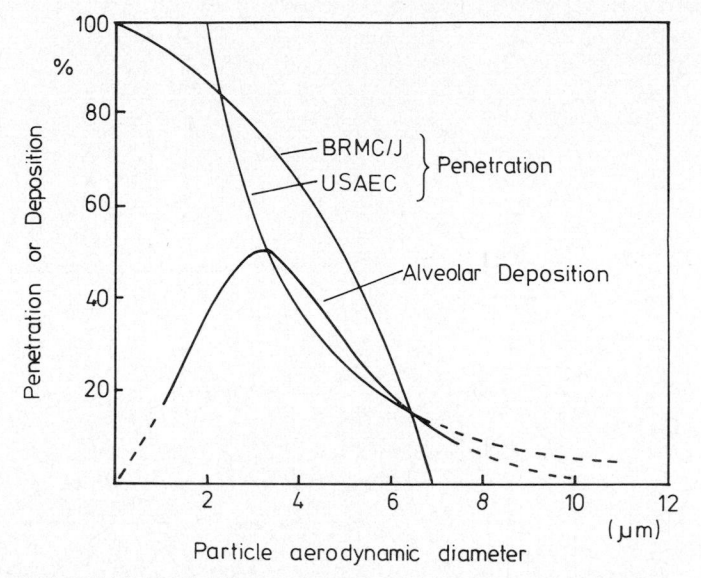

Figure 9–5. British Medical Research Council and Johannesburg and USAEC particle selection curves for respirable dusts compared with alveolar curve of Stahlhofen et al.[3]

belt-mounted pump to give a measure of personal exposure. The Casella cyclone[24] shown in Figure 9–8 operates at a flow rate of 1.9 L/min but higher volume static samplers are also available. Pulsations in the air flow from the pump must be smoothed to avoid affects on the size selection; dampers are often incorporated in the pump case for this purpose or they can be fitted externally in the air line. Both the cyclone and horizontal elutriator instruments must be operated at their specified flow rates, otherwise their size selection characteristics will be impaired.

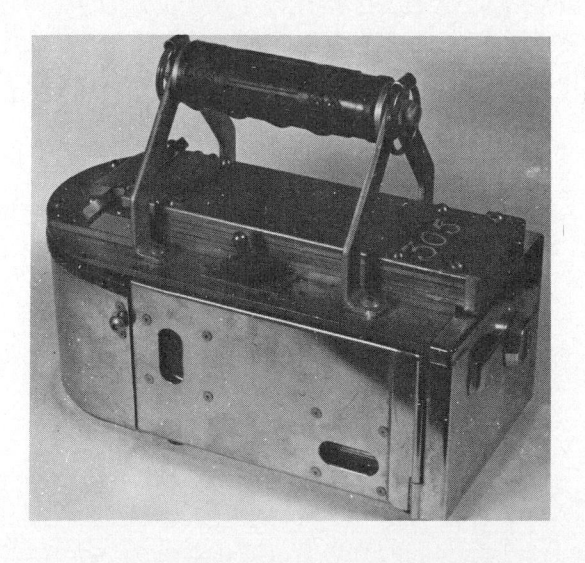

Figure 9–6. The MRE gravimetric sampler, Type 113A (Casella), for respirable dust.

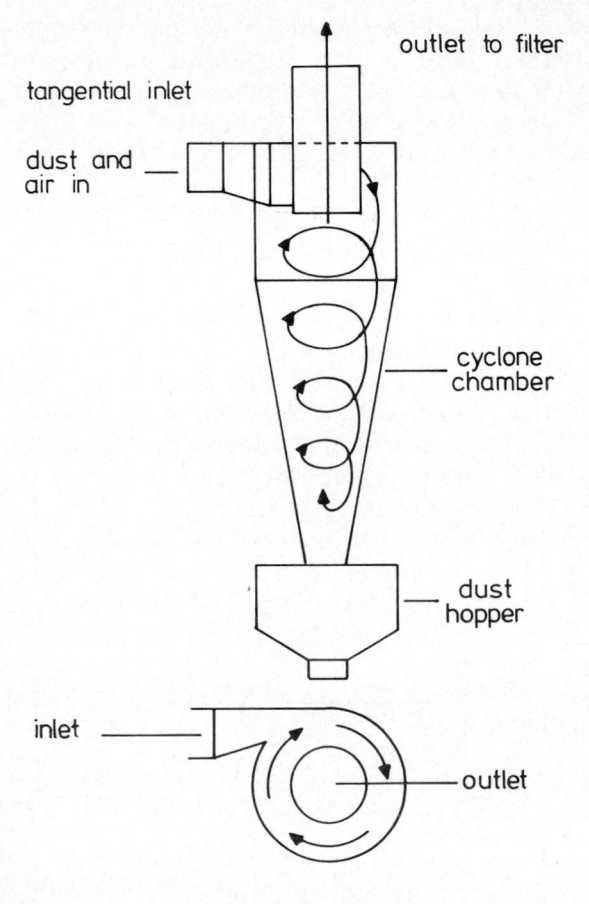

Figure 9–7. A schematic drawing of a typical cyclone size-selector for respirable dust.

Figure 9–8. The SIMPEDS cyclone dust sampler (Casella) for respirable dust.

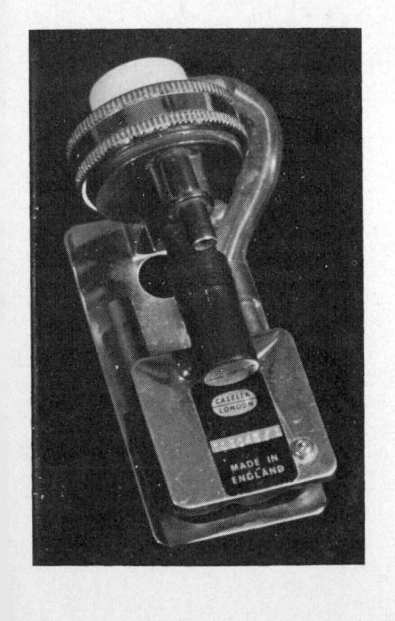

The filters chosen for use in cyclone or horizontal elutriator instruments must have a high filtration efficiency and be suitable for the measurement of mass and dust composition, if required. These requirements also apply to instruments used for total dust sampling and are discussed later.

Measurement of Inhalable Dust

The results of research into methods for measuring the total inhaled fraction of dust have been published recently.[25] Inertial effects largely control both the efficiency with which particles are inhaled and the efficiency of particle collection by blunt samplers. Coarse particles with a high inertia tend not to follow the air streams as they bend to enter the nose, mouth, or entry orifice of an instrument and may not be captured. These effects are important, particularly for particles of larger aerodynamic diameter, as may be seen in Figure 9–9. These results were derived from wind tunnel experiments using life-size model tailor's dummies[26–28] with simulated breathing and in which the entry efficiencies of particles through the nose and mouth were measured in a range of wind speeds

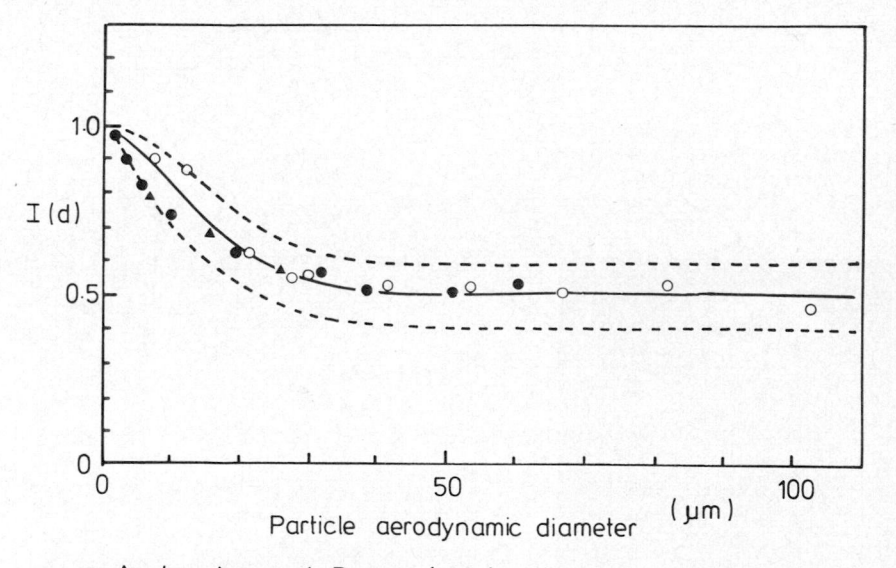

• Armbruster and Breuer (1981)
○ Vincent and Mark (1981)
▲ Ogden and Birkett (1977)

Figure 9–9. Inhalability [I(d)] of airborne dust measured as a function of particle aerodynamic diameter (d) averaged uniformly over all orientations of the model, normal work rate and wind speeds up to 8 m/s. The dotted lines indicate experimental tolerance limits. (Modified from Vincent, J. H., and Armbruster, L.: On the quantitative definition of the inhalability of airborne dust. Ann. Occup. Hyg., *24*, 245, 1981.)

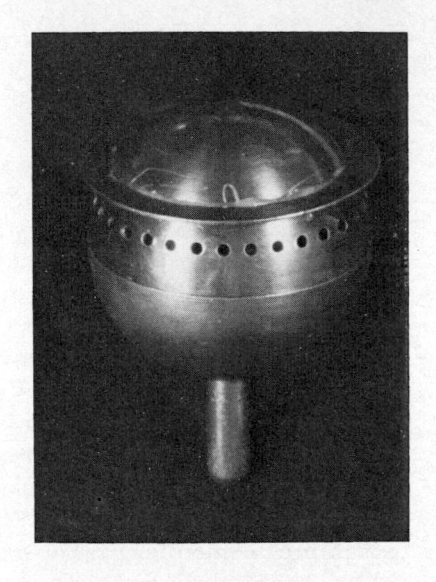

Figure 9–10. The ORB sampling head for inhalable dust.

and wind directions. The inhaled fraction falls from 1.0 to about 0.5 as particle size increases to a 40-micron aerodynamic diameter for results averaged for wind speed and orientation, and typical breathing rates. It then remains constant over the range of particle size measured up to about 100 microns. The effect is small for the fine, respirable subfraction of particles (<7 microns) but much larger for particles likely to settle in the nasopharyngeal or tracheobronchial regions.

The efficiencies of the blunt samplers commonly used by occupational hygienists to sample so called "total" dust (see Fig. 9–11) have been shown to depend on sampler design as well as on wind speed, location, and orientation.[27, 29] This can result in large differences of up to fivefold in measured mass concentration for samplers of different design, even when sampling simultaneously in the same environment.[30] It is desirable that sampling instruments should be designed with inlets that conform with the inhalability criteria demonstrated in Figure 9–9, and with subsequent means of separating the inhalable subfractions, if required. A prototype ORB sampler[29] has been developed for static sampling of inhalable dust but is not available commercially. This instrument is illustrated in Figure 9–10 and consists of a spherical sampling head with a series of circular holes drilled horizontally close to the equatorial plane. Samples are taken omnidirectionally at a flow rate of 2 L/min. Tests have shown that its entry characteristic agrees reasonably well with the inhalability criteria for dusts with an aerodynamic diameter up to 30 microns. Further development work is currently taking place. Since the efficiency of sampling the respirable subfraction is little affected by inertial effects, sampler design is relatively unimportant for these particles.

Measurement of Total Dust

The mass concentration of so called "total dust" has traditionally been measured by using a pump to draw a measured amount of dust-laden air through a filter or thimble mounted in a suitable holder, followed by weighing. A wide variety of pumps, filters, and filter holders are available; some typical devices are illustrated in Figure 9–11. These are all blunt samplers and subject to the limitations previously described. Interpretation of the results in relation to the quantity of dust actually inhaled needs to be made with these limitations in mind. If coarse dust is present, the method is only likely to be a useful comparative indicator of dust level where the same type of sampler is used repetitively in the same environment under identical operating and ambient wind conditions. Nevertheless, the method is widely used and will continue to be until satisfactory inhalable dust samplers are available commercially.

The equipment needed for *personal sampling* of dust exposure consists of a pump, a smoother (either separate or built within the pump), a filter holder for total dust or a cyclone for sampling respirable dust, and an appropriate filter together with tubing and a harness (belt, clips, etc.). The pump is usually fastened to a waist belt and the filter holder situated within the breathing zone, that is, within 30 cm of the nose or mouth.

The type of pump, filter, and filter holder selected will depend on the requirements of the investigation. When sampling respirable dust, the filter dimensions are determined by the cyclone selected, 37 mm in the case of the Casella SIMPEDS cyclone. This is also the case for static samplers in which the filter holder is incorporated within the instrument (e.g., the MRE gravimetric sampler, Type 113A). Methods for sampling

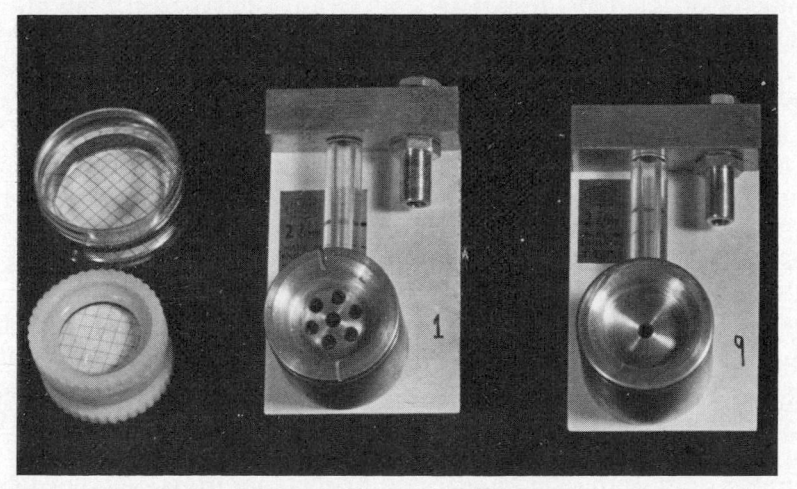

Figure 9–11. Typical total dust sampling heads. Gelman 25-mm diameter and Millipore 37-mm diameter open heads compared with 25-mm shielded sampling heads (Casella/ UKAEA Model T13032 single 4-mm port and modified seven-port head).

total dust or fume have not been closely defined, and a wide range of open or shielded filter holders are used, the most common being of either 25-mm, 37-mm, or 47-mm diameter.

Selection of Pumps. A wide range of lightweight, battery-powered, low-flow-rate pumps is available for personal sampling, though they can also be used for fixed-point, static sampling. These instruments use diaphragm, piston, and rotary pump systems, each with different physical characteristics, as indicated in Table 9–2. Flow rates vary with the type of pump from about 0.1 to 8.0 L/min. High-volume pumps or air movers capable of 100 L/min or more are also available for static sampling. The flow rate required will depend upon the likely dust concentration encountered, the amount of dust to be collected for accurate weighing, and other analytical requirements. Internal flowmeters or digital counters are incorporated in most pumps, but these need to be calibrated with an external flowmeter. It should be noted that the flow rate obtained with pumps varies with the resistance imposed by the filter system (see Fig. 9–12 and Table 9–5). For this reason flow rates should be checked during sampling and adjusted, if possible, or corrections applied to the volume of air sampled. Stabilized flow pumps that largely avoid this problem are now available. The performance of two such types is illustrated in Figure 9–12. In potentially explosive atmospheres (e.g., coal mines, chemical plants) intrinsically safe or flame-proof pumps must be used to minimize any risks.

Selection of Filters. Many different filter materials with markedly different physical and chemical properties are now available for dust

Table 9–2. CHARACTERISTICS OF PERSONAL SAMPLING PUMPS

Pump Type	Advantages	Disadvantages
Single-acting diaphragm	1. Highest efficiency low power consumption small battery low weight 2. Simple to repair 3. Cheapest to build	1. Pulsating flow, one pulse per rev. 2. Pressure drop limitation 500 mm water gauge 3. Valve leakage
Double-acting piston	1. Good efficiency medium power consumption medium weight 2. No pressure drop limitation	1. Difficult to repair 2. Mildly pulsating two pulses per rev. 3. Valve leakage
Dry-vane rotary	1. Smooth flow, three or four pulses per rev. 2. No valve leakage (no valves) 3. No pressure drop limitation 4. High reliability 5. Moderate cost	1. Low efficiency large battery high weight 2. Moderately difficult to repair

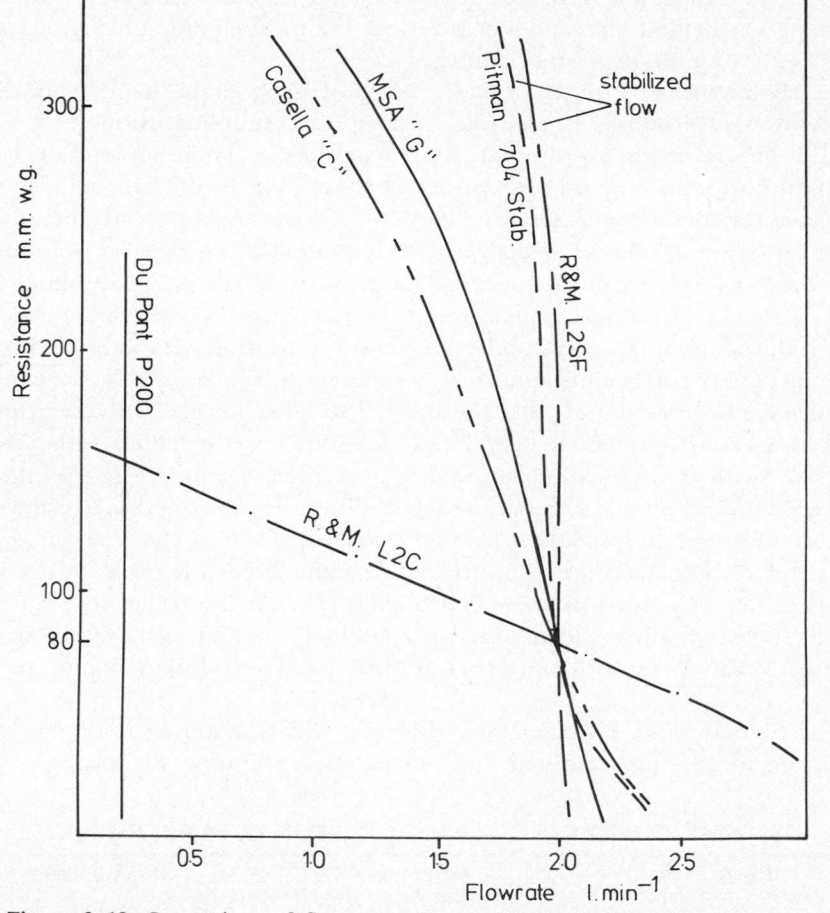

Figure 9–12. Comparison of flow-rate response to changing resistance of sampling pumps set at 2 L/min against 80 mm water gauge. (Du Pont set for 200 ml/min against 80 mm water gauge).

sampling. These include the polymer membrane, sintered, and fibrous filters listed in Table 9–3.

The filters are available in a range of diameters and pore sizes, the latter varying from about 0.1 to 10 microns, though the full range is not available in all materials. The main advantages of membrane filters are their relatively uniform pore size and their ability to retain efficiently dusts on the surface, as opposed to the in-depth filtration characteristics of fibrous filters. Considerable care is needed in selecting a filter for a particular purpose, since they are not all equally suitable for all sampling and analytical purposes.

The main *sampling requirements* are:

1. Physical robustness. Filters need to be sufficiently strong to avoid tearing in the filter holder or during handling.

2. High filtration efficiency. The values in Table 9–4 show that pore

Table 9–3. TYPES OF FILTERS

Membrane Filters	Fibrous Filters	Sintered Filter
Cellulose nitrate	Polystyrene (microsorban)	Silver
Cellulose acetate	Glass	
Cellulose mixed esters	Glass/binder	
Regenerated cellulose*	Paper	
Polyvinyl chloride (PVC)		
PVC (mineral filled)		
PVC/acrylonitrile (Copolymer)		
Polytetrafluoroethylene (PTFE)*		
PTFE/polypropylene*		
Nylon*		
Polycarbonate (Nuclepore)		

*Mainly used for liquid filtration.

size alone is less important than filter type in determining this characteristic for airborne particulates; submicron particles are efficiently trapped on some 5- or 8-micron pore size filters by virtue of the inertial and electrostatic forces that occur. It is usually desirable to use 5- to 10-micron pore size filters to minimize the loading on the sampling pump, as discussed below.

3. The appropriate size and type of filter should be selected so that it is compatible with flow characteristics of the pump if the required flow is to be maintained throughout the full sampling period. The flow resistance of the filter varies with flow rate, filter type, pore size, and filter diameter. The values shown in Table 9–5 for a range of filters and pore sizes were obtained at a flow rate of 2 L/min, but resistances at other flow rates may be obtained with reasonable accuracy by linear interpolation. Allowance should also be made for the added resistance imposed as dust builds up on the filter during sampling.

4. Filters with a relatively low electrical resistance should be used to minimize sampling losses due to electrostatic charging. Static eliminators should be utilized when weighing to limit errors due to this cause.

Table 9–4. COLLECTION EFFICIENCIES OF TYPICAL FILTERS, FOR AIRBORNE SUBMICRON PARTICLES*

Filter Type	Filtration Efficiency (%)
Cellulose nitrate membrane (8-micron pore size)	> 99
Mixed cellulose ester membrane (5-μm pore size)	> 99
Glass fiber (Whatman GF/A)	> 99
Silver membrane (3-micron pore size)	95
Whatman paper filters	> 90 (in general)

*Measured with methylene blue test cloud sampled at 1.9 L/min through 25-mm filters.

Table 9–5. VARIATION OF FILTER RESISTANCE WITH PORE SIZE AND FILTER DIAMETER

Filter Material	Pore Size (microns)	Filter Resistances for Diameters*			
		50 mm	47 mm	37 mm	25 mm
Sartorius cellulose nitrate or PVC	8.0	9.0	10	17	40
	1.2	40.0	46	78	196
	0.8	48	54	95	230
	0.2	276	320	530	>600
Millipore mixed esters	8.0	—	24	40	98
	1.2	—	88	150	360
	0.8	—	120	200	>600
	0.2	—	520	>600	>600
Gelman mixed esters	0.8	—	82	140	340
Gelman E glass fiber			24	40	100
Whatman GF/A glass fiber		13.6	17	27	64
Nuclepore	8.0	—	24	40	106
	0.8	—	44	78	190
	0.2	—	320	>600	>600
Flotronics silver membrane	5.0	—	19	32	78
	1.2	—	48	82	204
	0.8	—	70	117	290
	0.2	—	276	>600	>600

*At an airflow of 2 L/min in mm water gauge (W.G.).

The *analytical requirements* of filters depend on the nature of the analyses. For example, the weight stability of filters in air is of particular importance, since gravimetric assessments of dust samples are invariably required. If fiber counts on filters are required, it is essential that these can be rendered optically transparent for microscope evaluations. Direct on-the-filter measurements of mineralogical composition for quartz or other minerals are frequently carried out using infrared spectrophtometry (IR), x-ray diffraction (XRD), or scanning electron microscope and energy dispersive x-ray analyses (SEM/EDXA). X-ray fluorescence methods are often similarly used for elemental analysis. For these purposes, filters must allow good transmission of IR radiation or possess good surface filtration characteristics with low background scatter of radiation, in the case of XRD and SEM methods.

Filter samples may also be chemically extracted prior to analysis of the extract; for example, coal tar pitch volatiles are measured in coke oven fumes by benzene extraction. Similarly, dusts may be recovered by washing and ultrasonics for subsequent analysis. In these cases, the filter chosen must be compatible with the extraction or washing system used. They should be stable and not lose material by partial disintegration or solution. Direct incineration of filters to determine ash content and/or

mineralogical composition of the ash requires filters that combust gently without explosive loss; they should have a low inherent ash content. A list of recommended filters for various applications is provided in Table 9–6. Particle size variations are important in some analyses (e.g., IR, XRD), and size-selective samplers should be used in these cases, together with the appropriate filter, the standard dust and control filter.

The weight of filters in air can vary substantially, since they absorb varying amounts of water depending on the relative humidity. Changes of 1 mg or more can occur in the weight of cellulose nitrate filters with a change in relative humidity from about 10 to 75 per cent. Variations of up to 0.5 mg are frequently observed in practice with these and other cellulose ester filters. Much smaller variations occur with polyvinyl chloride (PVC), polycarbonate (Nuclepore), glass fiber, and silver filters. Control filters should be selected from each batch to monitor and correct for weight changes. Both control and sample filters should be allowed to stabilize overnight and reach equilibrium with the balance room atmosphere both before and after sampling. When mean control corrections (at least one control filter to ten sample filters is required) are applied in this way to sample weights, the error in weighing 25-mm-diameter cellulose nitrate filters is reduced to about 0.06 mg, with a standard deviation of 0.03 mg. The corresponding error for Nuclepore filters is 0.007 mg, with a standard deviation of 0.01 mg. Alternatively, a humidity-controlled atmosphere for both the filters and the balance can be used.

Measurement of Asbestos and Other Fibrous Dusts

Airborne concentrations of asbestos or other fibers are now generally measured using the "membrane filter method" first introduced by Britain's Asbestosis Research Council.[31] In practice this method utilizes the open filter holders, sampling pumps, and personal sampling procedures used for total dust sampling. Samples are usually collected on cellulose ester membrane filters of 0.8- or 1.2-micron pore size, since they are easily rendered optically transparent using triacetin, acetone/triacetin, or alternative treatments. This enables the number of fibers of defined size to be counted using phase-contrast microscopy. Fibers and other particles embedded within a cleared membrane filter are difficult to see because of the small differences in refractive index between the fibers and the filter matrix. The resulting small differences in optical path length through the particles and matrix produce small differences in the phase of light waves from these sources, which are converted by interference in the phase-contrast microscope into visible differences in the intensity of light. Detailed descriptions of the principles of phase-contrast microscopy may be found in standard texts.[32]

As with other microscope counting procedures, the method is based on counting the number of fibers on a small proportion of the filter

Table 9–6. SELECTION OF FILTERS FOR ANALYTICAL PURPOSES

Technique	Method of Measurement	Recommended Filter (Pore Size)	Remarks
Weighing of total or respirable dusts	Direct	Cellulose nitrate or acetate (8 microns, 5 microns) PVC (5 microns) Glass GFA Nuclepore (0.8 microns)	Accetable weight stability in air
Optical phase-contrast microscope for asbestos counts	Direct	Cellulose nitrate or other esters (0.8 or 1.2 microns)	Easily made transparent with acetone/triacetin, triacetin, etc.
SEM evaluations (number, size, mineralogical, elemental)	Direct	Nuclepore (0.4 microns, 0.8 microns)	Good, smooth surface
IR spectrophotometry (quartz, silicates)	Direct or after recovery or other treatment	PVC (5.0 microns) Nuclepore (0.8 microns) DM Copolymer	Good weight stability in air high IR transmission
XR diffraction (quartz, other minerals)	Direct or after recovery or other treatment	Silver (0.8 microns) Nuclepore (0.8 microns)	Good weight stability, low background scatter
XR fluorescence or atomic absorption spectrophotometry for elemental analysis	Direct or after recovery or other treatment	Paper (Whatman 41) Cellulose mixed ester (5 microns)	
Wash recovery of dusts (aqueous treatment with ultrasonics)	Direct	Cellulose nitrate (8.0 microns, 5.0 microns) Nuclepore (0.8 microns)	Robust, low residual ash
Ashing of filter dusts	Direct	PVC (5.0 microns), DM Copolymer Nuclepore (0.8 microns) Cellulose esters (5.0 microns)	Quantitative incineration possible, low residual ash/elemental contamination
Chemical digestion (e.g., for elemental analysis by atomic absorption spectrophotometry)	Direct	Cellulose esters (5.0 microns)	Low elemental contamination, easily digested
Solvent extraction	Direct	Silver (0.8 microns) Glass GFA	Robust and weight stable, solvent resistant

surface (about 0.5 per cent or less). A series of random field areas is selected for counting using a microscope graticule of the type shown in Figure 9–13.[33] Assuming that the area of filter examined is representative of the whole, the fiber concentration (f) may then be estimated from:

$$f = \frac{A \cdot N}{aV} \text{ fibers/ml}$$

where N = the number of fibers counted in area a (mm^2), A = the exposed area of filter (mm^2), and V = the volume of air sampled (ml).

Conventionally, only "respirable" fibers with a diameter less than 3 microns, a length greater than 5 microns, and a length to width ratio or "aspect ratio" greater than 3:1 are counted. The origin of this criterion has been recently reviewed by Walton.[34] The standard reflects the early evidence of the association of the asbestos hazard with longer fibers of respirable size that penetrate to the alveolar region. The aerodynamic diameter or settling speed is largely a function of fiber diameter, and the available evidence suggested that 3 microns was an appropriate upper limit in this respect. The aspect ratio of 3:1 was chosen simply to aid the discrimination between particles and fibers. While current evidence on the carcinogenicity of fibers supports the contention that these criteria should be revised to concentrate on longer (> 10 microns) and thinner (< 1.5 microns) fibers, the conventional criteria are now so widely used and embodied in national regulations that a major change is unlikely.

The counting of fibers in this way is not an exact science. Errors arise

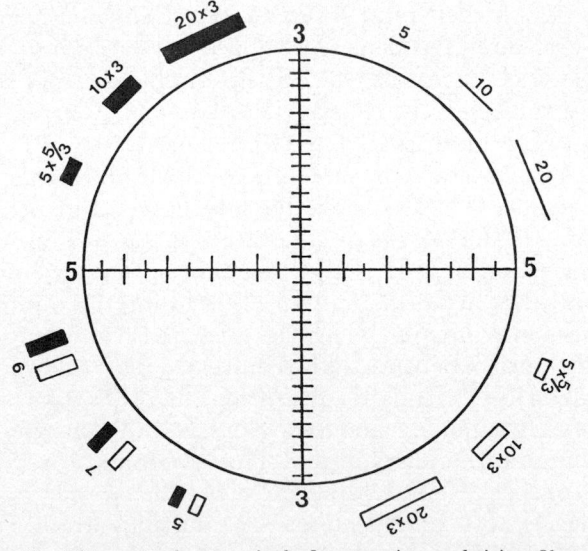

Figure 13. The Walton-Beckett graticule for counting and sizing fibrous particles.

from a number of sources, mainly: (1) the random nature of the fiber distribution on the filter, which gives rise to statistical errors that depend on the number of fibers counted; (2) technical differences in the method of evaluation (e.g., mounting medium used, microscope specifications, graticule types, fiber counting rules; and (3) subjective errors in manual counting. Such errors can be large. For example, comparisons between laboratories have shown threefold differences or more in asbestos count level.[34, 35] Reference methods have been introduced to standardize both sampling and evaluation procedures and so reduce errors associated with differences in method.[36–38] While their adoption will undoubtedly improve the situation, intensive investigations of counting variations in relation to both method differences and subjective effects have shown the latter to be much more important. While method differences can lead to overall differences in counts of ± 20 or 30 per cent, subjective differences between counters led to 10-fold random, two- or threefold systematic, and twofold temporal variations in counts even by experienced counters using nominally the same method.[35] These subjective errors can only be minimized and controlled by operating a reference scheme involving both training and regular counting check exercises within and between laboratories. Such quality assurance schemes are now in operation in several countries.[39]

Direct Reading Instruments

A range of direct reading instruments is now available for monitoring respirable or total dust. These instruments utilize one of several physical principles: the scattering of light by airborne dust particles (e.g., SIMSLIN II, Rotheroe & Mitchell Ltd.; ROYCO 220, Gelman Sciences Ltd.), the variation in oscillation frequency of a quartz crystal with deposited dust— the "piezo-electric" microbalance (TSI Respirable Aerosol Mass Monitor, Bristol Industrial Research Associates Ltd.), or the absorption of beta rays by dusts deposited on a mylar film (RDM Series 101, 201, 301, Analysis Automation Ltd.). Details of currently available instruments have been reviewed elsewhere.[40, 41] They have the advantage of giving shift average and immediate readings of mass concentration (or in some cases number count) during a working period so that short-term peak periods can be identified, and they avoid the tedium of weighing or counting. The data output of these instruments can also be recorded. Unfortunately, they are usually bulky and expensive and require regular calibration with the previously described standard measuring methods that are used for compliances with national standards. Nor are these instruments suitable for personal monitoring of exposure. They are mainly used for engineering control of background levels to alert the workers to potentially hazardous levels, for investigations of emissions from equipment or processes, and for other short-term studies.

References

1. Task Group on Lung Dynamics, Deposition and retention models for internal dosimetry of the human respiratory tract. Health Phys., *12*, 173, 1966.
2. Vincent, J. H., and Mark, D., The basis of dust sampling in occupational hygiene: a critical review. Ann. Occup. Hyg., *24*, 375, 1981.
3 Stahlhofen, W., Gebhart, J., and Heyder, J., Experimental determination of the regional deposition of aerosol particles in the human respiratory tract. Am. Ind. Hyg. Assoc. J., *41*, 385, 1980.
4. Mercer, T. T., The deposition model of the Task Group on Lung Dynamics: a comparison with recent experimental data. Health Phys., *29*, 673, 1975.
5. Ad-Hoc Working Group to Technical Committee 146—Air Quality, International Standards Organization, Recommendations on size definitions for particle sampling. Am. Ind. Hyg. Assoc. J., *42*, A64, 1981.
6. Walton, W. H., The nature, hazards and assessment of occupational exposure to asbestos dust: a review. Ann. Occup. Hyg., *25,* part 3, 187, 1982.
7. Le Roux, W. L., Recorded dust conditions and possible new sampling strategies on South African gold mines. *In* Shapiro, H. A., ed., Pneumoconiosis: Proceedings of the International Conference in Johannesburg. New York, Oxford University Press, 1969, p. 467.
8. BOHS Committee on Asbestos, Report from the Committee on Asbestos. A study of the health experience in two UK asbestos factories. Ann. Occup. Hyg., *27*, 1, 1983.
9. Kotze R. N., Final report of the Miners' Phthisis Committee GPSO, Pretoria, 1919.
10. Flugge de Smidt, A new konimeter. J. Chem. Metal. Mining Soc. S. Afr., *28*, 78, 1927.
11. Greenburg, L., and Smith, G. W., A new instrument for sampling aerial dust. Report of investigation, No. 2392. Washington, D. C., U. S. Bureau of Mines, 1922.
12. Littlefield, J. B., Feicht, F. L., and Shrenk, H. H., The Bureau of Mines midget impinger for dust sampling. Report of investigation, No. 3360. Washington, D. C., U.S. Bureau of Mines, 1937.
13. Owens, J. S., Suspended impurity in the air. Proc. R. Soc. Lond., *101A*, 18, 1922.
14. Watson, H. H., A system for obtaining from mine air, dust samples for physical, chemical and petrological examination. Trans. Inst. Mining Metal., *46*, 155, 1937.
15. Green, H. L., and Watson, H. H., Physical methods for the estimation of the dust hazard in industry. Special Report Series No. 199. London, Medical Research Council, 1935.
16. Kitto, P. H., and Beadle, D. G., A modified form of thermal precipitator. J. Chem. Metal. Mining Soc. S. Afr., *52*, 284, 1952.
17. Hamilton, R. J., A portable instrument for respirable dust sampling. J. Sci. Inst., *33*, 395, 1956.
18. Jacobsen, M., Rae, S., Walton, W. H., and Rogan, J. M., The relation between pneumoconiosis and dust exposure in British coal mines. *In* Walton, W. H., ed., Inhaled Particles III. London, Unwin Bros., 1971, p. 903.
19. Dunmore, J. H., Hamilton, R. J., and Smith, D. S. G., An instrument for the sampling of respirable dust for subsequent gravimetric assessment. J. Sci. Inst., *41*, 669, 1964.
20. Walton, W. H., Theory of size classification of airborne dust clouds by elutriation. Br. J. Appl. Phys., *5*, 529, 1954.
21. Hamilton, R. J., and Walton, W. H., The selective sampling of respirable dust. *In* Davies, C. N., ed., Inhaled Particles and Vapours. Oxford, Pergamon Press, 1961, p. 465.
22. Orenstein, A. J. (ed.), Proceedings of the Pneumoconiosis Conference in Johannesburg, 1959. London, J. & A. Churchill, 1960.
23. Lippmann, H., and Harris, W. B., Size-selective samplers for estimating "respirable" dust concentrations. Health Phys., *8*, 155, 1962.
24. Maguire, B. A., Barker, D., and Badel, D. A., Simpeds 70: an improved version of the Simpeds gravimetric dust-sampling instrument. *In* Walton, W. H., ed., Inhaled Particles III. London, Unwin Bros., 1971, p. 1053.
25. Vincent, J. H., and Armbruster, L., On the quantitative definition of the inhalability of airborne dust. Ann. Occup. Hyg., *24*, 245, 1981.
26. Ogden, T. L., and Birkett, J. L., The human head as a dust sampler. *In* Walton, W. H., ed., Inhaled Particles IV. Oxford, Pergamon Press, 93, 1977.

27. Vincent, J. H., and Mark D., Application of blunt sampler theory to the definition and measurement of inhalable dust. *In* Walton, W. H., ed., Inhaled Particles V. Oxford, Pergamon Press, 1982, p. 3.
28. Armbruster, L., and Breuer, H., Investigations into defining inhalable dust. *In* Walton, W. H., ed., Inhaled Particles V. Oxford, Pergamon Press, 1982, p. 21.
29. Ogden, T. L., and Birkett, J. L., An inhalable dust sampler for measuring the hazard from total airborne particulate. Ann. Occup. Hyg., *21*, 41, 1978.
30. Dodgson, J., Harrison, G. E., McCutcheon, G. T., et al., Problems in measuring the mass concentration of airborne man-made mineral fibres. *In* Proceedings of the Conference on the Biological Effects of Man-made Mineral Fibres, 1982. Copenhagen, World Health Organization. In press.
31. Asbestosis Research Council, Technical note 1: the measurement of airborne dust by the membrane filter method. Rochdale, England, ARC, 1971.
32. Bennett, A. H., Osterberg, H., Jupnik, H., and Richards, O. W., Phase Microscopy: Principles and Applications. New York, John Wiley & Sons, 1951.
33. Walton, W. H., and Beckett, S. T., A microscope eyepiece graticule for the evaluation of fibrous dust. Ann. Occup. Hyg., *20*, 19, 1977.
34. Walton, W. H., The nature, hazards and assessment of occupational exposure to airborne asbestos dust: a review. Ann. Occup. Hyg., part 2, *25*, 155, 1982.
35. Crawford, N. P., Effects of counting rule packages on the reproducibility of asbestos fibre counts. *In* Fourth International Colloquium on Dust Measuring Techniques and Strategy, Edinburgh. London, Asbestos International Association, 1982, p. 45.
36. Council of the European Communities, Council directive on the protection of workers from the risks related to exposure to asbestos at work. Official Journal of the European Communities *L263*, 25, 1983.
37. Asbestos International Association, Recommended technical method no. 1. Reference method for the determination of airborne asbestos fibre concentrations at workplaces by light microscopy (Membrane filter method). London, AIA Health and Safety Publication, 1979.
38. World Health Organization, Methods of monitoring and evaluating airborne man-made mineral fibres. Euro Report and Studies, No. 48. Copenhagen, WHO, 1981.
39. Ogden, T. L., Coping with subjective errors. *In* Fourth International Colloquium on Dust Measuring Techniques and Strategy, Edinburgh. London, Asbestos International Association, 1982, p. 60.
40. American Conference of Governmental Hygienists, Air Sampling Instruments, 6th ed., Cincinnati, Ohio, ACGH; 1983.
41. Gill, F. S., and Ashton, I., Dust. *In* Monitoring For Health Hazards at Work. London, Royal Society for the Prevention of Accidents, Grant McIntye Ltd., 1982.

10
RESPIRATORY PROTECTION

Brian Boehlecke

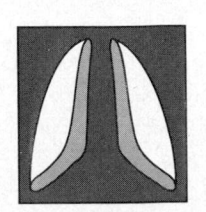

In workplace situations in which available environmental control technology cannot reduce airborne concentrations of toxic materials to safe levels, the use of personal respiratory protective devices (respirators) may be necessary. Respirators are especially useful for protection during brief or unusual exposures such as may occur during accidental release of toxic agents or short-term work in an area with unavoidably high concentrations of an inhalant. The use of respirators should not be considered an acceptable alternative to engineering control measures that prevent atmospheric contamination, such as enclosure of operations, exhaust ventilation, or substitution of less toxic materials, when these measures are feasible.[1] This chapter will present some basic considerations in providing an effective personal respiratory protection program. More comprehensive discussions can be found elsewhere.[2–5]

Determination of the need for a respirator program must be based on a thorough assessment of the potential respiratory hazards of the workplace. Information to be reviewed includes the toxicologic effects of all airborne contaminants, the relationship of airborne concentrations to established permissible exposure levels, and the projected duration of exposure. Work practices and engineering controls should be reviewed to determine if changes could reduce worker exposure to toxic materials to acceptable levels without the use of respirators. If this is not possible, an appropriate type of respirator should be sought. Selecting a respirator requires detailed information on the toxic agents involved and the legal requirements of governmental agencies that regulate the use of respiratory protective devices.[6, 7]

SELECTION OF A RESPIRATOR

Types of Respirators

The first step in developing an adequate respiratory protection program is to identify the type of respirator that, if used properly, is

239

capable of reducing exposure to toxic materials to acceptable levels. Air-purifying respirators simply remove contaminants from ambient air, usually by filtration or adsorption, while atmosphere-supplying respirators provide a separate source of breathable gas. Clearly, if the ambient air is deficient in oxygen, only atmosphere-supplying respirators provide sufficient protection. Various agencies concerned with respiratory protection have defined oxygen deficiency differently, with oxygen contents of from 16.5 to 19.5 per cent used as the lower limit for non-oxygen–deficient air. Even if the legal limit for oxygen deficiency in the applicable regulation is not exceeded, if the *potential* for reduced oxygen content exists, a medical judgment on the risk to the worker becomes necessary, which takes into account the duration of exposure and the physical exertion required during exposure. Atmosphere-supplying respirators should be used if a risk of adverse health consequences is judged to be present due to reduced oxygen content. If oxygen deficiency is not present, air-purifying respirators may provide adequate protection, depending on the nature of the contaminant and its concentration.

Air-purifying respirators remove contaminants by passing inhaled air either through a fibrous filter to remove particulates or through a chemical sorbent to remove gaseous substances, or through a combination of both. Particulate removal depends upon the deposition of the particles on the filter by impaction, interception, or diffusion. The efficiency of entrapment is increased by using smaller diameter fibers more densely packed, but this increases resistance to air flow, and thus makes inhalation more difficult. Excessive inspiratory efforts can be avoided by using powered respirators in which air is forced through the filter by a blower. Electrostatically charged resin coating of the fiber can also increase efficiency, but high temperatures and humidity or liquid aerosols (mists) destroy the effectiveness of this type of filter. Clearly, the size distribution and concentration of particles, as well as the volume of air inhaled per minute, influence the amount of particulate contaminant that passes through the filter. The removal efficiency of filters usually increases as the particulate load on the filter increases, but this also increases the resistance to air flow. Gases can be removed by chemical reaction, absorption, or adsorption. Activated charcoal is a commonly used sorbent, and other materials may be added to increase removal of specific contaminants, e.g., iodine to remove mercury vapor. The ability of sorbents to remove gases and vapors diminishes as saturation occurs, and eventually the contaminant "breaks through." Sorbent cannisters containing drying agents to protect the sorbent may have indicators which change color to warn of saturation of the drying agent, but the sorbent may become saturated before the drying agent. Warning of a breakthrough may occur if the worker notices an odor, a taste, or an irritative effect of the contaminant being inhaled. A contaminant is considered to have adequate warning properties if it can be detected in concentrations not greater than the permissible exposure limit (PEL). In the United States, federal regulations prohibit the use of

air-purifying respirators for protection from organic vapors if the threshold concentration for warning is greater than three times the PEL.[7] For compounds with warning thresholds between one and three times the PEL, air-purifying respirators are acceptable only if it is determined that serious or irreversible adverse health effects do not occur from undetected exposure.

Performance Specifications

The efficiency of contaminant removal by filters and sorbents is measured directly as part of standardized certification testing of respirators performed by the National Institute for Occupational Safety and Health (NIOSH) at its Appalachian Laboratory for Occupational Safety and Health in Morgantown, West Virginia. For example, filters designed to provide protection from relatively nontoxic dusts must remove 99 per cent of the suspended mass from 2.88 m^3 of air containing 50 mg/m^3 of silica dust, with particles averaging approximately 0.5 micron in aerodynamic diameter. High-efficiency filters for more toxic dusts must remove 99.97 per cent of a test aerosol, with an average diameter of 0.3 micron at a concentration of 100 $\mu g/m^3$. Sorbents are tested with single or multiple gases, depending on their intended use. For example, cartridges to remove organic vapors must allow penetration of less than 5 parts per million (ppm) of carbon tetrachloride for at least 50 minutes when air containing 1000 ppm is passed through the cartridge at 32 L/min. This certification provides a basis for judging the effectiveness of the filters and sorbents under specific conditions, but does not imply that the measured level of removal efficiency applies to all possible conditions under which the contaminants of concern may be encountered. The general effectiveness of solvents in removing organic vapors has recently been reviewed. The authors describe some of the limitations of the NIOSH testing program and the problems that occur when a respirator is assumed to be equally effective under varying conditions.[8]

To reduce the inhaled concentrations of a contaminant, a respirator must exclude nonfiltered air from being inhaled. Respirators may have quarter masks (covering the nose and mouth, but not extending below the chin), half masks (extending below the chin), or full masks (covering the entire face). Leakage of ambient air between the mask and face seal or through the one-way expiratory valve may occur during inspiration when pressure inside the mask is below ambient pressure. The amount of leakage depends on the effectiveness of the mask-to-face seal, the seating of the expiratory valve, and the pressure gradient across the mask. This gradient will be increased if resistance to inspiratory flow through the filter or sorbent cartridge is increased (e.g., due to dust loading or the use of more densely packed sorbent) or if inspiratory flow rate is increased, as it may be during exertion. Leakage can thus be minimized by maintaining low inspiratory flow resistance, maintaining proper expiratory valve

seating, and fitting respirator masks as closely as possible to individual users. Since masks are manufactured in a limited variety of sizes and shapes, a good match for the facial features of a given individual is not always possible. Crude but rapid fit testing can be done each time a respirator is used by having the wearer inhale gently with the inlet of the respirator occluded to detect gross leakage. With appropriate sorbents in place, qualitative fit testing can also be done by exposing the wearer to vapors from isoamyl acetate (banana oil) or aerosols of stannic chloride which form by sublimation when this material is exposed to air. Detection of the characteristic odor of the former or the irritative effects of the latter indicates leakage. NIOSH also performs fit testing as part of the certification testing procedure and publishes lists of equipment meeting the current standards.[9, 10]

The same considerations concerning inspiratory leakage of ambient air apply to supplied atmosphere–type respirators. These respirators may use a continuous flow of air from the source or air may be supplied on demand through a valve that opens when pressure inside the mask drops at the onset of inspiration. Inspiratory leakage can be essentially eliminated in these types of respirators by providing a continuous flow that exceeds the maximal inspiratory flow of the wearer or by using a pressure-demand valve that maintains a positive pressure inside the mask at all times. These methods of maintaining positive pressure inside the mask require more air from the source per minute than lower flow continuous or demand-type systems. If the source is a compressed cylinder, the useful life of the cylinder is thus reduced.

Protective Factors

The overall protective factor of a respirator is defined as the ratio of the concentration of an airborne contaminant outside the respirator mask to that inside the respirator. This factor reflects both filter or sorbent efficiency, and the effectiveness of exclusion of ambient air by valves and the mask-to-face seal. Quantitative fit testing and measurement of the protection factor achieved can be done by sampling from within the mask of specially adapted respirators during exposure to a known concentration of a test aerosol, such as sodium chloride, in a test chamber or hood. Protection factors have been measured directly for different types of respirators with the various mask configurations by using a panel of persons to represent the variety of facial configurations in the work force.[11]

Protection factors representative of various types of respirators are listed in Table 10–1. These factors should be considered only approximate guidelines for the capabilities of a given class of respirator. Some respirators have achieved desired protection factors in only 61 per cent of males and 22 per cent of females when tested under laboratory conditions.[12] A recent statement clarifies some of the terms used to describe

Table 10–1.   REPRESENTATIVE RESPIRATOR PROTECTION FACTORS*

Type of Respirator	Protection Factor
I. Air-Purifying Type	
A. For protection from particulates	
1. Single-use dust or quarter-mask dust	5
2. Half-mask dust or high efficiency	10
3. Full facepiece, high efficiency	50
B. For protection from gases or vapors	
1. Half-mask	10
2. Full facepiece	50
II. Atmosphere-Supplying Type	
1. Demand valve with half-mask	10
2. Demand valve with full facepiece	50
3. Pressure-demand valve with half-mask	1000
4. Pressure-demand valve with full facepiece	2000

*Modified from Pritchard, J. A.: A Guide to Industrial Respiratory Protection. NIOSH 79-189. Washington, D.C., U.S. Department of Health Education, and Welfare, 1976.

respiratory protection equipment and outlines the problems encountered when comparisons are made between potential protection in a laboratory setting and true protection in a work situation.[13] Other workers have found that certain demand-type atmosphere-supplying respirators performed poorly, giving protection factors less than 5 in some individuals.[14] Because the protection provided was less than that of air-purifying respirators for most of the respirators tested, the authors recommended that demand-type atmosphere-supplying respirators not be used.

Consideration of important factors in selecting the appropriate respiratory protective equipment for a given workplace condition can be done in a systematic manner by using the decision logic approach developed jointly by the Occupational Safety and Health Administration (OSHA) and NIOSH.[2] Current OSHA regulations should be consulted for applicable legal requirements, and detailed technical considerations are also available in the latest American National Standards Institute document on respiratory protection.[1, 5, 6] Important factors already discussed include the chemical and physical form of the hazard, its relative toxicity and warning properties, and the expected or measured workplace concentration.

A determination of whether the hazard poses an immediate danger to life or health (IDLH) must also be made. An immediate danger is present if an unprotected worker is at risk to suffer death, immediate or delayed irreversible adverse health effects, or severe eye or respiratory tract irritation that could hamper escape with less than 30 minutes of exposure.[7] Regardless of their protection factors, air-purifying respirators are not considered acceptable for use in IDLH conditions. The need for protection from less severe eye irritation or cutaneous absorption of systemic toxins should also be considered. Also important is the worker's

activity while wearing the respirator. Will respirator use be continuous or only for emergency escape? What is the duration of use and what type of physical exertion and mobility is required? Once this information is available, the decision logic referred to above can be used to assist in the selection of an appropriate type of respirator.

RESPIRATORY PROTECTION PROGRAM

Merely providing workers with respirators does not constitute an adequate respiratory protection program. Individual fitting should be done to be sure that facial deformities, eyeglasses, or facial hair does not prevent a proper mask-to-face seal. Conducting a training program, as outlined in Table 10–2, is important to achieve a high degree of worker acceptance, without which adequate protection cannot be achieved.

In situations in which the risk is from the cumulative effects of chronic exposure, the percentage of workers who use the respirators issued to them tends to be low.[15] Even in more immediately threatening conditions, use may be intermittent, with little or no actual protection achieved.[16] Worker compliance with procedures for use should be monitored and equipment periodically inspected. Monitoring of working conditions to detect changes that might necessitate an alteration in respiratory protection should also be done continuously. Important factors include changes in workplace concentrations of airborne contaminants, the addition of new contaminants, and changes in work practices such as longer durations of exposure or increased exertion during exposure. Naturally, these measures do not obviate the need for medical surveillance to detect adverse health effects indicating that protection is insufficient despite an apparently adequate respiratory protection program.

MEDICAL CONSEQUENCES OF RESPIRATOR USE

Wearing respiratory protective equipment is itself an added stress for the worker, and OSHA regulations require that a worker not be assigned to a task requiring a respirator unless the individual is physically able to perform the work and use the equipment.[1] However, it is left to the responsible physician to decide what health and physical conditions are pertinent and the criteria for the ability to use a respirator. The physiological consequences of wearing industrial respirators have recently been reviewed,[17] but it is clear that much of the information needed to establish guidelines for physicians making these decisions is not currently available.

The added resistance to breathing that results from wearing a respirator is likely to prolong the duration of the obstructed phase of respiration and decrease the minute ventilation of the wearer, both at rest and during exercise.[18–21] Whether this in turn leads to significant gas exchange abnor-

**Table 10–2. COMPONENTS OF WORKER TRAINING FOR USE OF
RESPIRATORS**

1. Explanation of the Need for Respirators
   a. Nature of the respiratory hazard
   b. Reasons that environmental controls are not sufficient
   c. Risks if protection not used properly
   d. Details of when respirators are to be used

2. Instruction in Use
   a. Bases for selection and capabilities of respirator used
   b. Limitations and detection of inadequate protection
   c. Basic operation and maintenance
   d. Fitting and periodic fit testing
   e. Recognition and procedures for emergencies
   f. Administrative structure for surveillance of the respiratory
      protection program

malities probably depends on the amount of added resistance to flow, the duration and intensity of exertion, the wearer's underlying respiratory capacity, and the functioning of the respiratory drive control system.[18, 19, 22–30] Transient reductions in arterial blood oxygen tension and more persistent elevations in arterial carbon dioxide content have been observed in normal subjects exercising with added external resistance to breathing. Maximal allowable levels for resistance to air flow are set forth in the NIOSH certification criteria for respirators.[7] Measured at a steady flow of 85 L/min., acceptable inspiratory resistance (measured as pressure) ranges from 5.0 cm H_2O for dust respirators to 8.5 cm H_2O for pesticide respirators. Expiratory resistance must be less than 2.0 cm H_2O for all types of air-purifying respirators. Requirements for atmosphere-supplying respirators are similar, but the pressure-demand type may have an expiratory resistance of 5.1 cm H_2O at 85 L/min. The pressure flow characteristics of respirators are such that higher flows cause a steep nonlinear increase in pressure drop, i.e., the resistance to flow increases at higher flows. Thus, higher flow rates, such as those used during heavy exertion, may be difficult to achieve wearing a respirator, even though breathing seems little affected at rest or with mild exertion. This is especially true for persons with airflow obstruction who have decreased expiratory flow rates and thus require more expiratory time during each breathing cycle to achieve the same tidal volume. As the respiratory rate is increased, the relative time for inspiration must be decreased, and thus inspiratory flow rates must be increased even more than would occur in a healthy person for the same total minute ventilation. This could result in a violation of the assumptions which have been used to determine acceptable levels of resistance for respiratory protective devices.[31] Adding external resistance has been shown to reduce the maximal voluntary ventilation (MVV) more for persons with airflow limitation than for healthy persons.[32] The percentage reduction in ventilation during exercise due to added resistance has been shown to be similar to the percentage reduction in MVV at rest

with the same added resistance.[21] Reductions in MVV of 18 to 32 per cent have been demonstrated, with respirator resistances of 8.5 cm H_2O for inspiration and 2.5 cm H_2O for expiration at 85 L/min., and this test was suggested as the test of choice for determining a worker's capability for wearing an industrial respirator.[33] While possibly useful, this test is not likely to be sufficient by itself. The physiological adaptations during exercise with added resistance are likely to be dependent on many factors, including respiratory drive, which may not be directly related to the ventilation achievable by a voluntary maximal effort.

Pulmonary Impairment and Respiratory Equipment

Federal regulations state that the wearer of a respirator "shall not experience undue discomfort because of airflow restriction. . . ."[7] The mechanism for unpleasant awareness of breathing is not clearly understood, but 10 per cent of men who exercised with added inspiratory resistance experienced this symptom when peak inspiratory pressure exceeded 14 cm H_2O.[34] This is higher than would be likely to occur with most respirators in use, unless very high inspiratory flow rates were necessary. Only 2 of 41 coal miners over the age of 45 years experienced respiratory symptoms while exercising for 15 minutes at moderately heavy work loads (6 to 7 times resting oxygen consumption), with added resistance equivalent to 20 cm H_2O at a flow of 85 L/min.[35] No symptoms occurred in 16 persons with "moderate" obstructive lung disease (ratio of forced expiratory volume in 1 second [FEV_1] to forced vital capacity [FVC] less than 0.70, but otherwise not specified) while exercising up to 63 per cent of their maximal capacity wearing an industrial respirator with an inspiratory resistance of 8.5 cm H_2O at a flow of 85 L/min.[36] However, symptoms have not been found to be sensitive indicators of gas exchange alterations during exercise with added resistance.[19, 25] Twelve subjects with a mean FEV_1/FVC ratio of 60 per cent showed small, but statistically significant reductions in minute ventilation and elevations of end-tidal carbon dioxide concentration during mild exercise (3 to 4 times resting oxygen consumption), with an inspiratory resistance of approximately 5.6 cm H_2O at a flow of 85 L/min., but none reported unpleasant respiratory sensations when asked standardized questions after the exercise.[37] Thus it appears that slight alterations in ventilation and gas exchange may occur as a consequence of wearing currently available industrial respirators, but even persons with mild pulmonary impairment are not expected to experience respiratory symptoms during short periods of exercise using this equipment.

Other potential effects which may limit a worker's ability to wear respiratory protective equipment have not been well studied.[17] The added dead space of respirators may lead to carbon dioxide retention, especially

at high work rates and in persons with a blunted respiratory drive. Cardiovascular effects due to altered intrathoracic pressures have not been well documented. Generally, heart rates have been similar during exercise with and without added respiratory resistance,[36, 37] but some researchers have reported higher rates with added resistance.[17] Systolic blood pressure has been reported to increase approximately 12 mm Hg both at rest and during exercise, when subjects wore respirators, with lesser effects on diastolic pressure.[36] Metabolic effects due to decreased oxygen uptake or alterations in blood pH have not been documented. Increased thermal stress and feelings of claustrophobia are potential adverse consequences that would seem to be more likely with a full facepiece or more complete enclosures. Skin irritation can occur from any device that forms a tight seal with the face.

No simple all-inclusive criteria can be given for deciding who can safely wear a respirator. Respirator wear should be considered a stress that is likely to cause some elevation in blood pressure and a reduction in minute ventilation. Alterations in gas exchange, with reduced arterial oxygen pressure and elevated carbon dioxide pressure, may occur in some individuals, especially those with impaired pulmonary function. The physician must use his or her overall medical judgment in determining whether workers with conditions such as chronic airflow limitation, hypertension, ischemic heart disease, diabetes, epilepsy, or psychological problems can safely tolerate the stress of respirator use. Workers assigned jobs requiring respirators should be monitored closely for signs of adverse reactions, since job pressures may prevent them from readily volunteering problems and ineffective intermittent use may result.

In summary, respirators are useful in providing adequate protection from respiratory hazards when engineering controls cannot reduce worker exposure to acceptable levels. Proper selection requires careful consideration of the nature of the hazard and the type of work to be performed while wearing the respirator. An adequate respiratory protection program must also include administrative and technical procedures to insure proper training of the workers and continued medical and industrial hygiene surveillance. Information on the medical consequences of respirator use is incomplete but suggests that current respirators can be worn for brief periods of moderate exertion without causing distress or adverse physiological effects in healthy persons. Use for longer durations, with more severe exertion, or by persons with chronic medical conditions has not been adequately investigated.

References

1. U. S. Code of Federal Regulations, Title 29, Part 1910.134(a)(1), Respiratory Protection.
2. Pritchard, J. A., A Guide to Industrial Respiratory Protection. NIOSH, 76-189. Washington, D.C., U.S. Department of Health, Education, and Welfare, 1976.

3. Douglas, D., Respiratory protective devices. *In* Clayton, G. D., and Clayton, F. E., eds., Patty's Industrial Hygiene and Toxicology. New York, John Wiley & Sons, 1978.
4. Lundin, A., Respiratory protective equipment. *In* Olishifski, J. B., ed., Fundamentals of Industrial Hygiene. Chicago, Ill., National Safety Council, 1979.
5. Standard Practices for Respiratory Protection. ANSI 88.2–1980. New York, American National Standards Institute, 1980.
6. U.S. Code of Federal Regulations, Title 29, Part 1910.1000(e), Air Contamination Standards.
7. U.S. Code of Federal Regulations, Title 30, Part II, Respiratory Protective Devices; Tests for Permissibility; Fees.
8. Moyer, E. S., Review of influential factors affecting the performance of organic vapor air-purifying respirator cartridges. Am. Ind. Hyg. Assoc. J., *44*, 45, 1983.
9. NIOSH Certified Equipment List. NIOSH 80-144. Washington, D.C., U.S. Dept of Health and Human Services, 1980.
10. Supplement to NIOSH Certified Equipment List. NIOSH 82-106. Washington, D.C., U.S. Dept of Health and Human Services, 1981.
11. Hack, A. L., Hyatt, E. C., Held, B., et al., Selection of respirator test panels representative of U.S. adult facial sizes. Los Alamos Scientific Laboratory Report, #LA-5488, March 1974.
12. Hyatt, E. C., Respirator protection factors. Los Alamos Scientific Laboratory Report, #LA-6084-MS, Jan. 1976.
13. Myers, W. R., Lenhart, S. W., Campbell, D., and Provost, G., Letter to the editor. Am. Ind. Hyg. Assoc. J., *44*, B25, 1983.
14. Hack, A. L., Bradley, O. D., and Trujillo, A., Respirator protection factors: Part II—Protection factors of supplied air respirators. Am. Ind. Hyg. Assoc. J., *41*, 376, 1980.
15. Cotes, J. E., Advances in respiratory protection (conference report). Ann. Occup. Hyg., *22*, 189, 1979.
16. Levine, M., Respirator use and protection from exposure to carbon monoxide. Am. Ind. Hyg. Assoc. J., *40*, 832, 1979.
17. Raven, P. B., Dodson, A. T., and Davis, T. O., The physiologic consequences of wearing industrial respirators: a review. Am. Ind. Hyg. Assoc. J., *40*, 517, 1979.
18. Zechman, F., Hall, F. G., and Hull, W. E., Effects of graded resistance to tracheal air flow in man. J. Appl. Physiol., *10*, 356, 1957.
19. Gee, J. B. L., Burton, G., Vassallo, C., and Gregg, J., Effects of external airway obstruction on work capacity and pulmonary gas exchange. Am. Rev. Respir. Dis., *98*, 1003, 1968.
20. Cerretelli, P., Sikand, R. S., and Farhi, L. E., Effect of increased airway resistance on ventilation and gas exchange during exercise. J. Appl. Physiol., *27*, 597, 1969.
21. Tabakin, B. S., and Hanson, J. S., Lung volume and ventilatory response to airway obstruction during treadmill exercise. J. Appl. Physiol., *20*, 168, 1965.
22. Tabakin, B. S., and Hanson, J. S., Response to ventilatory obstruction during steady-state exercise. J. Appl. Physiol., *15*, 579, 1960.
23. Demedts, M., and Anthonisen, N. R., Effects of increased external airway resistance during steady-state exercise. J. Appl. Physiol., *35*, 361, 1973.
24. Flook, V., and Kelman, G. R., Submaximal exercise with increased inspiratory resistance to breathing. J. Appl. Physiol., *35*, 379, 1973.
25. Silverman, L., and Billings, C. E., Pattern of airflow in the respiratory tract. *In* Davis, C. N., ed., Inhaled Particles and Vapours. New York, Pergamon Press, 1961, pp. 9–46.
26. Thompson, S. H., and Sharkey, B. J., Physiological cost and air flow resistance of respiratory protective devices. Ergonomics, *9*, 495, 1966.
27. Cherniack, R. M., and Snidal, D. P., The Effect of obstruction of breathing on the ventilatory response to CO_2. J. Clin. Invest., *35*, 1286, 1956.
28. Milic-Emili, J., and Tyler, J. M., Relation between work output of respiratory muscles and end-tidal CO_2 tension. J. Appl. Physiol., *18*, 497, 1963.
29. Clark, T. J. H., and Cochrane, G. M., Effect of mechanical loading on ventilatory response to CO_2 and CO_2 excretion. Br. Med. J., *1*, 351, 1972.
30. Flenley, D. C., Pengelly, L. D., and Milic-Emili, J., Immediate effects of positive-pressure breathing on the ventilatory response to CO_2. J. Appl. Physiol., *30*, 7, 1971.

31. Cooper, E. A., Suggested methods of testing and standards of resistance for respiratory protective devices. J. Appl. Physiol., *15*, 1053, 1960.
32. Zwi, S., Theron, J. C., McGregor, M., and Becklake, M. R., The influence of instrumental resistance on the maximum breathing capacity. Dis. Chest, *36*, 361, 1959.
33. Raven, P. B., Moss, R. F., Page, K., et al., Clinical pulmonary function and industrial respirator wear. Am. Ind. Hyg. Assoc. J., *42*, 897, 1981.
34. Bentley, R. A., Griffin, O. G., Love, R. G., et al., Acceptable levels for breathing resistance of respiratory apparatus. Arch. Environ. Health, *27*, 273, 1973.
35. Love, R. G., Muir, D. C. F., Sweetland, K. F., et al., Acceptable levels for breathing resistance of respiratory apparatus: results for men over the age of 45. Br. J. Ind. Med., *34*, 126, 1977.
36. Raven, P. B., Jackson, A. W., Page, K., et al., The physiologic responses of mild pulmonary impaired subjects while using a "demand" respirator during rest and work. Am. Ind Hyg. Assoc. J., *42*, 247, 1981.
37. Hodous, T., Petsonk, E. L., Boyles, C., et al., Effects of added resistance to breathing during exercise in obstructive lung disease. Am. Rev. Respir. Dis., *128*, 943, 1983.

11

SILICOSIS

Anthony Seaton

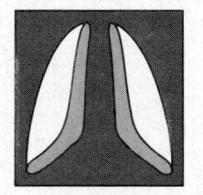

HISTORICAL ASPECTS

Silicosis is the name given to the fibrotic disease of the lungs caused by inhalation of dust containing crystalline silicon dioxide. As this compound forms the greater part of the earth's crust, the possibilities of exposure to the dust are numerous and have been since man first took to making tools and weapons from flint. Since almost any occupation involving the mining into or the cutting, shaping, or polishing of rock involves a risk of silicosis, it is curious that little mention of lung disease among such workers was made in classical times. Pliny the Elder, in his *Natural History* written in the first century A.D., mentions the dangers to miners of fumes and vapors, but not those of dust. Not until Agricola's major work on the mining and production of metals, *De re metallica*, was published in 1556[1] was an account given of the fatal effects of dust. In the sixth book, Agricola writes: "It remains for me to speak of the ailments and accidents of miners, and of the methods by which we can guard against them, for we should always devote more care to maintaining our health, that we may freely perform our bodily functions, than to making profits."

Unhappily the advice given here has not always been heeded, and the drive for profit both by individual miners and by their employers has over the succeeding four centuries resulted, by the neglect of safety precautions, in the production of untold ill health and premature death. Even in recent times, early widowhood has been the common lot of the women of mining areas, as it was in Agricola's day.

Agricola described the machinery necessary for ventilation of mines, though the emphasis was more on the removal of stale air that would not support combustion and of the fumes of fires used to crack the rocks than on the reduction of dust. Moreover, he described the responsibilities of the various mine officials in ensuring the safety of the workings.

A hundred and fifty years after Agricola, Ramazzini published *De morbis artificum diatriba*, describing in the first chapter the diseases afflicting

miners.[2] He emphasized the unpleasant and dangerous nature of mining by pointing out that the occupation was still, in the eighteenth century, considered a suitable punishment for malefactors, as it had been in Pliny's time. While Ramazzini mentioned cough and asthma as being recorded among miners by previous authors, he attributed most of their ill health to the absorption of the metals they were mining. He later mentions the use of powdered flint in pottery, but records that morbidity in this trade was due to lead posioning. Finally, in his chapter on stonecutters he records the inhalation of splinters leading to asthmatic afflictions, consumption, and cough. He quotes the pathological work of Diemerbroeck, who in studying the lungs of stonecutters who had died of asthma had found them full of sand. Ramazzini was aware that in this trade very small particles were suspended in the air, and quoted a master stonecutter who had told him of finding a handful of very fine sand inside an ox bladder hung in his workshop.

Over the eighteenth century there was a gradual realization of the hazards to health associated with work on millstones and grinding wheels in Europe, though the resultant disease was always assumed to be tuberculosis. Johnstone[3] in 1796 gave a paper to the Medical Society of London in which he described the frequency of premature death of needle pointers, from phthisis, attributing this to irritation of the lungs by inhaled particles of iron and stone. He advised the use of a gauze helmet to limit dust inhalation. He also noted that the work was so well known to be fatal that there was difficulty in employing labor and that the high wages paid to attract workers contributed to ill health by allowing them intemperance. By the time of the publication of Thackrah's great work on occupational health[4] in 1831, lung disease was known to cause premature death in knife grinding, the quarrying and cutting of sandstone as opposed to limestone, and the filing of cast iron as opposed to wrought iron. This work is particularly interesting because Thackrah made measurements of vital capacity on the workers he studied, comparing one group with another. While such tests form one of the bases of all studies of occupational lung disease nowadays, Thackrah's use of the technique antedated the development of the spirometer by Hutchinson in 1846.

In 1860, Peacock[5] produced an early example of a controlled mortality study when he compared the normal life span of wire basket makers with the typical 40-year life span of the makers of French burr millstones, though both groups were employed in the same factory and working conditions in terms of temperature, dampness, and light were, if anything, worse for the basket makers. He suggested the use of water and ventilation for dust suppression and the wearing of respirators. He examined the lungs by a technique of ashing and treatment with hydrochloric acid, and described the finding of siliceous matter similar to that found in the workshop. This technique was taken a little further by Greenhow,[6] who in 1865 published an investigation of a grinder's lung which contained small black and crystalline masses. These were not soluble in hydrochloric

acid, so they were not iron. The tissue was ashed and dissolved in hydrochloric acid and the residue examined. It included small angular masses that transmitted polarized light and dissolved in hydrofluoric acid, and thus seemed to be silica. The same author also described this disease in potters,[7] enumerating the particular aspects of that trade in which inhalation of silica and alumina could occur.

Silicosis made its appearance in the medical literature of the United States in the last quarter of the nineteenth century in isolated case reports and in the form of a "chronic disease of the air passages" among employees of a cutlery factory.[8] Early in the present century the disease was recognized among miners and rock crushers, and with the development of mechanization and the consequent increase in the prevalence of silicosis and silicotuberculosis, public concern began to be generated. In a survey by the U.S. Public Health Service in 1913–15, 60 per cent of 720 lead and zinc miners in Missouri were found to have these diseases.[9] Subsequent studies showed a very high prevalence of silicosis among Vermont granite workers and New York tunnelers, and by the 1930s the disease had been described in most of the trades in which it was known to occur in Europe.

The turning point in the history of silicosis in the United States came in the 1930s. Methods of dust suppression and dust avoidance were developed and their application spread, largely owing to the impetus of legal action for negligence taken against employers by many of the by then large population of silicotics. Public opinion was aroused particularly by the appalling episode at Gauley Bridge in southern West Virginia. This occurred when, in order to produce hydroelectric power, a tunnel was driven through a sandstone mountain. Cheap labor, largely brought in from the South, was used and no precautions were taken to diminish exposure to dust. Vigorous attempts were made to prevent the effects of this becoming public knowledge, but congressional hearings revealed that 476 workers had died in the course of the construction and a further 1500 had contracted silicosis.[10] Today a plaque celebrates the engineering achievement.

During the 1930s and 1940s the states began to introduce laws providing for compensation of victims of silicosis and many also established programs of industrial hygiene. Methods of dust control became more widely applied as the hazards became more fully known, though the application of these measures was slow, particularly in smaller industries and companies. The introduction of antituberculosis chemotherapy in the 1950s further revolutionized the management of that most serious complication of the disease, and there is little doubt that silicosis is much less prevalent now than a few decades ago.

SILICA AND INDUSTRY

Forms of Silica

Silicon dioxide, or silica, is the most abundant mineral in the earth's crust. It usually occurs as a tetrahedron, with a central atom of silicon

sharing four oxygen atoms with adjacent silicon atoms. The various arrangements of these atoms in space produce different forms of silica, which may be crystalline, microcrystalline, or amorphous. The commonest naturally occurring form of crystalline silica is quartz, which is a component of most rocks. While quartz is almost pure silicon dioxide, it usually contains traces of other elements that are responsible for the range of colors that it can assume and that give certain varieties, such as agate, onyx, and amethyst, value as gems or ornamental materials. Other crystalline forms of silica are cristobalite and tridymite, which occur naturally in volcanic rocks, for example, in California and Colorado, but which may also be produced by heating quartz or amorphous silica. There is some evidence that they are even more toxic than quartz itself. Of two other naturally occurring forms of crystalline silica, stishovite and coesite, the former has an octahedral structure and appears in experimental studies to be less toxic.

Microcrystalline, or cryptocrystalline, silica consists of minute crystals of quartz bonded together by amorphous silica as in flint and chert. Amorphous silica, which is noncrystalline and which is relatively nontoxic, occurs as diatomite (kieselguhr) and vitreous silica. The former consists of the skeletons of prehistoric marine organisms. Its usefulness largely depends on it being calcined, that is, heated either with or without alkalis. This process converts much of the amorphous material to cristobalite, which is probably responsible for its toxicity. Vitreous silica is formed when crystalline silica is melted, then cooled quickly. Again, heating above about 1000° C will ensure vitreous silica contains cristobalite.

All these forms of silicon dioxide are referred to as free silica to distinguish them from combined silica, or silicates. The latter compounds, which include asbestos, micas, and talc, imply different hazards to health, and are discussed in Chapters 12 and 13.

It can thus be seen that silica occurs in a wide range of rocks, though it is not always the main component. For example, sandstone and flint may contain almost 100 per cent silica, granite between 20 and 70 per cent, slate around 40 per cent, and certain types of fuller's earth and shales around 10 per cent. Negligible levels occur in the carbonate rocks, limestone, dolomite, and marble. A hazard to health should always be suspected whenever silica dust is likely to be liberated into the air, but the magnitude of the hazard can only be estimated by measurement of the dust levels and analysis of the content and type of free silica present.

Exposure to Silica

The importance of silica as a health hazard in industry today lies more in the fact that exposure may occur in a wide range of occupations than in the number of individuals suffering from silicosis. Early recognition of the disease has allowed preventive measures to be taken in many of the industries in which silicosis traditionally occurred, such as cutlery,

pottery, stone cutting, and flint work. Nevertheless, the manufacture of sandstone grindstones has recently been reported to cause silicosis in Northern Nigeria,[11] a limited amount of flint knapping still occurs in Suffolk (where Stone Age flint mines may still be visited), and new and unexpected outbreaks of silicosis are regularly being reported, for example, in coal mining[12] and the production of bentonite.[13] The occurrence of silicosis nowadays can be attributed to the failure to apply the considerable amount of accumulated knowledge on the subject, either through ignorance (as, for example, in underdeveloped countries or among unenlightened management) or through a willful disregard of the dangers. Recent reports of rapidly advancing silicosis among sandblasters[14] and silica flour workers[15, 16] are testimony that these factors operate even in highly developed industrial societies. The use of silica sand for sandblasting was abolished by law in the United Kingdom in 1949 and in the European community in 1955, yet persists in the United States.

A complete list of all industries in which silicosis may occur would not only be impracticable but meaningless in the absence of the sort of detail obtained in a careful occupational history. However, the major groups of industries in which a risk of exposure to silica dust may be suspected are as follows.

Quarrying, Stone Cutting, Mining, and Tunneling

Sandstone and granite are extensively used in building, as is slate, though now to a lesser extent. These materials may also be used in a ground or crushed form as fillers and abrasives, and in road building. While they are usually obtained by quarrying, slate may be mined. Exposure to silica in these industries depends on the amount of water suppression and the adequacy of ventilation, particularly in the sheds where the stones are shaped or crushed. The trades involved in the cutting, engraving, and polishing of these stones are clearly at risk, especially where sandblasting is used. Similarly, the cleaning and repair of stone public buildings, when not carried out as a wet process, may generate a dust hazard. Excavation, such as digging graves in sandstone, preparing foundations for buildings, and removing silica-containing overburden in open-cast, or strip mining for other minerals may also entail a silicosis risk.

Mining for metals usually involves the removal of quartz-rich ores, and silicosis may occur in gold, tin, iron, copper, nickel, silver, tungsten, and uranium mining. Other useful minerals, such as asbestos, mica, shales, barytes, fireclays, and fluorspar, are also mined in such a way that the dust may contain silica. Coal mining may involve exposure to silica in hardheading, driving shafts and tunnels, and using sand as a friction material on rails, and when intrusions of roof and floor are cut with the coal seam.

Tunneling through sandstone or granite constitutes an obvious risk,

especially with the use of modern machinery and the difficulties of providing effective ventilation. However, tunneling through limestone and the use of limestones with a low silica content to prevent explosion in coal mines (commonly called rock-dusting) do not entail a risk of silicosis.

Foundry Work

Foundries are the places where castings of iron, steel, and nonferrous materials such as bronze are made. The process involves the production of a mold into which the molten metal is cast. A core may also be used to produce a hollow casting. The solidified casting is then knocked out of the mold. Silica, predominantly cristobalite, and other contaminants from the mold that have burnt onto the surface of the casting need to be cleaned off. Exposure to silica can potentially occur in the production of the molds and cores, which are made of quartz sand bonded by clays or resins, in the knocking out of the castings, and especially in the process of cleaning and polishing of the product. This is often known as fettling and may be done with hammers, grinding wheels, mills, or abrasive blasting. Silicosis has resulted from the continued use of sandblasting in the southern United States in the production of large-scale castings for shipbuilding and oil platforms.[17]

Workers in foundries are therefore exposed to a wide range of possible hazards, including silica, iron oxides, and fumes from molten metals and from the bonding resins. The latter may include isocyanates, and occupational asthma is not unknown among such workers. Fettlers are at greatest risk of silica exposure, though true silicosis with progression to massive fibrosis is probably rare except when sandblasting is used. The radiographic abnormalities in these workers usually represent a more benign mixed dust pneumoconiosis, the principal cause of radiographic shadowing often being iron (see Chap. 5).

Other possible sources of exposure to silica in foundries include the cleaning and repairing of furnaces lined with silica brick (see below) and the general contamination of the workplace by dusty processes.

Ceramics

Powdered flint and clays containing free silica have traditionally been used in the manufacture of china and earthenware. China clay itself usually contains a relatively small proportion (less than 5 per cent) of silica, but crushed, calcined flint or other siliceous clays need to be added, usually in a wet process, prior to shaping and firing. The unfinished articles are then polished or fettled and may subsequently be glazed with a mixture also containing silica. Risks of exposure chiefly occur among those involved in crushing flint and in fettling. Significant exposure can occur from contaminated clothing. In the past, articles were baked in kilns on a bedding of powdered flint, and workers were exposed to this. More

recently, this has been replaced by alumina, while other substitutes for flint and siliceous clays in the clay mixture are being introduced. Thus the hazards of silicosis in this industry, which used to be appreciable, are now very much reduced. Historically, this used to be one of the very few industries in which women contracted silicosis. However, the increasing employment of women in jobs traditionally held by men has also widened their opportunities of getting this disease.

Production of refractory brickware for lining kilns, furnaces, boilers, and other places where fire resistance is required involves the crushing, shaping, and baking of sandstone. Exposure may occur in the initial mining, crushing, and milling processes; in shaping and laying the bricks; and especially in stripping, cleaning, and repairing of the linings of boilers and similar plants. It should be noted that men working as boilermakers or repairers may be exposed to a number of hazards, often in very confined spaces—silica from brick linings, asbestos from lagging, cement and occasionally filling between bricks, and, in the case of work on oil-fired boilers, vanadium from oil residues. The fly-ash residue of coal burning is probably not hazardous, since it has a low silica content, though there has been one rather dubious recent report of "fly-ash pneumoconiosis."[18]

Other Industries

Silicosis may also be encountered in a wide range of other trades. The use of finely ground quartz in sandblasting has already been referred to; it is hoped that substitution of other materials such as shot, slag, grit, and carborundum will soon eliminate this hazardous material. The abrasive properties of silica are also still made use of in some scouring powders, polishes, toothpastes, and sandpaper, although adequate and less toxic substitutes are available. Silica flour, or finely milled crystalline silica, is used in many of these products, and also as a filler in paints, woods, surfacing materials, rubbers, and plastics. Not only is it potentially very toxic, but it may be marketed and labeled incorrectly as amorphous silica.[19] Rapidly progressive silicosis has recently been described in the production of silica flour in the United States[15] and Australia.[16, 20]

Diatomaceous earth, being amorphous silica, is thought not to entail a great hazard; however, when calcined it is converted largely into cristobalite and tridymite. Extensive deposits occur in the western United States, where it is strip mined, crushed, and calcined. It is used in filters, abrasives, insulation materials, and absorbents. Exposure may therefore occur in many different and unexpected situations (see p. 10 for an example). It is probably only when exposure to calcined material occurs that there is a significant risk of silicosis.[21]

Other uses of silica in industry include glassmaking, where sand may be used both for polishing and as a component, and enameling, where quartz and other materials are crushed and melted together. Other small

industries employing forms of silica such as the use of slate in the production of furniture, billiard tables, and ornaments, and the manufacture of semiprecious stones from colored forms of quartz, survive in industrialized nations, while traditional crafts such as the manufacture of sandstone grinding wheels may still be found in less developed countries.

Numbers of Workers Exposed

Because exposure to silica can occur in a wide range of industries, it is clear that no reasonable estimate of the numbers of workers at risk of silicosis can be made. For example, it is not known how many coal miners are exposed to sufficiently high levels of silica in the mixed respirable dust and thus to the risk of silicosis rather than coal workers' pneumoconiosis; recent unpublished studies in Britain suggest it may be about 5 per cent of face workers. However, an enumeration of workers employed in the industries traditionally at risk has been obtained for the United States in 1970[22] (Table 11–1). It is to be noted that far from all of these individuals will be exposed to free silica; conversely there are many others, for example, workers in the shipbuilding, construction, and chemical and rubber industries, who are not included in the list.

EPIDEMIOLOGY

Prevalence of Silicosis

Owing to the large number of industries in which there is a risk of silicosis, the irregular employment and transient nature of the labor force, and differences in notification practices in different states and countries, it is difficult to get an idea of the prevalence of silicosis. Trasko[23] in 1954 obtained records of nearly 13,000 compensated cases in 26 states, a figure she considered a gross underestimate of the true prevalence. This figure, however, included subjects with coal workers' pneumoconiosis. In the United Kingdom, where because of smaller numbers and uniform notification practices the figures are more reliable, 721 cases were compensated in 1957 and the number had fallen to 162 new cases in 1969. In the

Table 11–1. NUMBERS OF WORKERS EMPLOYED IN INDUSTRIES WITH POTENTIAL EXPOSURE TO FREE SILICA, UNITED STATES, 1970

Coal mining	125,000
Metal mining	76,000
Nonmetal minerals	95,000
Stone, clay, and glass products	507,000
Iron and steel foundries	188,000
Nonferrous foundries	69,000

subsequent decade this figure has fluctuated between 170 and 110, with a general downward trend. The number of workers compensated for silicosis in some industries contrasted with the number of those compensated for asbestosis and coal workers' pneumoconiosis is shown in Table 11–2. It should be noted that these figures are for workers diagnosed as suffering disablement and therefore exclude those with radiological abnormalities but with no pulmonary impairment. The steady downward trend in all industries, while in part reflecting a reduced number of workers at risk, can also be taken as evidence of the general effectiveness of preventive measures.

The metal mining industry is the most important source of silicosis in the United States. A detailed survey of 76.6 per cent of the work force in 50 metal mines in this country was carried out by the U.S. Public Health Service and the Bureau of Mines[24] between 1958 and 1961. An overall prevalence of silicosis of 3.4 per cent was found and one third of this number had complicated disease. There was considerable variation in prevalence from mine to mine, and this was related to the silica content of the dust rather than the metal being mined. The other factors related to the development of silicosis were the subject's occupation—face workers and those in the most dusty jobs having the highest prevalence—and length of time in the industry. There was very little disease among workers who had been employed for less than 10 years, while the prevalence rose to 3 per cent at 20 years, 12 per cent at 30 years, and 16.6 per cent after 30 years. There was some evidence that the reduction in dust levels since 1935 had resulted in a prolongation of the period between exposure and when disease developed.

The prevalence in other industries is less sure. Trasko[23] estimated the total number of true silicotics in 20 of the states to be about 6000, with around 1600 being miners, a similar number working in foundries, and much smaller numbers employed in other trades (Table 11–3).

Table 11–2. NUMBERS OF SUBJECTS AWARDED INDUSTRIAL INJURY COMPENSATION FOR SILICOSIS IN CERTAIN TRADES IN BRITAIN, COMPARED WITH THOSE COMPENSATED FOR COAL WORKERS' PNEUMOCONIOSIS AND ASBESTOSIS

Disease	Year			
	1957–61	1962–66	1967–71	1972–76
Silicosis				
Slate quarry and splitting	161	238	158	152
Other mining and quarrying	293	139	109	62
Refractory	163	98	72	40
Pottery	699	329	147	96
Foundry	838	384	263	170
Coal workers' pneumoconiosis	16,228	14,426	3,515	2,938
Asbestosis	192	398	730	718

Table 11–3. WORKERS COMPENSATED FOR SILICOSIS IN 20 STATES*

Metal mining	1637
Mixed mining	854
Nonmetallic mining and quarrying	185
Tile and clay	150
Potteries	257
Glass	13
Stone cutting	485
Nonmetallic minerals	165
Foundries	1645
Refractory	89
Others	593

*Data from Trasko, V. M.: Some facts on the prevalence of silicosis in the United States. Arch. Ind. Health *14*, 379, 1956.

These figures, when considered with the likely number of employees in most of these industries, appear to suggest that the prevalence is not very high overall. However, it is admitted that the figures may well be an underestimate. That this may be the case is suggested when the number of 1645 foundrymen in that survey is compared with the figures from a detailed epidemiological survey of British foundrymen,[25] which revealed a 34 per cent prevalence of simple pneumoconiosis among fettlers and a 14 per cent prevalence among foundry floor men. These figures suggest that as many as 40,000 British foundrymen had radiographic evidence of simple pneumoconiosis. This survey also showed that around 9000 of these might be expected to have had category 2 or 3 pneumoconiosis, though complicated disease appears not to occur in this industry. Moreover, the radiographic category of disease correlated neither with symptoms nor with ventilatory dysfunction. However, there is a complicating factor in foundrymen's disease, in that substantial amounts of radiopaque material other than silica are inhaled, and the pneumoconiosis is better regarded as being mixed rather than true silicosis.

In other industries in which the prevalence of silicosis has been investigated, a steady decline has been noted. The original studies of Vermont granite workers in the 1920s showed that almost all workers in dusty areas developed the disease and a high proportion became tuberculous. Subsequent investigations of the industry, following the introduction of dust controls in 1937, have shown silicosis to be virtually absent.[26, 27] Granite workers have also been investigated in Europe. Monumental masons were studied in Scotland in 1951 and again in the 1970s.[28] Radiographic changes were found only in men exposed to dust over 20 years, the overall prevalence in the first survey being 10 per cent and in the more recent study 3 per cent. Complicated disease, not found in the recent survey, was present in 2 per cent of subjects in the original series. The disease in Scottish granite workers therefore appears relatively benign and progresses only slowly. On the other hand, a study in southwestern Britain[29] showed 17.6 per cent of granite workers to have silicosis, most being of category 2 or above, while a Swedish study[30] also has suggested that a more rapidly progressive disease, related to higher dust levels,

occurs in that country. Clearly, local conditions, including dust control measures, the silica content of the granite, the type of study, and the population sample studied, vary in most reports, and figures are not easily compared. A gratifying decline in the prevalence of silicosis, similar to that noted in American granite workers, has also been reported in workers involved in the production of diatomaceous earth.[21]

In some industries there has been complacency about dust levels, because the dust has been thought to contain unimportant amounts of silica. This had been the case among slate workers in North Wales, who were investigated by Jarman and colleagues in 1957.[31] They found an overall prevalence of radiographic nodulation of 8 per cent, and almost 1 per cent had massive fibrosis. Active, bacteriologically proven tuberculosis was found in 0.5 per cent of those surveyed, a figure four times that among coal miners. Twenty years later, a survey in this now much smaller industry showed a strikingly similar prevalence of pneumoconiosis, indicating that little improvement in dust control had occurred.[32] Similarly, an investigation of workers milling bentonite (sodium montmorillonite) in Wyoming in 1971 disclosed a number of subjects with disabling and fatal pneumoconiosis in an industry in which the hazard was not thought to exist.[13] Dust levels in this industry were found to be high, with a free silica content of about 10 per cent.

While classical silicosis in most industrial settings nowadays is a rather slowly progressive disease that affects only a minority of the work force, recent reports of rapidly progressive silicosis from a number of industries have shown not only that this disease still occurs but also that it may affect a substantial proportion of the work force. For example, 37 per cent of workers at two silica flour mills studied in 1981 showed silicosis, 11 per cent of them with massive fibrosis.[15] A survey by NIOSH of dust samples from 27 United States silica flour mills in the 1970s showed over half to have exceeded the current hygiene standard.[19] Studies of sandblasters in the Louisiana Gulf area, while not being able to estimate the prevalence of silicosis, suggest that acute progressive disease may not be as rare as has been supposed.[33]

Exposure-Response Relationships

Ideally, a hygiene standard aimed at controlling the incidence of occupational disease should be based on a knowledge of the relationships between the disease and the dose of noxious material. In practice, this ideal has rarely been achieved, and this unfortunately is the case with silicosis. Most epidemiological studies have not had adequate, or indeed any, measurements of dust exposure. The most recent studies of Vermont granite workers have attempted to fill this gap with estimates of exposure based on employment records and available measurements of dust in the sheds. Early radiological opacities have been estimated to be likely to occur

in 50 per cent of the work force after exposure to about 0.5 mg/m³ of respirable dust for 46 working years.[27] The respirable dust, however, only contains around 10 per cent quartz. Similar analyses of the relationships between dust exposure and decrement in FEV_1 have been carried out,[34] but subsequent studies of this population have cast serious doubt on the conclusions, suggesting that loss of FEV_1 is not a serious effect of the relatively low levels of dust exposure in the granite industry.[35]

Little other information on dose-response relationships is available. The British studies of slate workers have only provided information based on years of exposure.[32] One recent study of coal miners,[12] in which 21 men who had shown progression of simple pneumoconiosis over a 4-year period were matched with controls from the same mine who did not have progressive pneumoconiosis, has shown that the rapid progression is likely to be due to the relatively high quartz concentrations to which the men had been exposed. Figure 11–1 shows the cumulative quartz exposures of these men in relation to that of a hypothetical man exposed to 0.1 mg/m³ over his working life. Most men with rapid progression (and several controls) had received doses above this level, but three progressors fell just below the line. It should be noted that the 21 cases in this study were the only progressors found out of a total pit population of 623. This seems to indicate that a quartz standard of rather less than 0.1 mg/m³ for industries in which there is a silicosis risk would protect the majority of the work force. However, this work was carried out in an industry in which other minerals may interfere with the toxicity of silica and where relatively low proportions of quartz (probably below about 10 per cent) in the mixed dust can be regarded as less harmful.[36]

CLINICAL FEATURES

Chronic Silicosis

The most usual form of silicosis is that which occurs after many years of exposure to relatively low levels of dust. This disease resembles coal workers' pneumoconiosis in that the simple nodular form is not associated with any symptoms or physical signs. Such subjects may complain of cough, sputum, or breathlessness, but these symptoms are likely to be related to accompanying disease of the airways.[24] However, simple radiological silicosis is occasionally a progressive disease, even in the absence of further dust exposure,[37] and may sometimes develop into progressive massive fibrosis unless the exposure has been predominantly to mixed dust (as in foundrymen) or has been relatively limited.

When progressive massive fibrosis occurs, the patient develops symptoms related to reduction of lung volumes, distortion of bronchi, and, though to a lesser extent than in coal workers' pneumoconiosis, compensatory and bullous emphysema. The main symptom is shortness of breath, though cough and sputum production are usual also. The breathlessness

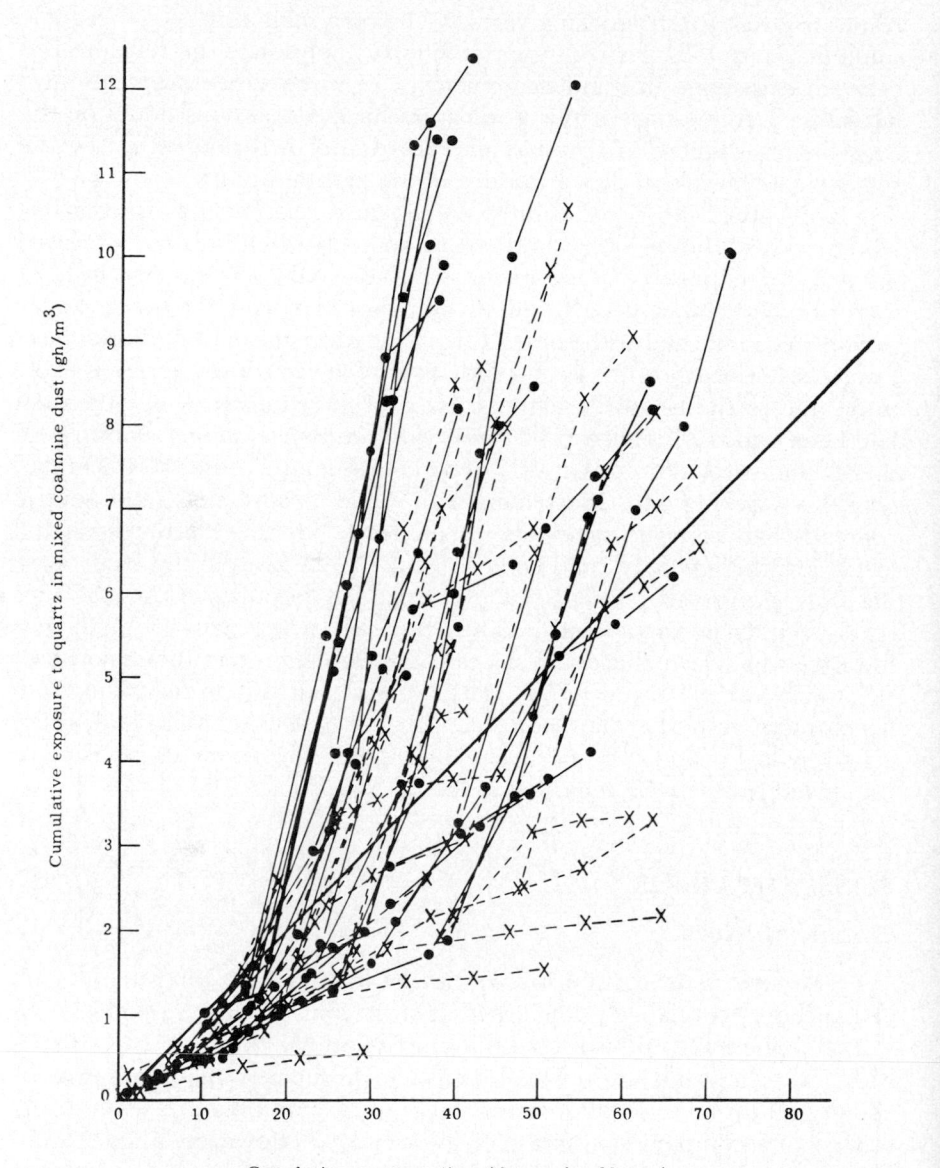

Cumulative exposure time (thousands of hours)

Figure 11–1. Cumulative exposure to quartz (gh/m³) of a group of British coal miners over 80,000 working hours. Men who showed rapid radiological progression of pneumoconiosis (● — ●) had received doses around or above the level, represented by a continuous 45° line, of an average exposure to 0.1mg/m³. Controls (×–––×) without rapid progression at the time of study had received a wide range of doses. (From Seaton, A., Dick, J. A., Dodgson, J., and Jacobsen, M., Quartz and pneumoconiosis in coal miners. Lancet, 2, 1272, 1981.)

is progressive and ultimately disabling. The final episode in the life of the silicotic is the development of cardiorespiratory failure. If the physiological effect of the silicosis has been predominantly restrictive, as is most usually the case, this tends to be of the hypoxic type, with electrocardiographic evidence of pulmonary hypertension but without overt cardiac failure. However, with the predominantly obstructive type of functional defect associated with bullous emphysema or complicating airways disease, clinical cor pulmonale may occur. The classical description of complicated silicosis, and one that was still accurate in many respects in the potteries of England when the author worked there in the 1960s, came from J. T. Arlidge, a distinguished physician who studied occupational medicine in that region during the latter half of the nineteenth century.[38] His book *The Hygiene, Diseases and Mortality of Occupations*, published in 1892, contains the following description of complicated silicosis, a description which is applicable to the disease in whatever occupation it occurs.

> The pulmonary mischief from the dust of potter's clay is slow but sure in its occurrence. The siliceous character of the clay lends it more potency for harm than almost any other dust. . . .It is much more irritant than coal dust and stands on a par with the worst kinds of stone dust. . . .When uncomplicated by tubercles, the potter's disease advances imperceptibly. Haemoptysis does not usher in the malady, and more frequently than not never makes its appearances. . . .There is no febrile reaction, no accelerated pulse, no hectic, and no rapid emaciation. . . .The cough is more paroxysmal and violent than that of phthisis, and the urgency of dyspnoea greater, and out of proportion to the ascertained extent of consolidated lung. The signs of condensation are not so specially limited to the infraclavicular spaces as in tuberculous lesions, and hence the sinking below the clavicles is not marked.
>
> Areas of dullness on percussion are often distributed at different parts particularly in the scapular region near the base of the lungs. Between these an emphysematous condition is discoverable; a phenomenon more common along the anterior margin of the lungs. There is not an equal shrinking and contraction of the thoracic cavity at large. . . .As might be foreseen from the increased strain on the pulmonary circulation, the heart gets frequently involved, the right side becomes dilated and the valves inefficient. Hence anasarca in prolonged cases is no infrequent occurrence before the scene closes. I would add that the general aspect and physiognomy differ from those of tubercular phthisis. . . .the lustrous eye, the often pink and transparent skin of phthisis, the clubbed finger ends, and the incurved nails are wanting. But in looking for these distinctive signs we must never forget how frequently tubercular deposit modifies the picture of fibrosis.

This description of a progressive disease causing breathlessness but few physical signs—no finger clubbing or crackles in particular—cannot be bettered. Fortunately this end point in the disease is now rare and, in general, chronic silicosis develops only after a prolonged period of exposure so that massive fibrosis, when it does occur, rarely does so early enough to shorten the patient's life or even to cause disability.

Accelerated Silicosis

In some occupations, such as sandblasting and production of silica flour and diatomaceous earth, exposure to high concentrations of silica over a relatively short period of a few years results in a more rapidly progressive form of the disease.[15, 17, 39] The symptoms are those of the more chronic disease, but clinical and radiographic progression is rapid, producing a more diffuse and irregular fibrosis. Hypoxic respiratory failure is the sequel, often after as little as 10 years from first exposure.

Acute Silicosis

An acute form of silicosis occurs in subjects exposed to very high concentrations of silica over periods of as little as a few weeks. This disease was first described by Middleton in 1929 as an occupational hazard for those involved in the production of abrasive soap powders.[40] The first cases in the United States were described by Chapman, also in workers involved in the mixing of alkali and finely ground crystalline silica to produce abrasive soap powders.[41] In spite of its dramatic course and general knowledge of the dangers of silica, acute silicosis has been described repeatedly even in the last few years, for example, in sandblasters,[14, 17] ceramic workers,[42] silica flour workers,[15, 16] and open-cast coal miners.[43] The history is typically one of progressive dyspnea, fever, cough, and weight loss after a heavy but relatively short exposure to silica. The exposure time may vary from a few weeks to four or five years. Death occurs in hypoxic respiratory failure,[44] and the fatal course of the disease is probably not influenced by steroids, bronchial lavage, or any other treatment, though there are anecdotal reports of temporary alleviation of symptoms by steroids.[45] Complication by mycobacterial infections is frequent, and nocardiosis and fungal infections have also been reported.[17]

Complications of Silicosis

Mycobacterial and Opportunist Infections. The major complication of silicosis is pulmonary tuberculosis. Early descriptions of lung disease in dusty industries did not distinguish between pneumoconiosis and tuberculosis, and undoubtedly before chemotherapy most fatal cases of silicosis were complicated by that disease. Although tuberculosis has come under increasing control in the developed world, reactivation of an old primary infection still remains a risk of silicotics. In endemic areas and among poorer people in the United States and other advanced countries the danger of tuberculosis in silicosis is very real. In South Africa, a necropsy series of gold, coal, and asbestos miners has shown a greater proportion of silicotics to have active tuberculosis than nonsilicotics.[46] Previous studies in that country showed that 20 per cent of silicotic gold miners had active

disease even in the 1960s,[47] though the overall prevalence of silicosis had fallen sharply following the introduction of dust controls. Over the same period tuberculosis was found to occur 30 times more frequently in silicotic than in nonsilicotic copper miners in Northern Rhodesia.[48] In United States metal miners in the early 1960s, 5.3 per cent of silicotics and 0.6 per cent of nonsilicotics showed radiographic evidence of active or quiescent disease,[23] while 0.5 per cent of British slate miners studied in the 1950s had bacteriologically proven active disease.[31] A recent study of these men has shown almost half to have radiological evidence of healed tuberculosis.[32] Even studies from Sweden in the 1960s and Switzerland in the 1950s have reported that 9 per cent and 21 per cent, respectively, of silicotics were found to have active disease.[49, 50]

It seems likely that tuberculosis is an even more frequent complication of accelerated and acute silicosis, though this is based on clinical observation of selected individuals rather than epidemiological study. Of 83 silicotic sandblasters in New Orleans, 10 had tuberculosis while 9 had infection with *Mycobacterium kansasii* and 3 with *Mycobacterium avium-intracellulare*. These latter two organisms have been reported as complications of silicosis in other studies,[51, 52] and probably occur whenever disease due to them is endemic, as in New Orleans.

Other opportunistic infections may occur in patients with accelerated or acute silicosis—nocardiosis, sporotrichosis, and cryptococcosis have been described,[17] and aspergillomata may complicate cavitating massive fibrosis.

The development of tuberculosis by a silicotic must result either from reactivation of an old primary infection or from recent infection in the presence of impaired lung defenses. Since silica is extremely toxic to macrophages and macrophages are the lung's main defense against *M. tuberculosis*, the connection between the two diseases is not surprising.[53]

Tuberculosis usually supervenes in a patient with chronic silicosis fairly late in the course of the disease. There may be no symptoms, but loss of weight, increased cough, hemoptysis, and rapid radiological change should alert the physician. In accelerated and acute silicosis, diagnosis may be even more difficult and repeated sputum culture is often the only reliable method.

Pneumothorax. Pneumothorax is a recognized complication of diffuse pulmonary fibrosis and bullous disease. It is therefore not likely to occur in excess in simple silicosis but may be anticipated in massive fibrosis complicated by bullous emphysema. It occurs frequently in accelerated and acute silicosis, in which it may prove a fatal complication.[17]

Rheumatoid and Other Collagen Diseases. Patients with silicosis show an increased prevalence of antinuclear antibodies,[54] though these probably reflect tissue damage rather than play a pathogenic role. Rheumatoid nodules, which may either calcify or cavitate, may appear in the lungs of silicotics with rheumatoid disease or with rheumatoid factor in their blood.[55] Silicotics are not, of course, immune to other manifestations of rheumatoid lung or pleuritis, though there is no evidence that they occur

in excess. Both the skin and visceral manifestations of systemic sclerosis or scleroderma have been described frequently in silicotics,[56] however, and there is little doubt that this disease occurs more commonly in individuals with silicosis than in the general population. Sandblasters with accelerated silicosis have been reported to have scleroderma, rheumatoid disease, or systemic lupus erythematosus in about 10 per cent of cases.[45] Focal glomerulonephritis has also been described in acute cases of silicosis.[16] This suggests that there is a real connection between the tissue damage of silicosis, the production of antinuclear antibodies, and the development of autoimmune disease, though the mechanisms remain a matter for speculation. In such cases some authors have observed an accelerated progression of the lung lesions and have suggested a therapeutic role for steroids.[45]

Other Complications. It is generally believed that silicosis does not predispose to lung cancer.[57] However, studies on the Swedish silicosis register have shown a small excess of lung cancer in silicotics from mining, the iron and steel industries, and quarrying and tunneling.[58] This excess may well have been related to factors, such as smoking habits or radiation exposure, that differed between those cases and the rest of the Swedish population. On balance it seems unlikely that silicosis itself predisposes to lung cancer. It should be remembered, however, that some miners may be exposed to radiation; uranium, fluorspar, tin, and hematite mining are occupations that have been described as having an increased risk of lung cancer (see Chap. 22). Gastric cancer is now well established as occurring more frequently than expected in coal miners,[59] and there is evidence that this is also the case in tin miners.[60] Again, this is less likely to be a complication of silicosis than to be a coincidental effect of exposure to dust or associated toxic substances underground.

Radiographic Changes

Chronic Silicosis

The radiographic appearances of chronic silicosis are similar to those of coal workers' pneumoconiosis. They may be described by the ILO classification, which is discussed in detail in Chapter 5. Essentially, simple silicosis is graded by its profusion, from 0/0 to 3/4, and according to the size of the majority of the opacities: p if less than 1.5 mm diameter, q if between 1.5 and 3 mm, or r if between 3 and 10 mm. Complicated silicosis, or progressive massive fibrosis, is said to be present when conglomerate masses greater than 1 cm diameter are present: if between 1 and 5 cm, these are called stage A; between 5 cm and a combined area of less than one third of the lung, stage B; and greater than this, stage C.

Certain radiographic features are characteristic of silicosis as opposed to coal workers' pneumoconiosis or other mixed dust pneumoconioses,

particularly the eggshell calcification of hilar lymph nodes (Fig. 11–2). This feature, which is not related to healed tuberculosis, is almost pathognomonic of silicosis, though it does occur rarely in sarcoidosis and tuberculosis. It may occur in the absence of obvious radiographic evidence of silicotic change in the lungs themselves. Another feature of simple silicosis is the tendency for individual nodules to increase in size. Thus the earliest radiographic sign of silicosis may be a few rather dense p-size lesions which within a few years will have become q or r nodules (Fig. 11–3). Such lesions characteristically occur in the upper zones of the lungs initially. Silicotic nodules therefore tend to be both larger and more dense than the usual lesions in coal workers' pneumoconiosis. A third feature of silicotic lesions is that they may calcify (Fig. 11–4). While this may be

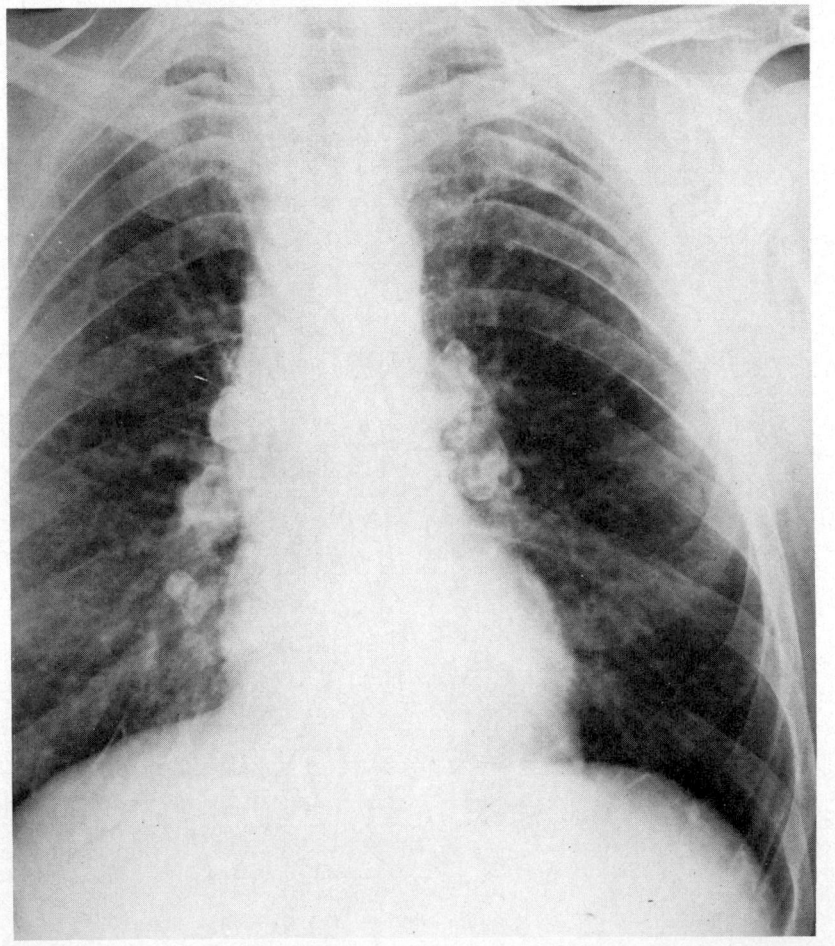

Figure 11–2. Chest radiograph of Welsh slate quarry worker showing category 1/2 simple silicosis with well-marked eggshell calcification of hilar lymph nodes. (Courtesy of Dr. J. Lyons.)

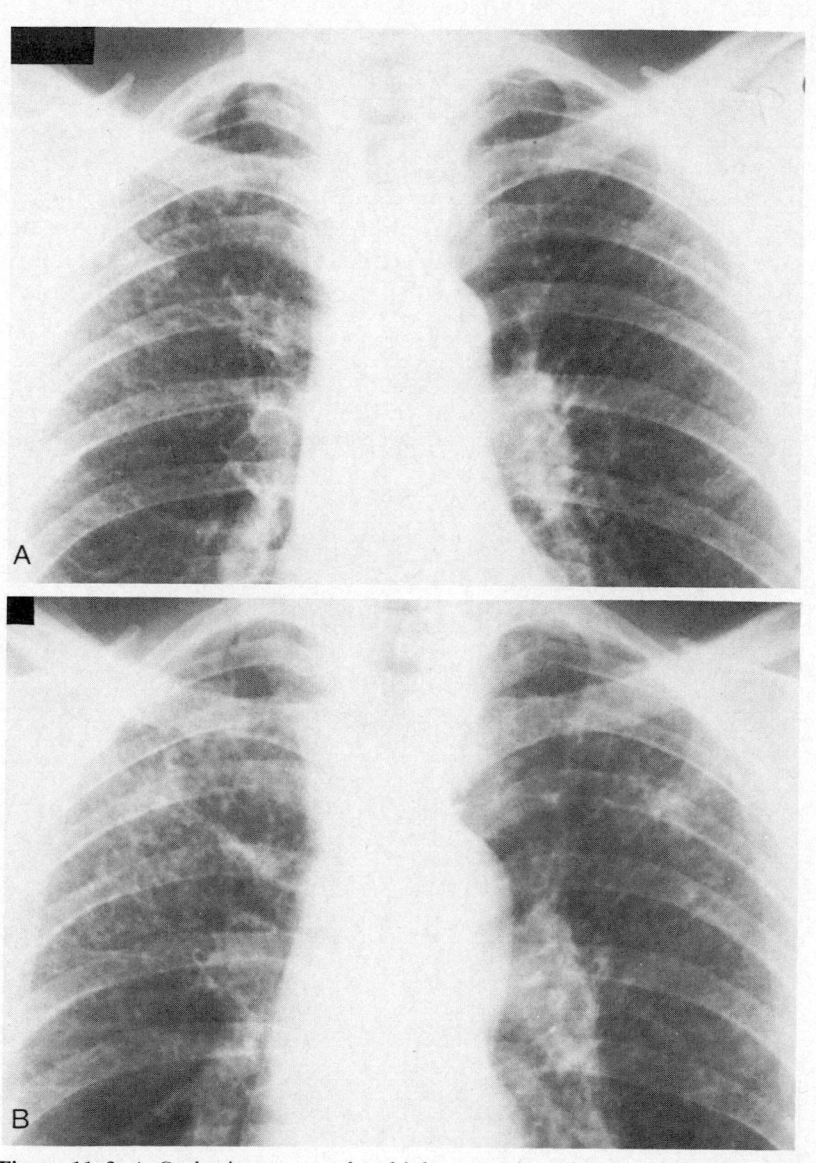

Figure 11–3. *A,* Coal miner exposed to high proportion of quartz in mixed coal mine dust. Film shows few dense p- and q-size nodules in upper lobes in 1974. *B,* Same subject 4 years later, showing increase in both size and profusion of nodules, with early bilateral agglomeration. (From Seaton, A., Dick, J. A., Dodgson, J., and Jacobsen, M., Quartz and pneumoconiosis in coal miners. Lancet 2, 1272, 1981.)

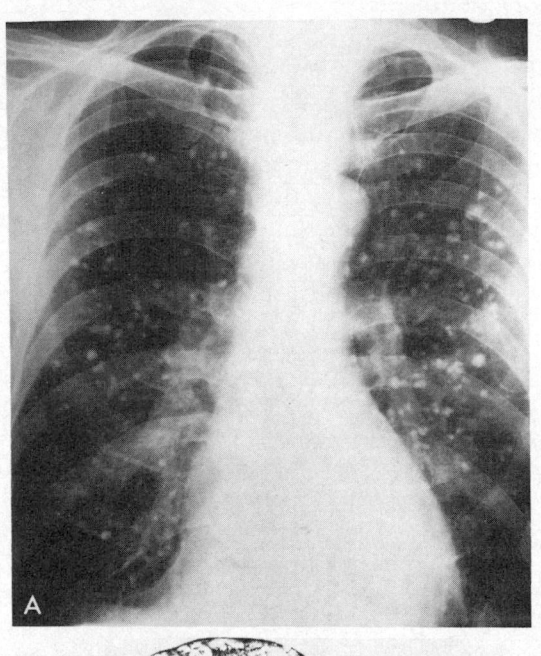

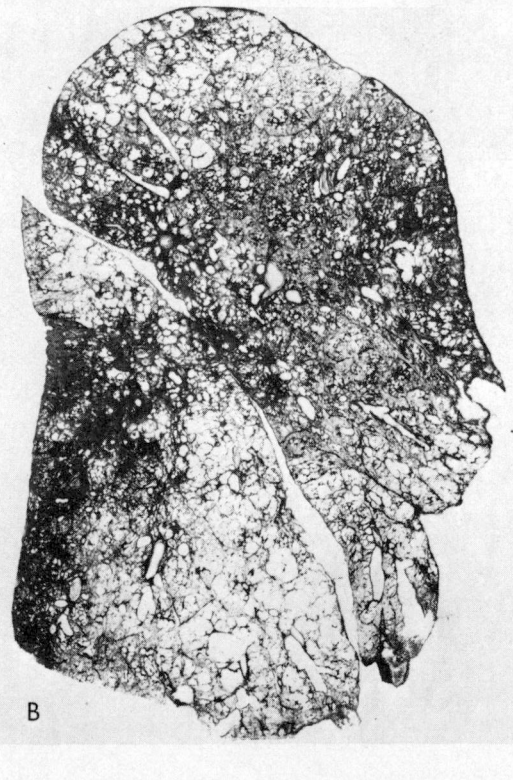

Figure 11–4. Calcified nodules in lungs of a Scottish granite quarry worker. At autopsy, those nodules were shown to be of the Caplan type. *A*, Chest radiograph. *B*, Gough paper section, showing lesions distributed particularly around the oblique fissure. (Courtesy of Dr. J. Lyons.)

evidence of Caplan's syndrome, it does occur in its absence, usually in very long-standing small silicotic nodules.

Complicated silicosis usually appears to arise as a result of aggregation of smaller lesions (Figs. 11–5 to 11–7), and may occur in one or several areas simultaneously. It is liable to involve any part of the lung, in contrast to coal workers' pneumoconiosis, in which the upper zones are most frequently affected first. These lesions grow in size and become more dense, though the rate of this change varies greatly. Nevertheless, silicotic lesions, both simple and complicated, may sometimes progress even in the absence of further dust exposure, and complicated silicosis not infrequently occurs for the first time after dust exposure has ceased.

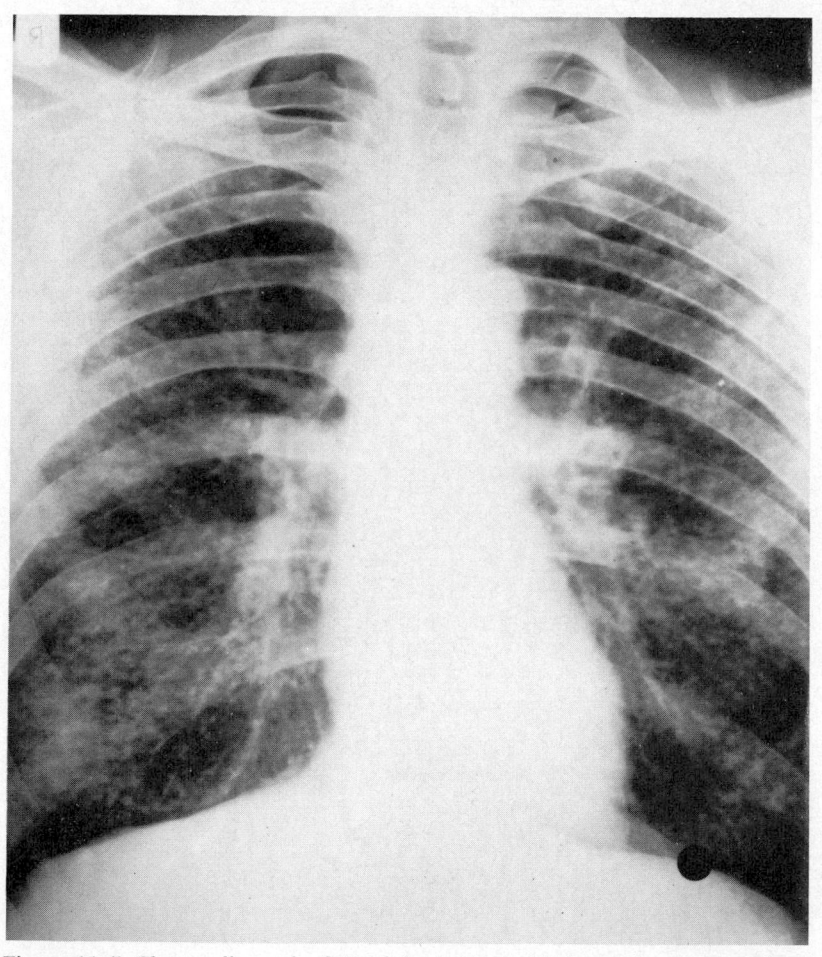

Figure 11–5. Chest radiograph of Welsh lead miner with heavy exposure to silica dust. Radiograph taken in 1952, showing category 3/3 simple silicosis. At this stage the man left the industry.

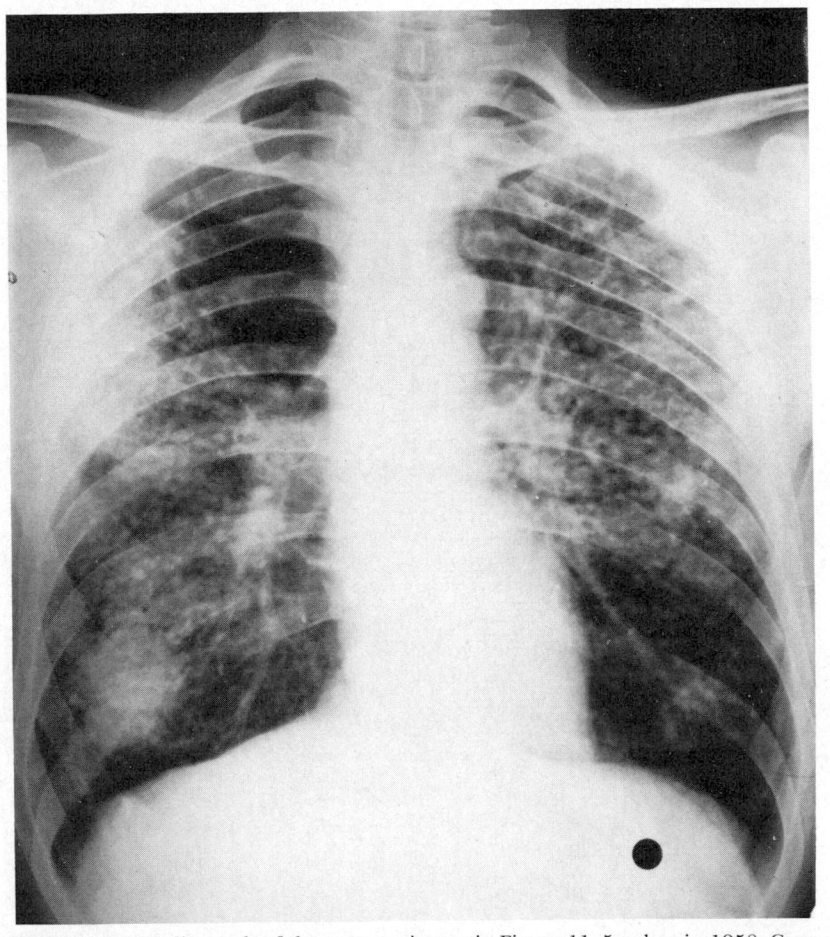

Figure 11–6. Radiograph of the same patient as in Figure 11–5, taken in 1958. Category B complicated silicosis has developed in right upper and lower zones.

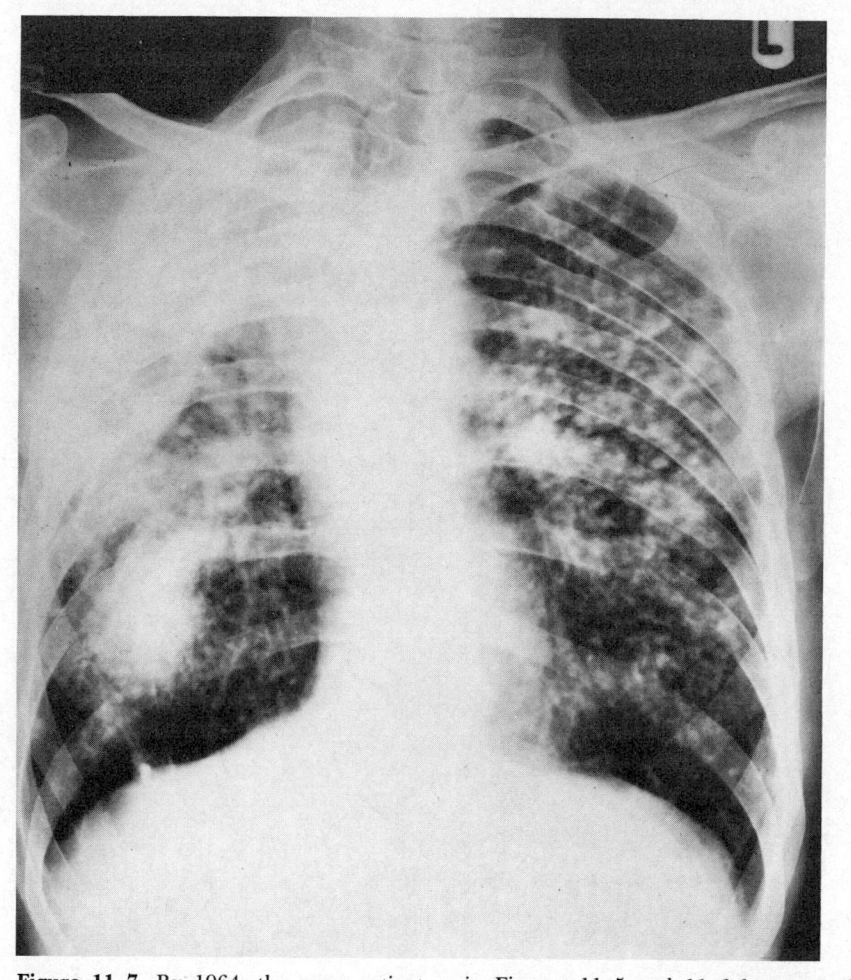

Figure 11–7. By 1964, the same patient as in Figures 11–5 and 11–6 has stage C complicated disease and conglomeration is beginning in the left lung. Marked fibrosis is present over the right upper lobe and bullous change at the right base. (Figures 11–5 to 11–7 courtesy of Dr. J. Lyons.)

The lesions of complicated silicosis cavitate less frequently than those of coal workers' pneumoconiosis. Nevertheless this does occur, usually due to ischemic necrosis but sometimes as a result of tuberculosis (Figs. 11–8 and 11–9). Compensatory emphysema is also seen as a result of complicated silicosis, usually at an advanced stage (Figs. 11–5 to 11–7). While complicated silicosis usually arises on a background of fairly advanced simple disease, it may occur as a result of enlargement of a few rather sparse lesions. In such cases, the absence of a nodular background may lead to confusion with tumors. The shape, which is often ovoid or sausage-like, the density, and the presence of surrounding emphysematous bullae may be helpful in differentiation.

Pleural fibrosis is of frequent occurrence in silicosis. This is usually diffuse, bilateral, and more marked over the upper zones. It may occasionally calcify, though not to the same extent as asbestos pleurisy (See Chap. 13).

As mentioned before, pneumothorax and tuberculosis may complicate silicosis. The former occurs as a result usually of a ruptured bulla. The

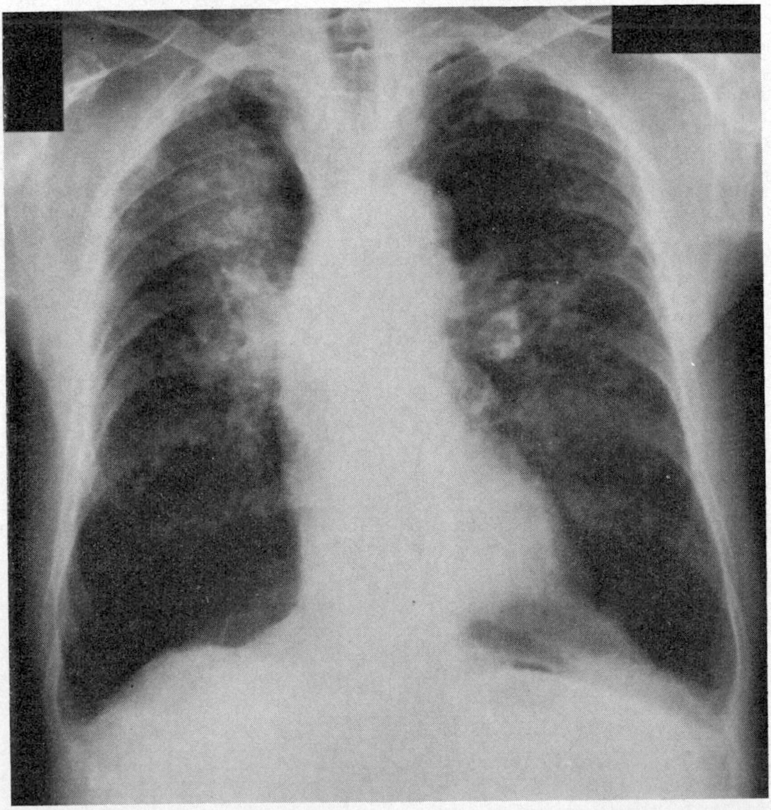

Figure 11–8. Radiograph of coal miner exposed to silica in tunneling, showing massive fibrosis and eggshell calcification of hilar nodes.

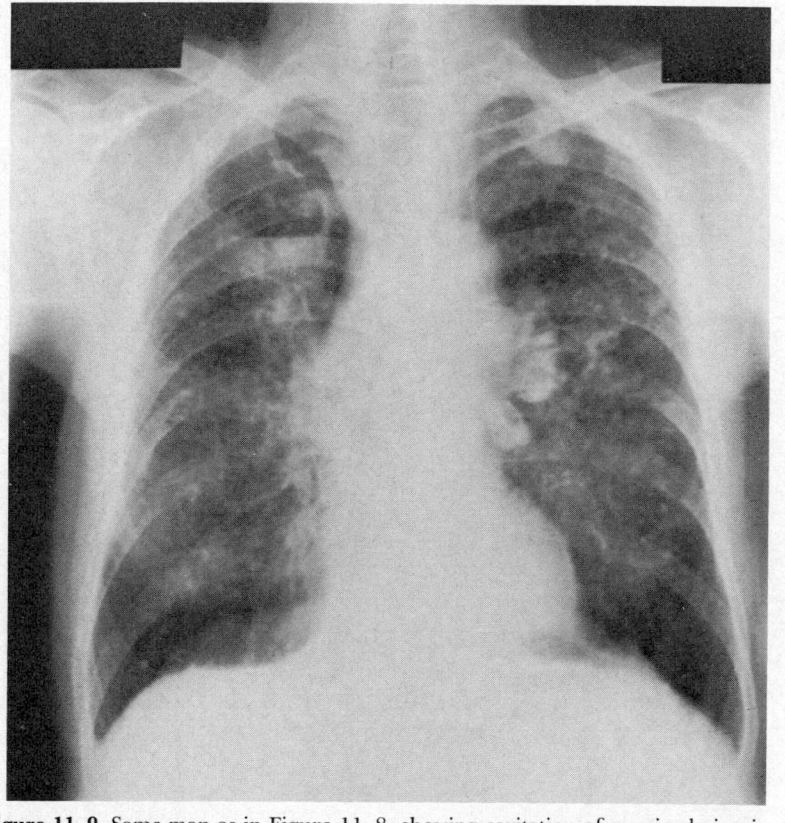

Figure 11–9. Same man as in Figure 11–8, showing cavitation of massive lesion in right upper lobe. Sputum culture proved positive for tubercle bacilli.

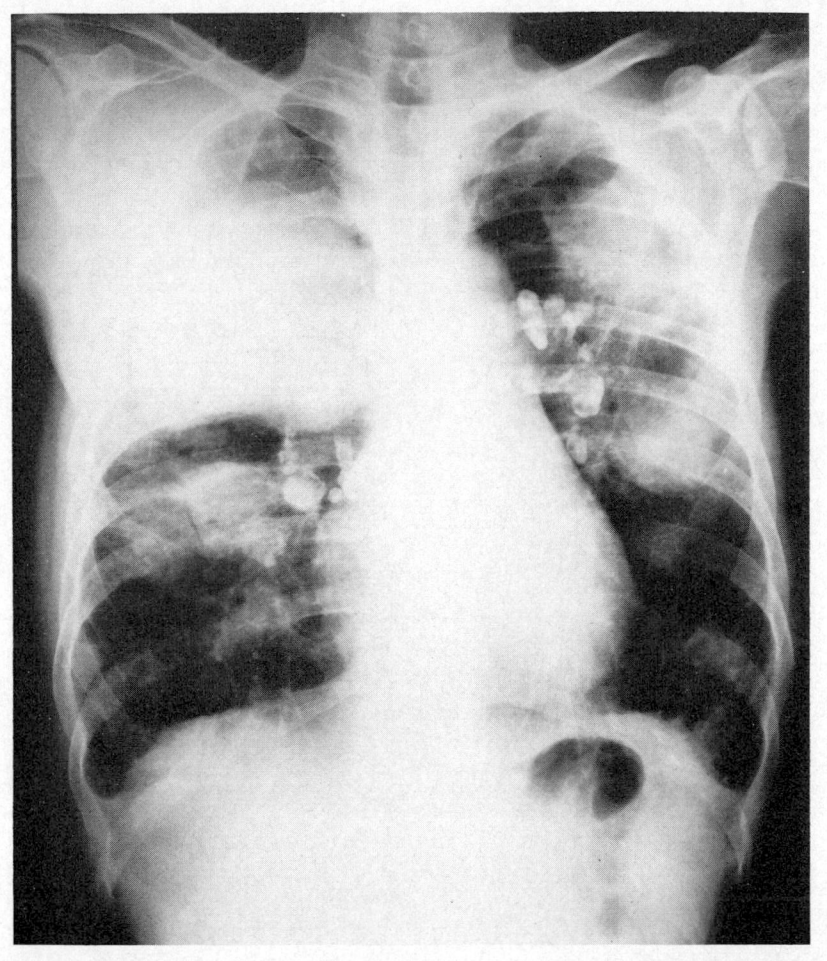

Figure 11–10. Chest radiograph of Welsh coal miner with heavy and prolonged exposure to silica in hardheading. Film shows stage C complicated disease, much of the rest of the lung being affected by compensatory emphysema. Eggshell calcification is also well seen.

latter may cause no radiographic change at all, but should be suspected if any rapid change in size of lesions occurs, if nodules cavitate, or if new softer or streaky fibrotic lesions develop (Figs. 11–8 to 11–10). The cornerstone of diagnosis of this disease in silicosis is bacteriology rather than radiology.

Caplan's syndrome occurs occasionally in silicosis as in coal workers' pneumoconiosis, the larger nodules usually appearing on a rather sparse background of simple silicosis and occasionally antedating the development of rheumatoid disease elsewhere. The nodules radiographically do not differ from those seen in coal workers' pneumoconiosis and may calcify or cavitate (See Chap. 16).

Accelerated Silicosis

The changes in accelerated silicosis are similar to those in chronic silicosis but appear earlier and progress more rapidly. They tend to start as a predominatly upper zone nodularity that progresses both to massive lesions and to irregular fibrosis and contraction of the upper lobes (Figs. 11–11 and 11–12). They make their first appearance within five or six years of first exposure and progress to massive fibrosis over a further similar period. In many cases the lesions are complicated by mycobacterial infection or pneumothorax[45]

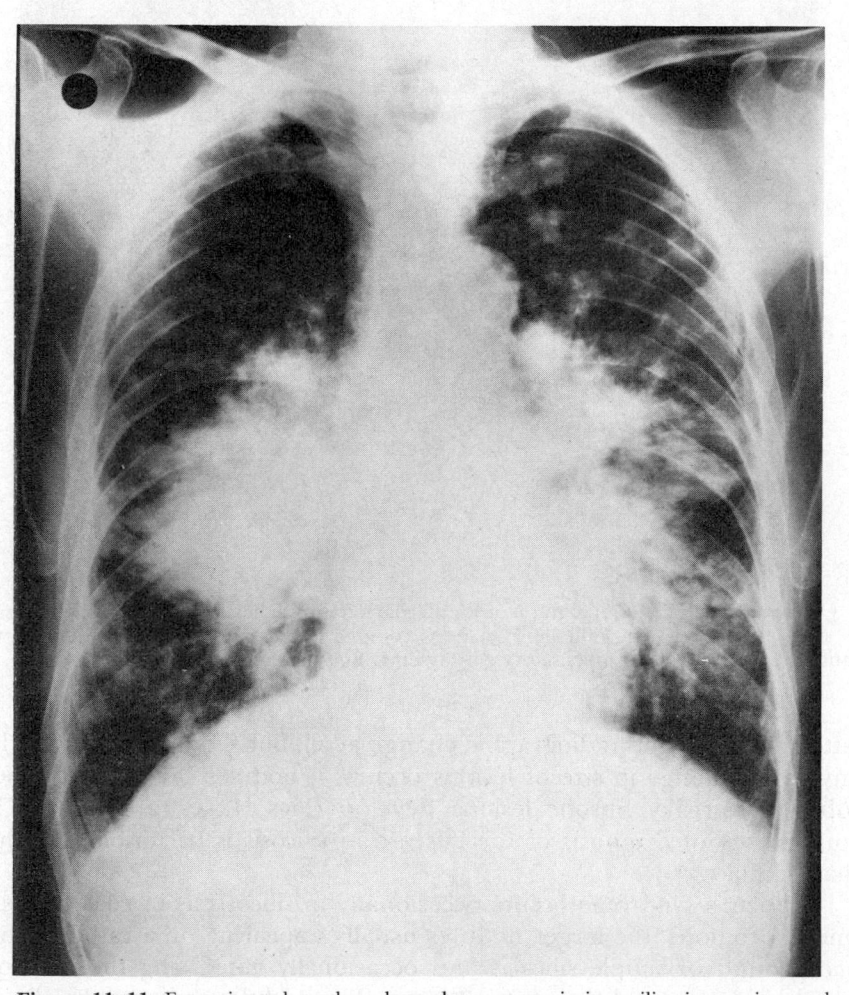

Figure 11–11. Extensive tuberculous bronchopneumonia in a silicotic granite worker. Rapid development of the midzone lesions and their unusual distribution suggested tuberculous infection. Patient recovered on triple therapy. (Courtesy of Dr. J. Lyons.)

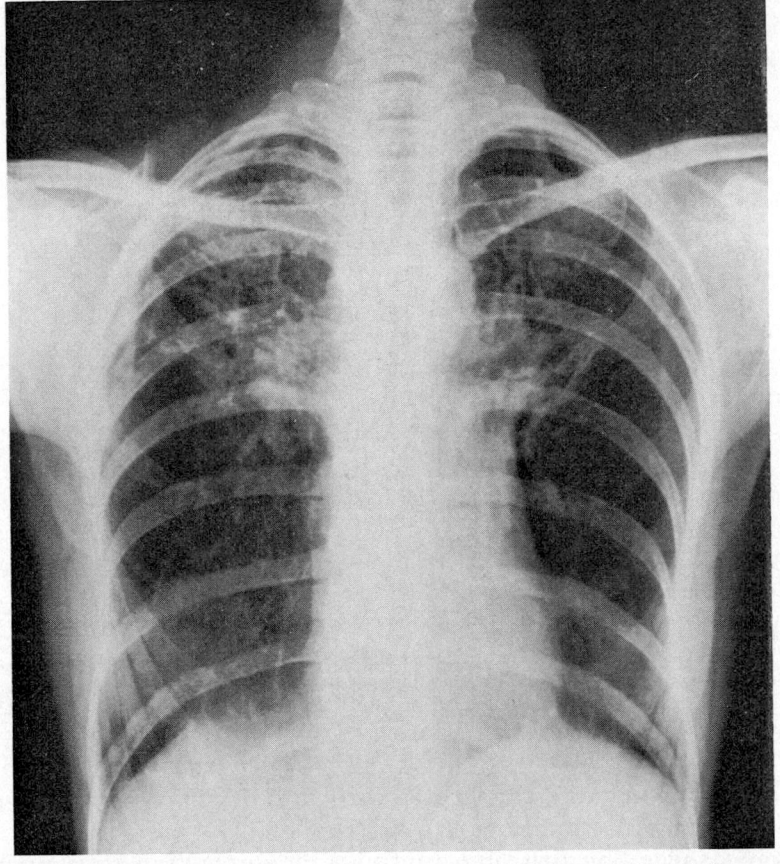

Figure 11–12. Radiograph of woman exposed to high levels of calcined diatomaceous earth in operating xerox camera, showing upper lobe fibrosis and lower lobe emphysema due to accelerated silicosis.

Acute Silicosis

In acute silicosis the nodular pattern is absent, the lungs showing a diffuse ground-glass appearance, similar to pulmonary edema (Fig. 11–13). The acute disease may, of course, be superimposed on previous chronic or accelerated disease, so mixed nodular and edematous patterns occur. In rare cases the diffuse pattern may resolve to leave irregular fibrosis, but usually the appearance persists until death, which occurs within a matter of months rather than years.

Pulmonary Function

The study of lung function in silicosis has been complicated by uncertainties in diagnosis (pure silicosis or mixed dust disease), the

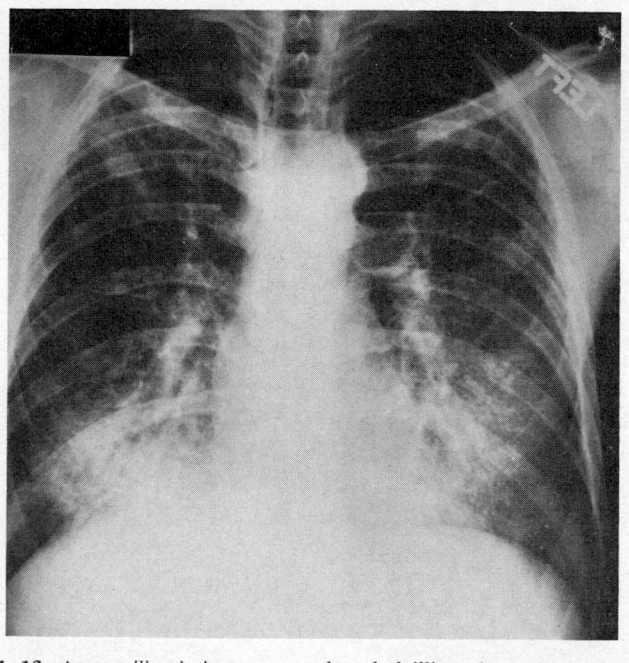

Figure 11–13. Acute silicosis in man employed drilling through overburden in strip mining for coal, showing bilateral acinar filling pattern most marked in lower zones. (From Banks, D. E., Bauer, M. A., Castellan, R. M., and Lapp, N. L.: Silicosis in surface coal mine drillers. Thorax, *38*, 275, 1983.)

presence of other diseases such as chronic bronchitis and emphysema, and differences in radiological categorization. However, a pattern has emerged suggesting that little functional abnormality occurs in simple nodular silicosis except possibly in ILO category 3 disease, whereas a mixed obstructive and restrictive pattern can be expected in more advanced complicated silicosis. Accelerated silicosis usually seems to produce a mixed restrictive and obstructive pattern and acute silicosis almost always causes severe and progressive restriction. None of these patterns of altered lung function is of diagnostic value, and considerable variation is found between individuals with similar radiographic appearance.

A detailed early study of South African gold miners showed that ventilatory function, exercise tolerance, and compliance were all lower in miners with advanced simple silicosis than in miners with normal radiographs, the two groups being matched for age and mining experience.[61] However, the differences for individual tests were not significant and could have been explained by an excess of bronchitics among the silicotics. Among British foundrymen, airways obstruction was not found in the absence of symptoms of chronic bronchitis, though there was a greater prevalence of these symptoms among these workers than among controls.[25] There was no relationship between pneumoconiosis and ventilatory capacity in this study.

More detailed studies of ventilatory mechanics have shown no differ-

ence between normal subjects and those with category 1 simple silicosis, but record a minor reduction in lung volumes and compliance in more advanced simple silicosis and a greater reduction in complicated silicosis.[62] This contrasts with findings in coal workers' pneumoconiosis, in which mechanical changes rarely occur in the absence of complicated disease.[63] This work has been supported by another study, which found that silicotics had lower vital capacity, physiological dead space, and exercise tolerance than controls with coal workers' pneumoconiosis and welders' siderosis, carefully matched for age and category of radiographic change.[64] Only the silicotics showed appreciable oxygen desaturation on exercise.

In order to distinguish the effects of silicosis from those of cigarette smoking or chronic bronchitis and other chest diseases, one study has been carried out in which 47 nonsmoking, nonbronchitic, unobstructed miners with silicosis were examined.[65] No abnormalities of diffusing capacity were found except in men with more extensive complicated disease, and no differences were found between those with p- and q-type opacities. Another study of South African gold miners has compared the lung function of miners with silicosis with that of those without the disease, in relation to their recorded dust exposures.[66] There were few significant differences that could be attributed to silicosis, the implication being that dust has two independent effects, one in causing a decrement in ventilatory capacity and the other in provoking silicosis. Although the FEV_1 and FEF_{25-75} were slightly lower in those with radiographic evidence of silicosis, the differences could be entirely accounted for by increased dust exposure.

Accelerated silicosis is more frequently associated with abnormalities of function. In sandblasters, these abnormalities are uncommon at the early nodular stage, but the development of either complicated disease or irregular fibrosis and lobar contraction is usually associated with earlier restriction, obstruction, or both.[67] Similar findings have been reported in the accelerated disease seen in diatomaceous earth workers,[68] though there is poor correlation between radiographic and functional abnormalities.

In acute silicosis, as would be expected, severe restrictive lung function abnormalities, with arterial hypoxemia and reduced diffusing capacity and compliance, are found.[14, 44]

Few longitudinal studies of lung function in silicosis have been reported. It would be anticipated that progression of simple disease would not be attended by an excess decline in function until massive fibrosis supervened. Progressive changes in keeping with radiological deterioration have been reported in accelerated silicosis of sandblasters, though there is considerable variation between individuals.[67]

Differential Diagnosis

Normally the diagnosis of silicosis presents no difficulties. The finding of diffuse radiographic shadowing in a patient known to have been exposed to silica is usually sufficient. Nonindustrial causes of diffuse

pulmonary mottling are almost always associated with a restrictive pattern and defects of gas diffusion on lung function testing. Such conditions, including sarcoidosis, cryptogenic fibrosing alveolitis, rheumatoid lung, carcinomatous lymphangitis, and pulmonary hemosiderosis, may of course occur in subjects who have been exposed to silica. If this is the case, the existence of previous radiographs is of great help. Moreover, the finding of restrictive lung function abnormalities and physical signs of pulmonary fibrosis (clubbing and basal crackles) suggest nonindustrial disease.

Difficulties commonly arise at the onset of progressive massive fibrosis, or less frequently Caplan's syndrome, in excluding carcinoma or tuberculosis. The latter must always be suspected and regular bacteriological testing of sputum is necessary. The former can usually be excluded by inspection of serial radiographs and, often, by the finding of several opacities. Very occasionally diagnosis of a newly arisen single peripheral opacity is impossible without lung biopsy or thoracotomy. Generally, however, a neoplasm is a better defined and more rapidly growing lesion than early massive fibrosis, and the distinction can be made radiographically.

The diagnosis of accelerated or acute silicosis may give rise to confusion if a careful industrial history is not taken. The former may progress to an irregular upper zone fibrosis that can be mistaken for tuberculosis, chronic sarcoidosis, chronic allergic alveolitis, or rare conditions such as ankylosing spondylitis lung (which may occur in the absence of clinical spondylitis) or histiocytosis X. The acute disease may resemble pulmonary edema, alveolar proteinosis, or acute allergic alveolitis. In all these cases the occupational history is paramount in leading to the diagnosis, and confirmation will often result from some quick inquiries at the workplace. As discussed in Chapter 2, further investigation of the patient is generally not necessary.

PATHOLOGY

Chronic and Accelerated Silicosis

Macroscopic Appearances. Inspection of the lungs commonly shows fibrous adhesions in the pleural cavity, with silicotic plaques visible over the pleural surfaces. The lungs tend to be more pigmented than usual. The hilar lymph nodes are often enlarged, containing fibrotic nodules, and sometimes calcified. When the lung is cut, grayish fibrotic nodules are seen, more profuse in the apical and posterior parts of upper and lower lobes (Fig. 11–14). These vary both in size, from a few millimeters to large conglomerate masses occupying most of a lobe, and in profusion. They are hard and occasionally calcified. Nodules that have been cut across show a characteristic whorled appearance both in the lung and in the lymph nodes. Several of these nodules may appear to have become confluent to produce very large lesions. These areas of massive fibrosis

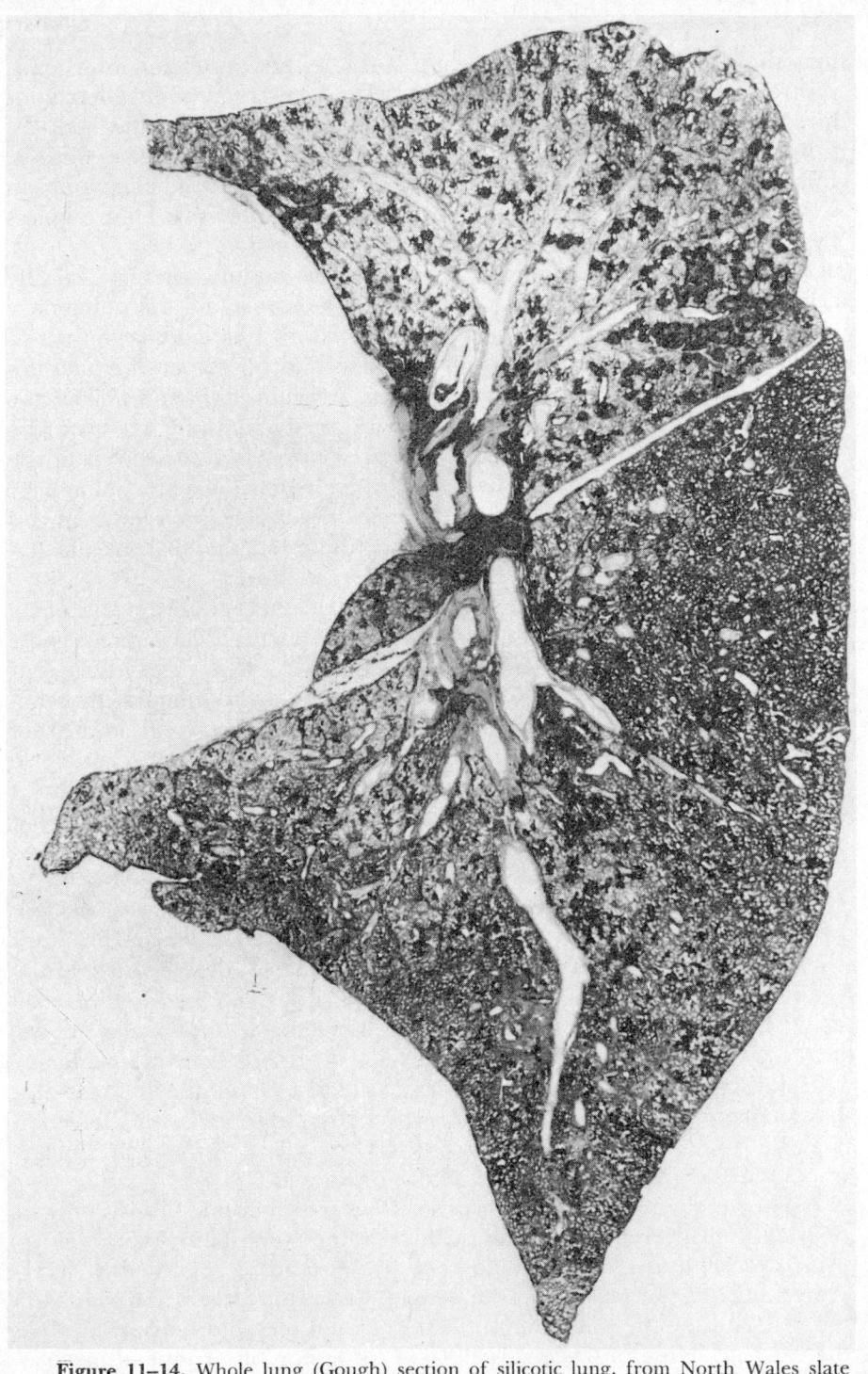

Figure 11–14. Whole lung (Gough) section of silicotic lung, from North Wales slate quarry worker, showing eggshell hilar calcification and silicotic nodules predominantly in the apical and posterior parts of both upper and lower lobes.

may show cavitation (Figs. 11–15 and 11–16), either in relation to ischemic central necrosis or, still quite commonly, in association with tuberculous infection. In the latter instance, caseation may be seen in the nodules. Emphysematous bullae often surround the areas of massive fibrosis. Enlargement of the right side of the heart occurs not uncommonly in advanced complicated silicosis, but evidence of congestive failure is less frequent in the absence of chronic airways obstruction.

Microscopic Appearances. The silicotic nodule characteristically arises in the region of the respiratory bronchiole, around the pulmonary arterioles and in paraseptal and subpleural tissues. The nodule consists of hyalinized collagen fibers centrally and reticulin fibers peripherally, the whole having a concentric arrangement and showing some fibroblastic activity at the edges in early lesions (Figs. 11–17 and 11–18). The respiratory bronchioles and small pulmonary vessels are involved in the progressing fibrosis and destroyed, and the elastic laminae of pulmonary arteries may sometimes be seen in the midst of a collagenous mass. In this respect the silicotic nodule differs markedly from the coal macule described in Chapter 14.

Particles of silica may be demonstrated in the nodules, occasionally by staining with toluidine blue to show metachromasia,[69] but more reliably by viewing the sections under polarized light when the birefringent particles can be seen (Fig. 11–19). Microincineration techniques, with hydrochloric acid treatment and dark-ground illumination, result in the best demonstration of these particles and allow those smaller than 1 micron to be seen.[70] Such methods have demonstrated that the amount of silica is variable and bears no relationship to the extent of the collagenous reaction. Final proof that quartz is the refractile material depends on the use of x-ray diffraction techniques.

The lesions of massive fibrosis consist of dense hyalinized collagen, often with necrosis in the center. The lesions are avascular and may not show the typical whorled appearance. These masses destroy the normal pulmonary architecture and the elastin ghosts of pulmonary vessels may again be demonstrated within them. Tuberculous infection may be detected by the finding of acid-fast bacilli and caseation in the center of nodules and by finding the characteristic tubercles of epithelioid cells and Langhans giant cells. Sometimes, however, the presence of this infection may be difficult to detect microscopically, since the histological appearances may be altered by the coexistence of silicosis.

The accelerated form of silicosis differs from chronic silicosis only in degree, the differentiation being clinical rather than pathological. However, descriptions of the pathology of what would be regarded as accelerated silicosis, for example, in diatomaceous earth workers and sandblasters,[14, 39] indicate that in addition to silicotic nodules and massive fibrosis, diffuse thickening of alveolar walls with proliferation of type II alveolar cells may be found. In addition, a granulomatous reaction with occasional giant cells may be a prominent feature. These cases typically show extensive upper zone fibrosis and lower zone emphysema.

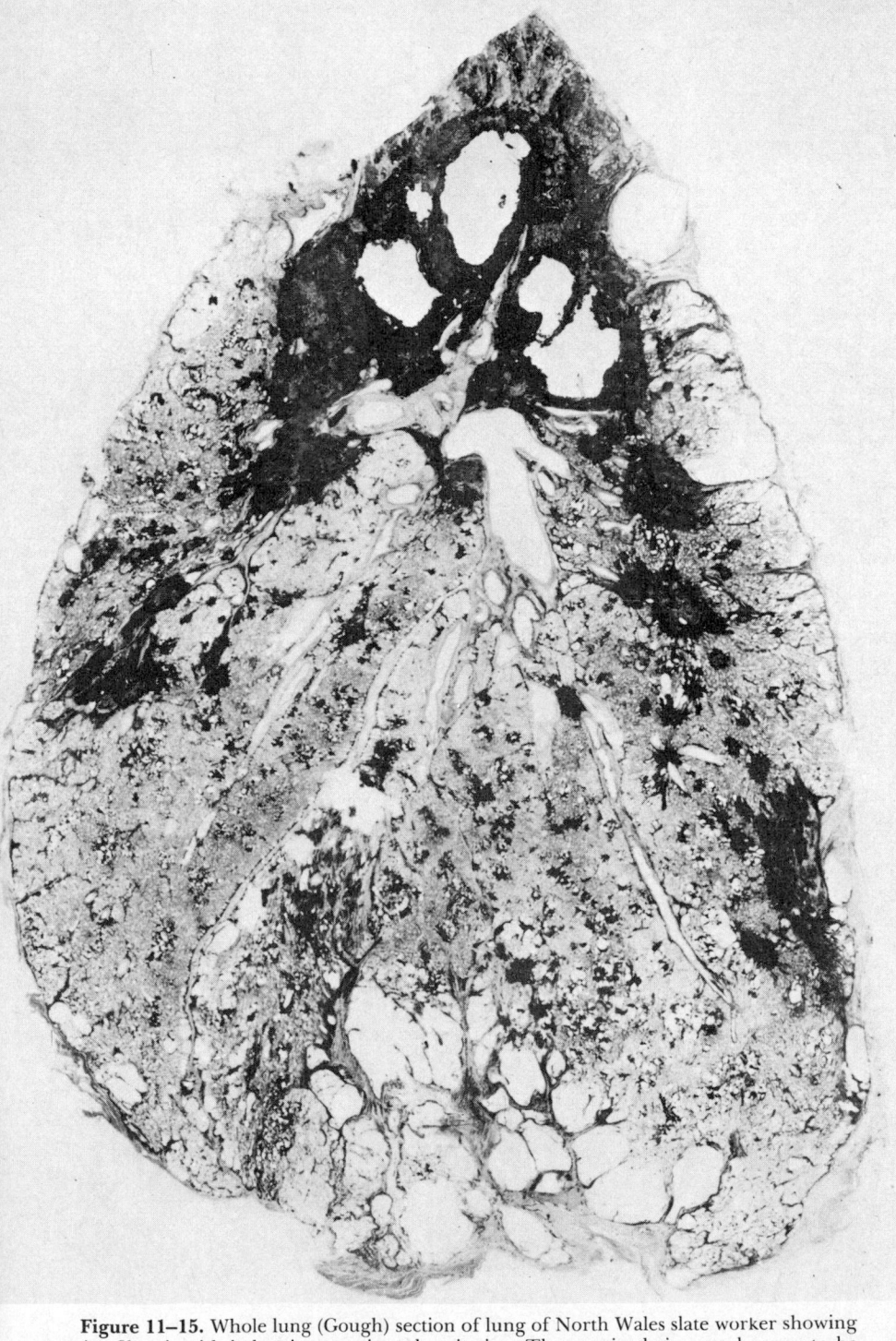

Figure 11–15. Whole lung (Gough) section of lung of North Wales slate worker showing massive fibrosis with ischemic necrosis and cavitation. The massive lesion can be seen to be composed of smaller silicotic nodules that have become confluent.

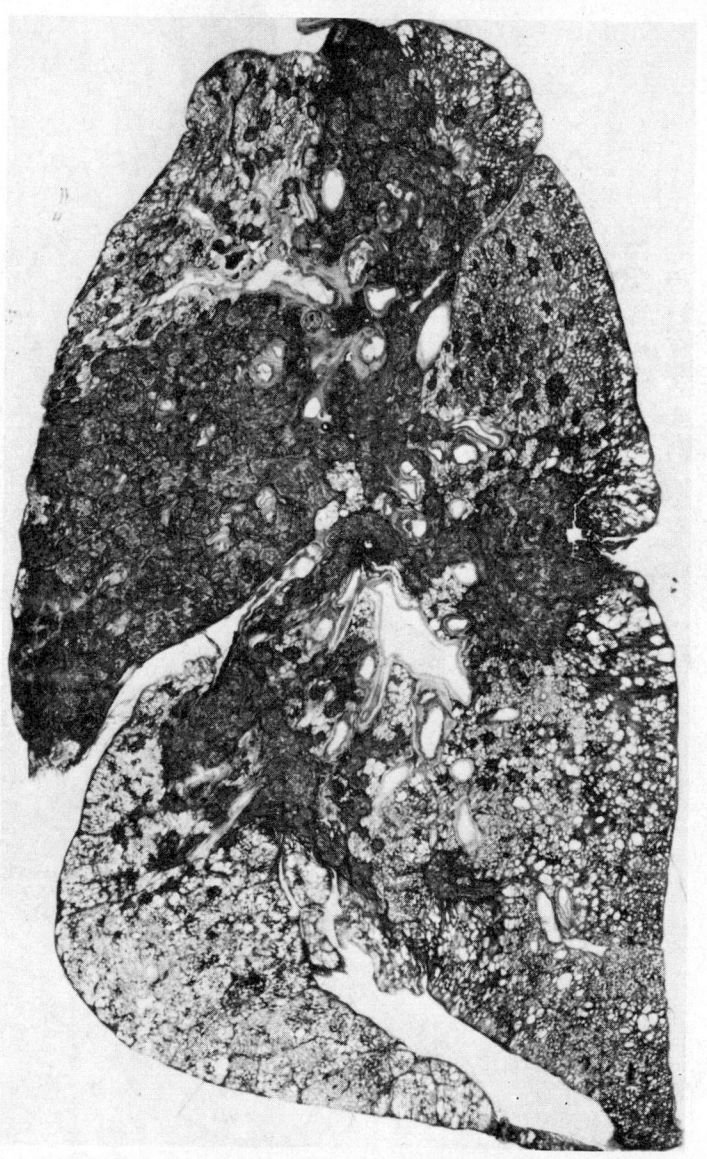

Figure 11–16. Whole lung (Gough) section from North Wales slate quarryman, showing extensive massive fibrosis due to conglomeration of smaller silicotic nodules.

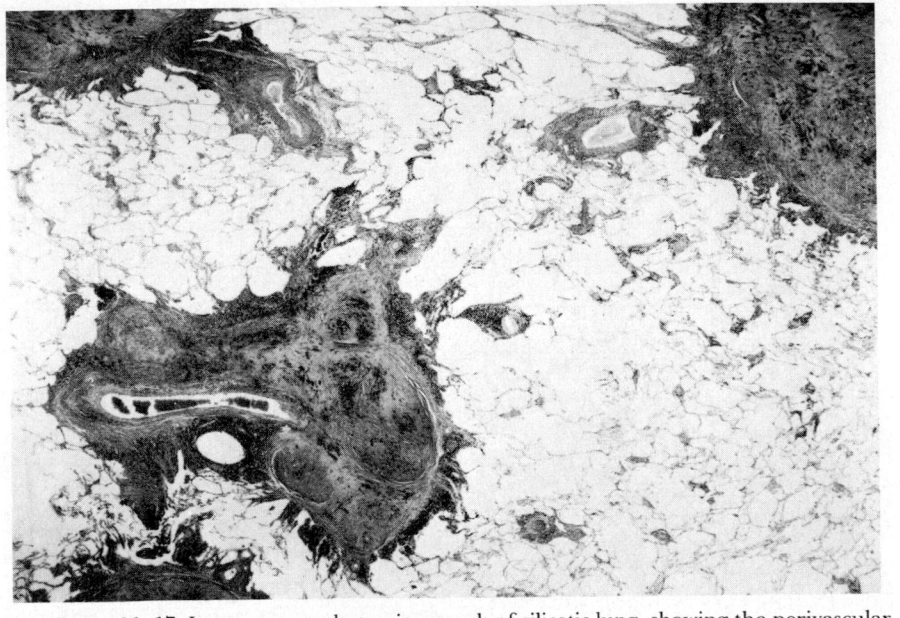

Figure 11–17. Lower power photomicrograph of silicotic lung, showing the perivascular location of the nodules and their whorled appearance.

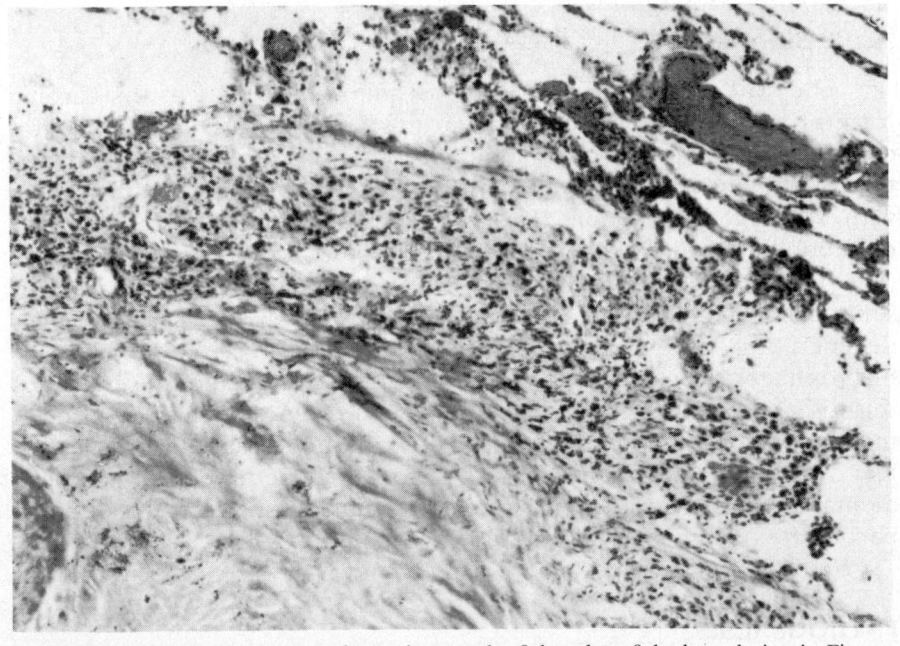

Figure 11–18. Higher power photomicrograph of the edge of the large lesion in Figure 11–17, showing dense acellular collagen (bottom left) surrounded by a rim of fibroblasts and macrophages.

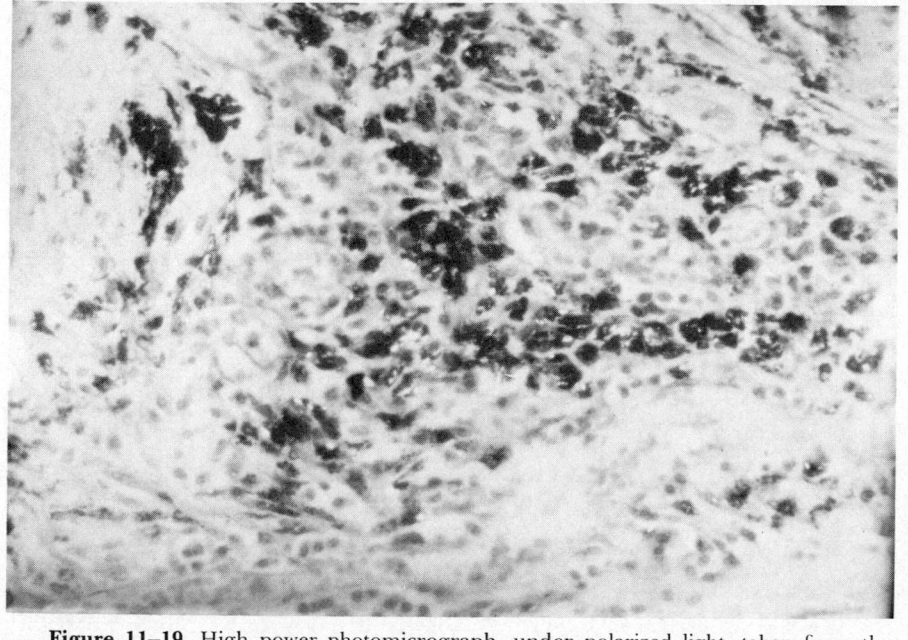

Figure 11–19. High power photomicrograph, under polarized light, taken from the peripheral rim of tissue in Figure 11–18, showing doubly refractile silica particles contained within macrophages.

Acute Silicosis

The pathology of acute silicosis is quite unlike that of the chronic form of the disease. The lungs are firm and edematous, and the pleural cavities may contain fibrinous adhesions. Microscopically, there is infiltration of the alveolar walls with plasma cells, lymphocytes, and fibroblasts with some collagenization. The alveoli themselves are filled with an eosinophilic coagulum that is postive to periodic acid–Schiff staining[16, 42, 44] (Fig. 11–20). Electron microscopy shows widening of alveolar walls with some collagen and clusters of type II cells. The alveolar spaces contain degenerating cells that are probably both type II alveolar cells and macrophages.[16] The presence of the interstitial pneumonitis differentiates this disease from pulmonary alveolar proteinosis. Although silica particles may be demonstrated in the lungs and lymph nodes, silicotic nodules are few or absent. The lesions of acute silicosis may be produced in experimental animals, usually by causing them to inhale concentrations of finely particulate quartz[71, 72] (Fig. 11–21).

PATHOGENESIS

Experimental studies have shown that silica, when ingested by macrophages, causes death and disruption of the cells. Tissue culture

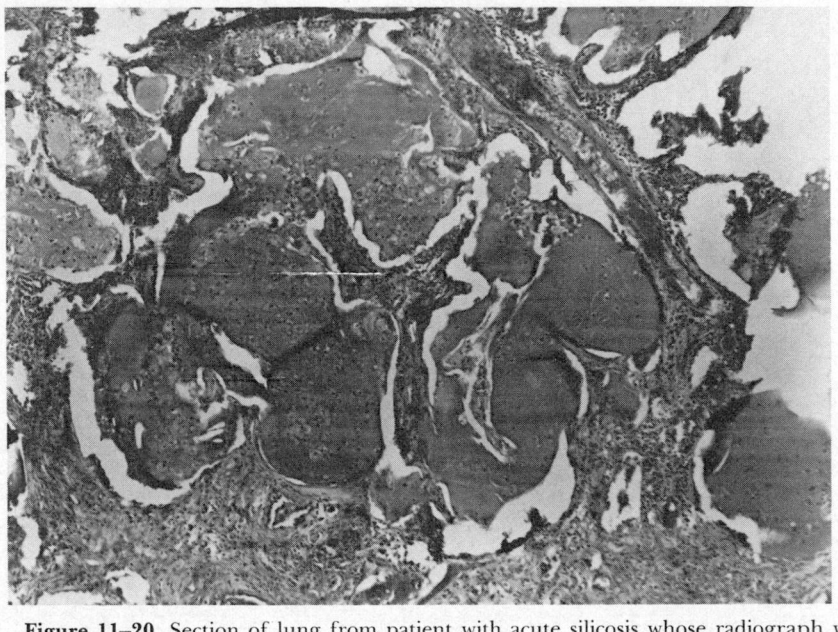

Figure 11–20. Section of lung from patient with acute silicosis whose radiograph was shown in Figure 11–13, showing interstitial fibrosis and alveoli containing macrophages and eosinophilic material staining with periodic acid–Schiff. (Courtesy of Dr. N. L. Lapp.)

experiments[73, 74] have demonstrated that initially the silica particles appear in phagosomes, which are then surrounded by lysosomes. These bodies then pour their enzymes into the phagosome, which becomes disrupted and liberates the silica particles into the cytoplasm, with subsequent death of the cell. In this, silica differs from carbon, which does not cause breakdown of the phagosomes or cell death. The mechanism whereby silica kills macrophages is uncertain.[75] Solubility is not a factor, since silica in a semipermeable diffusion chamber does not initiate fibrosis in the peritoneum of mice,[76] while different forms of silica induce fibrosis to a degree which bears no relationship to their solubilities.[77] The tetrahedral structure is important, as quartz, cristobalite, tridymite, and coesite are fibrogenic, whereas stishovite, which has an octahedral structure, and amorphous silica are not.

The fibrogenic reaction may be prevented by coating the silica with aluminium or by protecting the cell membranes with polyvinyl pyridine-N-oxide (PNO). A similar reaction seems to occur when quartz is inhaled in association with other silicates, which may protect the macrophage from the toxic effect of the silica. This may be responsible for the apparent absence of effect of low levels of quartz in mixed coal mine dust (see Chap. 16). It seems likely that the initial reaction occurs when silica, coated with protein from serum, is ingested into the macrophage and the lysosomal enzymes digest away the protein. The silica reacts with the lysosomal membrane, which becomes permeable and allows diffusion of

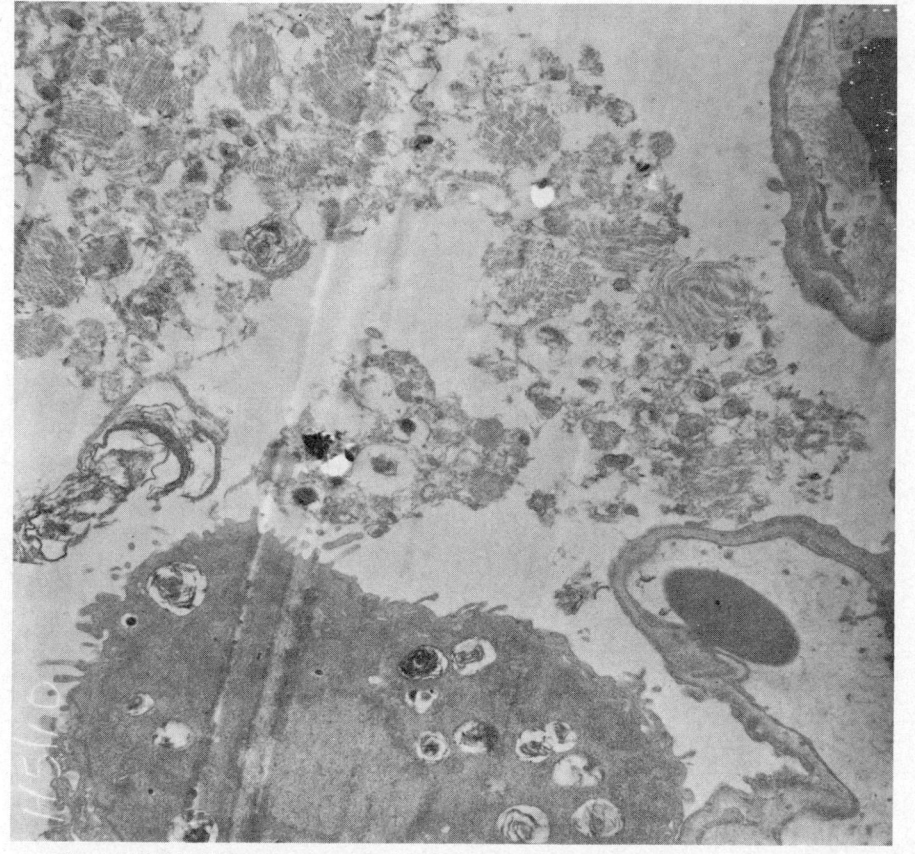

Figure 11–21. Electron micrograph of rat lung following exposure of the animal to quartz dust for 20 hours daily over six weeks. The cell at bottom left is a type II alveolar cell, showing lamellar bodies. Sphingomyelin inclusions from these structures are also present free in the air space, giving rise to the so-called proteinaceous material. Also present are small quartz particles with associated tearing of the tissue.

enzymes into the cell cytoplasm.[78] Recent work suggests that the cell membrane–silica reaction may result from peroxidation of membrane lipids.[79]

Once lung macrophages have been damaged, two things appear to happen. First, additional macrophages appear, ingest the liberated silica and die in their turn, and these macrophages are surrounded by a reticulin network that gradually occupies the alveolus and subsequently the respiratory bronchiole. Second, collagen is laid down, which then hyalinizes. The experimental work in this area has been summarized by Heppleston, who notes that four basic processes are involved and need to be explained by any hypothesis of the pathogenesis of silicosis:[80, 81] (1) the destruction of macrophages, (2) the production of more macrophages to continue ingesting liberated silica particles, (3) the stimulation of collagen formation,

and (4) the hyalinization of the collagen. He suggests, on the basis of observations that silica may produce an alveolar lipoproteinosis-like lesion in rats and humans, and may cause liberation of lipid factors from type II alveolar cells (the cells that secrete surfactant), that these lipid factors stimulate further production of macrophages from their probably blood-borne monocyte precursors in the marrow. Furthermore, the silica-induced death of macrophages has been shown to result in the liberation of nonlipid material that stimulates fibroblasts to form collagen.[80, 82, 83] The final episode, hyalinization of the collagen, seems to be related to the deposition of amyloid-like material among the collagen fibers.[84] This may be derived from immunoglobulins produced as part of the general stimulation of the reticuloendothelial system in silicosis.

The finding of antinuclear antibody and evidence of autoimmune disease in disproportionately large numbers of individuals with accelerated silicosis has already been mentioned. It seems likely that this is an effect of the lung damage caused by silica, possibly as a result of chronic liberation of nuclear material by the disruption of macrophages. There is no evidence that such antibodies play any role in the pathogenesis of the silicotic lesion except in rare cases of Caplan's syndrome.

Massive fibrosis in silicosis usually occurs as a result of coalescence of several smaller nodules, though in advanced stages this may not be apparent from inspection of the lesions. Diffuse fibrosis rather than massive lesions may also occur in the accelerated and acute forms of the disease, and mycobacterial infection may well play a part in the etiology and progression of some of these cases. This impaired resistance to infection is probably in turn related to the toxic effect of silica on macrophages, as reduced macrophage phagocytic ability has been shown to follow treatment of animals with silica.[85]

PREVENTION

Prevention of silicosis depends on recognition of the risk; currently, the chief danger lies in those industries in which silica appears in some disguise. This has been the case with abrasive soap powders and bentonite milling. Once the presence of particles of silica of respirable size has been recognized, the general measures of enclosure of processes, suppression of dust by water and ventilation, and protection of the worker by efficient respirators must be applied. Where heavy concentrations of silica occur, as in sandblasting, tunneling, or stripping of furnace linings, the only adequate protection is for the worker to be isolated from the dust by a protective helmet and suit with its own positive-pressure air supply. The importance of this measure has been emphasized by recent studies of sandblasters, in which high levels of silica were found *inside* respirators. Moreover, these individuals often worked without respirators when sandblasting had finished but while dust levels were still extremely high.[86] As

previously stated, suitable alternatives to silica should be introduced wherever possible.

In all industries in which a dust hazard is recognized, regular monitoring of levels of respirable dust should be carried out, and usually this is required by law. The current standard for silica-containing dusts in the United States and Britain is $\dfrac{10}{\% \text{ quartz} + 2}$ mg/m³. For dusts containing tridymite and cristobalite this value is divided by 2, whereas dusts with very low quartz levels (around 1 per cent) are controlled by a nuisance dust standard of 10 mg/m³. These figures are under review, but hard epidemiological evidence on which to base reliable standards is sparse.[22] Apart from careful control of the environment, workers exposed to silica should undergo chest radiography on a regular basis. A film every four to five years should be sufficient if silica levels are kept below the hygiene standard, but it should be remembered that radiographs will not help the work force if they are exposed to excessive dust levels.

MANAGEMENT

Once simple silicosis has developed, it is undesirable that the worker should continue to be exposed to the dust, since this will increase the likelihood of massive fibrosis occurring. The exception is foundry work, where this complication is very rare. However, in most cases nowadays, silicosis occurs toward the end of an individual's working life, and this advice may be modified in relation to the known risks in his particular industry.

Symptomatic measures in advanced disease include the provision of oxygen, antibiotics for acute respiratory infections, and cardiac drugs when cor pulmonale supervenes. It is not known whether steroids are of any use, either in preventing progression or in treating the disease at a late stage, as no controlled trials have been carried out. However, there is a possibility that they may slow down the accelerated form of the disease, and if they are to be used, prophylactic antituberculous drugs should also be given.

More specific measures that have been suggested for the treatment of silicosis include inhalation of aluminium powder and treatment with D-penicillamine or polyvinyl pyridine-N-oxide. The former has been shown in a careful controlled trial to be ineffective in the treatment of established silicosis, when given over a three-year period.[87] D-Penicillamine is a drug orginally introduced for chelating copper in Wilson's disease (hepatolenticular degeneration) that has been found to have a favorable action in severe rheumatoid arthritis.[88] One of its actions is to inhibit collagen synthesis and to allow soluble rather than insoluble collagen to be formed. It is possible that this action might be of use in the management of massive fibrosis and Caplan's syndrome, though clinical evidence so far is sparse.

Moreover, D-penicillamine has troublesome side effects on the stomach, skin, kidney, and blood, which will inevitably limit its use.

Polyvinyl pyridine-N-oxide is a polymer that carries a strong negative charge. It probably forms hydrogen bonds with polymerized silicic acid, thus preventing the latter substance from forming these bonds with the constituents of phagosomal membranes. Given by inhalation or by injection it protects animals from the toxic effects of silica.[89] However, because it has proved carcinogenic in animals, a search is under way for an effective but nontoxic related chemical that can be used in man.

Studies of the management of acute silicosis have been confined to case reports. By analogy with alveolar proteinosis, it would seem to be worthwhile to try bronchial lavage. The only alternative in this fatal disease is lung transplantation, which has not yet become a feasible proposition, though one such subject, a young sandblaster with acute silicosis, survived 10 months after replacement of his right lung.[90]

Tuberculosis in silicotics should be treated along standard lines, commencing with triple therapy until drug sensitivities are known.[91, 92] The other mycobacterial diseases, *Mycobacterium kansasii* and to a lesser extent *M. avium-intracellulare* infections, will also often respond to treatment with rifampicin, isoniazid, ethambutol, and ethionamide, even in the absence of *in vitro* sensitivity.[93] These diseases can often be cured with appropriate chemotherapy, although their onset may accelerate the progress of the silicotic fibrosis.[17]

References

1. Agricola, G., De re Metallica, 1556, Hoover, H. C., and Hoover, L. H., trans., The Mining Magazine (London), 1912.
2. Ramazzini, B., De morbis artificum diatriba, 1713, Wright, W. C., trans., New York, Hafner Publishing Co., 1964.
3. Johnstone, J., Some account of a species of phthsis pulmonalis, peculiar to persons employed in pointing needles in the needle manufacture. Mem. Med. Soc. London, 5, 89, 1799.
4. Thackrah, C. T., The effects of principal arts, trades and professions and of civic states and habits of living on health and longevity; with a particular reference to the trades and manufactures of Leeds. London, Longman, Rees, Orne, Brown and Green, 1831.
5. Peacock, T. B., On French millstone maker's phthsis. Br. Foreign Med. Chir. Rev., 25, 214, 1860.
6. Greenhow, E. H., Specimen of diseased lung from a case of grinder's asthma. Trans. Path. Soc. Lond., 16, 59, 1865.
7. Greenhow, E. H., Specimen of potter's lung. Trans. Path. Soc. Lond., 17, 36, 1866.
8. Trasko, V. M., Silicosis: a continuing problem. U.S. Public Health Reports, 73, 839, 1958.
9. Lanza, A. J., and Childs, S. B., Miners' consumption: a study of 433 cases of the disease among zinc miners in southwestern Missouri. Public Health Bulletin No. 85. Washington, D.C., U.S. Government Printing Office, 1917.
10. U.S. Congress House Committee on Labor Sub-Committee, An investigation relating to health conditions of workers employed in the construction and maintenance of public utilities, H. J. Res. 449, 74th Congress. Washington, D. C., U.S. Government Printing Office, 1936.

11. Warrell, D. A., Harrison, B. D. W., Fawcett, I. W., et al., Silicosis among grindstone cutters in the north of Nigeria. Thorax, *30*, 389, 1975.
12. Seaton, A., Dick, J. A., Dodgson, J., and Jacobsen, M., Quartz and pneumoconiosis in coalminers. Lancet, *2*, 1272, 1981.
13. Phibbs, B. P., Sundin, R. E., and Mitchell, R. S., Silicosis in Wyoming bentonite workers. Am. Rev. Respir. Dis., *103*, 1, 1971.
14. Suratt, P. M., Winn, W. C., Brody, A. R., et al., Acute silicosis in tombstone sandblasters. Am. Rev. Respir. Dis., *115*, 521, 1977.
15. Banks, D. E., Morring, K. L., Boèhlecke, B. A., et al., Silicosis in silica flour workers. Am. Rev. Respir. Dis., *124*, 445, 1981.
16. Xipell, J. M., Ham, K. N., Price, C. G., and Thomas, D. P., Acute silicolipoproteinosis. Thorax, *32*, 104, 1977.
17. Bailey, W. C., Brown, M., Buechner, H. A., et al., Silico-mycobacterial disease in sandblasters. Am. Rev. Respir. Dis., *110*, 115, 1974.
18. Golden, E. B., Warnock, M. L., Hulett, L. D., and Chruch, A. M., Fly ash lung: a new pneumoconiosis? Am. Rev. Respir. Dis., *125*, 108, 1982.
19. Banks, D. E., Morring, K. L., and Boehlecke, B. E., Silicosis in the 1980s. Am. Ind. Hyg. Assoc. J., *42*, 77, 1981.
20. Zimmerman, P. V., and Sinclair, R. A., Rapidly progressive fatal silicosis in a young man. Med. J. Aust., *2*, 704, 1977.
21. Cooper, W. C., and Cralley, L. J., Pneumoconiosis in diatomite mining and processing. Public Health Service Publication No. 601. Washington, D.C., Government Printing Office, 1958.
22. Criteria for a recommended standard: occupational exposure to crystalline silica. Washington, D. C., U.S. Department of Health, Education, and Welfare, 1974.
23. Trasko, V. M., Some facts on the prevalence of silicosis in the United States. Arch. Ind. Health, *14*, 379, 1956.
24. Silicosis in the Metal Mining Industry: A Re-evaluation, 1958–61. U.S. Public Health Service, Department of Health, Education and Welfare, and Bureau of Mines, Washington, D.C., Government Printing Office, Ch. 5.
25. Lloyd Davies, T. A., Respiratory Disease in Foundrymen: Report of a Survey. London, H. M. Stationery Office, 1971.
26. Ashe, H. B., and Bergstrom, D. E., Twenty-six years experience with dust control in the Vermont granite industry. Ind. Med. Surg., *33*, 973, 1964.
27. Theriault, G. P., Peters, J. M., and Johnson, W. M., Pulmonary function and roentgenographic changes in granite dust exposure. Arch. Environ. Health, *28*, 23, 1974.
28. Lloyd Davies, T. A., Doig, A. T., Fox, A. J., and Greenberg, M., A radiographic survey of monumental masonry workers in Aberdeen. Br. J. Ind. Med., *30*, 227, 1973.
29. Hale, L. W., and Sheers, G., Silicosis in West Country granite workers. Br. J. Ind. Med., *20*, 218, 1963.
30. Ahlmark, A., Bruce, T., and Nyström, Å., Silicosis from quarrying and working of granite. Br. J. Ind. Med., *22*, 285, 1965.
31. Jarman, T. F., Jones, J. G., Phillips, J. H., and Seingry, H. E., Radiological surveys of working quarrymen and quarrying communities in Caernarvonshire. Br. J. Ind. Med., *14*, 95, 1957.
32. Glover, J. R., Bevan, C., Cotes, J. E., et al., Effects of exposure to slate dust in North Wales. Br. J. Ind. Med., *37*, 152, 1980.
33. Hughes, J. M., Jones, R. N., Gilson, J. C., et al., Determinants of progression in sandblasters' silicosis. *In* Walton, W. H., ed., Inhaled Particles V. Oxford, Pergamon Press, 1983, p. 701.
34. Musk, A. W., Peters, J. N., Wegman, D. H., and Fine, L. J., Pulmonary function in granite dust exposure: a four-year follow-up. Am. Rev. Respir. Dis., *115*, 769, 1977.
35. Graham, W. G. B., O'Grady, R. V., and Dubuc, B., Pulmonary function loss in Vermont granite workers. Am. Rev. Respir. Dis., *123*, 25, 1981.
36. Walton, W. H., Dodgson, J., Hadden, G. G., and Jacobsen, M., The effect of quartz and other non-coal dusts in coalworkers' pneumoconiosis. *In* Walton, W. H., ed., Inhaled Particles IV, Vol. 2. Oxford, Pergamon Press, 1977, p. 669.
37. Fletcher, G. H., Silicosis and working capacity in Zambian miners. 4th International Pneumoconiosis Conference, Bucharest, 1971, p. 358.
38. Posner, E., John Thomas Arlidge (1822–99) and the potteries. Br. J. Ind. Med., *30*, 266, 1973.

39. Vigliani, E. C., and Mottura, G., Diatomaceous earth silicosis. Br. J. Ind. Med., 5, 148, 1945.
40. Middleton, E. L., The present position of silicosis in industry in Britain. Br. Med. J., 2, 485, 1929.
41. Chapman, E. M., Acute silicosis. J.A.M.A., 98, 1439, 1932.
42. Roeslin, N., Lassabe-Roth, C., Morand, G., and Batzenschlager, A., La silico-protéinose aiguë. Arch. Mal. Prof., 41, 15, 1980.
43. Banks, D. E., Bauer, M. A., Castellan, R. M., Lapp, N. L., Silicosis in surface coal mine drillers. Thorax, 38, 275, 1983.
44. Buechner, H. A., and Ansari, A., Acute silico-proteinosis. Dis. Chest, 55, 274, 1969.
45. Ziskind, M., Jones, R. N., and Weill, H., State of the art—Silicosis. Am. Rev. Respir. Dis., 113, 643, 1976.
46. Sluis-Cremer, G. K., Active pulmonary tuberculosis discovered at post-mortem examination of the lungs of black miners. Br. J. Dis. Chest, 74, 374, 1980.
47. Chatgidakis, C. B., Silicosis in South African white gold miners. A comparative study of the disease in its different stages. Med. Proc., 9, 383, 1963.
48. Paul, R., Silicosis in Northern Rhodesia copper mines. Arch. Environ. Health 2, 96, 1961.
49. Bruce, T., Silicotuberculosis. Scand. J. Respir. Dis. (Suppl.), 65, 139, 1968.
50. Burckhardt, P., Die Silikotuberkulose und uhre Prophylaxe. Schw. Med. Woch., 97, 980, 1967.
51. Dworski, M., Schepers, G. W. H., Wilson, G. E., et al., Fatal pulmonary disease in an industrial worker caused by an atypical acid-fast bacillus. Ind. Med. Surg., 26, 536, 1957.
52. Schepers, G. W., Smart, R. H., Smith, C. R., et al., Fatal silicosis with complicating infection by an atypical acid-fast photochromogenic bacillus. Ind. Med. Surg., 27, 27, 1958.
53. Snider, D. E., The relationship between tuberculosis and silicosis. (Editorial) Am. Rev. Respir. Dis., 118, 455, 1978.
54. Jones, R. N., Turner-Warwick, M., Ziskind, M., and Weill, H., High prevalence of antinuclear antibodies in sandblasters' silicosis. Am. Rev. Respir. Dis., 113, 393, 1976.
55. Gambini, G., Agnoletto, A., and Magistretti, M., Tre casi di sindrome di Caplan. Med. Lav., 55, 261, 1964.
56. Rodnan, G. P., Benedek, R. G., Medsger, T. A., and Cammarata, R. J., The association of progressive systemic sclerosis (scleroderma) with coal miners' pneumoconiosis and other forms of silicosis. Ann. Int. Med., 66, 323, 1967.
57. Rüttner, J. R., Silicosis and lung cancer in Switzerland. In Shapiro, H. A., ed., Pneumoconiosis. Proceedings of Interntional Conference in Johannesburg. New York, Oxford University Press, 1970.
58. Westerholm, P., Silicosis: observations on a case register. Scand. J. Work Environ. Health, 6(Suppl.), 2, 1980.
59. Jacobsen, M., Dust exposure, lung diseases and coalminers' mortality. Ph.D. thesis, University of Edinburgh, 1976.
60. Fox, A. J., Goldblatt, P., and Kinlen, L. J., A study of the mortality of Cornish tin miners. Br. J. Ind. Med., 38, 378, 1981.
61. Becklake, M. R., du Preez, L., and Lutz, W., Lung function in silicosis of the Witwatersrand gold miner. Am. Rev. Tuberc., 77, 400, 1958.
62. Teculescu, D. B., Stanescu, D. C., and Pilat, L., Pulmonary mechanics in silicosis. Arch. Environ. Health, 14, 461, 1967.
63. Seaton, A., Lapp, N. L., and Morgan, W. K. C., Pulmonary mechanics and frequency dependence of compliance in coalworker's pneumoconiosis. J. Clin. Invest., 15, 1203, 1972.
64. Marek, K., and Kujawska, A., L'influence des lésions pneumoconiotiques précoces sur la fonction respiratoire. Fourth International Pneumoconiosis Conference, Bucharest, 1971, p. 375.
65. Teculescu, D. B., and Stanescu, D. C., Carbon monoxide transfer factor for the lung in silicosis. Scand. J. Resp. Dis., 51, 150, 1970.
66. Irwig, L. M., and Rocks, P., Lung function and respiratory symptoms in silicotic and nonsilicotic gold miners. Am. Rev. Respir. Dis., 117, 429, 1978.

67. Jones, R. N., Weill, H., and Ziskind, M., Pulmonary function in sandblasters' silicosis. Bull. Physiopath. Respir., *11*, 589, 1975.

68. Motley, H. L., Smart, R. H., and Valero, A., Pulmonary function studies in diatomaceous earth workers. I. Ventilatory and blood gas exchange disturbance. Arch. Ind. Health, *13*, 265, 1956.

69. Curran, R. C., Observations on the formation of collagen in quartz lesions. J. Pathol. Bact., *66*, 271, 1953.

70. Gross, P., and Tolker, E. B., Dust particles in lung sections. Some notes on methods of their visualization. Arch. Environ. Health, *12*, 213, 1966.

71. Gross, P., and de Treville, R. T. P., Alveolar proteinosis: its experimental production in rodents. Arch. Pathol., *86*, 255, 1968.

72. Heppleston, A. G., Atypical reaction to inhaled silica. Nature, *213*, 199, 1967.

73. Allison, A. C., Harrington, J. S., and Birbeck, M., The examination of the cytotoxic effect of silica on macrophages. J. Exp. Med., *124*, 141, 1966.

74. Allison, A. C., Harrington, J. S., Birbeck, M., and Nash, T., Observations on the cytotoxic action of silica on macrophages. In Davies, C. N., ed., Inhaled Particles and Vapours II. Oxford, Pergamon Press, 1967, p. 121.

75. King, E. J., Mohanty, E. P., Harrison, C. V., and Nagelschmidt, G., The action of different forms of pure silica on the lungs of rats. Br. J. Ind. Med., *10*, 9, 1953.

76. Curran, R. C., and Rowsell, E. V., The application of the diffusion diameter technique to the study of silicosis. J. Pathol. Bact., *76*, 561, 1958.

77. Brieger, H., and Gross, P., On the theory of silicosis. III. Stishovite. Arch. Environ. Health, *15*, 751, 1967.

78. Allison, A. C., Mechanisms of macrophage damage in relation to the pathogenesis of some lung diseases. In Brain, J. D., Proctor, D. F., and Reid, L. M., eds., Lung Biology in Health and Disease. New York, Marcel Dekker, 1977, p. 1075.

79. Gabor, S., Arica, Z., Zugravu, E., et al., In vitro and in vivo quartz-induced lipid peroxidation. In Brown, R. C., Gormley, I. P., Chamberlain, M., and Davies, R., eds., The In Vitro Effects of Mineral Dusts. London, Academic Press, 1980, p. 13.

80. Heppleston, A. G., The fibrogenic action of silica. Br. Med. Bull., *25*, 282, 1969.

81. Heppleston, A. G., Observations on the mechanism of silicotic fibrogenesis. In Walton, W. H., ed., Inhaled Particles III. London, Unwin Brothers, 1971, p. 357.

82. Heppleston, A. G., and Styles, J. A., Activity of a macrophage factor in collagen formation by silica. Nature, *214*, 521, 1967.

83. Bateman, E. D., Emerson, E. J., and Cole, P., The use of diffusion chambers to examine the biological effects of mineral dusts. In Brown, R. C., Gormley, I. P., Chamberlain, M., and Davies, R., eds., The In Vitro Effects of Mineral Dusts. London, Academic Press, 1980, p. 289.

84. Vigliani, E. C., and Pernis, B., Immunological factors in the pathogenesis of the hyaline tissue of silicosis. Br. J. Ind. Med., *15*, 8, 1958.

85. Miller, S. D., and Zarkower, A., Alteration of murine immunologic responses after silica dust inhalation. J. Immunol., *113*, 1533, 1974.

86. Samini, B., Neilson, A., Weill, H., and Ziskind, M., The efficiency of protective hoods used by sandblasters to reduce silica dust exposure. Am. Ind. Hyg. J., *36*, 140, 1975.

87. Kennedy, M. C. S., Aluminium powder inhalations in the treatment of silicosis of pottery workers and pneumoconiosis of coal-miners. Br. J. Ind. Med., *13*, 85, 1956.

88. Andrews, F. M., Golding, D. N., Freeman, A. M., et al., Controlled trial of D-penicillamine in severe rheumatoid arthritis. Lancet, *1*, 175, 1973.

89. Barhad, B., Rotarn, G., Lazarescu, I., et al., Experience in polyvinyl pyridin-N-oxide action on experimental lung silicosis. 4th International Pneumoconiosis Conference, Bucharest, 1971, p. 315.

90. Derom, F., Barbier, F., Ringoir, S., et al., Ten-month survival after lung homotransplantation in man. J. Thorac. Cardiovasc. Surg., *61*, 835, 1971.

91. Medical Research Council/Miners' Chest Diseases Treatment Centre, Chemotherapy of pulmonary tuberculosis with pneumoconiosis. Tubercle, *48*, 1, 1967.

92. Dubois, P., Gyselen, A., and Prignot, J., Rifampicin-combined chemotherapy in coal-workers' pneumoconio-tuberculosis. Am. Rev. Respir. Dis., *115*, 221, 1977.

93. Hunter, A. P., Campbell, I. A., Jenkins, P. A., and Smith, A. P., Treatment of pulmonary infections caused by mycobacteria of the *Mycobacterium avium-intracellulare* complex. Thorax, *36*, 326, 1981.

12

SILICATES AND DISEASE

Anthony Seaton

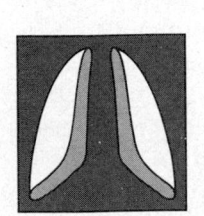

From a commercial point of view, the asbestos minerals are the most important of the silicates, and these are discussed separately in Chapter 13. Apart from asbestos, however, there are many naturally occurring silicates that have been found useful in industry that can have adverse effects on the health of the work force. In addition, recent interest has focused on environmental contamination by fibrous silicates in nonoccupational settings. Since this has important implications for preventive occupational medicine, a number of documented episodes will also be discussed in this chapter.

For convenience, the silicates of potential or actual medical importance will be considered under the separate headings of fibrous and nonfibrous types, since in general the effect of a silicate is likely to depend in part on its physical configuration. The nonfibrous silicates discussed include talc, kaolin, micas, fuller's earth and other clays, and cement. It should be noted that some of these may contain a proportion of fibers and that, while their potential health effects are generally similar to those of coal, when this fiber proportion is large they may cause effects similar to those of asbestos. The fibrous silicates may be regarded as those which predominantly consist of particles at least three times as long as they are broad and which contain a proportion that is potentially respirable, that is, of diameter less than 3 microns. Those that occur naturally include the amphiboles (some of which have sufficient commercial value to be grouped as asbestos), the zeolites, wollastonite, attapulgite, and sepiolite. In addition, fibrous silicates may be produced commercially by melting rock or other raw material—the so-called manmade vitreous fibers. In general, the health effects of the fibrous silicates can be expected to resemble those of asbestos should people be exposed to sufficient amounts of the respirable particles.

NONFIBROUS SILICATES

Talc

Talc is a hydrated magnesium silicate with the theoretical formula $Mg_6Si_8O_{22}(OH)_4$. It occurs as sheet crystals, easily cleaved into very thin plates, and this property, together with its softness, gives talc its value as a lubricant powder. It contains trace elements such as iron and nickel, which are responsible for its varying color. Talc has been produced geologically by alteration of magnesium-bearing rocks, especially serpentines and limestones, and when mined may often be contaminated by asbestos, such as tremolite or anthophyllite, by limestones, or by quartz.[1] Contamination by asbestos has given rise to confusion as to whether reports of adverse health effects are due to the talc or the contaminant. Moreover, talc viewed under the microscope may look fibrous, due to plates either being seen end on or being rolled, or to fractured plates appearing as needles.[2] Thus there remains some uncertainty about its potential health effects, though epidemiological studies are beginning to clarify this.

Deposits of talc are found in 10 of the United States, principally New York, Vermont, California, and Texas, as well as in Ontario, Manchuria, Italy, and the Pyrenees. Asbestos contamination appears to occur particularly in New York and Texas. The talc is mined as soapstone and is generally milled and calcined on the same site. Soapstone is used as French chalk by tailors, while the milled material is widely used in the production of paints, rubber, ceramics, pharmaceuticals, asphalt, roofing materials, paper, lubricants, insecticides, and cosmetics.[3] Its most familiar form is as a dusting powder. Exposure to talc may occur in any of these industries and, very occasionally, significant amounts may be inhaled by users of the commercial product. Talc as supplied commercially is rarely pure: that supplied for the cosmetic, food, and pharmaceutical industries may be up to 90 per cent pure, but industrial grades may contain less than 50 per cent talc. The residue is usually chlorite, carbonates, some quartz, and occasionally asbestos. Analyses in the 1960s of 22 commonly available talc powders showed a fiber content of between 8 and 30 per cent,[4] though many of these fibers may well not have been asbestos. More recently, the major cosmetic manufacturers have drawn up specifications for cosmetic talc that should ensure the virtual absence of asbestos.[5, 6]

Talc Pneumoconiosis. Dreesen and Dalla Valle investigated two Georgia talc mines and mills in 1935,[7] and found workers to be exposed to high concentrations of dust. Of 69 men examined, 14 were said to have slight pneumoconiosis, while 8 had advanced disease with disability. In the early 1940s several other investigators found evidence of disease among talc workers. Porro and co-workers[8] described 15 cases in detail and included 5 autopsy reports. They commented on the occurrence of cor pulmonale in these patients. Siegal and co-workers[9] investigated 221 miners and millers and found evidence of lung fibrosis in 32. Later follow-

up of these affected workers showed that they suffered a slow progression to disability.[10] A study in New York State of 220 miners and millers employed before 1940 and with 15 or more years' exposure to talc showed that by 1967, 91 had died.[11] Deaths from cardiac disease constituted the expected 27 per cent. Thirty-one per cent had died of pneumoconiosis and 21 per cent of neoplasms, including 9 individuals with lung cancer and 1 with a "fibrosarcoma" of the pleura. Eight of these 10 also had pneumoconiosis. A more recent follow-up of this population showed a marked fall-off in the number of deaths from pneumoconiosis, probably related to improved dust control.[12] Many of the earlier deaths had occurred in workers exposed to talc before wet drilling was introduced and who had undoubtedly worked in higher dust conditions than occur today.

It should be remembered that the New York talc miners were also exposed to the asbestos minerals tremolite and anthophyllite.[13] However, studies of other miners and millers in Vermont and Italy, where the talc is free of asbestos, have also shown pneumoconiosis and increased death rates from nonmalignant respiratory disease.[14-16] In general, over the last two decades simple pneumoconiosis has appeared in the United States only after prolonged exposure to the relatively low levels of dust now prevalent.[17] The same seems to be true of French talc millers in the Pyrenees, where both simple and complicated pneumoconiosis have been described after prolonged exposure to talc dust containing no asbestos and only trivial amounts of quartz.[18]

In addition to its occurrence in talc miners and millers, talc pneumoconiosis has been described occasionally in subjects exposed to the commercial product. One such patient worked as an inspector of talc aerosols,[19] while another appears to have had an obsession for applying the powder to himself.[20] Common to these reports is a history of unusually heavy exposure. One study of rubber workers using talc has shown no convincing evidence of pneumoconiosis.[21] Other studies are being conducted, but it seems likely that pneumoconiosis among users of talc is an extremely rare event.

The clinical features of talc pneumoconiosis resemble those of asbestosis, but in general seem to take rather longer to develop. The subject initially is symptom-free, but as the disease progresses cough and breathlessness develop. Digital clubbing, cyanosis, and basal crackles are features of the advanced case, and death from cor pulmonale occurs.[8, 22] The disease continues to progress slowly even in the absence of continued exposure to the dust.[10] Occasionally the disease may progress unusually rapidly, with death occurring within a few years of a very heavy exposure. A study of Italian miners had provided some evidence that tuberculosis may complicate talc pneumoconiosis.[15]

Commercial talc, when inhaled in high concentrations by small children, may provoke severe episodes of respiratory distress that can prove fatal.[23] These reactions seem to be of a bronchoconstrictive type and are

probably due to bronchial irritation. A granulomatous pulmonary arteritis is also being recognized more frequently in drug addicts who inject solutions of talc-containing tablets into their veins,[24, 25] and interstitial fibrosis has been described in a man who was prone to inhale the contents of pharmaceutical capsules prior to performing as a punk rock drummer.[26]

The initial radiographic appearance of talc pneumoconiosis is an ill-defined reticular and nodular lesion that appears preferentially in the mid zones. The nodules have a tendency to coalesce, and progressive massive fibrosis may occur (Fig. 12–1). The reticular lesions develop as a typical interstitial fibrosis and may involve the whole lung, though the apices are usually spared.[8] Calcified plaques may occur on the pleural surfaces.[17, 22] While these may often be due to asbestos contamination, they have also been described to occur frequently in individuals working with talc containing no true asbestos.[27]

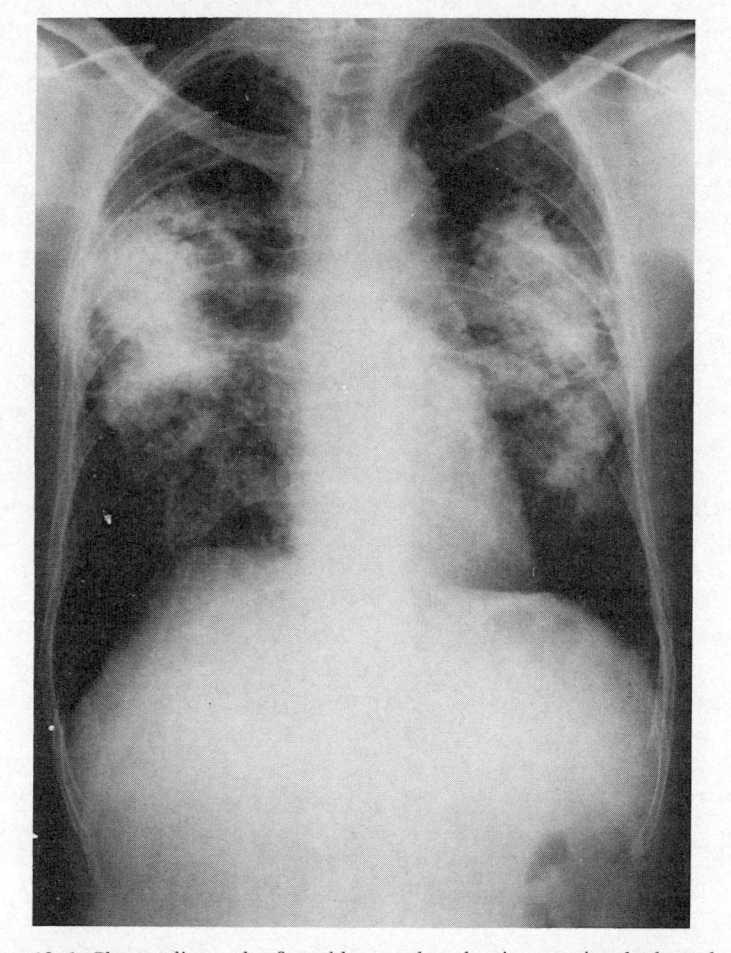

Figure 12–1. Chest radiograph of a rubber worker showing massive shadows due to talc pneumoconiosis.

Studies of lung function have shown reduction in lung volumes and diffusing capacity in the advanced disease.[28, 29] Comparison of workers exposed over similar periods to fibrous and nonfibrous talc has shown little difference either clinically or in terms of lung function, though more subjects with restrictive disease are found among those exposed to fibrous forms. There is some evidence of a dose-related decrease in lung volumes and flow rates in association with exposure to talc containing asbestos,[30] though not with exposure to asbestos-free talc.[28]

Macroscopic examination of the lungs in an established case of talc pneumoconiosis shows fibrous pleural adhesions. The cut surface is studded with small gray nodules, predominantly in the mid and lower zones. Conglomeration of nodules, leading to progressive massive fibrosis, occurs and these lesions may cavitate.

Microscopically, in an early case foreign-body granulomata containing doubly refractile particles engulfed in macrophages may be found[18, 19] (Fig. 12–2). Reticulin and collagen are laid down around the macrophages, resulting in interstitial fibrosis as the disease progresses. Hyperplasia of alveolar cells is seen, and endarteritis is found in small pulmonary arteries, particularly around confluent lesions.[8, 22] In addition to particles of talc, ferruginous bodies and fibers are usually visible. On the whole, the fibrous reaction to talc is less intense than that to silica. Nevertheless, with prolonged exposure sufficient fibrosis and endarteritis may occur, resulting in cor pulmonale.[8]

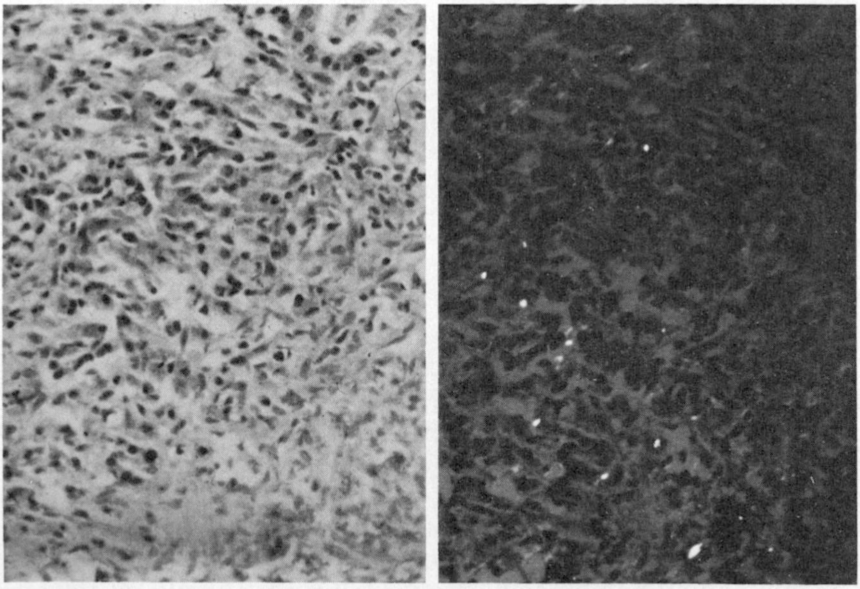

Figure 12–2. Area of fibrosis in lung of patient who inhaled the contents of medicinal capsules prior to performance as a punk rock musician. View on right shows talc particles visible by their transmission of polarized light.

Prevention of talc pneumoconiosis depends on institution of the same measures of industrial hygiene used in the prevention of other pneumoconiosis. Once a case is established, especially if it is of a subacute type, consideration should be given to steroid therapy in view of the results reported in the cases of a talc aerosol inspector[19] and an intravenous drug abuser.[31]

Talc and Lung Cancer. Following the early reports of an increased risk of lung cancer in New York talc miners,[11] concern has been expressed that talc itself may be carcinogenic. Further follow-up of the New York workers has confirmed their lung cancer risk to have been increased by about fourfold,[12] though another study in the same state suggested that earlier experience in other mines, possibly involving exposure to radon daughters, was a more likely cause than exposure in talc mines.[32] Studies of non-asbestos–exposed talc workers have failed to show an increased mortality risk from lung cancer in Italian miners or millers[15] or in Vermont millers.[16] A small excess risk was found in Vermont miners, though numbers were very small, and the dust exposures of the miners were generally lower than those of the millers.[16] Finally, to date no animal evidence that talc is carcinogenic by either inhalation or intrapleural inoculation has been produced,[33] nor has inoculation of cosmetic grade talc into the human pleural cavity (in the management of pneumothorax) been shown to result in mesothelioma between 14 and 40 years later.[34]

In conclusion, it is clear that talc exposure may cause pneumoconiosis. While this may be due to contamination of the material with asbestos or silica, there is sufficient evidence that the mineral itself is mildly fibrogenic and causes a disease more akin to coal workers' pneumoconiosis than to silicosis or asbestosis. However, the histological pattern will vary according to the composition of the dust inhaled. It seems clear that, under current working conditions, talc pneumoconiosis is rare. There does seem to be an increased risk of lung cancer in some talc miners and millers. However, it is most unlikely that this is due to talc, the evidence pointing either to contaminating asbestos or to coincidental exposure to other carcinogens.

Kaolin

Kaolin consists mainly of kaolinite, a hydrated aluminum silicate, $Al_2(Si_2O_3)(OH)_4$, found mainly in Georgia, North Carolina, southwestern England, Japan, Egypt, Czechoslovakia, and Germany. It is a clay mineral, found in association with quartz, mica, and feldspar, and used in ceramics, paper, paint, and cement manufacture, in soaps and toothpastes, and as a medicinal. It is normally obtained by quarrying, most processes involving washing the deposit away with jets of water. This floats the clay from the sand and mica and allows it to be pumped away as a slurry. This is filtered and the kaolin is then dried and may be milled and occasionally calcined. The latter process converts it into the aluminum silicate, mullite, and cristobalite. Drying, milling, and bagging entail the major risks of exposure

to kaolin dust, but some processes may also carry a risk of exposure to quartz or cristobalite.

Kaolin Pneumoconiosis. Middleton recorded the occurrence of radiographic changes in two china clay workers in 1936.[35] However, industrial exposure to kaolin was generally regarded as harmless until Lynch and McIver described the autopsy findings of two men who had died in their mid-thirties of massive fibrosis.[36] Both had been heavily exposed to kaolin and neither had evidence of concomitant tuberculosis. Both massive whorled nodules and fibrosis of alveolar walls were found in these men. Subsequently Hale and co-workers published a report of six subjects with kaolin pneumoconiosis, one of whom had massive fibrosis.[37] They measured the lung dust in one of their cases and in the lung of an American kaolin worker, and found between 20 and 40 gm of kaolin in them.

Several studies have been carried out on the prevalence of kaolin pneumoconiosis and have made the point that suppression of dust is particularly difficult in parts of this industry. A radiographic survey of an Egyptian plant in 1959 revealed five cases of pneumoconiosis, two with massive fibrosis and one with complicating tuberculosis, among 914 men examined.[38] All had a history of heavy exposure for more than 15 years, and one of the men with massive fibrosis died of cor pulmonale. In Britain a survey of 553 men in 1961 showed the prevalence of kaolin pneumoconiosis to rise from nil in workers employed for less than 5 years to 23 per cent in those exposed for more than 15 years.[39] It was felt that although simple pneumoconiosis was not associated with disability, it implied a risk of development into massive fibrosis, four such cases being found. A survey of 1130 kaolin workers in Georgia in the 1950s revealed pneumoconiosis in 44 men, including 13 with massive fibrosis.[40] The latter men showed progressive disease and clinical evidence of pulmonary dysfunction. A more recent survey of a large group of Georgia kaolin miners showed that simple kaolinosis had little effect on lung function and that even complicated disease produced little impairment.[40a]

The individual with kaolin pneumoconiosis would not be expected to show any clinical abnormality until advanced massive fibrosis with compensatory emphysema or cor pulmonale developed. The most usual radiological change is the presence of diffuse small nodules characteristic of types q and r of the ILO classification. Massive fibrosis also mimics that occurring in coal miners, with large ovoid lesions developing predominantly in upper and mid zones[37-40] (Fig. 12–3).

In kaolin pneumoconiosis the lungs show grayish nodular lesions, varying between 1 and 6 mm and softer than in classical silicosis. Fibrosis may be present, but under the microscope the nodules tend to be cellular and packed with dust. Nodules may become confluent, but the massive fibrosis has a diffuse appearance. Cavitation of massive fibrosis, interstitial alveolar wall fibrosis, and compensatory emphysema may all occur (Figs. 12–4 and 12–5).

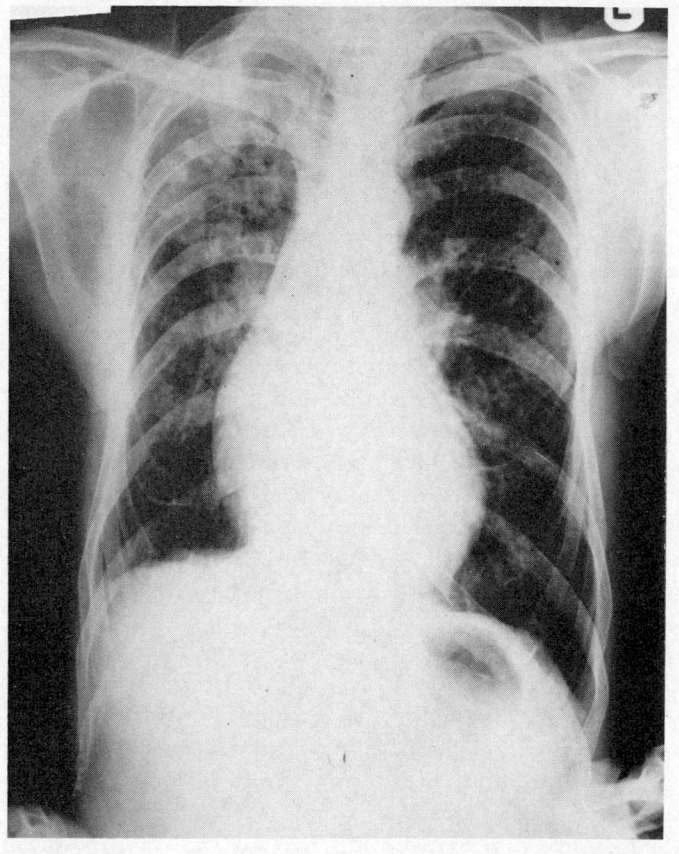

Figure 12–3. *A,* Chest radiograph of a Cornish china clay worker. His only industrial exposure, over 30 years, had been to china clay. He died of cor pulmonale. Radiograph shows a fine pinpoint pneumoconiosis with conglomerative changes in the right upper lobe and loss of volume in the right lung.

There is little doubt that kaolinite itself is responsible for these lesions rather than quartz or other contaminating minerals. Intratracheal injection of kaolinite into rats has indicated that it is mildly fibrogenic and produces cellular dust macules and some infiltration of alveolar walls.[41] The reaction resembles that to low-rank coals and to shale, both of which contain kaolinite. It seems likely that inhalation of a relatively large amount of kaolin is required to elicit a clinically detectable response.

Fuller's Earth

Fuller's earth is an absorbent clay, originally used in the process of fulling, or removing grease from wool, and now principally used in refining oils, as a binder of foundry moulding sands, as a filter, and as a filler in cosmetic preparations. The term fuller's earth is generally taken

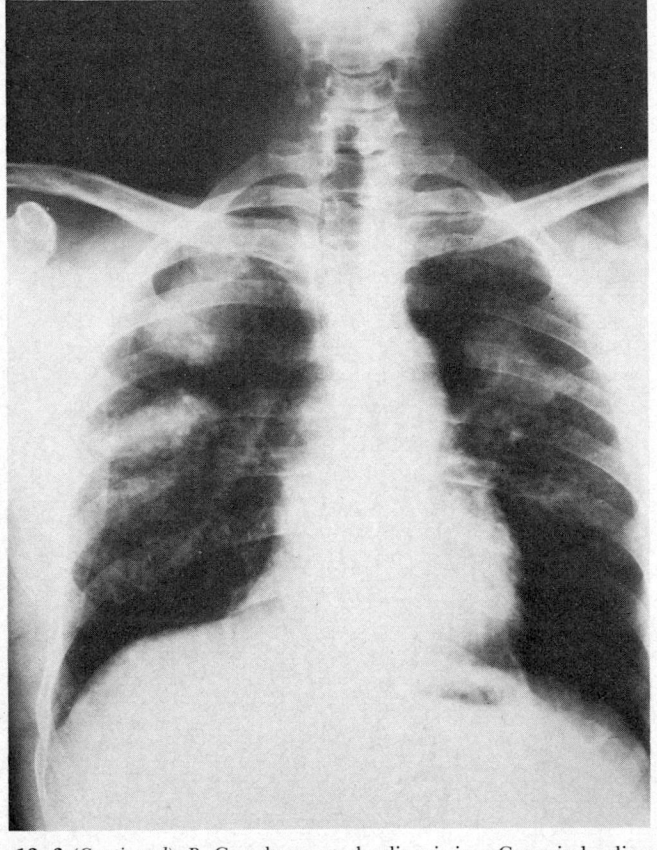

Figure 12–3 *(Continued). B,* Conglomerate kaolinosis in a Georgia kaolin worker.

to apply to calcium montmorillonite, an aluminum silicate, but it may also be used to describe other silicates such as bentonite (sodium montmorillonite). Calcium montmorillonite, found in Illinois, Arkansas, Mississippi, Britain, and Germany, is obtained mainly by strip mining methods. Drying, crushing, and milling take place on site.

Fuller's Earth Pneumoconiosis. Middleton originally drew attention to the occurrence of radiological changes in workers exposed to fuller's earth in 1938.[42] Subsequently, McNally and Trostler[43] studied the radiographs of 49 men engaged in the production and loading of the material and found an increase in bronchovascular markings in most. Two had advanced massive fibrosis and both these subjects had been unable to work because of dyspnea.

The pathology of the pneumoconiosis was described in one case by Campbell and Gloyne in 1942.[44] They found irregular, black, soft patches mainly in the upper zones. Microscopically, the air spaces contained many dust particles surrounded by reticulin, though with relatively little cellular

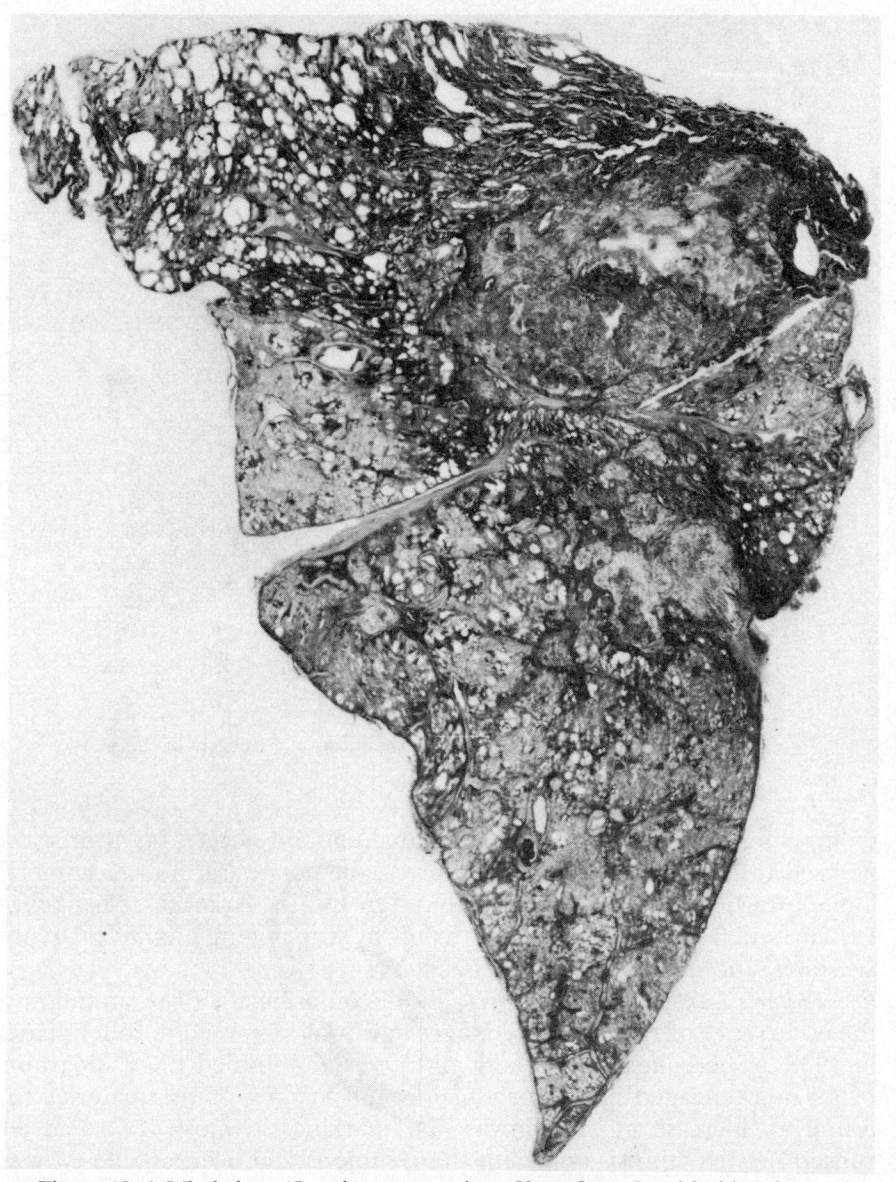

Figure 12–4. Whole-lung (Gough) paper section of lung from Cornish china clay worker, showing massive fibrosis in posterior part of upper lobe and large nodules throughout the rest of the lung. Interstitial fibrosis and cystic change are also present in the upper lobe.

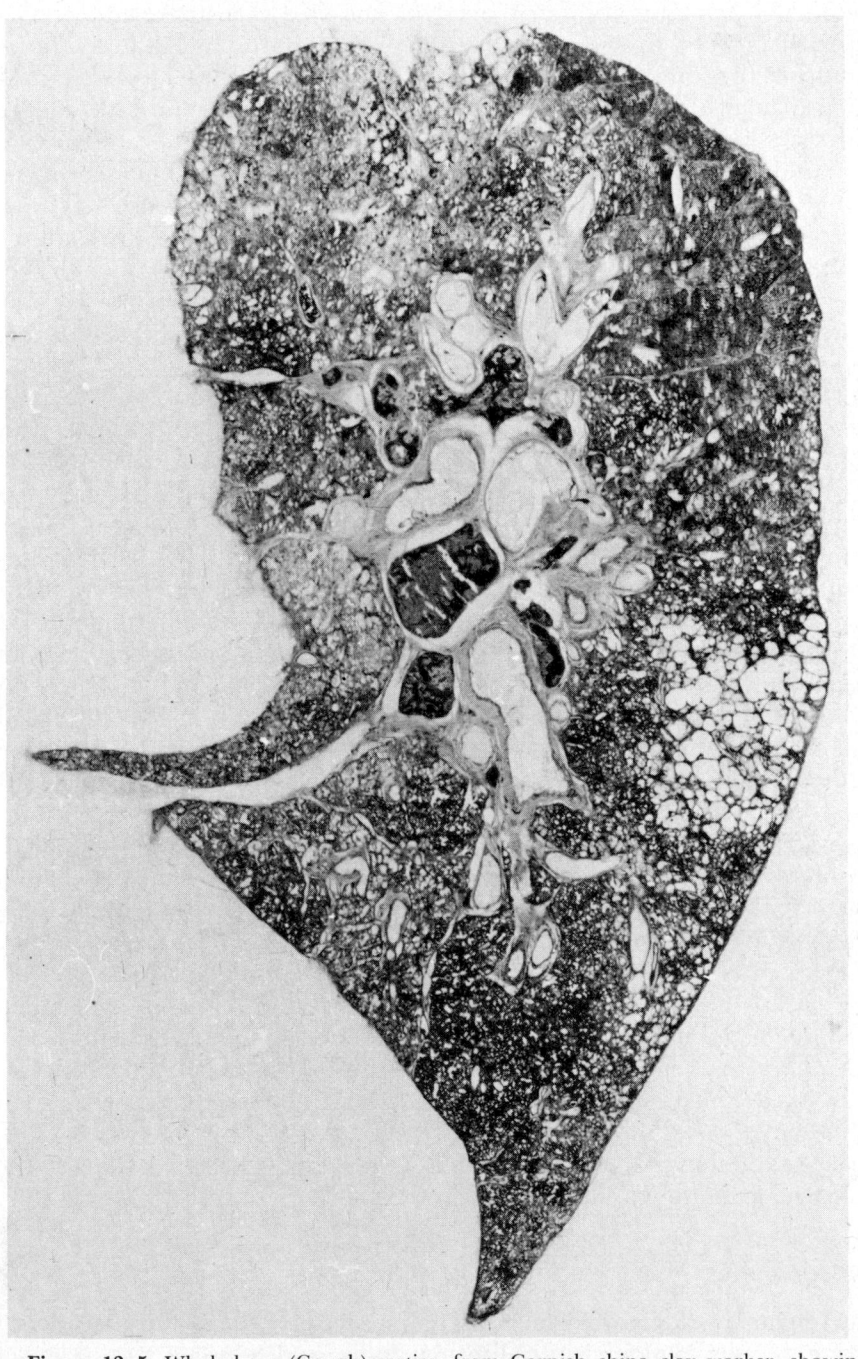

Figure 12–5. Whole-lung (Gough) section from Cornish china clay worker, showing diffuse interstitial fibrosis and some cystic areas, most marked in posterior part of lower lobe.

reaction. The relatively benign nature of the disease is illustrated by a report by Tonning[45] of a man aged 79 who died of a stroke and who had worked 50 years previously in the fuller's earth industry. His lungs showed multiple black nodules, consisting of dust-laden macrophages surrounded by reticulin, with some surrounding focal emphysema but little collagen formation. More recently Sakula[42] investigated British fuller's earth workers and found two with radiographic changes of simple pneumoconiosis. In one, an autopsy showed features similar to those previously described.

It seems to have been established that prolonged exposure to dust of fuller's earth can cause a relatively benign pneumoconiosis, though there is a risk of the development of more serious massive fibrosis. The pneumoconiosis appears similar to those caused by kaolin, some coals, and shale.

Other Clays and Pneumoconiosis. Pneumoconiosis has been described in Scottish shale miners.[46] This industry, now defunct in Scotland, was once an important producer of mineral oil. Shale oil was also produced in France, and the industry survives in Estonia. A new industry, with plans for massive oil production, will probably arise in Colorado and the mountain states, though at present this is only in a pilot stage. Scottish and Rocky Mountain shales differ, the former having a higher content of quartz and silicates and the latter containing more limestone. In the Scottish cases, radiological and pathological changes of both simple pneumoconiosis and massive fibrosis have been described, the lesions resembling those of kaolin pneumoconiosis (Figs. 12–6 to 12–8). Whether kaolin or other clay minerals in the shale were responsible has not been established.

Ball clays, used in ceramics, pottery and earthenware, bricks, and refractory products, consist of kaolinite with a relatively high quartz content. Pneumoconiosis appears to occur less in handling this material than in the production of china ware, where exposure to quartz has been higher. Nevertheless, pneumoconiosis with silicotic features has been described among workers milling ball clays.[47] A rapidly progressive form of silicosis has also been described among workers crushing and milling bentonite (sodium montmorillonite) in Wyoming.[48] This mineral is used as a filter, for refining oil and in drilling for oil, and as a bonding material for molds in foundries. It is associated with quartz and cristobalite and these minerals rather than bentonite itself are the likely cause of the disease. Bentonite had mild cytotoxicity *in vitro* but does not appear to be fibrogenic in animal inhalation experiments.[49, 50]

Sillimanite

Sillimanite is anhydrous aluminum silicate, a rock of high density commercially exploited in California, India, and South Africa. It is very resistant to heat and of low electrical conductivity, and is used in the manufacture of refractory materials and porcelain for electrical equip-

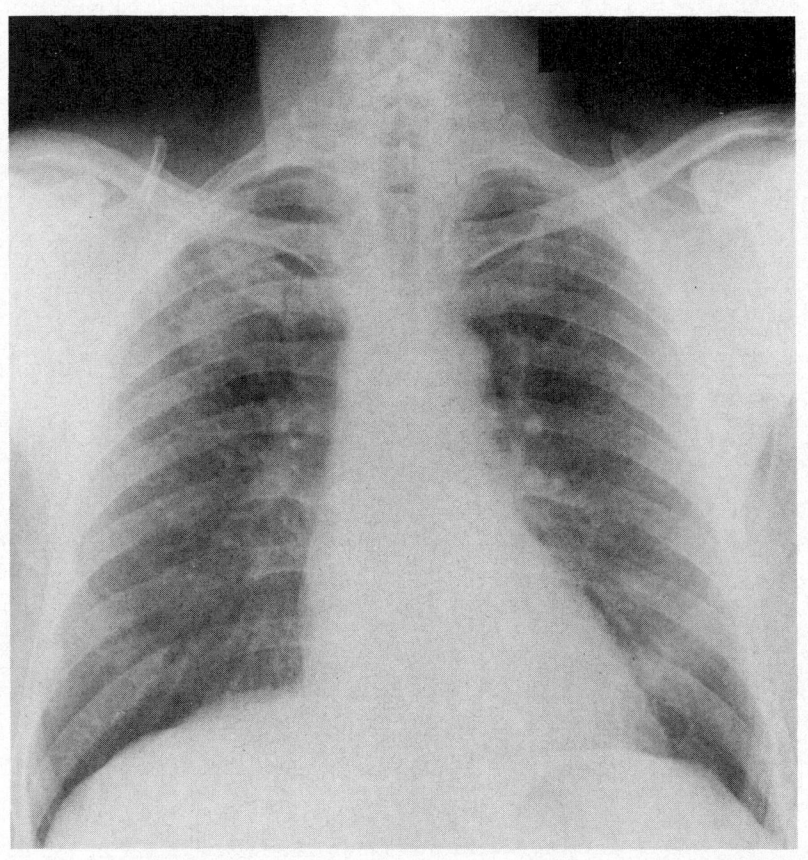

Figure 12–6. Radiograph of Scottish shale miner, showing lesion of massive fibrosis in right upper zone.

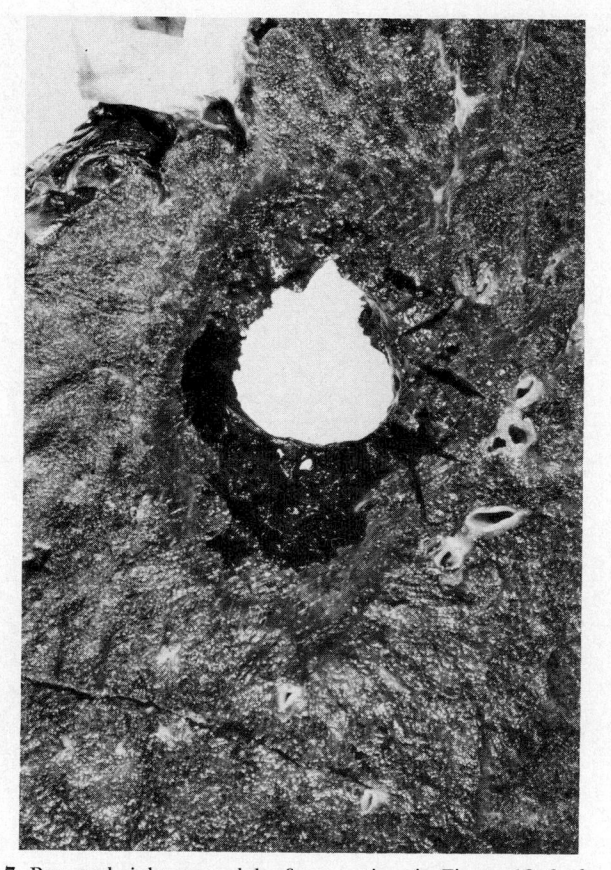

Figure 12–7. Resected right upper lobe from patient in Figure 12–6, showing cavitated massive fibrosis.

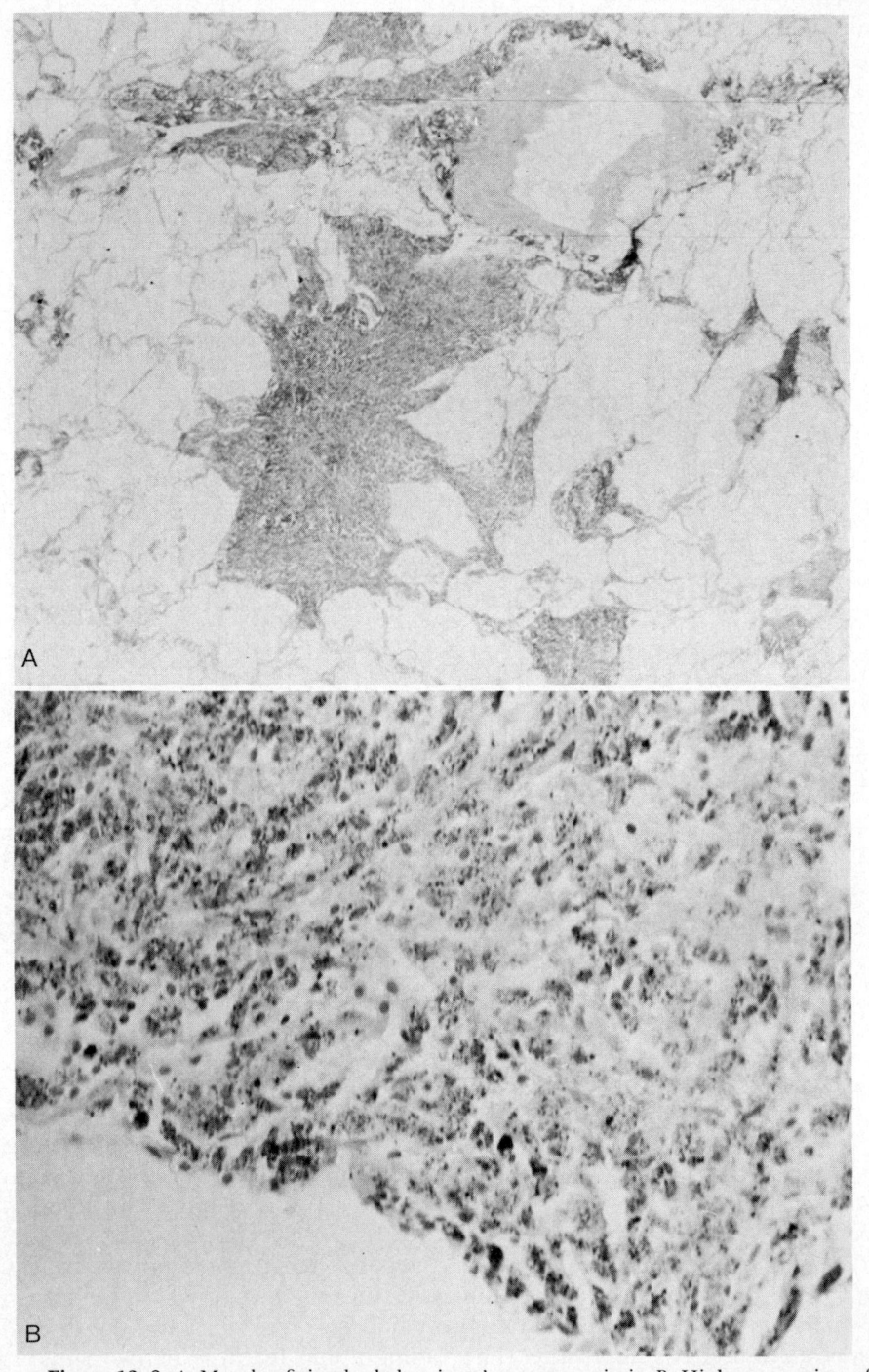

Figure 12–8. *A*, Macule of simple shale miners' pneumoconiosis. *B*, High-power view of lower part of same lesion, showing dust-filled macrophages.

Illustration continued on following page

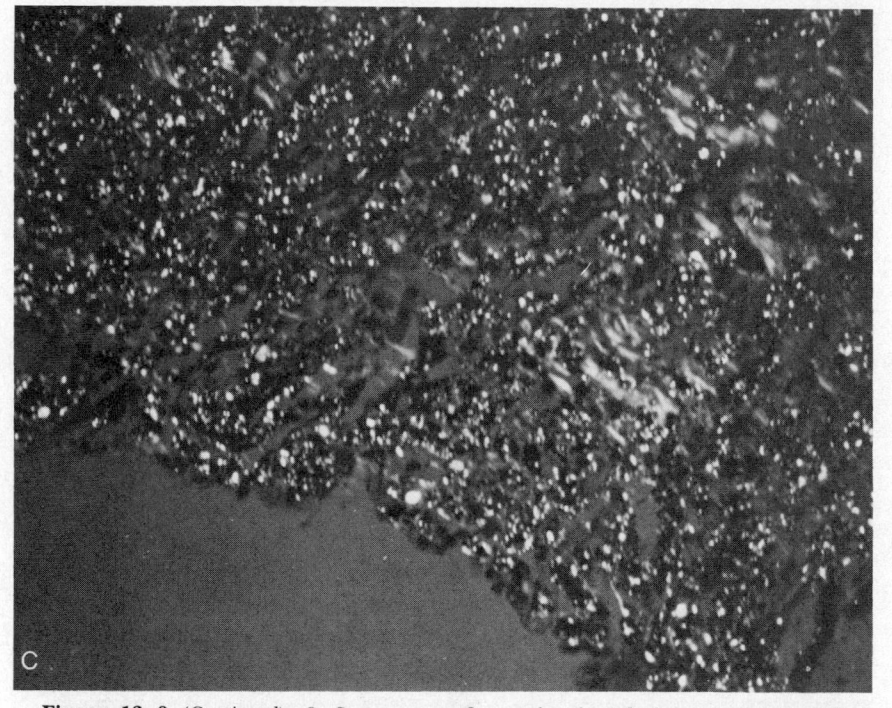

Figure 12–8 *(Continued)*. *C*, Same area of macule viewed through polarized light, showing doubly refractile silicate particles.

ment. It has a prismatic crystalline structure with fibrous form, but fractures easily when crushed, forming a powder rather than fine crystals. In 1936 Middleton examined 13 workers exposed to the dust and noted minimal radiographic changes without accompanying symptoms.[35] There is some evidence that exposure to sillimanite may cause interstitial pulmonary fibrosis both in exposed workers[51] and in experimental animals.[52] Whether these lesions in exposed workers are due to sillimanite itself or to contaminating mullite or cristobalite is not clear.

Nepheline

Nepheline is a hard rock consisting mainly of the feldspar albite. It is composed of sodium, potassium, and aluminum silicates and is mined in Canada. The rock is milled into a powder for use in glazing pottery. Deposits are uncommon and therefore few workers are exposed to the dust. Nevertheless, there has been a report of one man who was heavily exposed for four years in whom massive fibrosis developed.[53] The dust to which he was exposed apparently contained no free silica and the disease was attributed to nepheline. The radiographic features of two subjects from Ontario, Canada, with nepheline pneumoconiosis are shown in Figure 12–9.

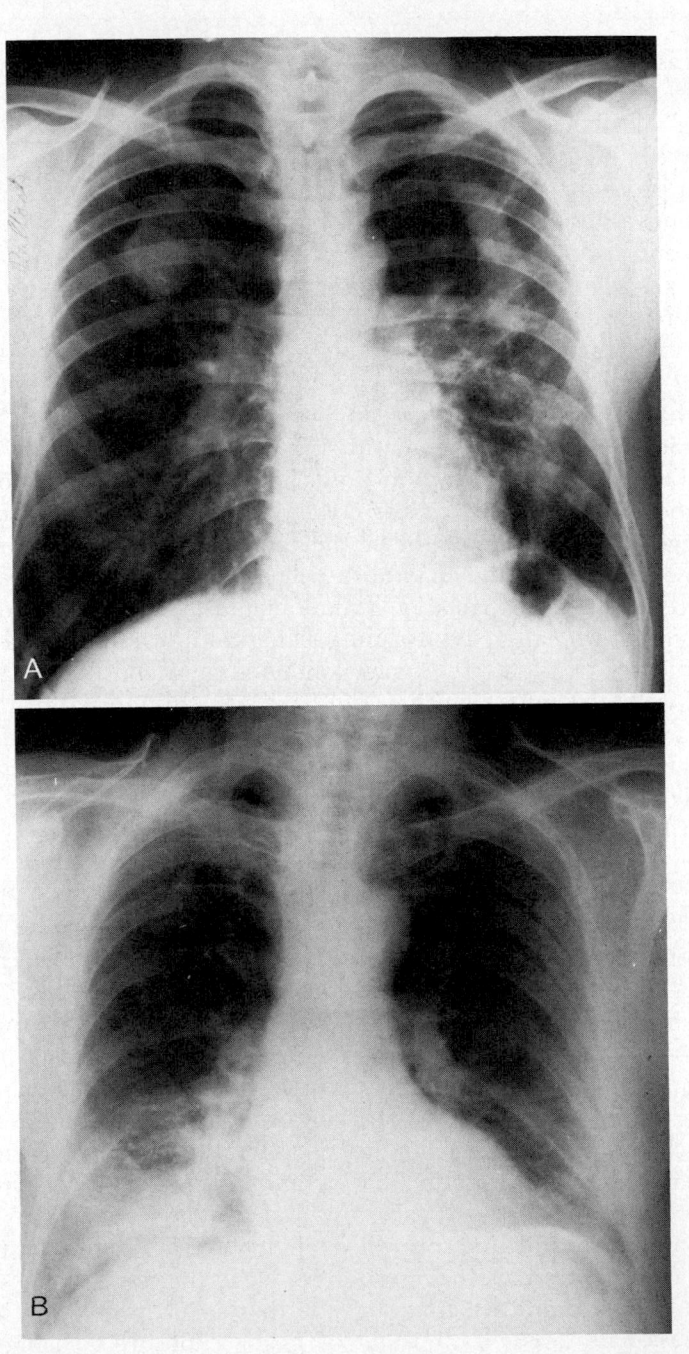

Figure 12–9. Two subjects with nepheline pneumoconiosis, one showing typical complicated disease *(A)*, the other a process appearing more like subacute silicosis *(B)*. (Courtesy of
Dr. D. L. Holness.)

Mica

Micas are complex aluminum silicates, two forms of which are commercially important. Muscovite is a potassium aluminum silicate, mined in India and the United States. It is transparent and highly resistant to heat and electricity. Sheets of it are used as windows in stoves and furnaces, while in ground form it is used in the manfacture of paper, wallpaper, and paints. Phlogopite, a magnesium aluminum silicate, is mined in Canada and used, because of its heat- and electricity-resisting properties, almost exclusively in the electricity industry.

There have been several reports of both symptomatic and radiological disease among mica miners or workers exposed to ground mica. Middleton reported some cases of pulmonary fibrosis in 1936,[35] and subsequent reports have recorded the disease in the United States.[54, 55] The U.S. Public Health Service found 10 men with pneumoconiosis among 57 workers exposed to hand-ground mica in 1940.[54] Smith found evidence of pleural calcification in 5 of 302 workers engaged in producing mica insulators and suggested that mica might be the cause.[56] However, in retrospect it seems more likely that they had unsuspected exposure to asbestos. A more recent report has described a granulomatous pulmonary and hepatic condition in a woman grinding and packing mica, who eventually died of cor pulmonale.[57] The granulomata contained mica and there was diffuse alveolar wall thickening, which would have been an unusual feature if the disease was sarcoidosis. It seems reasonable to assume that this was an unusual reaction to mica. However, studies in animals have only produced relatively benign, nonfibrotic dust granulomata, and in general mica can be regarded as a substance of low toxicity.[58]

Cement

Most cement is produced by the Portland process, in which calcareous rocks such as limestone or chalk and argillaceous materials (clay or shale) are crushed and ground, heated, and then calcined in a long rotary kiln. This produces a clinker, which is cooled rapidly and, mixed with gypsum and slag, ground in steel ball mills. The finished product contains little if any quartz, consisting largely of calcium silicates and aluminates. It may contain chromium derived from the ball mill rather than the raw materials. Many cements are mixed with asbestos, and in this production process the work force may be at risk of asbestosis and neoplasia.[59, 60]

No really satisfactory controlled epidemiological studies of cement production workers have been reported. Nevertheless, there is sufficient evidence in the literature that suggests that small radiological opacities may occasionally occur as a result of heavy exposure.[61, 62] One slightly bizarre case of pulmonary granulomatosis in a cement worker has been described pathologically.[57] It seems unlikely that inhalation of cement dust leads to a serious fibrosing type of pneumoconiosis, but there is some

evidence that heavily exposed workers may suffer a greater than expected deterioration in ventilatory capacity.[63, 64]

Mullite

Mullite is a crystalline aluminum silicate that may be found widely in nature or may be formed in various processes, such as the calcining of kaolin. A report of granulomatous pulmonary fibrosis in workers exposed to mullite has come from Australia, where alunite clays had previously been calcined to produce potash. The residue was being reclaimed, because of its highly absorbent properties, as a cat litter. Three men working in very dusty conditions had radiological evidence of interstitial lung disease, and a biopsy in one showed a fibrosing, granulomatous pneumonitis.[65]

FIBROUS SILICATES

Amphiboles

The most important amphiboles, amosite, crocidolite, and anthophyllite, are discussed in Chapter 13. Many closely related minerals occur in nature and several of these have attracted attention because of suspected health hazards. Tremolite, as previously mentioned, is an important contaminant of some talcs and is also found in the Quebec chrysotile deposits. It has been mined as asbestos in Korea and is present in the soil in parts of southeastern Europe and Turkey. In such areas pleural plaques may be endemic in agricultural communities. In southeastern Turkey epidemiological and pathological investigations have shown a high prevalence of pleural calcification, pulmonary fibrosis, mesothelioma, and lung cancer in certain villages where tremolite-containing rock is quarried by the men, ground by the women in their homes, and then used as a whitewash each year.[66]

Cummingtonite-grunerite is a term used for a group of amphibole minerals, including the asbestos amosite. A crystalline form which may cleave into fragments that fulfil the definition of fibers, being three times as long as they are broad, occurs in association with the iron ore taconite in Minnesota and Norway and in association with gold ore in South Dakota. Anxiety about possible health effects arose when asbestos-like minerals were found in the water of Lake Superior,[67] and were traced to the dumping of taconite tailings into the lake by a mining company (on the state's order). A large number of investigations, both epidemiological and experimental, followed, and although this particular form of cummingtonite-grunerite proved mildly cytotoxic *in vitro*, no particular harm came to rats fed large amounts of it,[68] and epidemiological studies of miners exposed to it at work showed no increased risk of cancer nor any excess of respiratory disease other than silicosis and tuberculosis.[69, 70] The

latter diseases would be an expected hazard, since the dust contains up to 40 per cent quartz. Not surprisingly, the lungs of taconite miners may contain cummingtonite-grunerite.[71] However, the present evidence suggests that the risk from exposure in the workplace is in no way comparable to that associated with asbestos, while it seems highly unlikely that contamination of the water supplies is of any biological significance.

Fibrous Erionite

Zeolites are hydrated aluminum silicates with substitution of alkaline metals and earths in their framework. Many different types have been described and even more are synthesized for their absorbent, filtration, and catalytic properties. A familiar use is as a molecular sieve, as in gas chromatography. It is important to realize that most zeolites do not have a fibrous form and are not known to have any toxic effects. One, however, has attracted much attention recently as the mineral almost certainly responsible for endemic lung disease in central Turkey. Two villages in particular have been shown to have extraordinarily high death rates from mesothelioma and lung cancer, with almost 40 per cent of the population dying of these two types of malignant disease.[72–75] In addition, pleural plaques, chronic pleural fibrosis, and pulmonary fibrosis are endemic in these villages.

It was initially thought that the lung disease must have been due to asbestos, as in other parts of Turkey,[66] but none was found in the environment. Subsequent investigations have shown that fibrous erionite is probably responsible. This mineral, much of which is of very fine diameter (less than 0.25 micron) but often quite long, forms part of the volcanic tuff on which the villages are situated.[76] This rock is quarried extensively by the villagers as building material and stucco, and many houses are in fact partly caves cut into the rock. Fibers of erionite have been found in the lungs of patients from the villages.[74] It is very likely that exposure to the erionite begins at an early age and that this is responsible for the relative youth of many of the victims of mesothelioma.[77]

The importance of these observations is considerable. First, they show that the "asbestos diseases" may be caused by other, unrelated fibers. Second, they show that fine fibers, often too small to be seen by optical microscopy, may be particularly dangerous, especially when combined with early environmental exposure. Third, they point to the need for caution when considering potential exploitation of the zeolites or when mining within volcanic tuffs. A particular risk might be expected, for example, when digging missile silos in parts of Nevada. Clearly in the future such ventures must be preceded by an examination of the potential liberation of respirable fibers, including those only visible by electron microscopy (Fig. 12–10). Any such fibers should be assumed to represent a health hazard to exposed workers. Animal studies would be likely to give further weight to this argument, as they have with fibrous erionite.[78]

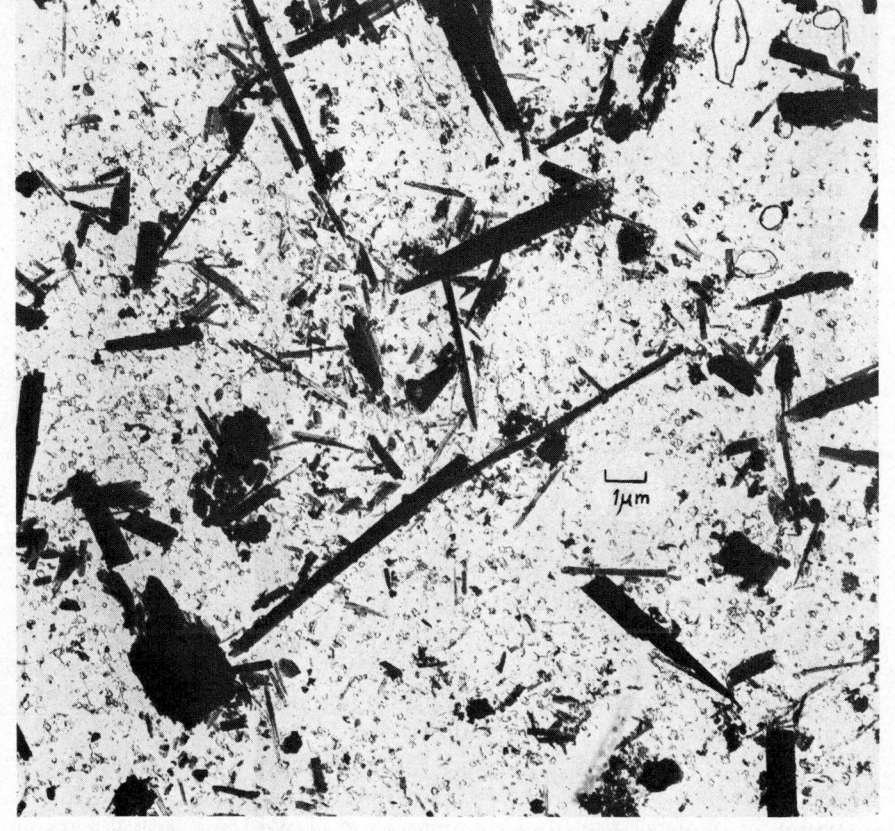

Figure 12–10. Electron microscopical view (×9257) of erionite from Nevada, showing many fine fibrous particles.

One final problem concerns what to do with people living in areas of endemic environmental contamination. In the case of the Turkish villages, plans are now well advanced to relocate the entire populations to areas of different geology, as this appears to be the only possible solution.

Other Natural Fibrous Minerals

A number of clay minerals occur naturally in a fibrous form. Of these, attapulgite (palygorskite) and sepiolite have important commercial applications, with production of over one million tons annually. They are used as absorbents and filters, and in pesticides, paints, medications, fertilizers, and cosmetics.[79] An important and familiar use is in cat litter. Major amounts are produced in Nevada, Spain, and Turkey. A limited number of studies of exposed workers has been carried out. One such study has attributed pulmonary fibrosis to inhalation of attapulgite,[80] and the same researchers have demonstrated that this material is as cytotoxic *in vitro* as

chrysotile.[79] However, the fibers, though extremely thin, are very short and it seems quite possible that they are not as toxic in the animal or human subject as might be feared. Some support for this comes from a study of Turkish sepiolite workers which did not produce any evidence of an excess of asbestos-type diseases over that which might have been anticipated in that area.[81] Nevertheless, caution is clearly necessary in handling these fibrous materials, and prospective epidemiology coupled with good industrial hygiene measurements are necessary.

Wollastonite is a fibrous calcium silicate used in ceramics and as a substitute for asbestos in boards, insulation, and brake linings. Some is mined in New York State. These fibers also are very fine but short. One cross-sectional survey has shown no evidence of pleural disease in the small work force.[82] However, further studies of larger numbers of exposed individuals and of fiber counts in this industry are necessary before the absence of a hazard can be assumed.

Manmade Vitreous Fibers

Although artificial fibers have been produced in some form since the middle of the nineteenth century, it is only since World War II that this has become a major industry. A number of different products and processes are involved and potential health implications may differ among them. Three broad categories of fiber can be distinguished: continuous filament, insulation wool, and special purpose fiber. The former is produced from glass, which is melted, extruded through pores and drawn on a drum. In general, the fiber diameters are above the respirable range, though some fibers less than 3 microns in diameter may be found in the air. Continuous filament fiber is used in fabrics and insulation materials, and as a reinforcement for plastics and cement. Insulation wool is made from various basic materials, such as metal slag, igneous rock, or glass, which are melted down and then blown by high-pressure steam or spun by rapid rotation into a fibrous mat. Most is used for thermal or acoustic insulation, usually after having been bound with a resin. A higher proportion of the fibers produced in these processes are less than 3 microns in diameter. Special purpose fibers include flame-attenuated glass fibers and ceramic fibers; the latter are made from molten kaolin or alumina and silica. These fibers may be very fine, with a high proportion in the respirable range, and are used in lightweight insulation, such as in aircraft and spacecraft, ear defenders, and filters. They have been in production only over the last 20 to 30 years.

A characteristic of manmade fibers is that they do not break longitudinally but transversely. This means that wear and tear results in shorter rather than finer fibers, which may be an important factor in their apparent lack of serious effects on the health of the work force. Another factor is undoubtedly the relatively low levels of respirable fibers found in association with the manfacturing process. Nevertheless, implantation

of fine glass fibers in the pleural cavity of rats has produced mesothelioma[83] and the evidence strongly suggests that manmade mineral fibers have the *potential* to cause mesothelioma, presumably if sufficiently large numbers of durable fibers of respirable size were to be inhaled by workers. This observation has stimulated a considerable amount of research into the health effects of these fibers.

In general, epidemiological studies have shown no increased risk of carcinoma of the lung in work forces exposed over prolonged periods to glass fiber or insulation fibers.[84–86] Moreover, there is no evidence of mesothelioma or pneumoconiosis occurring in workers in these industries. However, there is one clinical report of histologically proven pulmonary fibrosis in men exposed to high levels of rock wool in the lagging industry and in whom fibers were demonstrated in the lung biopsies.[87] There is some dispute about whether or not there is an increased risk of death from nonmalignant respiratory disease,[84, 86, 88] related partly to the comparison of populations from industrial areas with the population of the United States as a whole and partly to lack of information on smoking habits.[85] At present it seems unlikely that there is a seriously increased risk.

Animal studies have shown that mesothelioma results from implantation of fine, long fibers in serosal cavities,[83] but inhalation experiments have not produced an excess of pulmonary fibrosis or tumors.[89] Consistent with these findings, *in vitro* cell studies have shown fine, long fibers to be cytotoxic,[91] while studies of the lungs of exposed workers have demonstrated fibers but no important pathological reaction.[90]

In conclusion, it can be assumed that manmade fibers have the potential to cause mesothelioma and pulmonary fibrosis. They are not likely to do so in the manufacturing industry, where levels of respirable fibers are generally low, with the possible exception of the special purpose fibers. Further environmental and epidemiological investigations are needed in these workplaces. A risk should be assumed in the user industry and is likely to relate to the numbers of fibers below 3 microns in diameter and above 10 microns in length to which workers are exposed. Such industries should base their occupational hygiene on this assumption, and it is desirable that epidemiological investigations should also be carried out. Finally, further studies of fiber levels in the lungs of deceased workers are necessary, since it may be that manmade fibers are less durable in tissues than other natural fibers. If this proved to be true, it would give further reassurance that manmade fibers are relatively safe substitutes for asbestos.

Other Artificial Substitutes for Asbestos

Calcium silicate and carbon fiber are also produced on a large scale in industry and have been used as substitutes for asbestos. The use of each may produce airborne particles in the respirable range, some of

which fulfil the 3:1 ratio definition of fibers.[92, 93] However, no health effects have been described in the work force handling carbon fiber,[94] while calcium silicate seems only to have been studied in animals, in which it has produced some preliminary evidence of toxicity requiring further investigation.[93, 95]

Vermiculite

Vermiculite is composed of hydrated laminar crystals containing aluminum, iron, and magnesium silicates. About 20 varieties of vermiculite exist. It has a crystalline structure similar to that of mica and on heating expands into wormlike structures—hence its name. Deposits of vermiculite are found in Montana, Virginia, and South Africa. The deposits are often contaminated by quartz, talc, clay, and asbestos, the latter usually consisting of tremolite and actinolite. Vermiculite is fire resistant and is used in cement, plaster and hardboard. Pleural effusions and frank fibrosis have been reported in workers, but these are a consequence of the asbestos contained in the mineral.[96]

References

1. Pooley, F. D., and Rowlands, N., Chemical and physical properties of British talc powders. In Walton, W. H., ed., Inhaled Particles IV. London, Pergamon Press, 1977, p. 639.
2. Boundy, M. G., Gold, K., Martin, K. P., et al., Occupational exposures to non-asbestiform talc in Vermont. In Dement, J. M., and Lemen, R., eds., Dusts and Disease (Occupational and Environmental Exposures to Selected Particulate and Fibrous Dusts). Park Forest South, Ill., Pathotox Publishers Inc., 1979, p. 365.
3. van Ordstrand, H. S., Talc pneumoconiosis. Chest 58, 2, 1970.
4. Cralley, L. J., Key, M. M., Groth, D. H., et al., Fibrous and mineral content of cosmetic talc products. Am. Ind. Hyg. Assoc. J., 29, 350, 1968.
5. Phillipson, I. M., Talc quality. Lancet, 1, 48, 1980.
6. Hamer, D. H., Rolle, F. R., and Schelz, J. P., Characterization of talc and associated minerals. Am. Ind. Hyg. J., 37, 296, 1976.
7. Dreesen, W. C., and Dalla Valle, J. M., Effects of exposure to dust in two Georgia talc mills and mines. Pub. Health Rep., 50, 131, 1935.
8. Porro, F. W., Patton, J. R., and Hobbs, A. A., Pneumoconiosis in the talc industry. Am. J. Roent., 47, 507, 1942.
9. Siegal, W., Smith, A. R., and Greenburg, L., The dust hazard to tremolite talc mining, including roentgenological findings in talc workers. Am. J. Roent., 49, 11, 1943.
10. Kleinfeld, M., Messite, J., and Tabershaw, I. R., Talc pneumoconiosis. Arch. Ind. Health, 12, 66, 1955.
11. Kleinfeld, M., Messite, J., Kooyman, O., and Zaki, M. H., Mortality among talc miners and millers in New York State. Arch. Environ. Health, 14, 663, 1967.
12. Kleinfeld, M., Messite, J., and Zaki, M. H., Mortality experiences among talc workers: a follow-up study. J. Occup. Med., 16, 345, 1974.
13. Dement, J. M., and Zumwalde, R. D., Occupational exposures to talc containing asbestiform minerals. In Dement, J. M., and Lemen, R., eds., Dusts and Disease (Occupational and Environmental Exposures to Selected Particulate and Fibrous Dusts). Park Forest South, Ill., Pathotox Publishers Inc., 1979, p. 287.
14. Rubino, G. F., Scansetti, G., Piolatto, G., and Romano, C. A., Mortality study of talc miners and millers. J. Occup. Med., 18, 186, 1976.

15. Rubino, G. F., Scansetti, G., and Piolatto, G., Mortality and morbidity among talc miners and millers in Italy. *In* Dement, J. M., and Lemen, R., eds., Dusts and Disease (Occupational and Environmental Exposures to Selected Particulate and Fibrous Dusts). Park Forest South, Ill., Pathotox Publishers Inc., 1979, p. 357.

16. Selevan, S. G., Dement, J. M., Wagoner, J. K., and Froines, J. R., Mortality patterns among miners and millers of non-asbestiform talc: preliminary report. *In* Dement, J. M., and Lemen, R., eds., Dusts and Disease (Occupational and Environmental Exposures to Selected Particulate and Fibrous Dusts). Park Forest South, Ill., Pathotox Publishers Inc., 1979, p. 379.

17. Gamble, J. F., Fellner, W., and Dimeo, M. J., An epidemiologic study of a group of talc workers. Am. Rev. Respir. Dis., *119*, 741, 1979.

18. Léophante, P., Fabre, J., Potts, J., et al., Les pneumoconioses par le talc. Arch. Mal. Prof., *37*, 513, 1976.

19. Moskowitz, R. L., Talc pneumoconiosis: a treated case. Chest, *58*, 37, 1970.

20. Nam, K., and Gracy, D. R., Pulmonary talcosis from cosmetic talcum powder. J.A.M.A., *221*, 492, 1972.

21. Fine, L. J., Peters, J. M., Burgess, W. A., and Di Berardinis, L. J., Studies of respiratory morbidity in rubber workers. IV. Respiratory morbidity in talc workers. Arch. Environ. Health, *31*, 195, 1976.

22. Kleinfeld, M., Giel, C. P., Majernowski, J. M., and Messite, J., Talc pneumoconiosis. Arch. Environ. Health, *7*, 101, 1963.

23. Gould, S. R., and Barnardo, D. E., Respiratory distress after talc inhalation. Br. J. Dis. Chest, *66*, 230, 1970.

24. Wendt, V. E., Puro, H. E., Shapiro, J., et al., Angiothrombotic pulmonary hypertension in addicts—"blue velvet" drug addiction. J.A.M.A., *188*, 755, 1964.

25. Waller, B. F., Brownlee, W. J., and Roberts, W. C., Self-induced pulmonary granulomatosis. A consequence of intravenous injection of drugs intended for oral use. Chest, *78*, 90, 1980.

26. Buchanan, D. R., Lamb, D., and Seaton, A., Punk rocker's lung: pulmonary fibrosis in a drug-snorting fire-eater. Br. Med. J., *283*, 1661, 1981.

27. Gamble, J., Greife, A., and Hancock, J., Cross-sectional epidemiologic and industrial hygiene survey of talc workers mining ore from Montana, Texas, and North Carolina. *In* Proceedings of the National Workshop on Substitutes for Asbestos. Environmental Protection Agency Publication No. EPA-560/3-80-001. Washington, D.C., Government Printing Office, 1980, p. 570.

28. Kleinfeld, M., Messite, J., Shapiro, J., and Swencicki, R., Effect of talc dust inhalation on lung function. Arch. Environ. Health, *10*, 431, 1965.

29. Kleinfeld, M., Messite, J., Shapiro, J., et al., Lung function in talc workers. Arch. Environ. Health, *9*, 559, 1964.

30. Gamble, J., Fellner, W., and DiMeo, M. J., Respiratory morbidity among miners and millers of asbestiform talc. *In* Dement, J. M., and Lemen, R., eds., Dusts and Disease (Occupational and Environmental Exposures to Selected Particulate and Fibrous Dusts). Park Forest South, Ill., Pathotox Publishers Inc., 1979, p. 307.

31. Smith, R. H., Graf, M. S., and Silverman, J. F., Successful management of drug-induced talc granulomatosis with corticosteroids. Chest, *73*, 552, 1978.

32. Stille, W. T., and Tabershaw, I. R., The mortality experience of upstate New York talc workers. J. Occup. Med., *24*, 480, 1982.

33. Wagner, J. C., Berry, G., Hill, R. J., and Skidmore, J. W., An animal model for inhalation exposure to talc. *In* Dement, J. M., and Lemen, R., eds., Dusts and Disease (Occupational and Environmental Exposures to Selected Particulate and Fibrous Dusts). Park Forest South, Ill., Pathotox Publishers Inc., 1979, p. 389.

34. Research Committee of the British Thoracic Association and the Medical Research Council Pneumoconiosis Unit, A survey of the long-term effects of talc and kaolin pleurodesis. Br. J. Dis. Chest, *73*, 285, 1979.

35. Middleton, E. L., Industrial pulmonary disease due to the inhalation of dust. Lancet, *2*, 59, 1936.

36. Lynch, K. M., and McIver, F. A., Pneumoconiosis from exposure to kaolin dust: kaolinosis. Am. J. Pathol., *30*, 1117, 1954.

37. Hale, L. E., Gough, J., King, E. J., and Nagelschmidt, G., Pneumoconiosis of kaolin workers. Br. J. Ind. Med., *13*, 251, 1956.

38. Warraki, S., and Herant, Y., Pneumoconiosis in china-clay workers. Br. J. Ind. Med., *20*, 226, 1963.
39. Sheers, G., Prevalence of pneumoconiosis in Cornish kaolin workers. Br. J. Ind. Med., *21*, 218, 1964.
40. Edenfield, R. W., A clinical and roentgenological study of kaolin workers. Arch. Environ. Health, *1*, 392, 1960.
40a. Kennedy, T., Rawlings, W., Jr., Baser, M., and Tockman, M., Pneumoconiosis in Georgia kaolin workers. Am. Rev. Respir. Dis., *127*, 215, 1983.
41. Martin, J. C., Daniel, H., and LeBouffant, L., Short and long-term experimental study of the toxicity of coal-mine dust and some of its constituents. *In* Walton, W. H., ed., Inhaled Particles IV. London, Pergamon Press, 1977, p. 361.
42. Sakula, A., Pneumoconiosis due to fuller's earth. Thorax, *16*, 176, 1961.
43. McNally, W. D., and Trostler, I. S., Severe pneumoconiosis caused by inhalation of fuller's earth. J. Ind. Hyg., *23*, 118, 1941.
44. Campbell, A. H., and Gloyne, S. R., A case of pneumoconiosis due to the inhalation of fuller's earth. J. Pathol. Bact., *54*, 75, 1942.
45. Tonning, H. O., Pneumoconiosis from fuller's earth. Report of a case with autopsy findings. J. Ind. Hyg., *31*, 41, 1949.
46. Seaton, A., Lamb, D., Rhind Brown, W., et al., Pneumoconiosis of shale miners. Thorax, *36*, 412, 1981.
47. Thomas, R. W., Silicosis in the ball-clay and china-clay industries. Lancet, *1*, 133, 1952.
48. Phibbs, B. P., Sundin, R. E., and Mitchell, R. S., Silicosis in Wyoming bentonite workers. Am. Rev. Respir. Dis., *103*, 1, 1971.
49. Adamis, Z., and Timar, M., Studies on the effects of quartz, bentonite and coal dust mixtures on macrophages *in vitro*. Br. J. Exp. Pathol., *59*, 411, 1978.
50. Timar, M., Kendrey, G., and Juhasz, Z., Experimental observations concerning the effects of mineral dust on pulmonary tissue. Med. Lav., *57*, 1, 1966.
51. Gärtner, H., and van Marwych, C., Lungenfibrose durch Sillimanit. Deutsch. Med. Woschr., *72*, 708, 1947.
52. Jötten, K. W., and Eickhoff, F. W., Lung changes from sillimanite dust. Arch. Gewerbepath, *12*, 223, 1944.
53. Barrie, H. J., and Hosselin, L., Massive pneumoconiosis from a rock dust containing no free silica. Nepheline lung. Arch. Environ. Health, *1*, 109, 1960.
54. Dreesen, W. C., Dalla Valle, J. M., Edwards, T. I., et al., Pneumoconiosis among mica and pegmatite workers. Pub. Health Bull. No. 250. Washington, D.C., U.S. Public Health Service, 1940.
55. Vestal, T. F., Winstead, J. A., and Joliet, P. V., Pneumoconiosis among mica and pegmatite workers: a supplementary study. Ind. Med., *12*, 11, 1943.
56. Smith, A. R., Pleural calcification resulting from exposure to certain dusts. Am. J. Roent., *67*, 375, 1952.
57. Pimental, J. C., and Menezes, A. P., Pulmonary and hepatic granulomatous disorders due to the inhalation of cement and mica dusts. Thorax, *33*, 219, 1978.
58. Goldstein, B., and Rendall, R. E. G., The relative toxicities of the main classes of mineral. *In* Shapiro, H. A., ed., Pneumoconiosis. Proceedings of an International Conference in Johannesburg. New York, Oxford University Press, 1969, p. 429, 1970.
59. Finkelstein, M. M., Asbestosis in long-term employees of an Ontario asbestos-cement factory. Am. Rev. Respir. Dis., *125*, 496, 1982.
60. Thomas, H. F., Benjamin, I. T., Elwood, P. C., and Sweetnam, P. M., Further follow-up study of workers from an asbestos cement factory, Br. J. Ind. Med., *39*, 273, 1982.
61. Scansetti, G., Coscia, G. C., Pisani, W., and Rubino, G. F., Cement, asbestos, and cement-asbestos pneumoconioses. A comparative clinical-roentgenographic study. Arch. Environ. Health, *30*, 272, 1975.
62. Bazas, T., Effects of occupational exposure to dust on the respiratory system of cement workers. J. Soc. Occup. Med., *30*, 31, 1980.
63. Kalacic, I., Chronic nonspecific lung disease in cement workers. Arch. Environ. Health, *26*, 78, 1973.
64. Kalacic, I., Ventilatory function in cement workers. Arch. Environ. Health, *26*, 84, 1973.
65. Musk, A. W., Greville, H. W., and Tribe, A. E., Pulmonary disease from occupational exposure to an artificial aluminium silicate used for cat litter. Br. J. Ind. Med., *37*, 367, 1980.

66. Yazicioglu, S., Ikayto, R., Balci, K., et al., Pleural calcification, pleural mesotheliomas and bronchial cancers caused by tremolite dust. Thorax, *35*, 564, 1980.

67. Cook, P. M., Glass, G. E., and Tucker, J. H., Asbestiform amphibole minerals: detection and measurement of high concentrations in municiple water supplies. Science, *185*, 853, 1974.

68. Hilding, A. C., Hilding, D. A., Larson, D. M., and Aufderheide, A. C., Biological effects of ingested amosite asbestos, taconite tailings, diatomaceous earth and Lake Superior water in rats. Arch. Environ. Health, *36*, 298, 1981.

69. McDonald, J. C., Gibbs, G. W., Liddell, F. D. K., and McDonald, A. D., Mortality after long exposure to cummingtonite-grunerite. Am. Rev. Respir. Dis., *118*, 271, 1978.

70. Clark, T. C., Harrington, V. A., Asta, J., et al., Respiratory effects of exposure to dust in taconite mining and processing. Am. Rev. Respir. Dis., *121*, 959, 1980.

71. Gylseth, B., Norseth, T., and Skaug, V., Amphibole fibers in a taconite mine and in the lungs of the miners. Am. J. Ind. Med., *2*, 175, 1981.

72. Baris, Y. I., Sahin, A. A., Ozesmi, M., et al., An outbreak of pleural mesothelioma and chronic fibrosing pleurisy in the village of Karain/Ürgüp in Anatolia. Thorax, *33*, 181, 1978.

73. Baris, Y. I., Artvinli, M., and Sahin, A. A., Environmental mesothelioma in Turkey. Ann. N.Y. Acad. Sci., *330*, 423, 1979.

74. Artvinli, M., and Baris, Y. I., Malignant mesotheliomas in a small village in the Anatolian region of Turkey: an epidemiologic study. J. Natl. Cancer Inst., *63*, 17, 1979.

75. Artvinli, M., and Baris, Y. I., Environmental fiber-induced pleuropulmonary diseases in an Anatolian village: an epidemiologic study. Arch. Environ. Health, *37*, 177, 1982.

76. Pooley, F. D., Evaluation of fiber samples taken from the vicinity of two villages in Turkey. *In* Dement, J. M., and Lemen, R., eds., Dusts and Disease (Occupational and Environmental Exposures to Selected Particulate and Fibrous Dusts). Park Forest South, Ill., Pathotox Publishers Inc., 1979, p. 41.

77. Baris, Y., The clinical and radiological aspects of 185 cases of malignant pleural mesothelioma. *In* Wagner, J. C., ed., Biological Effects of Mineral Fibres, Vol. 2. Lyon, International Agency for Research on Cancer, Scientific Publications No. 30, 1980, p. 937.

78. Suzuki, Y., Carcinogenic and fibrogenic effects of zeolites: preliminary observations. Environ. Res., *27*, 433, 1982.

79. Bignon, J., Sebastien, P., Gaudichet, A., and Jurand, M. C., Biolõgical effects of attapulgite. *In* Wagner, J. C., ed., Biological Effects of Mineral Fibres, Vol. 1. Lyon, International Agency for Research on Cancer, Scientific Publications No. 30, 1980, p. 163.

80. Sors, H., Gaudichet, A., Sebastien, P., et al., Lung fibrosis after inhalation of fibrous attapulgite. Thorax, *34*, 695, 1979.

81. Baris, Y. I., Sahin, A. A., and Erkan, M. L., Clinical and radiological study in sepiolite workers. Arch. Environ. Health, *35*, 343, 1980.

82. Shasby, D. M., Petersen, M., Hodous, T., et al., Respiratory morbidity of workers exposed to wollastonite through mining and milling. *In* Dement, J. M., and Lemen, R., eds., Dusts and Disease (Occupational and Environmental Exposures to Selected Particulate and Fibrous Dusts). Park Forest South, Ill., Pathotox Publishers Inc., 1979, p. 251.

83. Stanton, M. F., Layard, M., Tegeris, A., et al., Carcinogenicity of fibrous glass: pleural response in the rat in relation to fiber dimension. J. Natl. Cancer Inst., *58*, 587, 1977.

84. Enterline, P. E., and Marsh, G. M., Mortality of workers in the man-made mineral fibre industry. *In* Wagner, J. C., ed., Biological Effects of Mineral Fibres, Vol. 2. Lyon, International Agency for Research on Cancer, Scientific Publications No. 30, 1980, p. 965.

85. Gross, P., Man-made vitrous fibers: present status of research on health effects. Int. Arch. Occup. Environ. Health, *50*, 103, 1982.

86. Robinson, C. F., Dement, J. M., Ness, G. O., and Waxweiler, R. J., Mortality patterns of rock and slag mineral wool production workers: an epidemiological and environmental study. Br. J. Ind. Med., *39*, 45, 1982.

87. Ciaccia, A., Pusinanti, F., Beltrami, A., and Fasano, E., Pneumoconiosis da fibre di lana di roccia. Riv. Pat. Clin. Tuberc. e Pneumol., *49*, 305, 1978.

88. Bayliss, D. L., Dement, J. M., Wagoner, J. K., and Blejer, H. P., Mortality patterns among fibrous glass production workers. Ann. N.Y. Acad. Sci., *271*, 324, 1976.

89. Gross, P., The biologic characterisation of inhaled fiber glass dust: a critical review of pertinent studies and reports. Arch. Environ. Health, *31*, 101, 1976.
90. Gross, P., Lungs of workers exposed to fiber glass. A study of their pathologic changes and their dust content. Arch. Environ. Health, *23*, 67, 1971.
91. Brown, R. C., Chamberlain, M., and Skidmore, J. W., *In vitro* effects of man-made mineral fibres. Ann. Occup. Hyg., *22*, 175, 1979.
92. Holt, P. F., and Horne, M., Dust from carbon fibre. Environ. Res., *17*, 276, 1978.
93. Davis, J. M. G., Addison, J., Bolton, R. E., et al., Toxicology of calcium silicate insulating materials. Institute of Occupational Medicine Technical Memorandum, TM/83/1. Edinburgh, 1983.
94. Jones, H. D., Jones, T. R., and Lyle, W. H., Carbon fibre: results of a survey of process workers and their environment in a factory producing continuous filament. *In* Walton, W. H., ed., Inhaled Particles V. Oxford, Pergamon Press, 1982, p. 861.
95. Richards, R. J., Tetley, T. D., and Hunt, J., The biological reactivity of calcium silicate composites: *in vivo* studies. Environ. Res., *26*, 243, 1981.
96. Lockey, J. E., and Brooks, S. M., Health Effects of Vermiculite. *In* Proceedings of the National Workshop on Substitutes for Asbestos. Environmental Protection Agency Publication No. EPA 560/3-80-001. Washington, D.C., Government Printing Office, 1980.

13

ASBESTOS-RELATED DISEASES

Anthony Seaton

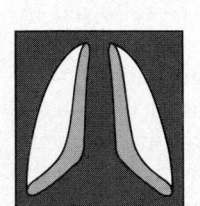

Asbestos is the name given to a number of naturally occurring fibrous silicates with the common property of great resistance to destruction by chemical and physical means. Their fibrous configuration allows them to be woven into cloth and to be used as a strengthener in cement and other materials. The minerals known collectively as asbestos belong to one of two mineralogical groups, the serpentines and the amphiboles. The only type of asbestos that is a member of the former group is chrysotile, or white asbestos, which has as curly fibers that sheer into many smaller fibrils. Its chemical composition ($Mg_3Si_2O_5(OH)_4$) is similar to that of micas and kaolinites, but its fibrous structure is due to rolled sheets of silicate with outer magnesium and hydroxide ions. The amphiboles include amosite, or brown asbestos ($(MgFe^{++})_7Si_8O_{22}(OH)_2$), crocidolite, or blue asbestos ($Na_2(MgFe^{+++}Fe^{++})Si_8O_{22}(OH)$), anthophyllite ($(MgFe^{++})_7Si_8O_{22}(OH)_2$), tremolite ($Ca_2(MgFe^{++})_5Si_8O_{22}$), and actinolite ($Ca_2(MgFe^{++})_5Si_8O_{22}(OH)_2$). These minerals differ from chrysotile in that their crystals are arranged in straight double chains rather than curled plates.

HISTORICAL ASPECTS

Anthophyllite fibers have been found in the clay of pots dating from 2500 B.C., and were presumably added to give increased strength to the finished article. Asbestos was used in classical times for weaving into funeral shrouds and wicks for lamps. Pliny in A.D. 50 mentioned that the weavers producing wicks for the lamps of the vestal virgins wore masks to avoid inhaling the dust.[1] The name asbestos comes from the Greek word meaning "unquenchable" in reference to its use in lamps, while the French word, *amiante,* probably derives from a village in Cyprus now known as Amiandos, near to where asbestos is still mined. Intermittent

use was made of asbestos in Europe in the eighteenth century and before, but its large-scale use followed the exploitation of the Quebec deposits in the 1860s and the South African deposits in the 1890s.

Suspicion as to the harmful effects of asbestos on health probably arose in Britain and Italy at the turn of the century.[2] In 1907 Murray reported a case of pulmonary fibrosis in an asbestos worker to a British governmental committee on compensation for industrial diseases[3] and in 1917 Pancoast and colleagues reported the radiological features.[4] The detailed description of the clinical and pathological features followed in 1927.[5, 6] An increasing awareness of the hazards of asbestos culminated in Merewether and Price's report to the British Parliament in 1930,[7] which resulted in the introduction of safety measures for asbestos factories and in the medical supervision of the workers. The first indication that patients with asbestosis might die of bronchial carcinoma came in a review of 100 cases by Wood and Gloyne in 1934,[8] and in 1949, following a number of other papers reporting the association of the two diseases, Merewether established that there was an excess of deaths due to lung cancer among asbestotics.[9] He found that 13.2 per cent of asbestotics died of lung cancer, as opposed to 1.3 per cent of silicotics. In a study of 113 asbestos textile workers in 1955, Doll found 11 to have died from lung cancer, compared to the statistically expected number of 0.8.[10] However, continuation of this study for a further 10 years showed that the improvements in industrial hygiene following the introduction of the British asbestos regulations in 1931 had been accompanied by a considerable reduction in the risk of asbestosis and carcinoma.[11] Meanwhile, in a study of 632 New York insulation workers, Selikoff and co-workers found an excess mortality of 99 due largely to bronchial carcinoma, but also in part to gastrointestinal neoplasms.[12, 13]

Mesothelioma, the other malignant tumor associated with asbestos exposure, was known to pathologists and had been reported in association with asbestosis in the 1930s.[2] However, it was not until 1960, when Wagner and his colleagues reported 33 cases from the North-West Cape of South Africa,[14] that the relationship became clear. Twenty-eight of these cases had worked or lived in the Cape asbestos field and 4 had worked in other parts of the asbestos industry. The geographic distribution of the cases suggested exposure to the North-West Cape crocidolite, since cases were not found in the amosite mining areas of South Africa. Shortly afterwards, similar tumors were described in relation to asbestos exposure in Britain and the United States as well as in the crocidolite mining area of Australia.

PRODUCTION AND USES OF ASBESTOS

The major producers of asbestos are Canada, South Africa, and the U.S.S.R. The Quebec mines are the Western world's most important producers of chrysotile, which constitutes about 70 per cent of all com-

mercially produced asbestos. South Africa produces most of the world's amosite and crocidolite. The U.S.S.R. is the world's major overall asbestos producer, its chrysotile being used almost exclusively within the Eastern bloc. Much smaller amounts of chrysotile are produced in the United States (mostly in Vermont), Italy, Cyprus, China, South America, and Zimbabwe, while some crocidolite has been produced in Australia. Anthophyllite comes only from Finland. Current annual output of the major producers is estimated to be 1.6 million tons from Canada, 780 thousand tons from South Africa, and 2.6 million tons from the U.S.S.R. All other production accounts for about 16 per cent of the total 6.2 million of annual world output, some 150 thousand tons being produced in the United States.

Initially asbestos was produced by surface mining, but most is now obtained from underground mines. Although the process, which includes drilling and blasting, may be dusty, much of the asbestos at this stage is bound to the parent rock, and this, together with dust suppression measures in the mines, makes the actual mining of asbestos less hazardous to health than might be expected. Exposure to silica is an additional hazard of mining in South Africa, but not apparently in Canada. The raw asbestos is then crushed in mills, usually at the mine, to release the fibers, which may then be carded to produce material containing parallel fibers suitable for spinning or incorporating into asbestos products. These processes, and the attendant cleaning and maintenance of the machinery, may generate large amounts of dust. Subsequently, the asbestos is transported in impermeable plastic bags (jute bags, being porous, have now been replaced) to the users. Asbestos is attractive to industry because of its strength and resistance to the effects of heat, acid, and sound. In the case of chrysotile it can also be woven. It is therefore mainly used to strengthen materials such as cement and plastics; as insulation, on boards, tiles, and various fillers and paints; and as friction material in brakes. The major current use is in cement for building and for pipes. This is a use in which crocidolite has advantages, and the production of large-diameter pressure pipes is probably a major justification for the continued use of this type of asbestos. Amosite is particularly useful in friction materials, but like chrysotile is also widely used in many of the 3000 or so current applications of asbestos.

Approximately a million tons of asbestos are used annually in the United States. Three quarters of this is used in the construction industry, most of it previously incorporated into cements, tiles, felts, and so on. However, these materials may need to be cut, drilled, or handled in some way that has the potential to liberate dust. Perhaps 8 per cent of the asbestos used in construction is in the obviously dangerous free form. Spraying of asbestos-containing materials has been banned in several contries including the United States. Insulation, or lagging, of boilers, pipes, and electric lines in factories, houses, and ships is commonly performed by covering them with asbestos. Originally the asbestos was

mixed with water by the lagger and applied while wet, but most insulation is now done by cutting and shaping pre-formed materials. Plumbers, demolition workers, and workers employed in dockyards, railroad workshops, and power stations may therefore be at risk of asbestos exposure.

Outside the construction industry, risks of exposure occur in the production and application of the materials just mentioned and also in their repair and removal. There is also some risk that workers may carry asbestos home on their clothing, thus causing their families to be exposed. Exposure of the general public may occur as a result of atmospheric pollution around an asbestos mine or works, the dumping of asbestos wastes, or the deterioration of asbestos materials in buildings. The risks attached to such exposures are discussed in the following section.

EPIDEMIOLOGY

Relationships Between Exposure and Risk of Disease

The early studies of Merewether,[7, 9] Doll,[10] and Wagner[14] established that asbestos exposure entailed a risk of the development of three diseases: asbestosis, bronchial carcinoma, and mesothelioma. Subsequent work has concentrated on determining the type of relationship between exposure and risk of disease, the ultimate objective being to provide information upon which an appropriate hygiene standard could be based. This objective has been difficult to achieve largely because of uncertainty concerning the dose, and often the type, of asbestos to which workers had been exposed. Furthermore, it is possible to use many different measures of response, including radiological and clinical assessments with their inherent variabilities, and mortality studies with their problems associated with the reliability of death certification and selection of appropriate control statistics. Nevertheless, several important longitudinal studies of exposed workers have been carried out and information has been obtained which is not likely to be bettered in the near future.

A major problem has been the large-scale use in industry of three different types of asbestos and of the strong suggestion that these might have differing degrees of pathological effect. In particular, it has seemed likely that the risk of mesothelioma is much higher in people working with crocidolite than in those working with chrysotile, with amosite occupying an intermediate position. Studies of populations exposed to single types of asbestos have now largely confirmed this. Groups of workers employed in Canada and the United Kingdom during World War II making filters for military gas masks out of crocidolite, in conditions that were not thought to be especially dusty, have shown very high death rates from mesothelioma.[15, 16] These workers characteristically had relatively brief exposures to asbestos, often for less than 12 months. Similar results are now being found in Australian crocidolite miners and millers.[17] In the

United States, a group of workers who were employed for a relatively short period using only amosite in the production of insulation for naval vessels was identified.[18] In contrast to the conditions in the gas mask factories, this work was thought to be very dusty. The occurrence of mesothelioma was less frequent (4.1 per cent of all deaths over 35 years, compared with 16 per cent of the Canadian and 10 per cent of the British crocidolite deaths over a similar period), but still occurred much more frequently than in a long-term follow-up of Canadian chrysotile miners and millers.[19] Finally, the occurrence of mesothelioma in the latter study has been slightly greater than would have been expected from the background incidence of the disease in Canada. It can therefore be stated with reasonable confidence that the risk of mesothelioma is greatest following exposure to crocidolite, somewhat less after exposure to amosite, and much less though still increased after exposure to chrysotile. To date, the tumor has not been described in association with exposure to anthophyllite in Finland.

In spite of these studies, it is not possible to relate a level of exposure to such fibers to risk of mesothelioma, because fiber counts were not made. The closest approximation to such a dose-response study comes from recorded occupational histories and from counts of asbestos in the lungs of deceased workers. From the British gas mask study, it is clear that work with crocidolite in what were apparently relatively clean conditions for a period of between 6 months and 4 years was sufficient to cause the disease. The lungs of these workers with mesothelioma contained large numbers of crocidolite fibers, comparable to the amount found in other mesothelioma patients exposed for much longer in other industries.[15] Thus, the time of exposure is a poor guide to its level and it seems that the only sensible policy with crocidolite is to avoid using it altogether.

Information on a dose-response relationship between exposure to amosite and the development of mesothelioma is even less reliable. Evidence from the only study to shed light on this matter suggests a dose-response relationship, with those employed for the longest times having the greatest risks.[18] In this study, which relied solely on occupational histories, heavy exposures seemed to reduce the interval between exposure and appearance of the tumor. Prolonged exposures were not necessary, however, with mesotheliomas appearing in individuals who had worked little more than six months in the factory. By contrast, mesothelioma is relatively rare in chrysotile workers and usually has occurred only after prolonged exposure.[19, 20] In addition, the intensity of the initial exposure seems to make little difference as a risk factor, suggesting that the passage of time may allow chrysotile to be eliminated from the lungs more readily than the amphiboles.[21]

A similar, but probably not so steep, gradient exists between the liabilities of the three main types of asbestos that cause lung cancer. Prolonged exposure to chrysotile seems to increase the risk by a factor of about two to three, being rather higher in millers than in miners.[19, 20, 22]

In one long-term prospective study of Quebec chrysotile miners and millers, a clear dose-response relationship has been demonstrated, as dust counts had been made over a considerable period.[23] The risks of lung cancer were not increased, even with high exposure, in men employed for less than five years. Thereafter, they increased with increasing exposure levels and durations up to about 2.5 times that of the unexposed population. While lung cancer occurred in nonsmokers in this population, the two factors of smoking and asbestos exposure clearly increase the risk in either an additive[23] or a multiplicative manner.[24] Exposures to amosite seem to entail a higher risk of lung cancer,[18] doubled after brief exposure and 6.5 times that expected following more than two years' exposure. In gas mask workers, crocidolite exposure has been associated with a risk of around double that expected after exposures of only several months.[15] After prolonged exposure, anthophyllite miners and millers in Finland have also been shown to have a risk of lung cancer two to three times that of the unexposed population.[25]

Asbestosis may result from exposure to any type of asbestos. Demonstration of dose-response relationships has been complicated not only by the difficulty of assessing the exposure dose but also by problems in measuring the response, especially at an early stage. There is considerable interobserver variability in recording lung crackles or early irregular basal radiological shadows, for example. Nevertheless, many studies have addressed this problem and useful information, at least with respect to chrysotile asbestos, has been obtained. Even the best of these studies, however, have had to accept inevitable imperfections in their data that result in an inability to draw other than rather broad conclusions as to dose-response relationships. For example, the important study of Quebec miners and millers[26, 27] has included valuable information on dose, but measured in particle counts that can be converted into fiber counts only with the introduction of considerable loss of reliability of the measurements. Moreover, this study, which was primarily designed to study mortality and which clearly showed increased risk of mortality with increasing dose, confined itself to the study of current employees. This is likely to have resulted in an underestimate of the risk of acquiring significant radiological or functional abnormalities, which the authors concluded to be about 1 per cent for exposures between 100 and 200 million particles per cubic foot-year, a dose they estimated to be equivalent to about 200 fiber-years per cubic centimeter. Another important study, that of workers in asbestos cement manufacturing plants in the United States,[28] suffered from similar uncertainties of measurement, because of the need to convert from particle counts to fiber counts, and also was confined to current workers. This study found no clear evidence of a dose-response relationship for exposure below an estimated 200 fiber-years per cc. A third study, of a British asbestos textile factory, attempted to avoid these problems by studying workers who had left the industry as well as those remaining. In addition, for most of the period of exposure, measurements of asbestos were made directly as fiber counts.[29] An early

report of this research,[30] in which only current workers had been studied, suggested a 1 per cent risk of asbestosis for an exposure of 100 fiber-years per cc. However, the later and more complete follow-up used differing criteria for the response, from crackles alone to possible asbestosis (essentially, when the diagnosis was suspected by the factory doctor) to certified asbestosis (when the British Pneumoconiosis Medical Boards certified the disease on the basis of legal criteria, a situation in which mortality risks are known to be increased).[31] The relationships are illustrated in Figure 13–1. The authors concluded that in order for no more than 1 per cent of workers to develop possible asbestosis over a 40-year exposure period, the fiber concentration should be somewhere between 1.1 and 0.3 fibers per cc. They felt that this uncertainty could not be reduced until data on workers exposed to lower fiber levels become available.

Risks in Specific Occupations

A number of other investigations have examined risks in specific occupations involving exposure to asbestos. Many of these have involved exposure to more than one fiber type. Insulation workers have been studied extensively in the United States, where exposure has been predominantly to chrysotile and amosite, and have been shown to have increased mortality from bronchial carcinoma, mesothelioma, asbestosis, and some gastrointestinal neoplasms.[32] These increases in mortality only became apparent some 15 to 20 years after exposure commenced. Asbestos weaving has been studied in Britain[29, 30] and workers have shown an increased mortality rate related to exposure, mainly to chrysotile. However, where crocidolite was used in asbestos factories, a substantial increase also in the risk of dying of mesothelioma of both pleura and peritoneum was found.[33, 34, 35] Similar risks have been shown in the manufacture of asbestos cement and its products.[28, 36] Work in railroad repair sheds and dockyards, where exposure to crocidolite and amosite is likely to occur, has been shown to lead to increased risks, particularly of mesothelioma and asbestosis.[37–41] One study of a cohort of workers producing purely chrysotile papers and board has shown a relatively low risk of disease.[42] The risks associated with other, presumably low, exposures, as encountered in power stations and brake lining maintenance work, remain to be determined, though in the latter work, much of the asbestos may be converted to nonfibrous forsterite by the heat of friction.[43]

Nonoccupational Risks

Much public anxiety has been generated by reports that the effects known to occur from occupational exposure to asbestos may also result from nonoccupational and environmental exposure. Clearly, some people

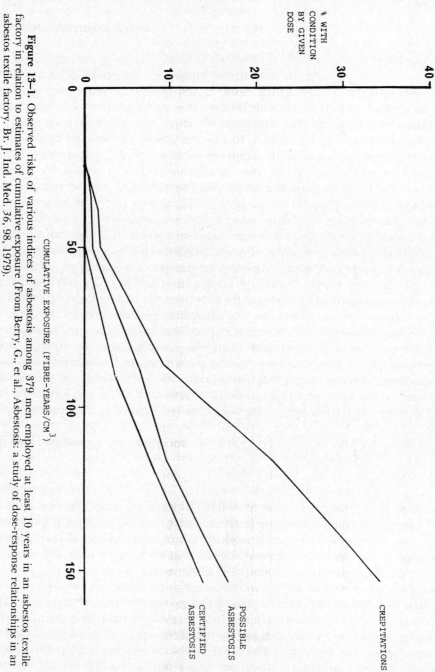

Figure 13–1. Observed risks of various indices of asbestosis among 379 men employed at least 10 years in an asbestos textile factory in relation to estimates of cumulative exposure (From Berry, G., et al., Asbestosis: a study of dose-response relationships in an asbestos textile factory. Br. J. Ind. Med. 36, 98, 1979).

Asbestos-Related Diseases

not using asbestos directly may nevertheless be exposed to relatively high doses, for example, other workers close to the site of asbestos spraying or stripping, housewives washing overalls, and people living next to asbestos mills and factories in which hygiene is unsatisfactory. It is reasonable to assume that such people run risks similar to those of workers. In the absence of such exposure, it seems unlikely that a measurable increase in risk of asbestosis, lung cancer, or mesothelioma is likely to occur. However, this statement needs qualification, since exposure to asbestos may occur but not be recognized. For example, it seems likely that large numbers of people are at risk of mesothelioma in parts of the Cape Province in South Africa because of environmental contamination by crocidolite mine waste.[44] Furthermore, it has recently been recognized that mesotheliomas may occur in certain parts of the world where fibrous minerals are found naturally in the rock and may be used for building and whitewash. Two such endemics have been described in separate parts of Turkey. In one, mesotheliomas and pleural plaques seemed to occur in relation to exposure to erionite, a very fine naturally occurring fibrous mineral[45, 46] (see Chap. 12, p. 314), while in the other, the diseases were related to the use of whitewash and stucco containing tremolite.[47] Such episodes point to the need for care and vigilance in the use and disposal of any material containing respirable fibers. Nevertheless, there seems little cause for anxiety in situations in which airborne asbestos levels are known to be low, as in public buildings,[48] or in which minerals containing fibers are dumped or erode from pipes into drinking water. In these latter cases, an increased risk of gastrointestinal cancer among the users has been feared. Specific studies, however, showed no excess risk where asbestos cement pipes have been used for delivering the water supply[49, 50] nor after cummingtonite-grunerite, a fibrous amphibole forming parts of the tailings from iron ore mining, was dumped in large quantities in Lake Superior.[51, 52]

How Common is Asbestos-Related Lung Disease?

In most countries it is impossible to provide anything other than a crude guess as to the prevalence or incidence of asbestos-related disease. Estimates have varied from the overconfident to the overcautious, depending on the bias of the writer. In Britain an independent, government-run insurance system covers all employed people and provides, among other things, disability and death benefits for people suffering from recognized occupational diseases. Asbestosis, defined by strict criteria including the presence of some disablement, and mesothelioma have been included in this list of occupational diseases since 1931 and 1966, respectively. While clearly many factors determine whether a worker or his widow seeks and obtains such benefit, and also bearing in mind that the total number of workers and ex-workers at risk of the disease is not known

and has undoubtedly altered as time has passed, these figures nevertheless give some idea of the overall risk of serious disease in a population of some 50 million workers in an industrialized country. They therefore put such diseases into perspective. Figure 13–2 illustrates the certifications for asbestosis since 1964. It can be seen that the level has remained fairly static, around 120 to 150 per annum. The same figure also illustrates the number of deaths occurring in Britain in which asbestosis was mentioned on the medical certificate; there is a suggestion that a peak of around 200 per year may have been reached. Finally, the figures for death certificates mentioning mesothelioma reveal a steep climb from around 150 in 1968 to over 400 by 1978.[53] It is to be hoped that these figures will show a slower rate of climb within the next decade, reflecting the much tighter control over the importation and use of crocidolite in Britain since 1970.

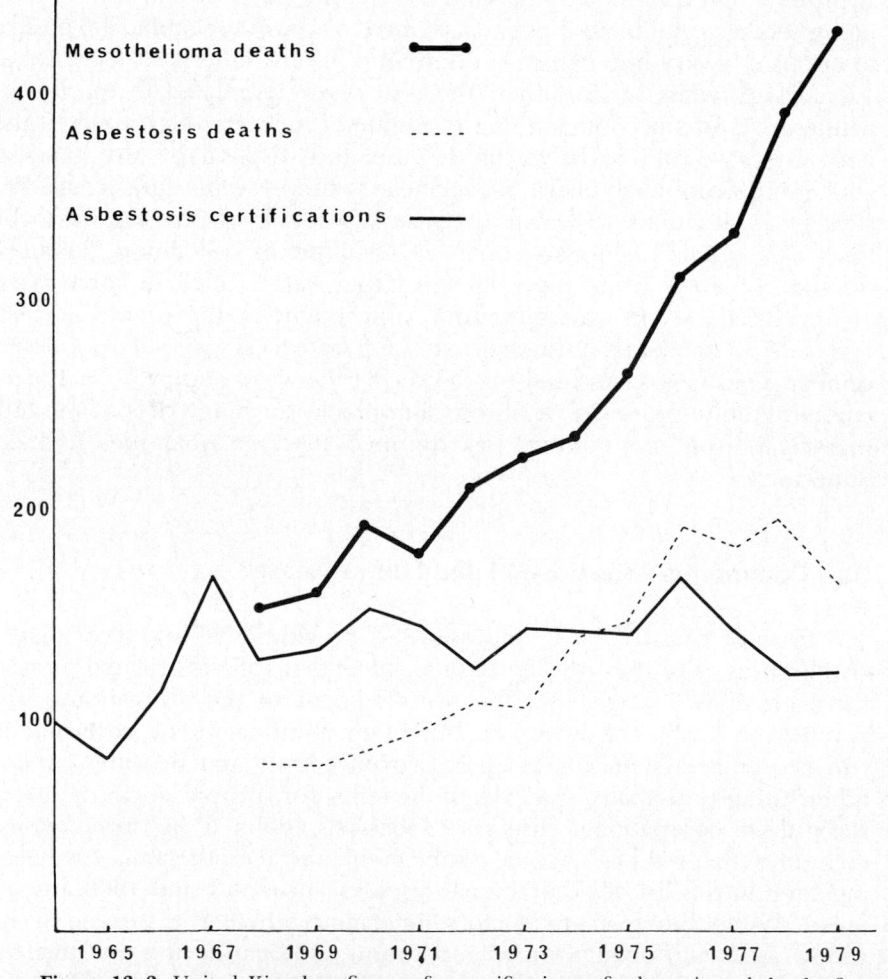

Figure 13–2. United Kingdom figures for certifications of asbestosis and deaths from asbestosis and mesothelioma, 1964–79.

Other trends in asbestos-related disease have been observed. After initial recognition of the disease, the average age of death from asbestosis in Britain was about 30 and this had risen to 41 in the 1930s and 57 by 1965;[54, 55] it is currently in the mid 60s. The prevalence of asbestosis after 20 years of exposure in one factory in Britain fell from 80 to 3 per cent between 1929 and 1957.[55]

It seems reasonable to suppose that through control of dust levels in the industry and medical surveillance of the work force at risk, together with reduced use of asbestos and increasing employment of substitute materials, asbestosis and asbestos-related lung cancer will become increasingly uncommon in the developed world. No such predictions can be made in the case of mesothelioma, except in countries where the use of crocidolite and amosite is to be abandoned.

ASBESTOSIS

Clinical Features

The initial symptom of asbestosis is shortness of breath on exertion, often accompanied by a dry cough. This symptom develops only after several years of progressive pulmonary fibrosis. The dyspnea progresses even when the patient is removed from contact with asbestos, usually resulting in the development of cor pulmonale and death within 15 years of the onset of the disease. In the later stages, cough, sputum, and loss of weight are frequently present and the patient is often subject to recurrent respiratory infections. Before the advent of chemotherapy, tuberculosis and bronchopneumonia were responsible for a high proportion of deaths among patients with asbestosis, but this is no longer the case. The complications of bronchogenic, gastrointestinal, and pleural neoplasms are frequent causes of death, the patient's pulmonary fibrosis making these tumors even less likely to be resectable than in otherwise well patients.

Though in many instances asbestosis will progress even after cessation of exposure, there is some evidence that very early detection may prevent progression to a serious stage of fibrosis.[56, 57] The early detection of the disease is therefore a matter of great importance. Among workers exposed regularly to asbestos, the disease might be expected to develop within 15 to 20 years, though this clearly depends on dust levels, cases having been recorded as progressing from first exposure to death within 10 years. In some occupations, such as spraying, an exposure of as little as three years may result in the development of asbestosis. The cornerstones of early diagnosis are clinical examination, chest radiography, and lung function testing, and all three have at times been claimed to provide the most consistent chance of early, presymptomatic diagnosis.

The first physical sign of asbestosis is the presence of repetitive end-inspiratory crackles in the dependent parts of the lungs.[58, 59] These aus-

cultatory findings are probably related to abnormal lung deflation[60-62] and are indistinguishable from those heard in other forms of pulmonary fibrosis. It is possible, though not proved, that the height of lung over which the crackles may be heard is an indication of the severity of the fibrosis. As the disease progresses, tachypnea, cyanosis, and frequently clubbing of the digits may be found.[63, 64] Movements of the chest wall may become restricted and latterly signs of cor pulmonale, with tall jugular "a" waves, a right ventricular heave, and epigastric third and fourth heart sounds may be detected.

Radiographic Features

The inhalation of asbestos is associated with changes both in the lung and in the pleura. There has been difficulty in the classification of the lung changes because they are predominantly linear and irregular, as opposed to the characteristically nodular changes found in silicosis and coal workers' pneumoconiosis. However, as a result of the suggestions of Bohlig[65] and Sluis-Cremer and Theron,[66] international agreement has been reached on an adaptation of the ILO classification to include the irregular and pleural lesions of asbestos exposure in a general classification of radiological changes in pneumoconiosis. The resulting UICC/Cincinnati classification and the latest version of the ILO classification (1980)[67, 68] are described in Chapter 5, and the symbols of this classification are used in the following description.

As in any diffuse lung disease, the earliest radiographic signs of asbestosis are undefinable and little interobserver agreement may be obtained on their presence or absence. Such fine, irregular, linear shadows are classified as 0/1 or 1/0 for profusion and as type s. Larger irregular and linear opacities are classified as t and so-called coarse blotchy lesions as u. Whether there is any pathological significance attached to the differentiation of these opacities is not known, but this classification does provide a basis for further epidemiological and physiological studies, and one such prospective study has validated them as predictors of mortality.[69]

Increasing profusion of the irregular shadows is indicated by an increased number up the scale from 1/0, 1/1, 1/2, 2/1, and so on, up to 3/+. At the stages between 2/2 and 3/3 the normal pulmonary vascular markings become obscured by the opacities. This classification avoids the use of terms implying pathological processes, such as fibrosis or honey-combing, and simply grades the film according to the size and profusion of the irregular opacities present. Standard films of the irregular opacities are available, and these are clearly necessary in order to achieve any form of international reproducibility.

Early evidence of asbestosis consists of linear shadows of varying thickness between less than 1 mm and 3 mm, most marked in the lower zones (Fig. 13–3). Increasing profusion of these markings results in a gradual obscuring of the vascular pattern and of the cardiac and diaphrag-

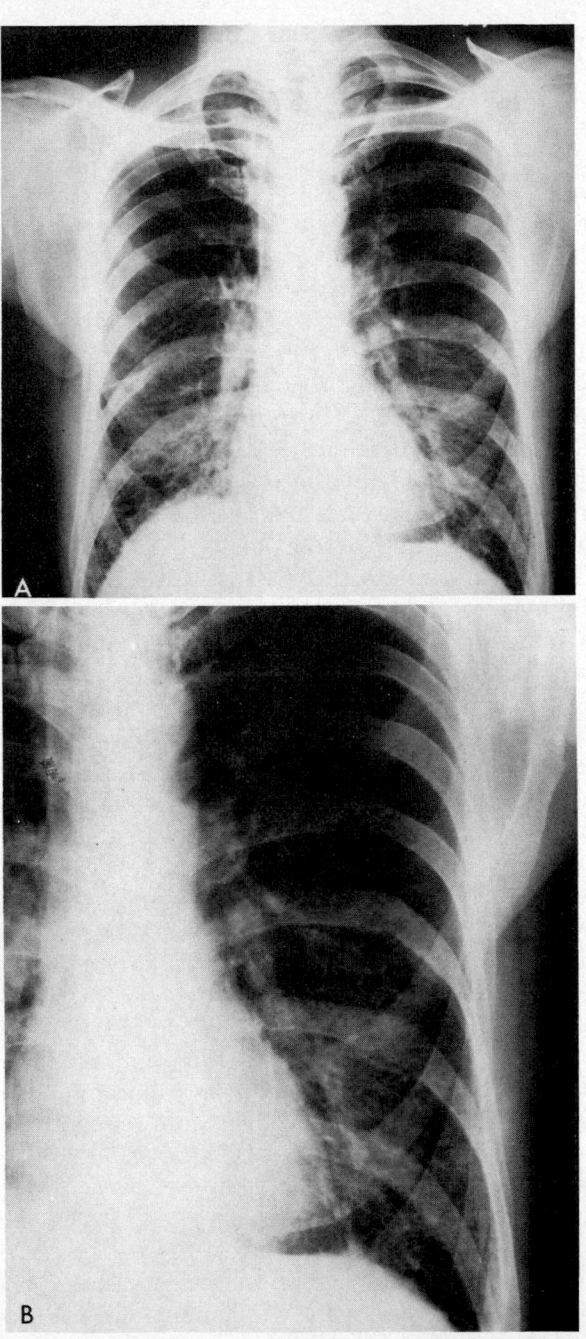

Figure 13–3. *A*, Chest radiograph of dock worker engaged for 20 years in repair work in ships' engine rooms, showing early changes of basal asbestosis and loss of volume, shown by depressed horizontal fissure, in right lower lobe. (Courtesy of Dr. J. Lyons.) *B*, Close-up view of left base of *A*, showing fine linear opacities of type S.

matic borders (Fig. 13–4). To a lesser extent nodular shadows may be present, and these may occasionally be the predominant opacity at an early stage. Ultimately there is a reduction in radiographic lung volume and the formation of cysts or honeycombing, combined with gradual increase in the cardiac size and dilatation of the proximal pulmonary arteries as cor pulmonale supervenes (Fig. 13–5). Throughout the course of the disease, with relatively few exceptions, the opacities are more profuse in the lower lung zones.

Only very occasionally do large masses, similar to those in complicated coal workers' pneumoconiosis, occur. In asbestosis, however, they have no particular predilection for the upper zones, being found in all parts of the lung.[70] The rare cases described in relation to rheumatoid disease have been basal in distribution.[71, 72] In the case of one of these patients, a follow-up report after his death 18 years later cast doubt on the role of asbestos in what appeared to have been widespread autoimmune disease.[73]

Additional radiographic evidence of asbestos exposure, though not necessarily of asbestosis, may be obtained from the presence of pleural thickening[74] and pleural calcification[75] (Fig. 13–6). Most characteristically, bilateral obliteration of costophrenic angles and calcification on the diaphragm and in plaques overlying the posterior ribs may be found in asbestos-exposed subjects. In some investigations, conducted in areas where there is a known source of asbestos exposure, pleural plaques demonstrated at autopsy have been invariably associated with asbestos bodies in the lungs.[75] However, other investigations in areas where there is less of an asbestos hazard have failed to demonstrate a greater frequency of radiographic pleural lesions in asbestos-exposed subjects than in the control population.[76] Clearly there are other causes of pleural thickening and calcification, such as previous empyema, hemothorax, or pleurisy. If these conditions have been excluded, asbestos exposure is the most likely cause of pleural abnormalities and this is particularly so if the changes are bilateral.[77]

As implied previously, the radiological appearances of asbestosis usually progress after exposure ceases, and in some cases may appear for the first time at this stage.[78] The rate of progression presumably depends on a combination of individual susceptibility and retained dose of dust in the lungs.[79]

Pulmonary Function

The characteristic functional abnormalities in asbestosis are progressive reduction in vital capacity and total lung capacity, a normal or sometimes slightly raised residual volume, and reduction in diffusing capacity for carbon monoxide. As the disease advances, an increase in minute ventilation and arterial hypoxemia occur. Increased static recoil pressures and a decrease in lung compliance may be found. Exercise tests show hyperventilation and arterial desaturation. These changes do not

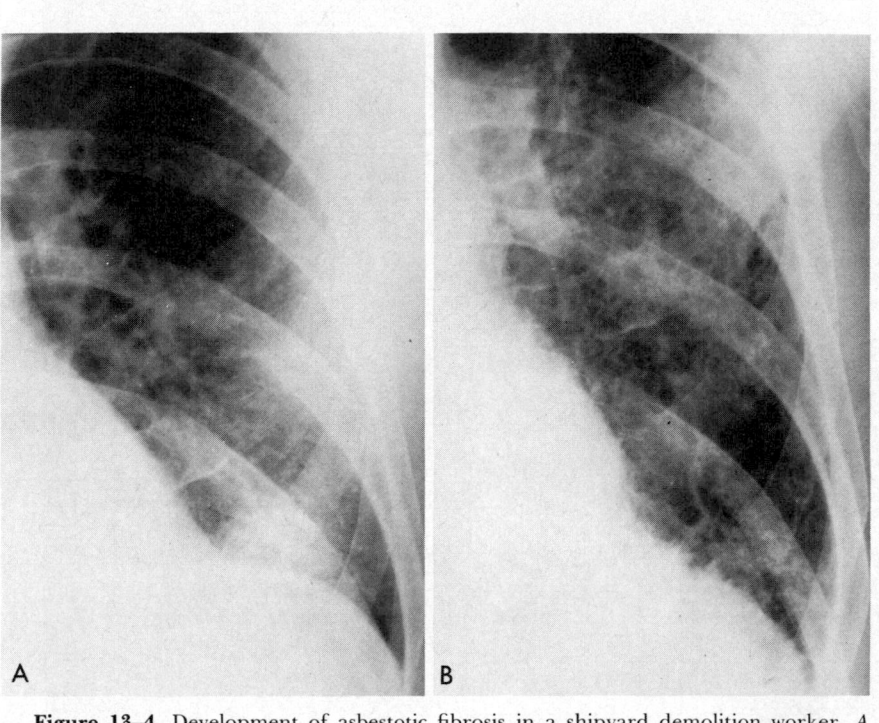

Figure 13–4. Development of asbestotic fibrosis in a shipyard demolition worker. *A*, Radiograph taken in 1967, showing only minimal linear and nodular changes at the bases. *B*, Radiograph taken in 1973, showing extensive basal fibrosis and honeycomb change. (Courtesy of Dr. J. Lyons.)

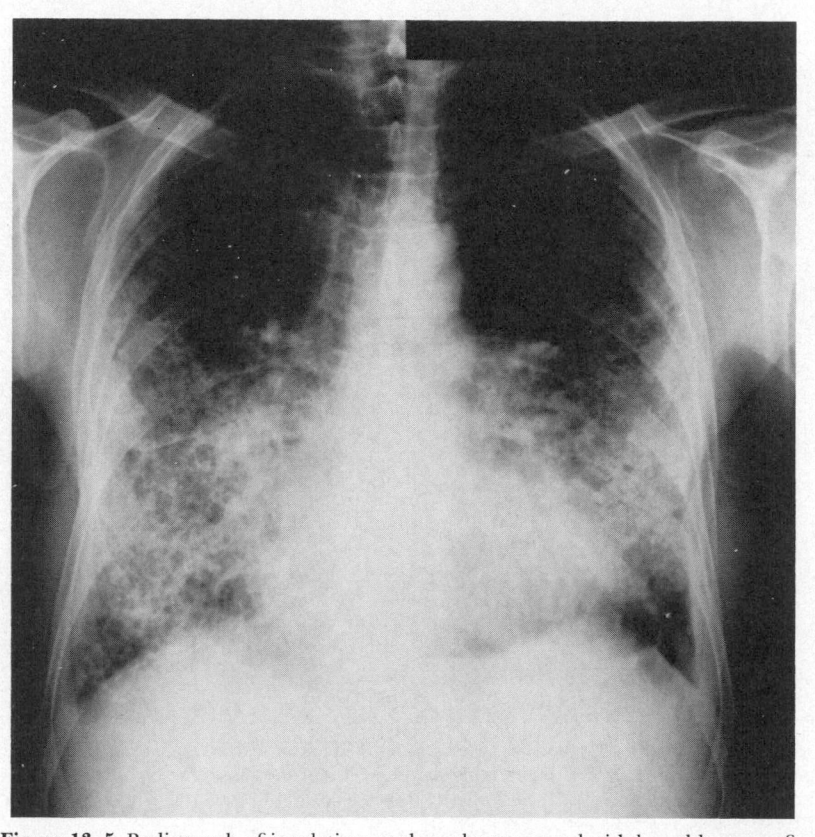

Figure 13–5. Radiograph of insulation worker who presented with breathlessness, finger clubbing, and evidence of cor pulmonale, showing advanced asbestos fibrosis, obliterated costophrenic angles, and calcification over right hemidiaphragm.

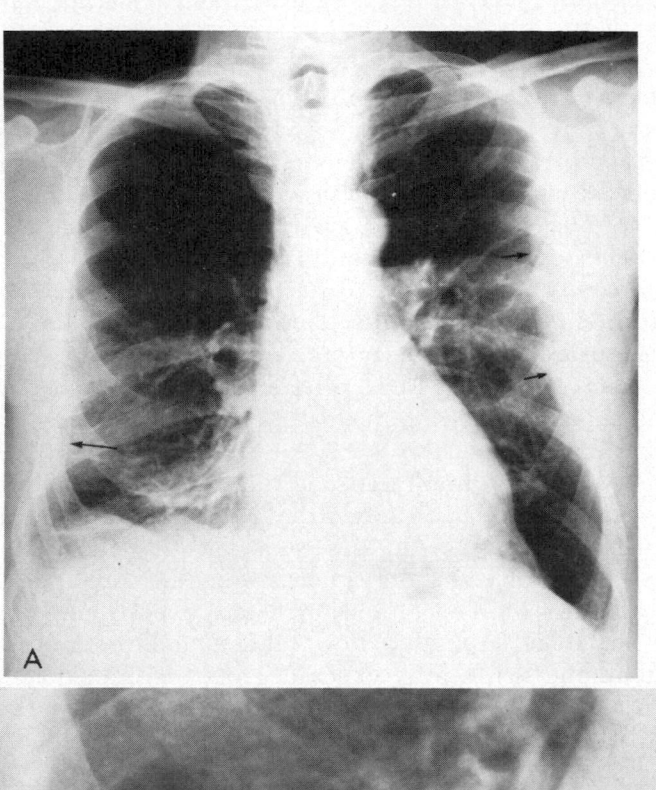

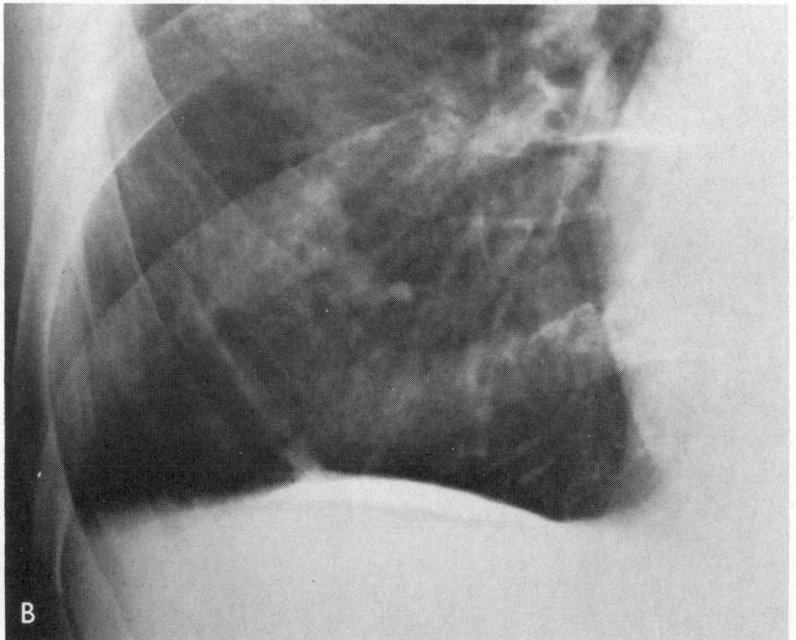

Figure 13–6. *A,* Large, noncalcified plaques (arrowed) in a shipyard worker exposed to asbestos. In addition, scant parenchymal asbestotic lesions are present. (Courtesy of Dr. J. Lyons.) *B,* Close-up view of the right lower zone of chest film of another subject. A well-delineated calcified pleural plaque is present on the right diaphragm.

differ from those found in other industrial and nonindustrial forms of pulmonary fibrosis.[58, 80]

More important than the functional definition of advanced disease is its detection at an early stage. Diffusing capacity seems to relate most closely to the degree of disability from asbestosis,[64] and attempts to detect the disease at a presymptomatic stage have concentrated on measurement of this and of vital capacity. Studies of lung function in relation to radiographic category[81, 82] have suggested that decrease in vital capacity and increase in exercise ventilation are the most sensitive tests. Those studies compared the steady state diffusing capacity with the vital capacity and found the former less sensitive, but since it is affected by hyperventilation, the steady state test may not be as useful as the single breath technique. In contrast, other workers have demonstrated a fall in diffusing capacity at an early stage of the disease.[57, 58] Fall in lung compliance parallels that in vital capacity.[82]

Detailed studies of lung mechanics[83] in asbestos miners with normal chest radiographs have shown a reduction in vital capacity and an increase in static lung recoil pressures in those subjects with the heaviest exposure to asbestos. These subjects still had normal single breath and steady state diffusing capacities. Moreover, the more heavily exposed miners in general had lower maximal expiratory flow rates at a given transpulmonary pressure than the less heavily exposed group, indicating an increased upstream airways resistance requiring a higher pressure to achieve an equal flow. This work is in line with pathological studies that show that the early lesions in asbestosis are around the respiratory bronchioles, where they might be expected to cause obstructive disease of the small airways of the lung.[84] Indeed, a study of 23 workers exposed to high levels of chrysotile over a period of only five months has documented the development of airways obstruction rather than restriction as the dominant initial response in both smokers and nonsmokers.[85]

The subject exposed to asbestos may therefore be expected to show a slight reduction in vital capacity and diffusing capacity and an increase in the static transpulmonary pressures at a relatively early stage in the disease process. Subsequent clinical deterioration will then be accompanied by further changes in these measurements, increase in resting and exercise ventilation, and decrease in total lung capacity. Arterial hypoxemia, initially on exercise and subsequently at rest, will appear, leading to the development of the complete picture of progressive alveolocapillary block and eventually cor pulmonale.

Pathology

The important pathological features of asbestos exposure are pulmonary fibrosis, the presence of asbestos bodies and fibers, and pleural plaques. In addition, massive fibrosis and chronic pleural thickening may be present, as may the complicating diseases, bronchial carcinoma and mesothelioma.

Asbestos Fibrosis

Macroscopically the appearance is of gray-white fibrosis, most extensive in the lower zones of the lungs (Fig. 13–7). Retraction of uninvolved bronchi and bronchioles may cause an appearance of honeycombing and sometimes bronchiectasis. Occasionally areas of massive fibrosis occur, and sometimes these cause retraction of and bullous formation in surrounding lung. This may be present in any part of the lung. The rounded nodules of Caplan's syndrome have occasionally been described[72, 86] and seem to occur in the lower zones. The distribution of the fibrosis predominantly in the lower parts of the lungs in asbestosis helps in the differential diagnosis,[87] most other forms of pulmonary fibrosis being either more generalized, as in fibrosing alveolitis, or predominantly in the upper zones, as in sarcoidosis, tuberculosis, and allergic alveolitis. Further help in the differentiation may come from associated pleural thickening and calcification. Occasionally, however, cases of mixed asbestosis and silicosis may be found, as in some South African miners, where the fibrosis may be misleadingly distributed mainly in the upper zones.

Microscopically, the earliest lesion in both human and experimental asbestosis appears to be an alveolitis in relation to asbestos fibers deposited in alveoli, principally around respiratory bronchioles (Fig. 13–8). These alveoli fill with large cells which electron microscopical studies have shown to be the phagocytic lung macrophages.[88] These cells, some of which disintegrate, become organized, at first by deposition of fibrin and subsequently by collagen formation. Initially the more peripheral air spaces are uninvolved but eventually the fibrosis spreads out into distal air sacs and alveoli. Eventually intrabronchiolar spread results in a widespread network of fibrosis through the lungs, more marked at the bases, with dilatation of the uninvolved small airways.[89] Histologically, massive fibrosis differs from the more usual type only in being more confluent and extensive.

Asbestos Fibers and the Asbestos Body

The feature that most obviously differentiates asbestosis from other forms of lung fibrosis is the presence of asbestos bodies. These structures are yellow-brown in color and measure about 20 to 150 microns in length and 2 to 5 microns in width (Fig. 13–9). They have clubbed ends and a segmented or beaded appearance.[90] They appear to develop, at least initially, within lung macrophages, where there is an aggregation of small, 60Å granules around the phagocytosed part of the asbestos fiber. These granules probably consist of ferritin.[88] In addition, under the electron microscope there appears to be deposition of a lighter and nongranular material on the asbestos fiber. The coating of ferritin forms clumps and may eventually produce a body up to 5 microns thick.[91]

Such asbestos bodies may be found in the sputum of people exposed to asbestos, though they do not necessarily indicate asbestosis. They may also be demonstrated to be present in a high proportion of normal lungs at routine necropsy,[92] by the use of ashed sections or special concentrating techniques, though routine hematoxylin and eosin staining reveals far

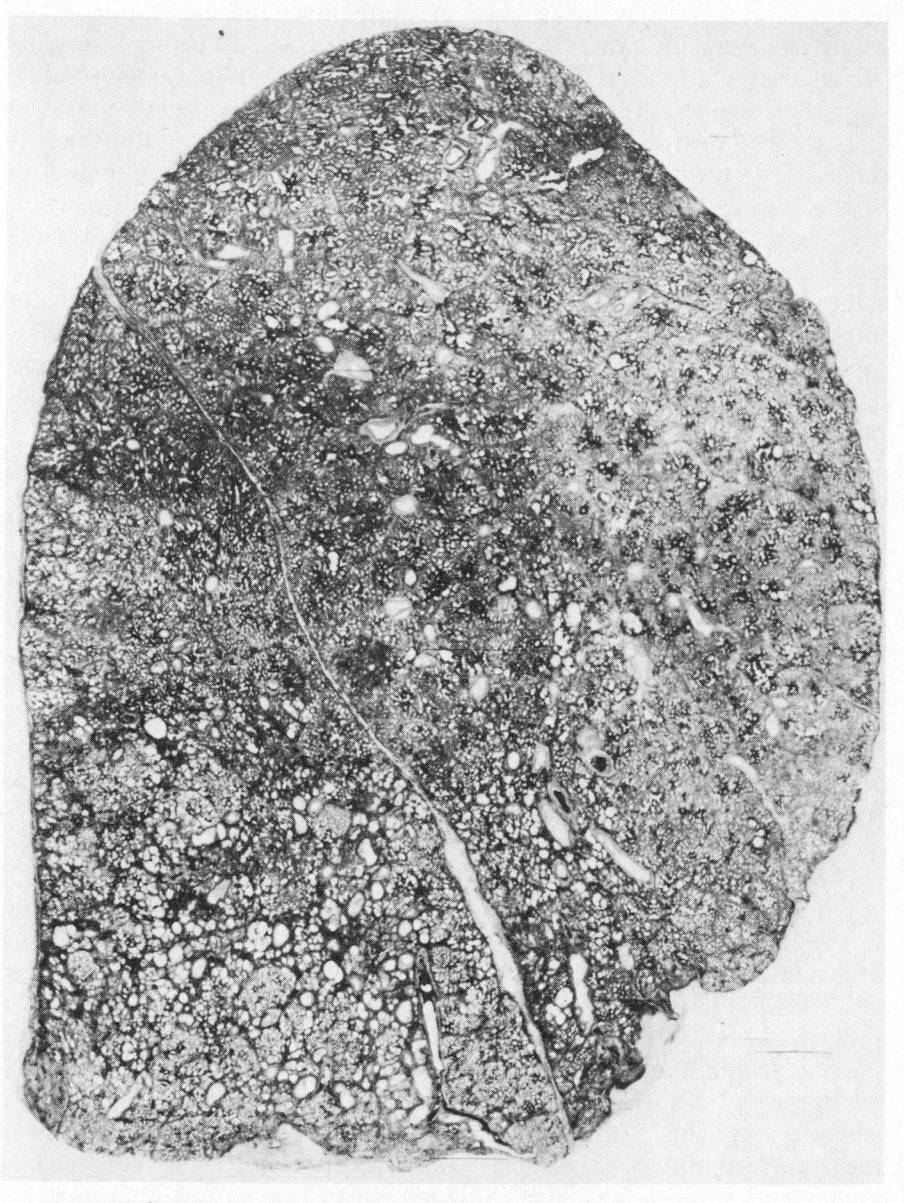

Figure 13–7. Whole-lung (Gough) section from patient with asbestosis, showing fibrotic changes and cyst formation in the lower lobe, with less marked changes in the lingula.

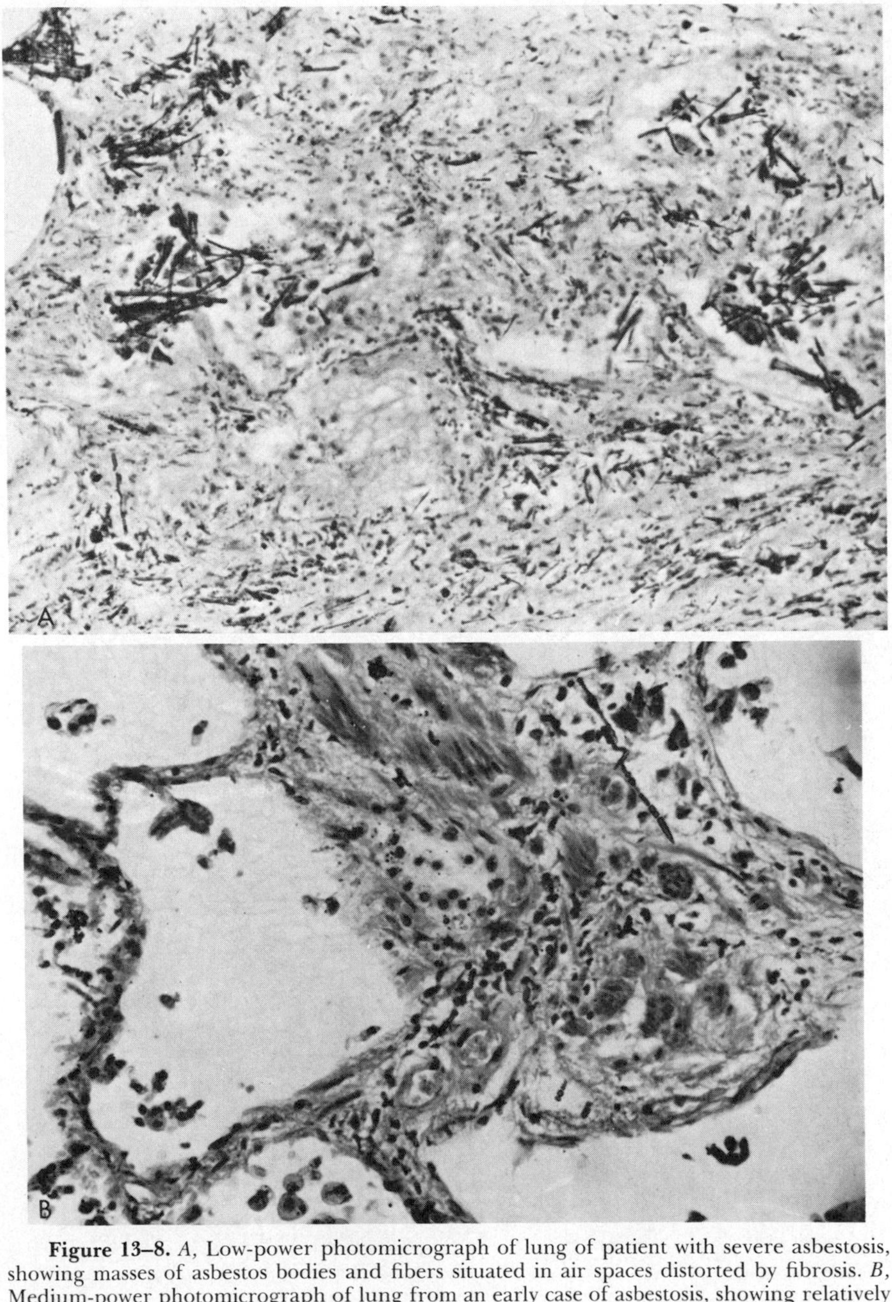

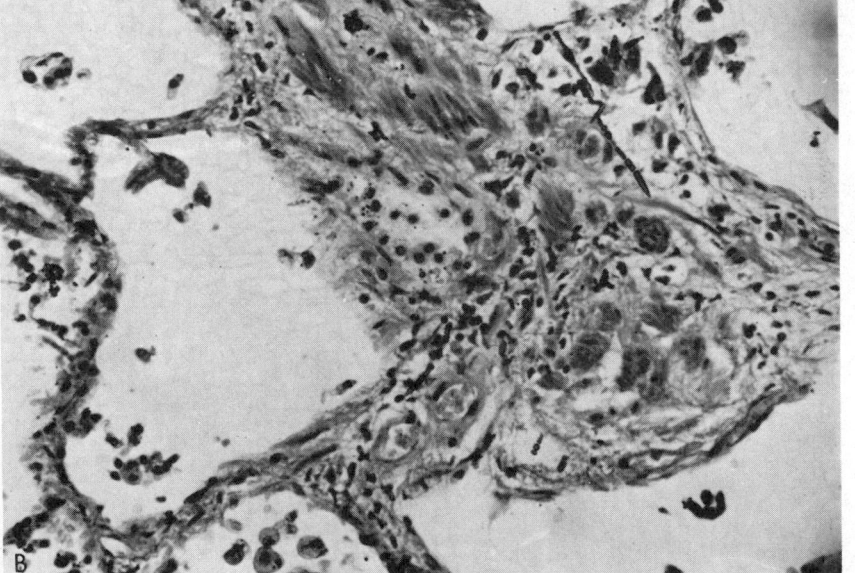

Figure 13–8. A, Low-power photomicrograph of lung of patient with severe asbestosis, showing masses of asbestos bodies and fibers situated in air spaces distorted by fibrosis. B, Medium-power photomicrograph of lung from an early case of asbestosis, showing relatively few asbestos bodies in a focus of interstitial fibrosis.

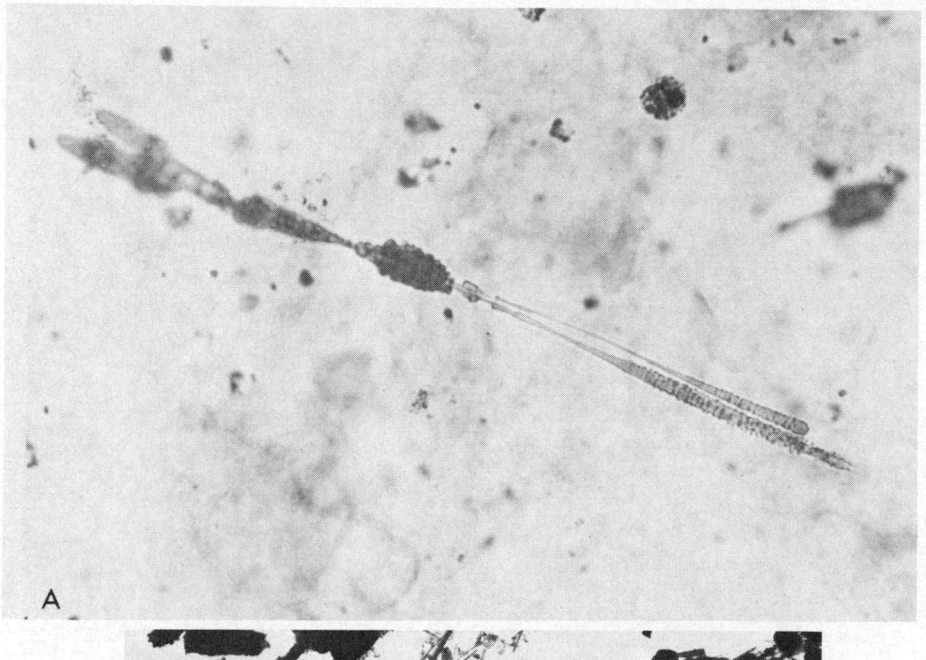

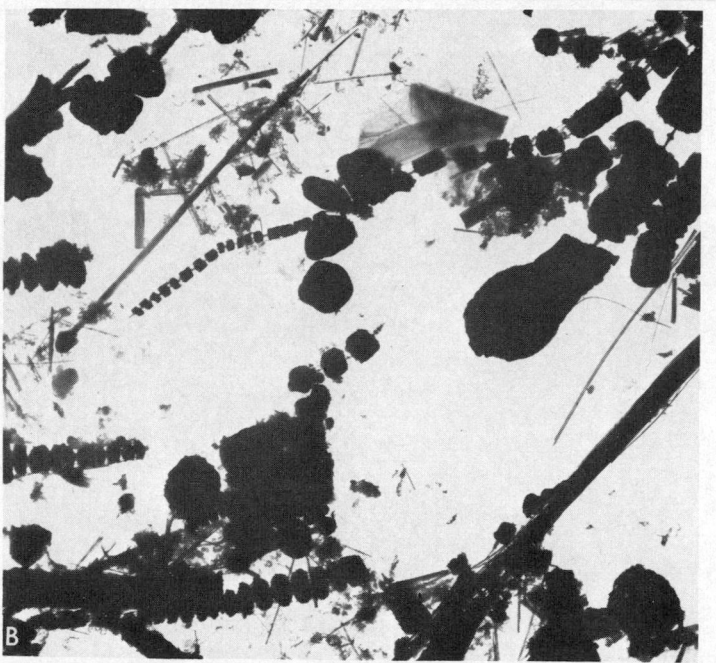

Figure 13–9. *A*, Two asbestos fibers, approximately 100 microns long, coated by iron-protein complex, from sputum of patient exposed to asbestos dust. *B*, Electron micrograph (×5000) showing asbestos bodies and fibers in lung tissue. Note the relative thinness of the fibers as compared to the bodies. Many fibers are seen to be uncoated, and their diameters would put them beyond the power of resolution of light microscopy.

fewer. There has been some dispute as to whether asbestos fibers invariably form the core of these bodies, as many other potentially respirable vegetable and mineral fibers may be found in the atmosphere.[93] However, electron microscopical studies with the use of microprobe analysis has confirmed that most such typical bodies do indeed contain asbestos, usually of the amphibole types, even in lungs obtained from the general population. Nevertheless, atypical or pseudo–asbestos bodies may form round a variety of other fibrous particles. It appears that in nonoccupationally exposed men, amosite and crocidolite most commonly form the cores of these bodies, while in women, tremolite, most likely from cosmetic talc, is found more frequently.[94–96] Asbestos bodies may also be found in other parts of the body besides the lungs, forming round fibers transported by lung lymphatics into the circulation.[97] Studies of the frequency with which asbestos bodies may be found in the general necropsy population have shown no increase over 30 years in New York,[98] though there is evidence of an increase in Britain in relation to a cumulative increase in asbestos usage.[99] These differences may be related to differences in the amount of bonded, as opposed to potentially free, asbestos constituting the increase in usage.

Histological studies in patients with asbestosis show asbestos bodies aggregated together in areas of fibrosis (Fig.13–8), and elastic staining can demonstrate that these were originally intra-alveolar.[89] Moreover, in areas of fibrosis, naked asbestos needles are also found, and are most easily demonstrated by polarized light. These average around 0.5 micron in diameter and 15 microns in length. Electron microscopy has shown them to be much more numerous than was originally suspected on the basis of light microscopy, and they can be shown in regions of fibrosis where asbestos bodies are not demonstrable (Fig. 13–9).[100] It is likely that the coating of fibers to form asbestos bodies renders them less liable to provoke fibrosis.[101] Experimental studies on guinea pigs show that inhaled asbestos dust causes fibrosis, whereas asbestos bodies do not.[102]

The use of an electron microscope reveals large numbers of asbestos fibers, even in the lungs of apparently nonexposed individuals. In one series from 21 urban dwellers, an average of 130 thousand fibers per gram of wet lung was found.[100] Most of these fibers are too small to form bodies or to be seen by light microscopy. Studies using light microscopy have shown that counts below 20,000 to 30,000 per gram dried lung represent the background level in people with no recorded exposure to asbestos, while counts above 100,000 can usually be related to a history of exposure.[104] Patients with mesothelioma usually have fiber counts of greater than 100,000 per gram dried lung, while in those with asbestosis the counts are usually over 3 million per gram.[105]

Management

In view of the irreversible and often progressive nature of asbestosis, it is clear that the objective of industry and legislators should be to prevent

the disease. There is no evidence that asbestosis is curable, though early detection may be consistent with a relatively benign course. Industry should therefore institute regular screening of the work force, aimed at removing workers with early signs of disease from further exposure. Once the disease has developed, treatment can only be supportive, using symptomatic oxygen therapy and a cardiac failure regimen in the late stages. Smoking should be discouraged in view of the very high risks of lung cancer in smoking asbestotics. Where it is available, the patient should be encouraged to claim industrial injuries benefit as partial compensation for his disability. If the disease can be shown to be a consequence of the negligence of an employer (and this is by no means always possible), the patient or surviving relative may be in a position to claim compensation under the law of tort (see Chap. 1).

CARCINOMA AND ASBESTOS

As stated previously, workers exposed to asbestos have an increased risk of developing bronchial carcinoma. This risk appears to be related to the exposure dose as well as to the type of asbestos, being greater among workers exposed to crocidolite and amosite than among those exposed to chrysotile or anthophyllite. The evidence suggests that there is an interaction between asbestos exposure and cigarette smoking. Selikoff and co-workers found no cases of bronchial carcinoma in nonsmokers, whereas the risk increased with increasing categories of exposure and cigarette smoking, such that a heavily exposed smoker had a risk 9 times that of a nonexposed smoker.[13] It has been calculated that the effects of the two carcinogens act in a multiplicative manner.[106]

Many studies have also shown an increased risk of other neoplasms in asbestos workers, though the risks differ in different studies.[107] There does seem to be an excess of intestinal carcinoma in some circumstances,[108] but the association of asbestos exposure with laryngeal carcinoma is dubious.[109]

Compared with bronchial carcinoma in the general population, the tumors occurring in an asbestos-exposed group seem to include an excess of the adenocarcinoma cell type. As both asbestosis and lung cancer are related to the exposure dose, the two occur together frequently. The percentage of patients with asbestosis who die of carcinoma has in fact risen from 17 per cent at the time of Merewether's report[9] to over 50 per cent.[110] However, it is possible that the carcinoma could develop before clinical evidence of asbestosis became apparent. Such cases may give rise to problems in deciding whether compensation is due, in life, to the subject and, after death, to his relatives. The presence of a history of exposure and radiographic features of asbestosis would be required in life, and, after death, the demonstration with relative ease of asbestos bodies or fibers and also asbestotic fibrosis. Clearly there is an ill-defined

borderland here, each case having to be decided on its merits (Fig. 13–10 and 13–11). Management of the carcinoma should be along standard lines. The presence of asbestosis will reduce the likelihood of resectability, but surgery probably remains the treatment of choice for all resectable tumors. Chemotherapy may eventually establish a place for itself in the management of oat-cell tumors, though to date it has only shown itself capable of prolonging life at a price of not inconsiderable side effects. In many cases, especially with oat-cell and epidermoid tumors, radiotherapy is the treatment required for symptomatic relief.

MESOTHELIOMA

In 1960, Wagner and his colleagues[14] from the North-West Cape of South Africa reported 33 cases of the rare pleural or peritoneal tumor, mesothelioma. The geographical distribution suggested an environmental factor, in particular, exposure to North-West Cape crocidolite asbestos. Cases were not found in the chrysotile or amosite mining areas of South Africa nor in the crocidolite area adjacent to the amosite deposits. Development of the tumor was not apparently related to the dose of asbestos inhaled, mesotheliomata being found in subjects with or without asbestosis, as well as in people who had been exposed in an environmental rather than an occupational setting. An interesting finding was the very long latent period, a mean of 40 years, between initial exposure and subsequent development of the tumor.

Shortly afterward, similar tumors were shown to occur in relation to asbestos exposure in Britain and the United States, as well as in the crocidolite-producing area of Australia. The relationship between mesothelioma and asbestos exposure has been investigated by two different epidemiological approaches. First, studies of populations of asbestos textile, shipyard, and insulation workers have shown a higher than expected number of cases, and second, surveys of patients with mesothelioma have shown that a high proportion give a history of asbestos exposure, albeit often for a short period, in the past. Elmes and Wade[111] found 45 cases of mesothelioma in Belfast, a shipbuilding and repairing area, and noted that there was a significantly higher exposure to asbestos among patients than among controls. Moreover, the lungs of 75 per cent of the patients, as opposed to 25 per cent of the controls, contained asbestos bodies. Most of these patients had been exposed to asbestos intermittently rather than continuously. Selikoff and co-workers[112] described 22 cases of mesothelioma, 6 pleural and 16 peritoneal, among New York insulation workers, the figure representing about 6 per cent of all deaths. It was shown that these workers would have had little if any exposure to crocidolite, since chrysotile and amosite had been used almost exclusively in the insulation trade. More recent work, discussed previously, has shown reasonably convincingly that there is a gradient from crocidolite to amosite to

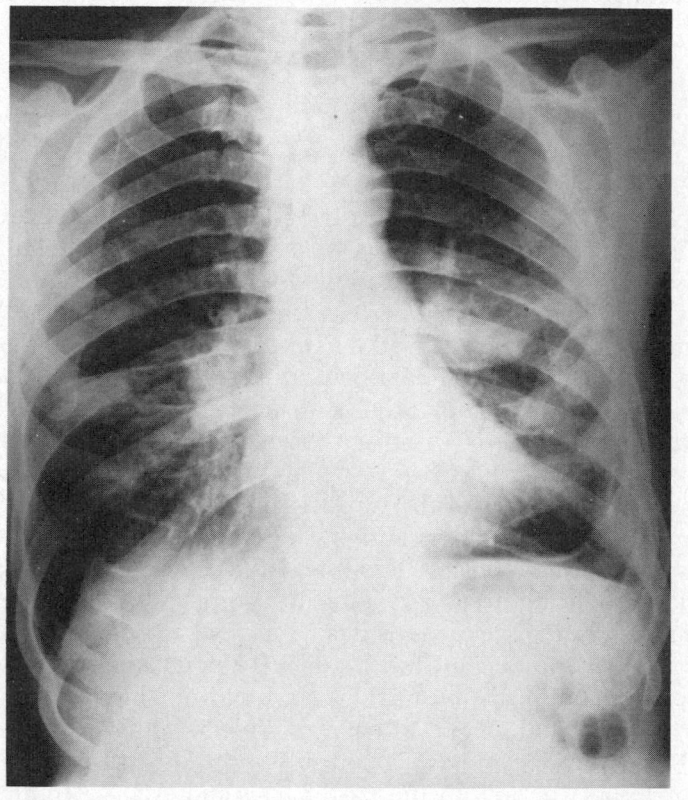

Figure 13–10. Chest radiograph of a man employed for 20 years in the steel industry. His job had involved frequent removal of asbestos lining from boilers and pipes, often in confined spaces. The radiograph shows a bronchial neoplasm in the left midzone, nodular and linear shadows suggestive of asbestosis in the lower zones, and pleural thickening at the left base.

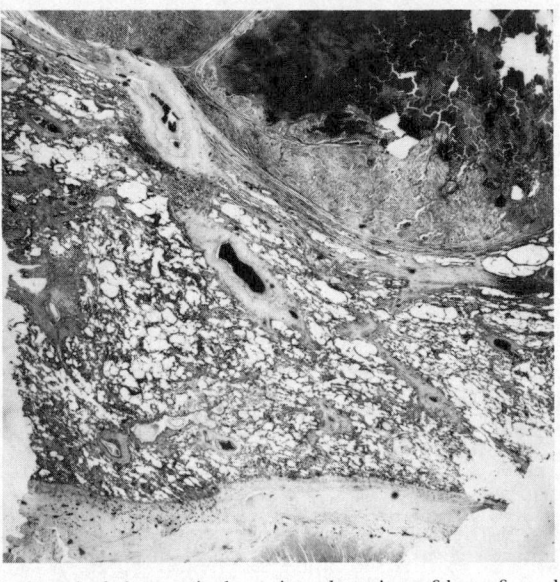

Figure 13–11. Two-inch by two-inch projected section of lung from left lower lobe of patient in Figure 13–10, showing (1) necrotic carcinoma at top right, (2) moderate degree of diffuse interstitial fibrosis, and (3) parietal pleural plaque of asbestos type at bottom. Large numbers of asbestos bodies were found. The patient was not diagnosed as having asbestosis in life, and whether the carcinoma, pulmonary fibrosis, and asbestos exposure were related is a matter for conjecture.

chrysotile in the potential to cause mesothelioma with crocidolite being the most dangerous.[112a]

In about 15 to 20 per cent of subjects with mesothelioma, there is no history of asbestos exposure. This, in addition to the occasional occurrence of mesothelioma in a child, is strong evidence that asbestos is not always responsible for the development of the tumor.

Clinical Features

The usual presenting complaints of patients with pleural mesothelioma are chest pain and breathlessness. The pain may be localized, often related to nerve or bone involvement, or of a diffuse generalized type.[113] It is as often of a dull, aching character as of a pleuritic type, but it may become severe. Virtually all patients complain of pain sooner or later, and it frequently becomes a most distressing symptom. The shortness of breath is progressive and is related to lung compression and restriction of respiratory movements by the tumor and associated pleural effusion. Mesothelioma of the peritoneum usually presents with diffuse abdominal pain, swelling, and loss of weight, but symptoms of obstruction of bowel or other organs may occur.

The findings on examination in the case of pleural tumor are the signs of pleural effusion, though frequently the mediastinum is pulled to

the side of the lesion rather than pushed the other way. In addition, tumor may be found growing through the chest wall to present as subcutaneous lumps. This is not uncommonly a sequel to pleural aspiration or thoracotomy, sufficiently so for repeated chest paracentesis to be ill advised. Clinical evidence of metastasis to other organs is rarely present, and the finding of this suggests that the pleural lesion is itself a metastasis from some other primary tumor, usually bronchial. Not uncommonly, however, local spread occurs to involve bones, lymph nodes, mediastinum, and pericardium, and thus enlarged supraclavicular nodes, rib tumors, superior vena caval obstruction, and cardiac tamponade are occasional findings. Peritoneal mesothelioma is usually detected clinically as ill-defined abdominal masses, and ascites is almost always present. This tumor may also spread into the pleural cavities, causing bilateral pleural effusions.

The diagnosis of mesothelioma is based on the findings of physical examination, radiology, and pleural aspiration and biospy. In all cases of pleural effusion a history of asbestos exposure should be assiduously sought. In many cases this will have occurred 20 to 40 years previously and will have been in a situation, such as in a dockyard or in insulation work, in which the use of crocidolite or amosite was likely. The differential diagnosis is usually between pleural metastasis, commonly from the lung, stomach, colon, breast, pancreas, or ovary, and tuberculous pleurisy. The latter, being treatable, should be excluded with great care, and if there is any doubt, antituberculous treatment should be given. Rheumatoid disease may also mimic mesothelioma, though rheumatoid pleurisy is more frequently bilateral and normally associated with the other features of the disease. In its earlier stages mesothelioma may be confused with any of the many causes of pleural effusion. Likewise, peritoneal mesothelioma is usually confused initially with one of many intra-abdominal syndromes, the diagnosis being made only at laparotomy.

The clinical course of mesothelioma is distressing for the patient and his or her attendants. Breathlessness and pain increase steadily in severity. Attempts to aspirate the effusion, which is often blood-stained, result only in its rapid reaccumulation. Extension of tumor through the thoracic cavity increases the patient's discomfort, as does involvement of mediastinal structures. The patient usually loses his appetite and weight. Fifty per cent of patients with pleural disease are dead within 12 months of diagnosis and very few survive more than two years.[113-115] The prognosis of the peritoneal tumor is, if anything, even worse.

Radiographic Features

Pleural mesothelioma presents either as a pleural effusion, a nodular pleural thickening, or more usually a combination of the two (Fig. 13–12). The lesion is almost always unilateral, a point of differentiation from rheumatoid disease, though in its later stages it may spread across the

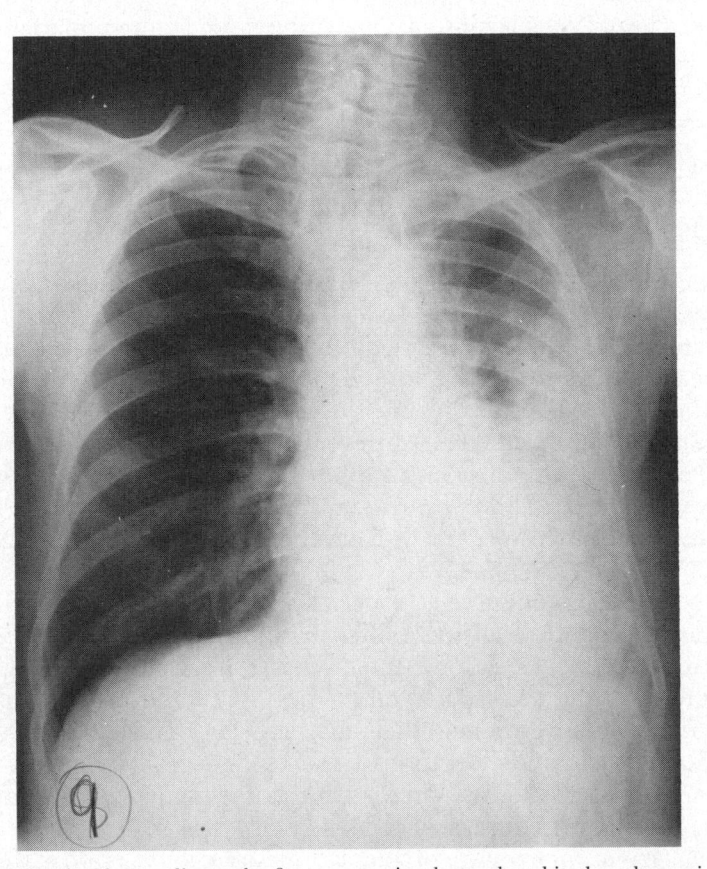

Figure 13–12. Chest radiograph of a man previously employed in the asbestos insulation trade. In addition to signs of a left pleural effusion, nodular peripheral shadowing is seen and the trachea is deviated to the left. Subsequent investigations confirmed the diagnosis of malignant mesothelioma.

mediastinum, and a peritoneal mesothelioma may spread through the diaphragm to both pleural cavities. Hydropneumothorax may occur, either spontaneously or as a result of aspirations, and when it does the collapsed lung and the under surface of the rib cage can be seen to be covered with thick nodular pleural deposits (Figs. 13–13 and 13–14). The fissures are often infiltrated (Fig. 13–15). The lesions are progressive and frequently the end result is an opaque hemithorax.

Occasionally other radiographic evidence of exposure to asbestos is present. Pleural calcification may be visible, as may the pulmonary lesions of asbestosis. The tumor itself may infiltrate the lung, producing large nodular lesions, while invasion of hilar and paratracheal nodes may make these structures visible radiographically. In these circumstances differentiation from primary bronchial carcinoma may be very difficult.

Pathology

The pathologist is usually first presented with aspirated pleural fluid. This may or may not be blood-stained. Cytologic examination of the fluid is sometimes helpful when carried out by a pathologist with considerable experience with the disease. Normal mesothelial cells do, however, have a reputation for looking malignant to the inexperienced. Electron microscopy may be helpful in their differentiation.[116] Hyaluronic acid may be found, and if so, this is strong supporting evidence for the diagnosis.[117] However, this is not always present, and since it may occasionally be found in pleural effusions associated with other tumors, it is not a pathognomonic finding.[118]

Pleural biopsy specimens, especially those obtained by needles, may be difficult to interpret owing to the variable histology of mesotheliomata. Increasing experience with the tumor can, however, lead to a high degree of diagnostic accuracy. In general, if the clinical and histological appearances are suggestive of mesothelioma, it is ill advised to repeat pleural biopsies and aspiration because of the tendency of the tumor to grow along needle tracks. For the same reason thoracotomy is highly undesirable as a diagnostic procedure.

The gross appearance of pleural mesothelioma is of a thick gray-white mass of tumor encasing the lung (Fig. 13–16). It often appears to have originated in the visceral pleura and may appear to be multicentric in development. Thomson[119] recognizes two types. The more frequent scirrhous type is harder and less bulky, and has more of a tendency to spread by lymphatics and occasionally by the blood stream. The encephaloid type is softer and presents as large tumor masses compressing the lung. Both types have a marked tendency to invade local mediastinal and chest wall structures as well as to infiltrate the diaphragm and, through it, the liver and peritoneum (Fig. 13–17). Spinal spread is often found if looked for. The lung is invaded either directly, into peripheral alveolar spaces, or by spread into septal and perivascular lymphatics, leading to

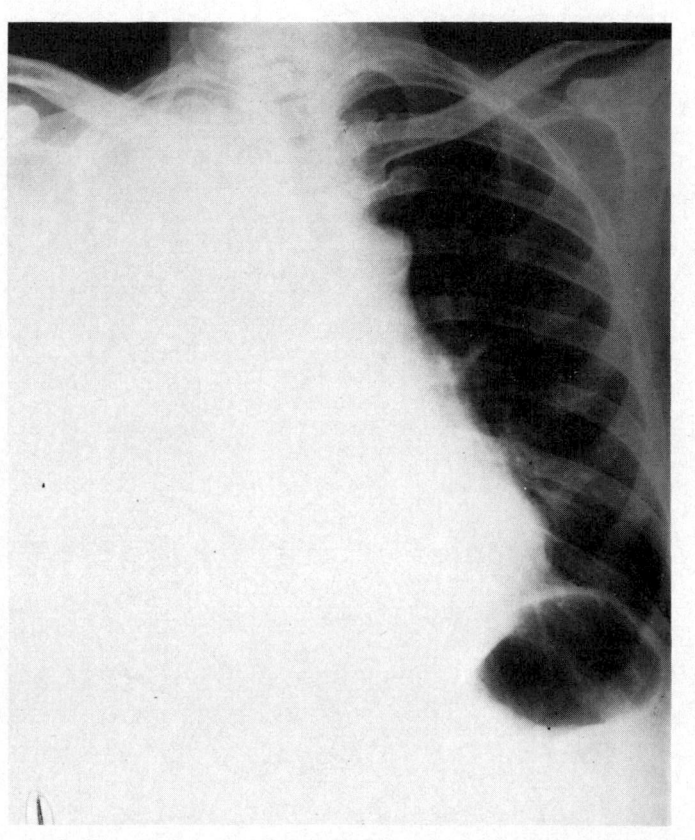

Figure 13–13. Chest radiograph of a man who had worked for 30 years as a marine engineer, with intermittent slight exposure to asbestos lagging in ships' engine rooms, showing massive right pleural effusion.

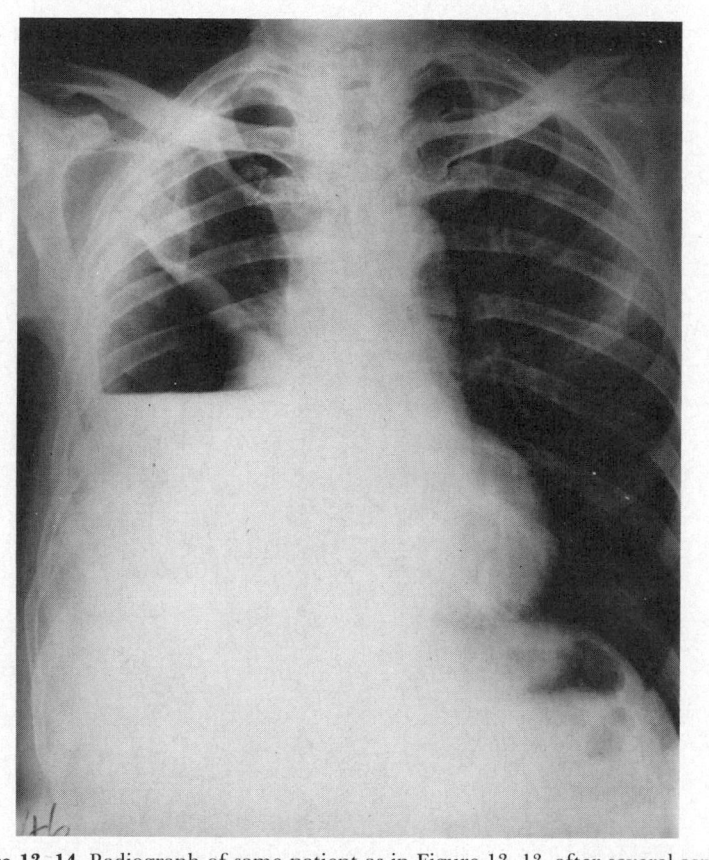

Figure 13–14. Radiograph of same patient as in Figure 13–13, after several aspirations, showing hydropneumothorax with tumor forming a layer over the collapsed lung and beneath the chest wall. This patient lived 10 months from presentation to death from malignant mesothelioma.

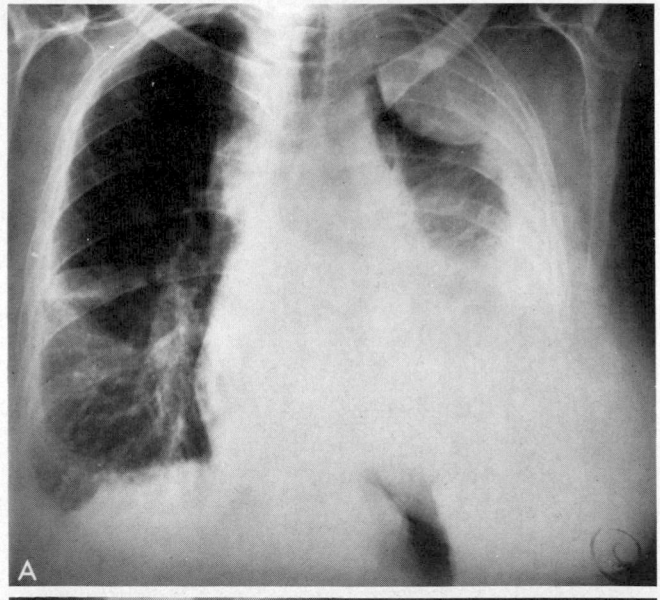

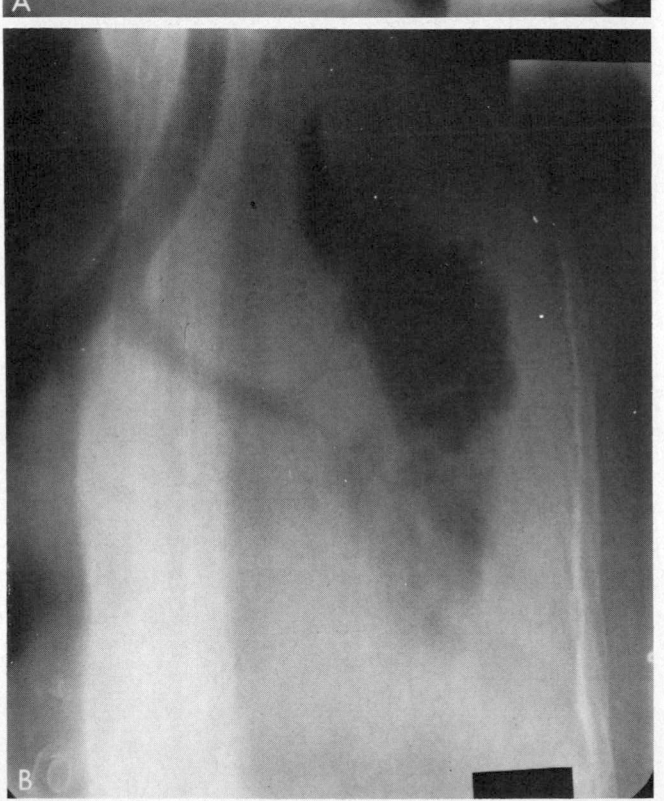

Figure 13–15. *A,* Radiograph of 60-year-old woman who denied any exposure to asbestos, either occupationally or environmentally. Nevertheless, large numbers of asbestos bodies and typical asbestos-type pleural plaques were found at autopsy, after her death from malignant mesothelioma. *B,* Tomogram showing tumor masses encasing left lung and compressing lobar bronchi.

Illustration continued on following page

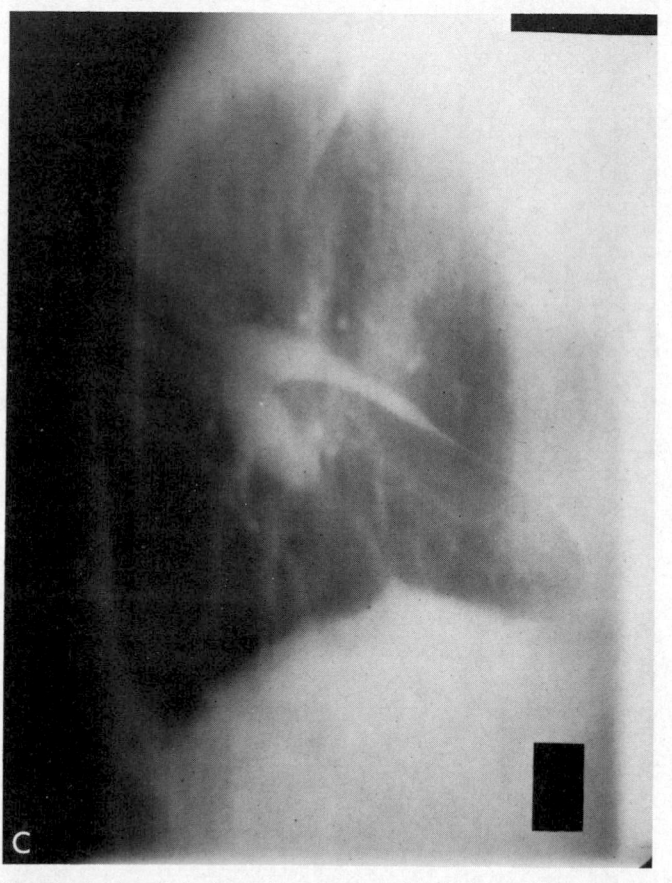

Figure 13–15 *(Continued). C,* Lateral tomogram of right lung. This tumor spread across the upper mediastinum, causing superior vena caval obstruction, and infiltrated the fissures in the right lung.

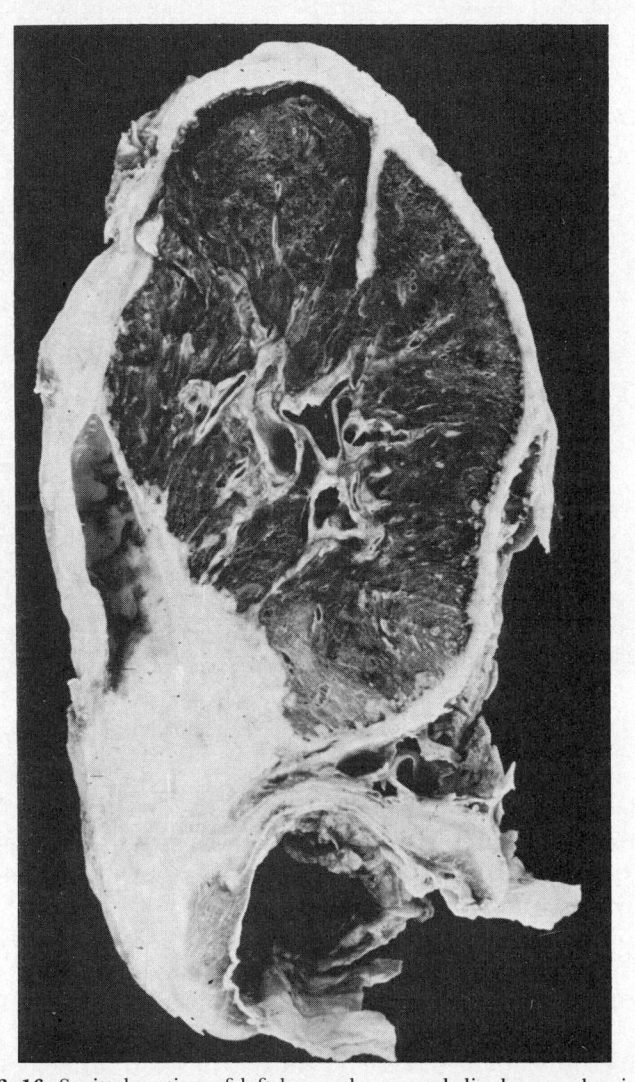

Figure 13–16. Sagittal section of left lung, pleura, and diaphragm showing symphysis of both pleural layers by a malignant mesothelioma. The fissure and diaphragm are also involved.

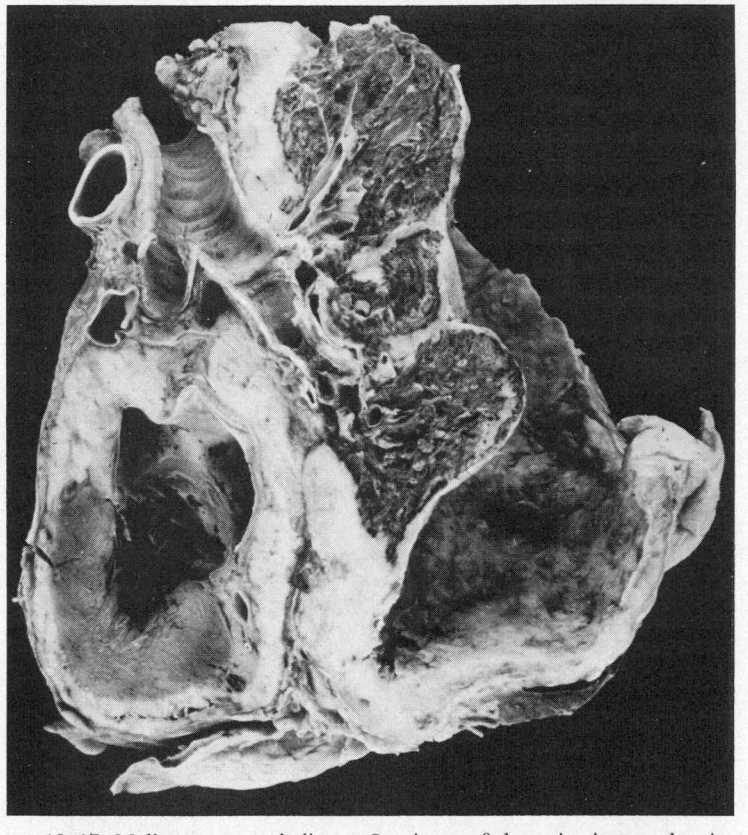

Figure 13–17. Malignant mesothelioma. Specimen of thoracic viscera, showing a loculated pleural effusion on the right, extensive tumor invasion of parietal and less of visceral pleura, and extension of the tumor around the pericardium.

hilar node involvement in some cases. Distant metastasis, though rarer than in bronchial carcinoma, does occasionally occur, blood-borne deposits having been described in brain, liver, lung, kidneys, and adrenals.[119] These are usually relatively few in number.

Peritoneal mesothelioma spreads more by direct invasion than by lymphatic or blood-borne metastasis.[120] This tumor may, however, spread through the diaphragm and cause bilateral pleural and pulmonary infiltration.

The mesothelial cell has the potential to develop either as an epithelial-like lining cell or as a mesenchymal stromal cell. Histological examination may therefore reveal either or both of these cell types.[118, 121] Most commonly both are present, though usually separated in different parts of the tumor mass. The epithelial cells are usually cuboidal or flattened, with uniform, often vacuolated nuclei. The cells tend to form tubular and papillary structures, separated by a matrix that varies both in abundance and in cellular content, from closely packed spheroidal cells to fibrous

tissue (Fig. 13–18). In some of these tumors it may be possible to demonstrate an acid mucopolysaccharide that can be removed by prior digestion of the tissue with hyaluronidase. This feature, together with a negative periodic acid–Schiff reaction may help in differentiation of the tumor from adenocarcinoma.[122]

The mesenchymal type of mesothelioma appears as a spindle cell sarcoma, though sometimes containing clefts and also areas of epithelial and tubular structure (Fig. 13–19). The mixed type of tumor may often consist of large masses of collagen arranged in bundles or in a complex network. Clefts are often present and these are lined by tumor cells. Areas of both epithelial and spindle cell types may be found in different parts of the lesion. It is this variability of the histological pattern that is the most characteristic feature of mesothelioma.

Management

Curative treatment of mesothelioma has been uniformly unsuccessful. In spite of expressions of enthusiasm by some radiotherapists and oncologists, neither radiation nor chemotherapy can be recommended at present for either attempts at cure or palliation. There is, however, a case for carefully controlled clinical trials.[123, 124] A few patients have survived several years after surgical excision of an early lesion,[125, 126] though in most instances thoracotomy has revealed a tumor well beyond resection. Some

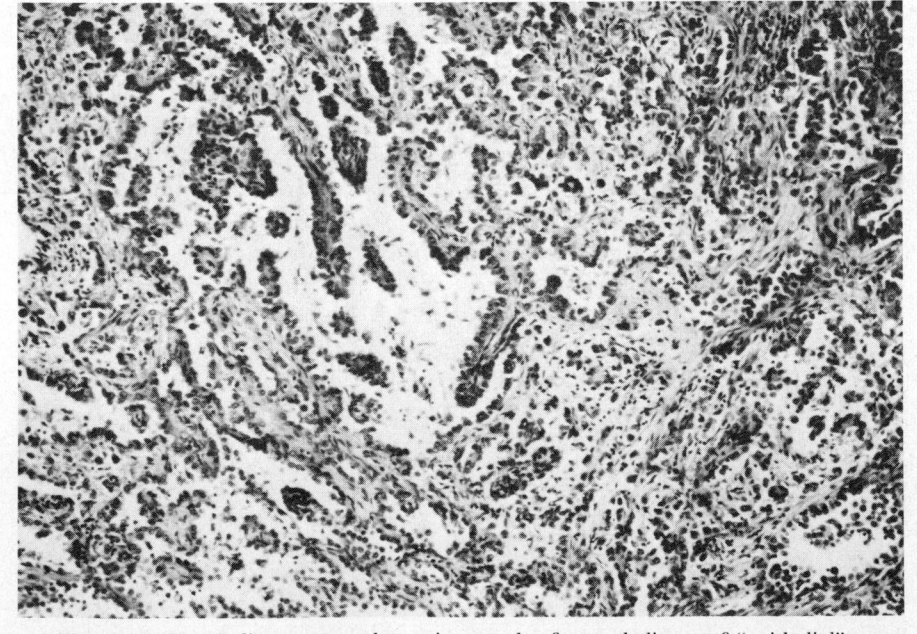

Figure 13–18. Medium-power photomicrograph of mesothelioma of "epithelial" type, showing the tubopapillary structure.

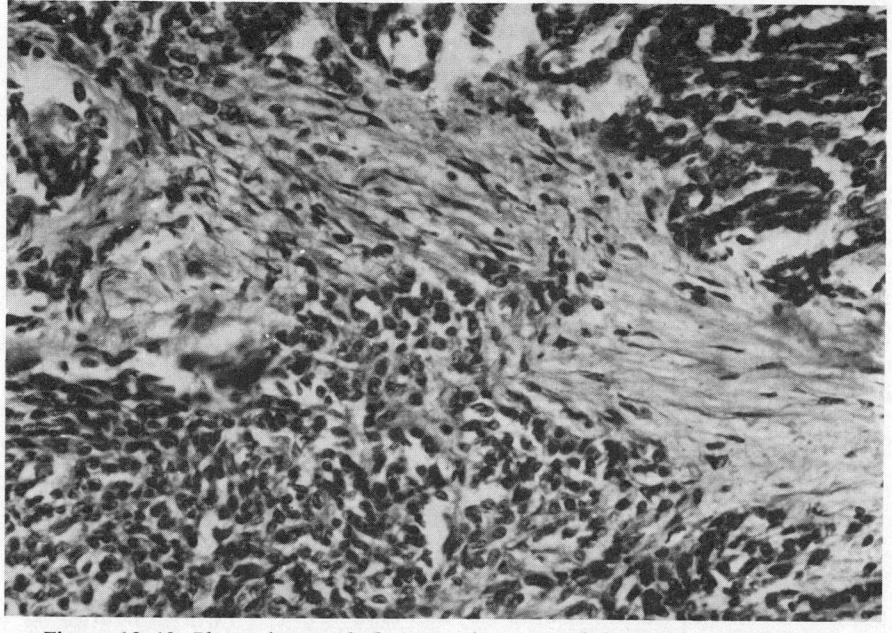

Figure 13–19. Photomicrograph from another part of the same mesothelioma as in Figure 13–18, showing a point of transition from the tubopapillary area (top right) to a sarcoma-like area below.

evidence suggests that the epithelial type of tumor, when resected at an early stage while still encapsulated by the parietal pleura, may respond better than others.[126] Most studies of surgical treatment, however, report a high operative mortality and very low five-year survivals.

Bearing these matters in mind, the humane physician will usually consider that the risks and side effects of aggressive treatment in most cases outweigh the rather dubious potential benefits. All treatment should be planned on the merits of the individual case, but in most, management will consist of appropriate use of analgesics, given sufficiently frequently to keep pain at bay, antidepressants, and aspiration of pleural effusion. Since the tumor has a tendency to grow along chest wall incisions and occasionally needle tracks, the latter should be kept to a minimum. With this in mind, measures to prevent reaccumulation of fluid are worth a trial, and the use of *Corynebacterium parvum* for this purpose holds considerable promise as an effective and relatively nontoxic method.[127, 128]

PLEURAL PLAQUES

The pleural plaques associated with asbestos exposure have a characteristic distribution. They are found on the parietal pleura and tend to be more frequent on the posterolateral and basal parts and on the central tendon of the diaphragm, where they appear as shiny, smooth, raised

yellowish areas (Fig. 13–20). They are distributed particularly beneath the surfaces of the ribs, whence they spread out over the intercostal spaces. Their characteristic radiological appearances have previously been described (Fig. 13–6).

Histologically, pleural plaques consist of fibers of collagen arranged parallel to the pleural surface, giving a basket-weave appearance. The deeper layers contain some fibroblasts and sometimes a few lymphocytes and plasma cells (Fig. 13–21). Calcification, when present, occurs in the center of the plaque on degenerated collagen and is probably related to the age of the lesion. Asbestos bodies are not found in plaques, though fibers have occasionally been seen.

Pleural plaques are covered with an intact layer of mesothelium, though this is not usually visible in necropsy specimens. Careful studies have shown that they are not associated with mesothelial proliferation, suggesting that when such changes are found in needle biopsies, the possibility of adjacent malignant disease should be suspected.[129]

Pleural plaques are a benign condition, indicating exposure to asbestos in the past. They probably occur more frequently after exposure to amphiboles than to chrysotile, since they do not occur frequently in all parts of Quebec.[130] They should not be taken to imply any more serious disease and should not prompt further investigation or follow-up, which will only needlessly alarm the patient. They can be regarded as a mild reaction to fibers that have reached the pleura by piercing lung tissue

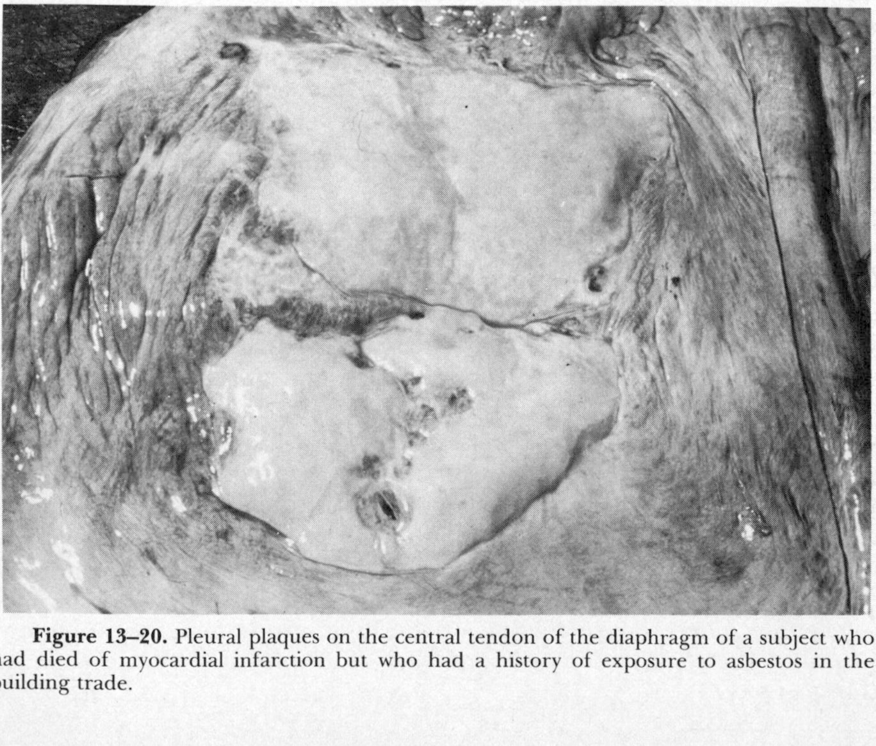

Figure 13–20. Pleural plaques on the central tendon of the diaphragm of a subject who had died of myocardial infarction but who had a history of exposure to asbestos in the building trade.

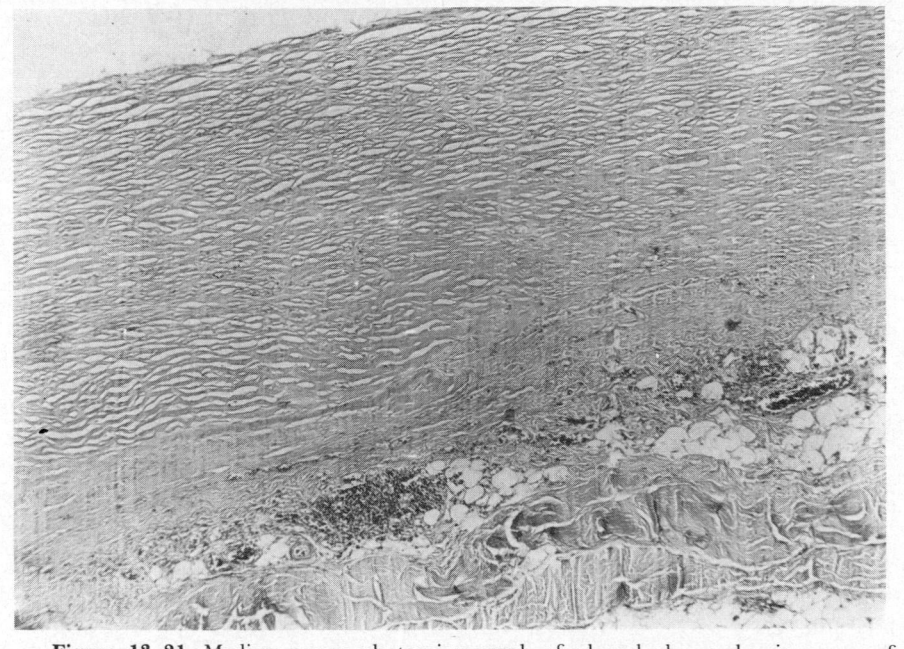

Figure 13–21. Medium-power photomicrograph of pleural plaque showing rows of collagen fibers lying parallel to the surface. The deeper layers contain a few lymphocytes and plasma cells.

under the influence of mechanical forces within the lung and lymphatic drainage in the parietal pleura.[131] It is likely that the aerodynamic properties of asbestos fibers also play a role in determining whether they reach the pleura and whereabouts in that tissue they will be deposited. They become arrested only when they reach impenetrable tissue such as bone or the central tendon of the diaphragm, where they set up a mild inflammatory reaction that leads to fibrosis.

OTHER PLEURAL CONDITIONS

Aside from plaques and mesothelioma, a number of other pleural syndromes may be seen in asbestos-exposed individuals.[132] Bilateral obliteration of the costophrenic angles is a frequent finding and is usually associated with pleural plaques elsewhere. Diffuse fibrosis of the visceral pleura often accompanies asbestosis and may also be a sequel to asbestos pleural effusion. This latter event may result in extensive irregular pleural calcification (Fig. 13–22). Thickening of the parietal pleura in the interlobar fissures may be an isolated response to asbestos exposure or may occur with other radiological signs.[132] Occasionally, diffuse visceral pleural thickening may produce folding of the lung, giving a radiographic appearance that mimics tumor[133] and that often provokes an unnecessary thoracotomy.

From a practical point of view, the most troublesome nonmalignant pleural syndrome is asbestos pleural effusion.[134, 135] This condition occurs in people currently working with asbestos and often appears within 10 years after beginning to work with asbestos. While it may be asymptomatic, in many cases it is associated with pleuritic pain and occasionally with fever or dyspnea. The effusion is usually small and commonly blood-stained, and a leukocytosis and raised sedimentation rate may be present. Understandably it always causes anxiety lest it be a mesothelioma. Tuberculous, carcinomatous, and rheumatoid effusions also need to be considered in the differential diagnosis. It occasionally recurs, often on the other side, and it may progress to diffuse pleural thickening after the fluid has been absorbed (Fig. 13–23). This in turn may cause a restrictive lung function defect sufficient to require treatment by pleurectomy.[136]

It does not seem likely that any of these pleural diseases predisposes to the development of mesothelioma, and relatively limited follow-up of such patients has not shown such a risk.[135] However, it is reasonable to suppose that individuals with one type of asbestos-related disease must be

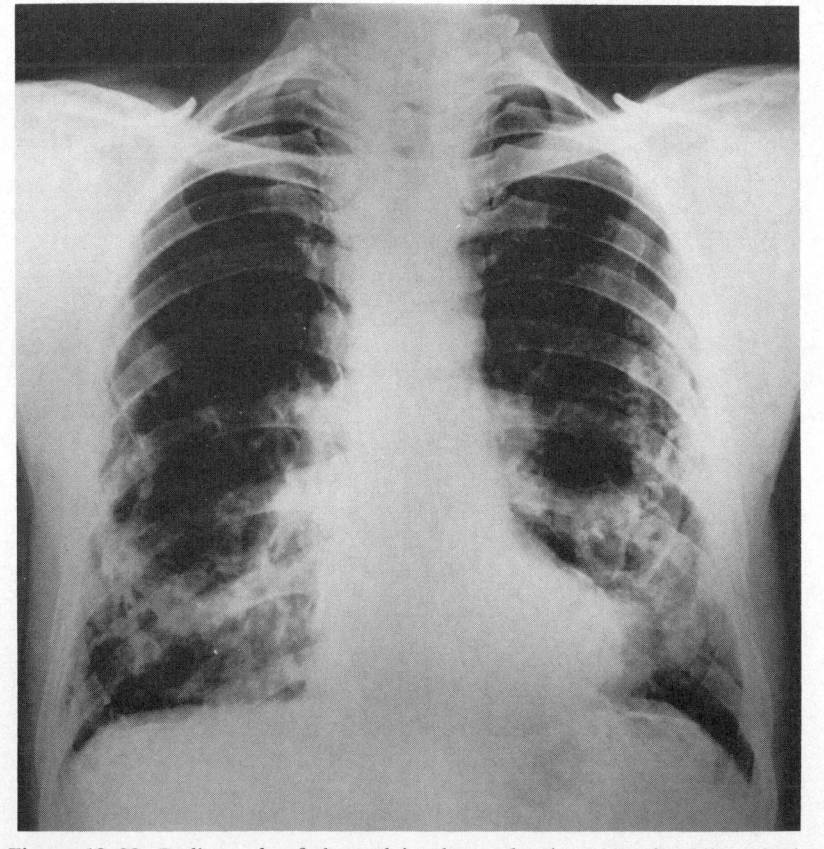

Figure 13–22. Radiograph of thermal insulator, showing extensive bilateral pleural calcification which was associated with a reduction in vital capacity and total lung capacity.

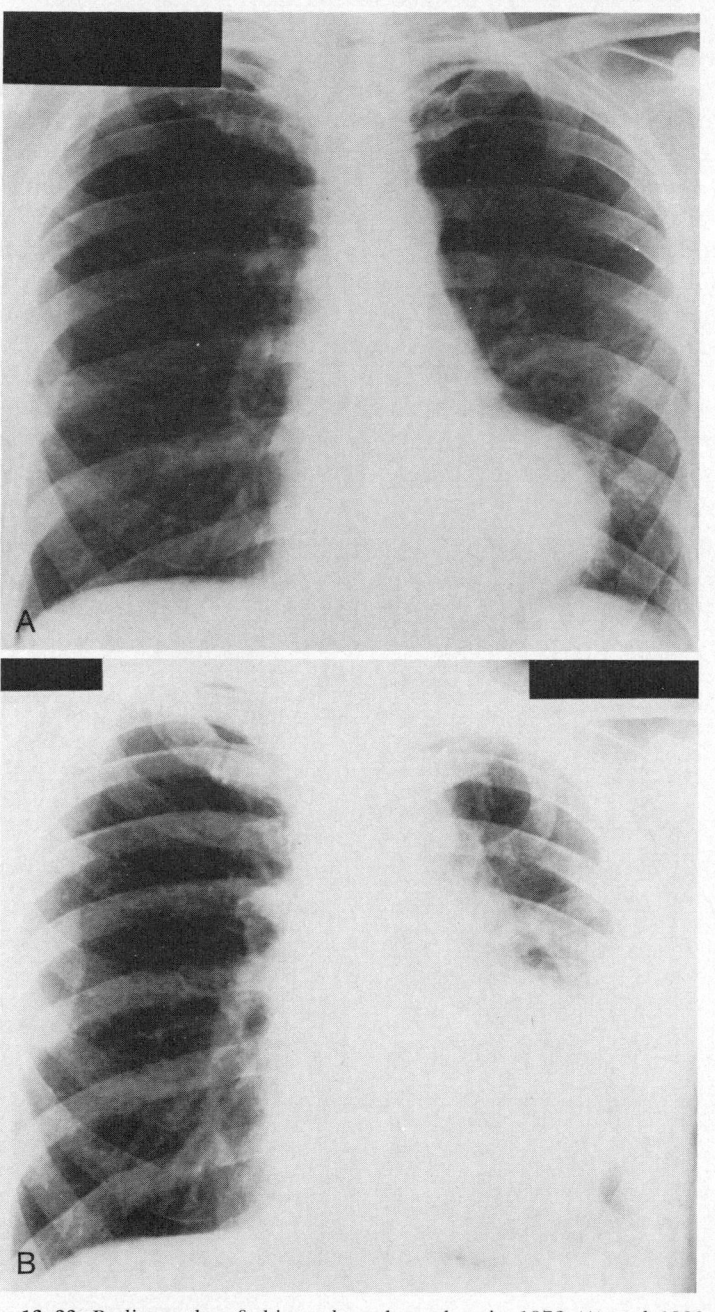

Figure 13–23. Radiographs of shipyard worker taken in 1976 (A) and 1980 (B). He ceased work in 1977, but the left pleural fibrosis, proven by multiple biopsies, continued to progress.

at some risk of developing others. This is no reason for unjustifiably investigating or causing alarm to such patients.

PATHOGENESIS OF ASBESTOS-RELATED DISEASES

Lung Penetration and Retention of Fibers

At first sight it seems surprising that fibers of 20 microns or more in length are found in the alveoli. However, it has been shown that the falling speed of a fiber is proportional to the square of its diameter, and length is less important. The falling speed of a particle is the factor of importance in determining whether the particle will be deposited in the larger airways by gravity or inertial impaction.[137] Only in the smallest airways does fiber length become important, resulting in interception of fibers at the level of the respiratory bronchioles.

Of the two major types of asbestos, the amphiboles (crocidolite, amosite, anthophyllite) are needle-like in shape, normally of less than 3 microns in diameter, and penetrate deeply into the lung (Fig. 13–24). More of these fibers are retained in the lungs of experimental animals than of chrysotile, which has a serpentine configuration and a relatively higher effective fiber diameter. Timbrell,[137] using hollow lung casts sawn off at the respiratory bronchiole level, has confirmed that the amphiboles penetrate to this level in much larger amounts than chrysotile. Those fibers that do not penetrate as far as the alveolated airways are removed by the ciliary mechanism. The finer, more penetrative fibers then depend on macrophage and lymphatic mechanisms for their removal. Thus it seems likely that the shortest fibers, less than about 10 microns in length, can be ingested and removed by macrophages leaving the longer, fine fibers behind. The lung's defenses then rely on two other mechanisms for removal of fibers. One, the formation of asbestos bodies as described previously, seems to involve only a small proportion, principally of the longer fibers. The other is the gradual degradation of the fibers *in situ,* and this seems to be relatively effective only with chrysotile, which has been shown to be capable of being broken down into short fibrils when retained in lung tissue. These fibrils can then be removed by macrophages. This mechanism explains the repeated observation that less chrysotile is found in the lung post mortem than would be anticipated from the exposure history of the patient in life and by comparison with the amphiboles.[138, 139] It should be mentioned, however, that several studies have shown more chrysotile to be retained in the pleura than the lung, though it may be that these fibers lose their carcinogenicity by leaching of their surface ions.[140, 141]

Fibrogenesis

All types of asbestos can produce lung fibrosis. The fibers, having reached the respiratory bronchioles, excite a macrophage response. *In vitro* studies have shown that asbestos is toxic to macrophages, though

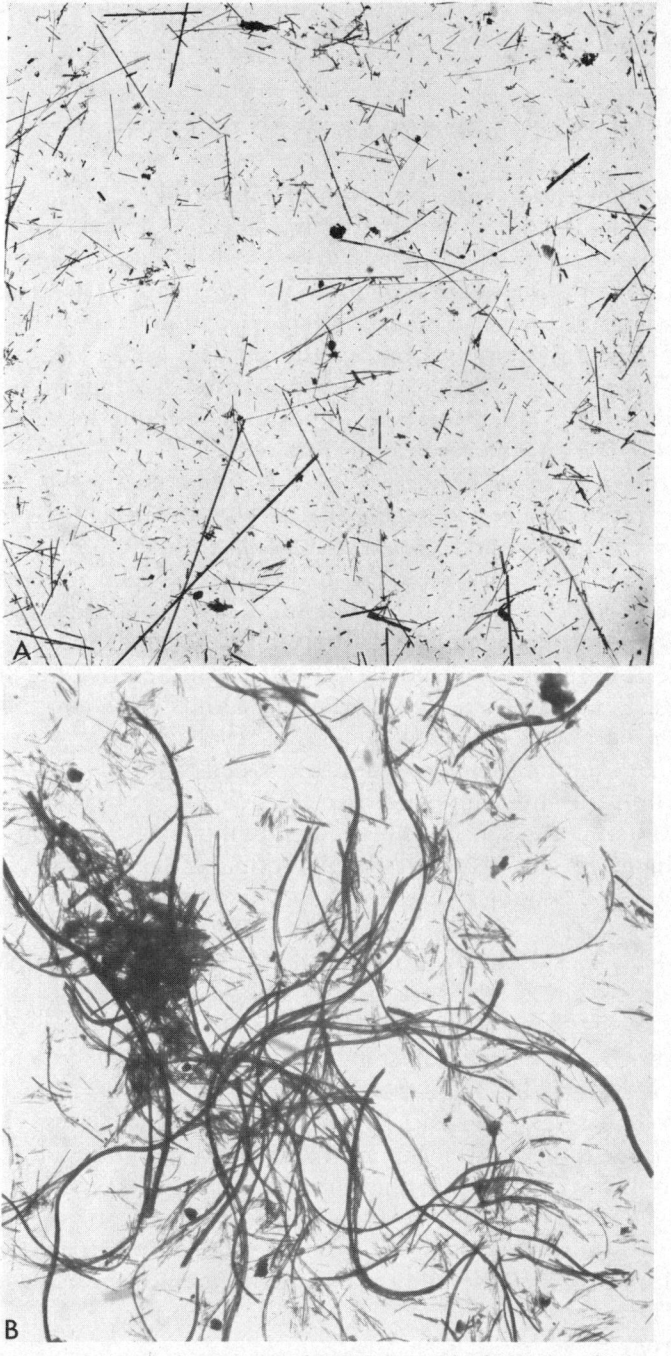

Figure 13–24. Electron micrographs of U.I.C.C. standard samples of asbestos. ×3750. *A*, Crocidolite. *B*, Chrysotile.

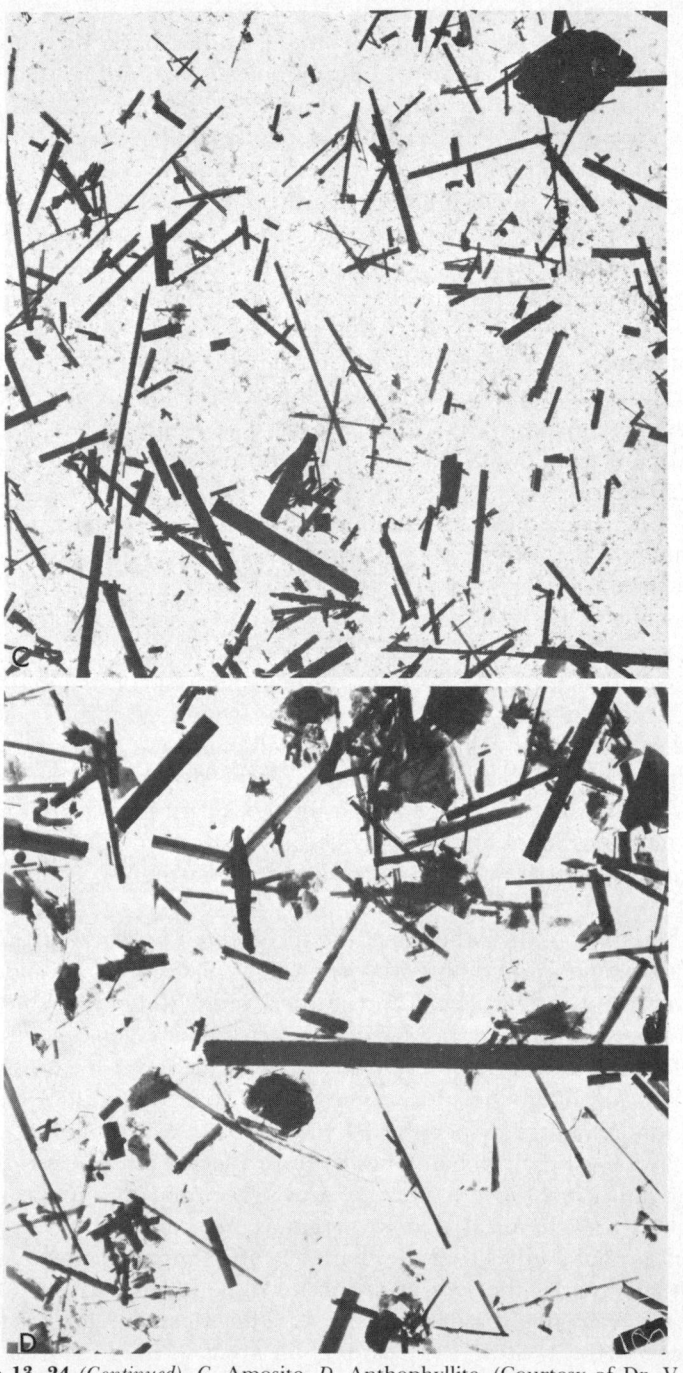

Figure 13–24 *(Continued). C,* Amosite. *D,* Anthophyllite. (Courtesy of Dr. V. Timbrell and Mr. M. Griffiths.)

curiously several such studies have shown the amphiboles to be less toxic than chrysotile.[142] Some animal inhalation studies have also shown chrysotile to be more toxic than the amphiboles,[143] a finding that contrasts with the human exposure evidence. The mechanisms of cell damage and ultimate fibrosis are still unclear, but it seems possible that the initial stage involves an interaction between the macrophage cell wall and either magnesium ions or surface charge on the incompletely ingested fiber. It is suggested that this immobilizes cell wall glycoproteins and allows the membrane to become leaky. Subsequent interaction between macrophage contents, presumably lysosomal enzymes, and the fibroblast initiates the formation of collagen.[144] It should be stressed that this hypothesis, though based on much experimental research, is very likely to be refined and modified as understanding of these cellular mechanisms increases.

Carcinogenesis

Bronchial carcinoma occurs in response to all types of asbestos in humans, though there appears to be a scale of increasing risk from chrysotile to crocidolite. To date, *in vitro* studies and animal inhalation experiments have failed to explain the cellular mechanisms involved. Recent work on differential effects on cells by carcinogenic and fibrogenic dusts has given rise to hope that some advances in understanding are on the horizon. It seems reasonable to suppose that damage to the cell nucleus without cell death may be a factor in the eventual production of a line of neoplastic cells; tests have been developed which examine the ability of fibers to induce giant cell formation in cells in tissue culture to a degree that correlates with the carcinogenicity of the fibers in animal studies.[155] Apart from holding out hope of leading to an understanding of mechanisms, such tests also find a practical application in the testing of new fibrous materials that are being produced or considered as substitutes for asbestos.

With respect to mesothelioma, the differences between different types of asbestos in neoplastic potential are not explained by animal or intraperitoneal or intrapleural injection studies, which in general show all such fibers to be potent producers of mesothelioma, even suggesting that chrysotile is the most toxic.[142] The observed differences in exposed human populations are likely therefore to be related to a combination of reduced penetration, and shorter persistence in the tissues of unaltered chrysotile. There has been much debate about the properties of asbestos that make it carcinogenic, but there is now general agreement that it is the physical rather than the chemical structure that is most important. It has been shown in animal studies that the diameter and length of fibers are crucial and that manmade fibers of appropriate dimensions can produce mesothelioma as effectively as asbestos.[146, 147] The most dangerous manmade fibers appear to be those of greater than about 8 microns in length and less than 1.5 microns in diameter, and this probably also holds true for asbestos.[148] However, this is an area of considerable research activity and it seems unlikely that the final word has yet been said.

PREVENTION

The essential factor in preventing asbestos-related diseases is control of the amount of asbestos to which the workers are exposed. Ultimately it is up to the legislators to decide how to weigh the value of asbestos to society against its apparent risks to health. In some ways this decision is being made easier by the increasing production of substitutes, though it should be remembered that the more closely such substitutes resemble asbestos, the more likely they are to have similar adverse effects.

It will be understood from the foregoing discussion that a precise dose-response relationship has not been described for asbestos and its effects on health. There is therefore no precise evidence on which a dust standard can be based. However, the best evidence available would suggest that a standard between 2 and 0.5 chrysotile fibers per cc is consistent with an asbestosis risk of approximately 1 per cent over a working lifetime. Clearly, the lower this standard is set, the smaller the risk, assuming the ability of industry to comply and of government to monitor compliance.

With regard to mesothelioma, it is fortunate that the amphiboles, which pose the most serious threat to human populations, are the least used forms of asbestos. It does not seem likely that any standard for crocidolite can be confidently expected to protect exposed workers against mesothelioma. Several countries, including Britain, have recognized this by imposing a crocidolite standard that effectively prevents its use. While amosite is probably not quite as toxic as crocidolite, an increasingly tight standard for this material would certainly be desirable from a health point of view.

Having a sensible standard for asbestos levels in the workplace is, of course, only part of the battle against these diseases. The standard has to be adhered to. There are considerable problems here, as the counting of fibrous particles is subject to very marked variability between individuals, laboratories, and countries. Variations occur with the sampling technique, the absolute dust counts, the microscopic technique, the method of mounting the slide, and the personality and fatigability of the counter. Also the counting rules (what is asbestos, which fibers to count?) are crucial factors. With all these sources of variability it is encouraging to note that active steps are now being taken by governments in Europe and North America to standardize techniques and to introduce central reference laboratories, the first of which is based in the Institute of Occupational Medicine in Scotland.

A further complicating factor in fiber counting results from incomplete knowledge of the range of fiber size that leads to the pathogenic effects. In theory it is only necessary to control exposure to fibers of the appropriate size range, but we still do not know for sure what this range is. In particular, do fibers that are too small to be seen with the light microscope pose a threat? If so, electron microscopy may be necessary on a wide scale and this would clearly pose major problems. Some hope for

future simplification of these difficulties attends the development of computer-based automatic counting machines.

Assuming that standards ensure limited exposure to chrysotile and prevent exposure to amphiboles, further measures to protect the work force include the wearing of approved respirators in places where dust levels may be high and regular surveillance of exposed workers. Anyone showing early evidence of the disease ("possible asbestosis") should be removed from further exposure and encouraged not to smoke. Indeed, education on the potentially harmful effects of both smoking and asbestos should be given to all asbestos workers.

Industrial hygiene measures taken where asbestos is produced or used should include efforts to ensure that people other than the work force are not exposed either: for example, the dusty air should be filtered and not discharged into the outside air: the filters should be disposed of with considerable care: asbestos waste should not be dumped where fibers can be released into the air; and asbestos workers should not be able to carry asbestos home on their clothes.

The widespread appreciation of the risks of asbestos has led to much greater care being taken with this valuable, and in many cases life-saving, material. It is to be hoped that there will soon be a downward trend in the numbers of people suffering from asbestosis. Unfortunately, because of the long latent period between exposure and the development of mesothelioma, many people will still die from this disease, but tight control of the amphiboles in some countries should show some effect in the next decade or two. National lung cancer statistics are unlikely to show any appreciable changes with further control of asbestos, since cigarette smoking is the overwhelmingly important cause of this disease.

References

1. Hunter, D., The Diseases of Occupations, 4th ed. London, English Universities Press, 1969, p. 1009.
2. Lee, D. H. K., Historical background to the asbestos problem. Environ. Res., 18, 300, 1979.
3. Murray, M., Departmental Committee for Compensation for Industrial Diseases, Cmd 3495 and 3496. London, H.M. Stationery Office, 1907.
4. Pancoast, H. K., Miller, T. G., and Landris, H. R. M., A roentgenologic study of the effects of dust inhalation on the lung. Trans. Soc. Am. Physicians, 32, 97, 1917.
5. Cooke, W. E., Pulmonary asbestosis. Br. Med. J., 2, 1024, 1927.
6. McDonald, S., Histology of pulmonary asbestosis. Br. Med. J., 2, 1025, 1927.
7. Merewether, E. R. A., and Price, C. W., Report on effects of asbestos dust on the lungs and dust suppression in the asbestos industry. London, H. M. Stationery Office, 1930.
8. Wood, W. B., and Gloyne, S. R., Pulmonary asbestosis: a review of 100 cases. Lancet, 2, 1383, 1934.
9. Merewether, E. R. A., Asbestosis and carcinoma of the lung. In Annual Report of the Chief Inspector of Factories for the Year 1947. London, H.M. Stationery Office, 1949.
10. Doll, R., Mortality from lung cancer in asbestos workers. Br. J. Ind. Med., 12, 81, 1955.

11. Knox, J. F., Doll, R. S., and Hill, I. D., Cohort analysis of changes in incidence of bronchial carcinoma in a textile asbestos factory. Ann. N.Y. Acad. Sci., *132*, 526, 1965.

12. Selikoff, I. J., Churg, J., and Hammond, E. C., Asbestos exposure and neoplasia. J.A.M.A., *188*, 22, 1964.

13. Selikoff, I. J., Hammond, E. C., and Churg, J., Asbestos exposure, smoking and neoplasia. J.A.M.A., *104*, 106, 1968.

14. Wagner, J. C., Sleggs, C. A., and Marchand, P., Diffuse pleural mesothelioma and asbestos exposure in the North-West Cape Province. Br. J. Ind. Med., *17*, 260, 1960.

15. Jones, J. S. P., Smith, P. G., Pooley, F. D., et al., The consequences of exposure to asbestos dust in a wartime gas-mask factory. *In* Wagner, J. C., ed., Biological Effects of Mineral Fibres. Lyon, International Agency for Research on Cancer, 1980, p. 637.

16. McDonald, A. D., Mesothelioma after crocidolite exposure during gas mask manufacture. Environ. Res., *17*, 340, 1978.

17. Hobbs, M. S. T., Woodward, S. D., Murphy, B., et al., The incidence of pneumoconiosis, mesothelioma and other respiratory cancer in men engaged in mining and milling crocidolite in Western Australia. *In* Wagner, J. C., ed., Biological Effects of Mineral Fibres. Lyon, International Agency for Research on Cancer, 1980, p. 615.

18. Seidman, H., Selikoff, I. J., and Cuyler Hammond, E., Short-term asbestos work exposure and long-term observation. Ann. N.Y. Acad. Sci., *300*, 61, 1979.

19. McDonald, J. C., and Liddell, F. D. K., Mortality in Canadian miners and millers exposed to chrysotile. Ann. N.Y. Acad. Sci., *330*, 1, 1979.

20. Nicholson W. J., Selikoff, I. J., Seidman, H., et al., Long-term mortality experience of chrysotile miners and millers in Thetford Mines, Quebec. Ann. N.Y. Acad. Sci., *330*, 11, 1979.

21. Peto, J., The incidence of pleural mesothelioma in chrysotile asbestos textile workers. *In* Wagner, J. C., ed., Biological Effects of Mineral Fibres. Lyon, International Agency for Research on Cancer, 1980, p. 703.

22. Rubino, G. F., Piolatto, G., Newhouse, M. L., et al., Mortality of chrysotile asbestos workers at the Balangero Mine, Northern Italy. Br. J. Ind. Med., *37*, 187, 1979.

23. McDonald, J. C., Liddell, F. D. K., Gibbs, G. W., et al., Dust exposure and mortality in chrysotile mining, 1910–1975. Br. J. Ind. Med., *37*, 11, 1980.

24. Saracci, R., Asbestos and lung cancer: An analysis of the epidemiological evidence on the asbestos-smoking interaction. Int. J. Cancer., *20*, 323, 1977.

25. Meurman, L. O., Kiviluoto, R., and Hakama, M., Combined effects of asbestos exposure and tobacco smoking on Finnish anthophyllite miners and millers. Ann. N.Y. Acad. Sci., *330*, 491, 1979.

26. McDonald, J. C., McDonald, A. D., Gibbs, G. W., et al., Mortality in the chrysotile asbestos mines and mills of Quebec. Arch. Environ. Health, *22*, 677, 1971.

27. McDonald, J. C., Becklake, M. R., Gibbs, G. W., et al., The health of chrysotile asbestos mine and mill workers of Quebec. Arch. Environ. Health, *28*, 61, 1974.

28. Weill, H., Hughes, J., and Waggenspack, C., Influence of dose and fiber type on respiratory malignancy risk in asbestos cement manufacturing. Am. Rev. Resp. Dis., *120*, 345, 1979.

29. Berry, G., Gilson, J. C., Holmes, S., et al., Asbestosis: a study of dose-response relationships in an asbestos textile factory. Br. J. Ind. Med., *36*, 98, 1979.

30. British Occupational Hygiene Society, Hygiene standards for chrysotile asbestos dust. Ann. Occup. Hyg., *11*, 47, 1968.

31. Berry, G., Mortality of workers certified by pneumoconiosis medical panels as having asbestosis. Br. J. Ind. Med., *38*, 130, 1981.

32. Selikoff, I. J., Hammond, C. E., and Seidman, H., Mortality experience of insulation workers in the United States and Canada, 1943–1976. Ann. N.Y. Acad. Sci., *330*, 91, 1979.

33. Newhouse, M. L., A study of the mortality of workers in an asbestos factory. Br. J. Ind. Med., *26*, 294, 1969.

34. Newhouse, M. L., Berry, G., Wagner, J. C., and Turok, M. E., A study of the mortality of female asbestos workers. Br. J. Ind. Med., *29*, 134, 1972.

35. Newhouse, M. L., and Berry, G., Predictions of mortality from mesothelial tumours in asbestos factory workers. Br. J. Ind. Med., *33*, 147, 1976.

36. Henderson, V. L., and Enterline, P. E., Asbestos exposure: factors associated with excess cancer and respiratory disease mortality. Ann. N.Y. Acad. Sci., *330*, 117, 1979.
37. Selikoff, I. J., Lillis, R., and Nicholson, W. J., Asbestos disease in United States Shipyards. Ann. N.Y. Acad. Sci., *330*, 295, 1979.
38. Mostert, C., and Meintjes, R., Asbestosis and mesothelioma on the Rhodesia railways. Cent. Afr. J. Med., *25*, 72, 1979.
39. Rossiter, C. E., and Coles, R. M., HM Dockyard, Devonport: 1947 mortality study. *In* Wagner, J. C., ed., Biological Effects of Mineral Fibres. Lyon, International Agency for Research on Cancer, 1980, p. 637.
40. Sheers, G., and Coles, R. M., Mesothelioma risks in a naval dockyard. Arch. Environ. Health, *35*, 276, 1980.
41. Rossiter, C. E., and Harries, P. G., UK Naval Dockyards Asbestos Study: survey of sample population aged 50–59 years. Br. J. Ind. Med., *36*, 281, 1979.
42. Weiss, W., Mortality of a cohort exposed to chrysotile asbestos. J. Occup. Med., *19*, 737, 1977.
43. Lorimer, W. V., Rohl, A. N., Miller, A., et al., Asbestos exposure of brake repair workers in the United States. Mt. Sinai J. Med. (NY), *43*, 207, 1976.
44. Flynn, L., South Africa blacks out blue asbestos risk. New Scientist, *94*, 237, 1982.
45. Baris, Y. I., Sahin, A. A., Ozesmi, M., et al., An outbreak of pleural mesothelioma and chronic fibrosing pleurisy in the village of Karain/Ürgüp in Anatolia. Thorax, *33*, 181, 1978.
46. Baris, Y. I., Saracci, R., Simonato, L., et al., Malignant mesothelioma and radiological chest abnormalities in two villages in Central Turkey. Lancet, *2*, 984, 1981.
47. Yazicioglu, S., Ilcayto, R., Balci, K., et al., Pleural calcification, pleural mesotheliomas, and bronchial cancers caused by tremolite dust. Thorax, *35*, 564, 1980.
48. Le Guen, J. M., and Burdett, G., Asbestos concentrations in public buildings—a preliminary report. Ann. Occup. Hyg., *24*, 185, 1981.
49. Harrington, J. M., Craun, G. F., Meigs, J. W., et al., An investigation of the use of asbestos cement pipe for public water supply and the incidence of gastrointestinal cancer in Connecticut, 1935–1973. Am. J. Epidemiol., *107*, 96, 1978.
50. Meigs, J. W., Walter, S. D., Heston, J. F., et al., Asbestos cement pipe and cancer in Connecticut, 1955–1974. J. Environ. Health, *42*, 187, 1980.
51. Clark, T. C., Harrington, V. A., Asta, J., et al., Respiratory effects of exposure to dust in taconite mining and processing. Am. Rev. Resp. Dis., *121*, 956, 1980.
52. Sigurdson, E. E., Levy, B. S., Mandel, J., et al., Cancer morbidity investigations: Lessons from the Duluth study of possible effects of asbestos in drinking water. Environ. Res., *25*, 50, 1981.
53. Health and Safety Executive, Health and Safety Statistics 1978–1979. London, H.M. Stationery Office, 1981.
54. Bamblin, W. P., Dust control in the asbestos textile industry. Ann. Occup. Hyg., *2*, 54, 1959.
55. Gilson, J. C., Problems and perspectives: the changing hazards of exposure to asbestos. Ann. N.Y. Acad. Sci., *132*, 696, 1965.
56. McVittie, J. C., Asbestos in Great Britain. Ann. N.Y. Acad. Sci., *132*, 128, 1965.
57. Hunt, R., Routine lung function studies on 830 employees in an asbestos processing factory. Ann. N.Y. Acad. Sci., *132*, 405, 1965.
58. Leathart, G. L., Pulmonary function tests in asbestos workers. Trans. Soc. Occup. Med., *18*, 49, 1968.
59. Murphy, R. L. H., and Sorensen, K., Chest auscultation in the diagnosis of pulmonary asbestosis. J. Occup. Med., *15*, 272, 1973.
60. Forgacs, P., Lung sounds. Br. J. Dis. Chest, *63*, 1, 1969.
61. Mori, M., Kinoshita, K., Morinari, H., et al., Waveform and spectral analysis of crackles. Thorax, *35*, 843, 1980.
62. Murphy, R. L., Auscultation of the lung: past lessons, future possibilities. Thorax, *36*, 99, 1981.
63. Smithers, W. J., Secular changes in asbestosis in an asbestos factory. Ann. N.Y. Acad. Sci., *132*, 166, 1965.
64. Wilson, R., and Hugh-Jones, P., The significance of lung function changes in asbestosis. Thorax, *15*, 109, 1960.

65. Bohig, H., Radiological classification of pulmonary asbestosis. Ann. N.Y. Acad. Sci., *132*, 338, 1965.
66. Sluis-Cremer, G. K., and Theron, C. P., A proposed radiological classification of asbestosis. Ann. N.Y. Acad. Sci., *132*, 373, 1975.
67. U.I.C.C./Cincinnati, Classification of the radiographic appearances of pneumoconioses. Chest, *58*, 57, 1970.
68. International Labour Organisation, International Classification of Radiographs of the Pneumoconioses. Geneva, ILO, 1980.
69. Liddell, F. D. K., and McDonald, J. C., Radiological findings as predictors of mortality in Quebec asbestos workers. Br. J. Ind. Med., *37*, 257, 1980.
70. Solomon, A., Radiology of asbestosis. *In* Shapiro, H. A., ed., Pneumoconiosis. Proceedings of the International Conference in Johannesburg. London, Oxford University Press, 1970, p. 243.
71. Telleson, W. G., Rheumatoid pneumoconiosis (Caplan's syndrome) in an asbestos worker. Thorax, *16*, 372, 1961.
72. Rickards, A. G., and Barrett, G. M., Rheumatoid lung changes associated with asbestosis. Thorax, *13*, 185, 1958.
73. Greaves, I. A., Rheumatoid "pneumoconiosis" (Caplan's syndrome) in an asbestos worker: a 17 years' follow-up. Thorax, *34*, 404, 1979.
74. Caplan, A., Gilson, J. C., Hinson, K. F. W., et al., A preliminary study of observer variation in the classification of radiographs of asbestos-exposed workers. Ann. N.Y. Acad. Sci., *132*, 379, 1965.
75. Hourihane, D. O'B., Lessof, L., and Richardson, P. C., Hyaline and calcified pleural plaques as an index of exposure to asbestos. Br. Med. J. *1*, 1069, 1966.
76. British Thoracic and Tuberculosis Association/M.R.C. Pneumoconiosis Unit, A survey of pleural thickening. Its relation to asbestos exposure and previous pleural disease. Environ. Res., *5*, 142, 1972.
77. Hillerdal, G., Non-malignant asbestos pleural disease. Thorax, *36*, 669, 1981.
78. Becklake, M. R., Liddell, F. D. K., Manfreda, J., and McDonald, J. C., Radiological changes after withdrawal from asbestos exposure. Br. J. Ind. Med., *36*, 23, 1979.
79. Gregor, A., Parkes, R. W., du Bois, R., and Turner-Warwick, M., Radiographic progression of asbestosis: preliminary report. Ann. N.Y. Acad. Sci., *330*, 147, 1979.
80. Bader, M. E., Bader, R. A., and Selikoff, I. J., Pulmonary function in asbestosis of the lung: an alveolar-capillary block syndrome. Am. J. Med., *30*, 235, 1961.
81. Becklake, M. R., Fournier-Massey, G. G., McDonald, J. C., et al., Lung function changes in relation to radiographic changes in Quebec asbestos workers. *In* Shapiro, H. A., ed., Pneumoconiosis. Proceedings of the International Conference in Johannesburg. London, Oxford University Press, 1970, p. 233.
82. Bader, M. E., Bader, R. A., Tierstein, A. S., and Selikoff, I. J., Pulmonary function in asbestosis: serial tests in a long-term prospective study. Ann. N.Y. Acad. Sci., *132*, 391, 1965.
83. Jodoin, G., Gibbs, G. W., Macklem, P. T., et al., Early effects of asbestos exposure on lung function. Am. Rev. Respir. Dis., *104*, 525, 1971.
84. Mead, J., The lung's "quiet zone." N. Engl. J. Med., *282*, 1318, 1970.
85. Harless, K. W., Watanabe, S., and Renzetti, A. D., The acute effects of chrysotile asbestos exposure on lung function. Environ. Res., *16*, 360, 1978.
86. Morgan, W. K. C., Rheumatoid pneumoconiosis in association with asbestosis. Thorax, *19*, 433, 1964.
87. Gough, J., Differential diagnosis in the pathology of asbestosis. Ann. N.Y. Acad. Sci., *132*, 368, 1965.
88. Davis, J. M. G., Electron microscope studies of asbestosis in man and animals. Ann. N.Y. Acad. Sci., *132*, 98, 1965.
89. Webster, I., The pathogenesis of asbestosis. *In* Shapiro, H. A., ed., Pneumoconiosis. Proceedings of the International Conference in Johannesburg. London, Oxford University Press, 1970, p. 117.
90. Goldstein, B., and Rendall, R. E. G., Ferruginous bodies. *In* Shapiro, H. A., ed., Pneumoconiosis. Proceedings of the International Conference in Johannesburg. London, Oxford University Press, 1970, p. 92.
91. Das, R. M., Holt, P. F., and Horne, M. C., The formation of asbestos bodies. Med. Lav., *68*, 431, 1977.

92. Utidjian, M. D., Gross, P., and deTreville, R. T. P., Ferruginous bodies in human lungs. Arch. Environ. Health, *17*, 327, 1968.
93. Cralley, L. J., Inhalable fibrous material. *In* Shapiro, H. A., ed., Pneumoconiosis. Proceedings of the International Conference in Johannesburg. London, Oxford University Press, 1970, p. 70.
94. Churg, A., and Warnock, M. L., Analysis of the cores of ferruginous (asbestos) bodies from the general population. I. Patients with and without lung cancer. Lab. Invest., *37*, 280, 1977.
95. Churg, A. W., Warnock, M. L., and Green, N., Analysis of the cores of ferruginous (asbestos) bodies from the general population. II. True asbestos bodies and pseudoasbestos bodies. Lab. Invest., *40*, 31, 1979.
96. Churg, A. W., and Warnock, M. L., Analysis of the cores of ferruginous (asbestos) bodies from the general population. III. Patients with environmental exposure. Lab. Invest., *40*, 622, 1979.
97. Auerbach, O., Conston, A. S., Garfinkel, L., et al., Presence of asbestos bodies in organs other than the lung. Chest, *77*, 133, 1980.
98. Selikoff, I. J., and Hammond, E. C., Asbestos bodies in the New York City population in two periods of time. *In* Shapiro, H. A. ed., Pneumoconiosis. Proceedings of the International Conference in Johannesburg. London, Oxford University Press, 1970, p. 99.
99. Pooley, F. D., Oldham, P. D., Chang-Hyum U., and Wagner, J. C., The detection of asbestos in tissues. *In* Shapiro, H. A. ed., Pneumoconiosis. Proceedings of the International Conference in Johannesburg. London, Oxford University Press, 1970, p. 108.
100. Churg, A., and Warnock, M. L., Asbestos fibers in the general population. Am. Rev. Respir. Dis., *122*, 669, 1980.
101. Gough, J., and Heppleston, A. G., The pathology of the pneumoconioses. *In* King, E. J., and Fletcher, C. M., eds., Symposium on Industrial Pulmonary Diseases. London, Churchill, 1960.
102. Vorwald, A. J., Durkam, J. M., and Pratt, P. C., Experimental studies of asbestos. Arch. Ind. Hyg., *3*, 1, 1951.
103. Arul, K. J., and Holt, P. F., Clearance of asbestos bodies from the lung: a personal view. Br. J. Ind. Med., *37*, 273, 1980.
104. Stovin, P. G. I., and Partridge, P., Pulmonary asbestos and dust content in East Anglia. Thorax, *37*, 185, 1982.
105. Whitwell, F., Scott, J., and Grimshaw, M., Relationships between occupations and asbestos-fibre content of the lungs in patients with pleural mesothelioma, lung cancer and other diseases. Thorax, *32*, 377, 1977.
106. Berry, G., Newhouse, M. L., and Turok, M., Combined effects of asbestos exposure and smoking on mortality from lung cancer in factory workers. Lancet, *2*, 476, 1972.
107. Liddell, F. D. K., Asbestos and the public health. Thorax, *36*, 241, 1981.
108. McDonald, J. C., Asbestos-related disease: an epidemiological review. *In* Wagner, J. C., ed., Biological Effects of Mineral Fibres. Lyon, International Agency for Research on Cancer, 1980, p. 587.
109. Newhouse, ML., Gregory, M. M., and Shannon, H., Etiology of carcinoma of the larynx. *In* Wagner, J. C., ed., Biological Effects of Mineral Fibres. Lyon, International Agency for Research on Cancer, 1980, p. 687.
110. Buchanan, W. D., Asbestosis and primary intrathoracic neoplasms. Ann. N.Y. Acad. Sci., *132*, 507, 1965.
111. Elmes, P. C., and Wade, O. L., Relationship between exposure to asbestos and pleural malignancy in Belfast. Ann. N.Y. Acad. Sci., *132*, 549, 1965.
112. Selikoff, I. J., Hammond, E. C., and Churg, J., Mortality experiences of asbestos insulation workers. *In* Shapiro, H. A., ed., Proceedings of the International Conference in Johannesburg. London, Oxford University Press, 1970, p. 180.
112a. Berry G., and Newhouse, M. L., Mortality of workers manufacturing friction materials using asbestos. Br. J. Ind. Med., *40*, 1, 1983.
113. Elmes, P. C., and Simpson, M. J. C., The clinical aspects of mesothelioma. Quart. J. Med., *45*, 427, 1976.
114. Newhouse, M. L., and Thompson, H., Epidemiology of mesothelial tumours in the London area. Ann. N.Y. Acad. Sci., *132*, 579, 1965.

115. Oels, H. C., Harrison, E. G., Carr, D. T., and Bernatz, P. E., Diffuse malignant mesothelioma of the pleura: a review of 37 cases. Chest, 60, 564, 1971.
116. Butler, E. B., and Johnson, N. F., The use of electron microscopy in the diagnosis of diffuse mesotheliomas using human pleural effusions. In Wagner, J. C., ed., Biological Effects of Mineral Fibres. Lyon, International Agency for Research on Cancer, 1980, p. 409.
117. Arai, H., Kang, K-Y., Sato, H., et al., Significance of the quantification and demonstration of hyaluronic acid in tissue specimens for the diagnosis of pleural mesothelioma Am. Rev. Respir. Dis., 120, 529, 1979.
118. McCaughey, W. T. E., Criteria for the diagnosis of diffuse mesothelial tumors. Ann. N.Y. Acad. Sci., 132, 603, 1965.
119. Thomson, J. G., The pathological diagnosis of malignant mesothelioma of pleura and peritoneum. In Shapiro, H. A., ed., Pneumoconiosis. Proceedings of the International Conference in Johannesburg. London, Oxford University Press, 1970, p. 150.
120. Winslow, D. J., and Taylor, H. B., Malignant peritoneal mesotheliomas. A clinicopathological analysis of 12 fatal cases. Cancer, 13, 127, 1960.
121. Churg, J., Rosen, S. H., and Moolten, S., Histologic characteristics of mesothelioma associated with asbestos. Ann. N.Y. Acad. Sci., 132, 614, 1965.
122. Arai, H., Endo, M., Sasai, Y., et al., Histochemical demonstration of hyaluronic acid in a case of pleural mesothelioma. Am. Rev. Respir. Dis., 111, 699, 1975.
123. Brady, L. W., Mesothelioma—the role for radiation therapy. Semin. Oncol., 8, 329, 1981.
124. Aisner, J., and Wiernik, P. H., Chemotherapy in the treatment of malignant mesothelioma. Semin. Oncol., 8, 335, 1981.
125. Hourihane, D. O'B., A biopsy series of mesotheliomata, and attempts to identify asbestos within some of the tumors. Ann. N.Y. Acad. Sci., 132, 647, 1965.
126. Butchart, E. G., Ashcroft, T., Barnsley, W. C., and Holden, M. P., The role of surgery in diffuse malignant mesothelioma of the pleura. Semin. Oncol., 8, 321, 1981.
127. Miller, J. W., Hunter, A. M., and Horne, N. W., Intrapleural immunotherapy with Corynebacterium parvum in recurrent malignant pleural effusions. Thorax, 35, 856, 1980.
128. Felletti, R. and Ravazzoni, C., Intrapleural Corynebacterium parvum for malignant pleural effusions. Thorax, 38, 22, 1983.
129. Sheldon, C. D., Herbert, A., and Gallagher, P. J., Reactive mesothelial proliferation: a necropsy study. Thorax, 36, 901, 1981.
130. Gibbs, G. W., Etiology of pleural calcification: a study of Quebec chrysotile asbestos miners and millers. Arch. Environ. Health, 34, 76, 1979.
131. Hillerdal, G., The pathogenesis of pleural plaques and pulmonary asbestosis: possibilities and impossibilities. Eur. J. Respir. Dis., 61, 129, 1980.
132. Solomon A., Irwig, L. M., Sluis-Cremer, G. K., et al., Thickening of pulmonary interlobar fissures: exposure-response relationship in crocidolite and amosite miners. Br. J. Ind. Med., 36, 195, 1979.
133. Hillerdal, G., Non-malignant asbestos pleural disease. Thorax, 36, 641, 1981.
134. Harries, P. G., A report on the effects and control of diseases associated with exposure to asbestos in Devonport dockyard. Royal Naval Clinical Research Working Party, C.R.W.P./71. Gosport, England, Institute of Naval Medicine, 1970.
135. Robinson, B. W. S., and Musk, A. W., Benign asbestos pleural effusion, diagnosis and course. Thorax, 36, 896, 1981.
136. Wright, P. H., Hanson, A., Kreel, L., and Capel, L. H., Respiratory function changes after asbestos pleurisy. Thorax, 35, 31, 1980.
137. Timbrell, V., The inhalation of fibers. In Shapiro, H. A., ed., Pneumoconiosis. Proceedings of the International Conference in Johannesburg. London, Oxford University Press, 1970, p. 3.
138. Rowlands, N., Gibbs, G. W., and McDonald, A. D., Asbestos fibres in the lungs of chrysotile miners and millers—a preliminary report. In Walton, W. H., ed., Inhaled Particles V. Oxford, Pergamon Press, 1982, p. 417.
139. Wagner, J. C., Pooley, F. D., Berry, G., et al., A pathological and mineralogical study of asbestos-related deaths in the United Kingdom in 1977. In Walton, W. H., ed., Inhaled Particles V. Oxford, Pergamon Press, 1982, p. 423.
140. Sebastien, P., Janson, X., and Gaudichet, A., Asbestos retention in human respiratory

tissues: comparative measurements in lung parenchyma and in parietal pleura. *In* Wagner, J. C., ed., Lyon, International Agency for Research on Cancer, 1980, p. 237.

141. Jaurand, M. C., Bignon, J., Sebastien, P., and Goni, J., Leaching of chrysotile asbestos in human lungs. Correlation with *in vitro* studies using rabbit alveolar mecrophages. Environ. Res., *14*, 245, 1977.

142. Bolton, R. E., Davis, J. M. G., Donaldson, K., and Wright, A., Variations in the carcinogenicity of mineral fibres. *In* Walton, W. H., ed., Inhaled Particles V. Oxford, Pergamon Press, p. 569.

143. Davis, J. M. G., Beckett, S. T., Bolton, R. E., et al., Mass and number of fibres in the pathogenesis of asbestos-related lung disease in rats. Br. J. Cancer, *37*, 673, 1978.

144. Bateman, E. D., Emerson, R. J., and Cole, P., Mechanisms of fibrosis. *In* Weill, H., and Turner-Warwick, M., eds., Occupational Lung Diseases: Research Approaches and Methods. New York, Marcel Dekker, 1981.

145. Chamberlain, M., Brown, R. C., and Griffiths, D. M., The correlation between carcinogenic activities *in vivo* and the cytopathic effects *in vitro* of mineral dusts. *In* Brown, R. C., Gormley, I. P., Chamberlain, M., and Davies, R., eds., The *In Vitro* Effects of Mineral Dusts. London, Academic Press, 1980, p. 345.

146. Stanton, M. F., and Wrench, C., Mechanisms of mesothelioma induction with asbestos and fibrous glass. J. Natl. Cancer Inst., *48*, 797, 1972.

147. Stanton, M. F., Layard, M., Tegeris, A., et al., Carcinogenicity of fibrous glass: pleural response in the rat in relation to fiber dimension. J. Natl. Cancer Inst., *58*, 587, 1977.

148. Brown, R. C., Chamberlain, M., Griffiths, D. M., and Timbrell, V., The effect of fibre size on the *in vitro* biological activity of three types of amphibole asbestos. Int. J. Cancer, *22*, 721, 1978.

14

COAL WORKERS' PNEUMOCONIOSIS

W. Keith C. Morgan

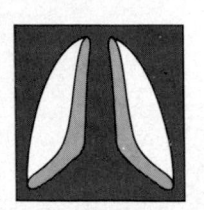

The first reference to coal mining in Great Britain, and, as far as is known, elsewhere, was made in A.D. 852 and is to be found in the *Saxon Chronicle of Peterborough*.[1] Further reference is made in Bishop Pudsey's Boldon Book (A.D. 1180), and mention is to be found of the digging of coal from Newcastle and Scotland in the thirteenth century.[2] As far as Scotland is concerned, the earliest miners were probably the monks of Newbattle Abbey. At first coal was dug only from surface outcroppings and it was not until the advent of the mechanical pump and the introduction of ventilation that underground mining became possible. Underground mines are subject to flooding, and it was the invention of the steam engine that provided the means to keep them dry. The first steam engines were constructed by Savery and Newcomen at the turn of the seventeenth century; however, a further 50 years elapsed before the steam-driven pump was used in a Scottish coal mine. Nonetheless, by 1840 Britain was producing between 30 and 40 million tons of coal a year, and such was the demand that a mere 15 years later, production had climbed to 100 million tons.[2] At that time about a third of a million men were employed as coal miners.

In the United States, coal mining started to become a major industry in the 1830s. The earliest mines were established in eastern Pennsylvania and western Maryland and what is now West Virginia. Those in Pennsylvania were located in the anthracite area, the anthracite often being removed from surface outcroppings. However, as in Britain, effective ventilation and pumping machines led to the development of deep underground mines. In the latter part of the nineteenth century, underground bituminous mines came into existence in western Pennsylvania, southern West Virginia, Kentucky, and Virginia. Without road access, their development was almost entirely dependent on the railways. Many coal towns of southern West Virginia, Kentucky, and eastern Virginia had

no road connections to the remainder of the state until the 1920s. In the late nineteenth and early twentieth centuries, large underground coal deposits were found in Illinois, Indiana, Utah, and Colorado.

In Britain, the advent and growth of the iron and steel industry brought with it an increasing demand for coal. As a result, many of the early coal mines developed near to iron and steel foundries. This was especially true of South Wales, where many of the valleys in Monmouth and Glamorgan were found to contain rich deposits of anthracite and steam coal. As the production of iron and steel increased, so did the demand for coal. The coal fire became the main source of heating in Britain and this further increased demand. Although there was much industrial unrest in the industry in the latter part of the nineteenth century, and perhaps even more in the early twentieth century, the industry continued to expand. In 1948, when the coal mines were nationalized, there were well over 700,000 coal miners in Britain.[3] Since that time the use of coal has not kept pace with that of other sources of energy and there are now just over 210,000 miners. However, the introduction of mechanization has boosted production to well over that which was mined with twice the number of miners.

A somewhat similar train of events took place in the United States. In the late nineteenth and early twentieth centuries the huge demand for coal that the steel companies of Pittsburgh and Cleveland generated, plus a dire shortage of labor in the Appalachian mines, led to the importation of many Europeans. Thousands of Central Europeans who were fleeing from Poland, Germany, and Austro-Hungary because of famine or religious persecution were herded into boats and carried across the Atlantic as "steerage" passengers. From New York, they were taken by train to the mining areas of West Virginia, Kentucky, and Pennsylvania.[4] Once in the mining town, they were lodged in company houses, or rather shacks, made to pay an excessive rent, and compelled to patronize the one store in the town, this being run by the company. As a result, most miners were in debt to the store and hence the company, and thus were unable to move. Trade unions were forbidden and attempts to unionize the miners led to the firing and blacklisting of any man suspected of being a union supporter. If the men went on strike, they were turned out of their company houses, and they and their families were allowed to starve. Between 1900 and 1930 several pitched battles, in which rifles and machine guns were used, were fought in West Virginia and eastern Kentucky. These took place between striking miners and a private army of thugs employed by the companies and hired from what was then known as the Baldwin Felts Agency. Black laborers used as strikebreakers were brought up from Alabama and the South in chartered trains, but since the latter were often machine-gunned by union supporters, armored trains became necessary. A strike in northern West Virginia in the 1920s lasted four years and resulted in numerous deaths from starvation among the miners and their families. During the strike, a bomb was thrown down a nonunion

The Underground Work Force

In order to understand the several health hazards to which miners are exposed, it is necessary to have some idea of the various jobs involved in coal mining. Any man who works underground is classified as a coal miner; however, the environmental conditions vary greatly according to the job. The most dusty area of the mine is the coal face, where the cutting machines and continuous miners are in operation. The cutting machine operator and his helper are usually exposed to the highest dust concentrations. Only slightly less exposed are the roof bolter, continuous miner operator, loading machine operator, and shot firer. Workers in these occupations are usually considered face workers (Figs. 14–1 to 14–3).

After the coal has been cut and detached from the seam, it is then loaded on a conveyor belt or other transportation system prior to being moved from the face. This is usually effected with a shuttle car. From the shuttle car the coal is then loaded into a small "train," which in the United States is usually powered by electricity. In Europe, diesel engines or

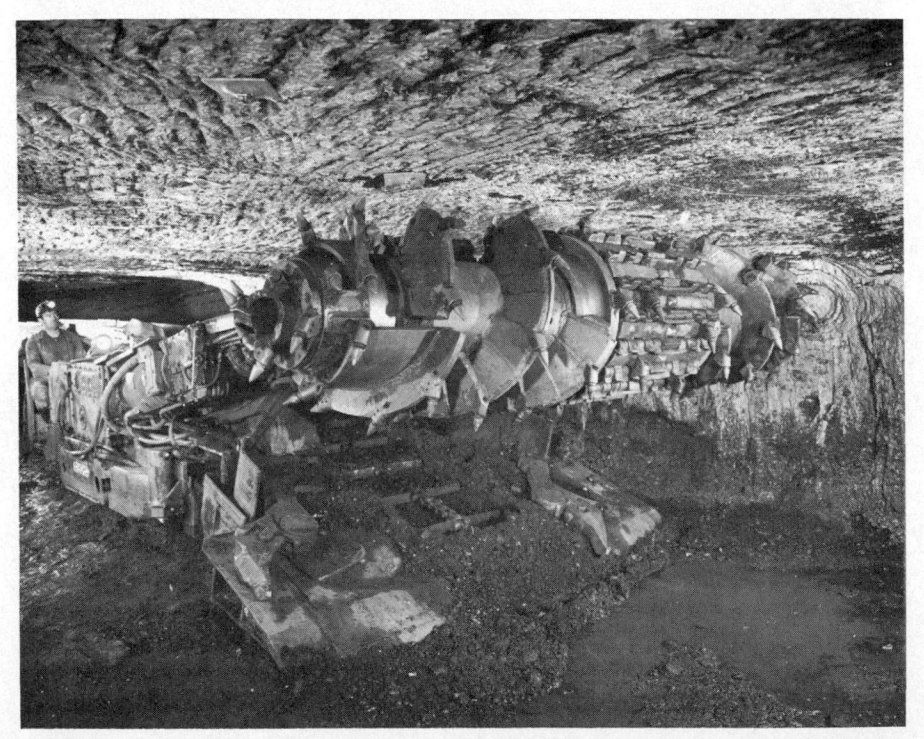

Figure 14–1. Continuous miner. The cutting head of this Joy Continuous Miner is designed to cut automatically an arched roof, thereby making the roof more stable and lessening the chance of roof falls. Coal is ripped from the seam and falls to the floor whence it is collected by gathering arms and a conveyor belt which are built into the machine. (Courtesy of Joy Manufacturing Co.)

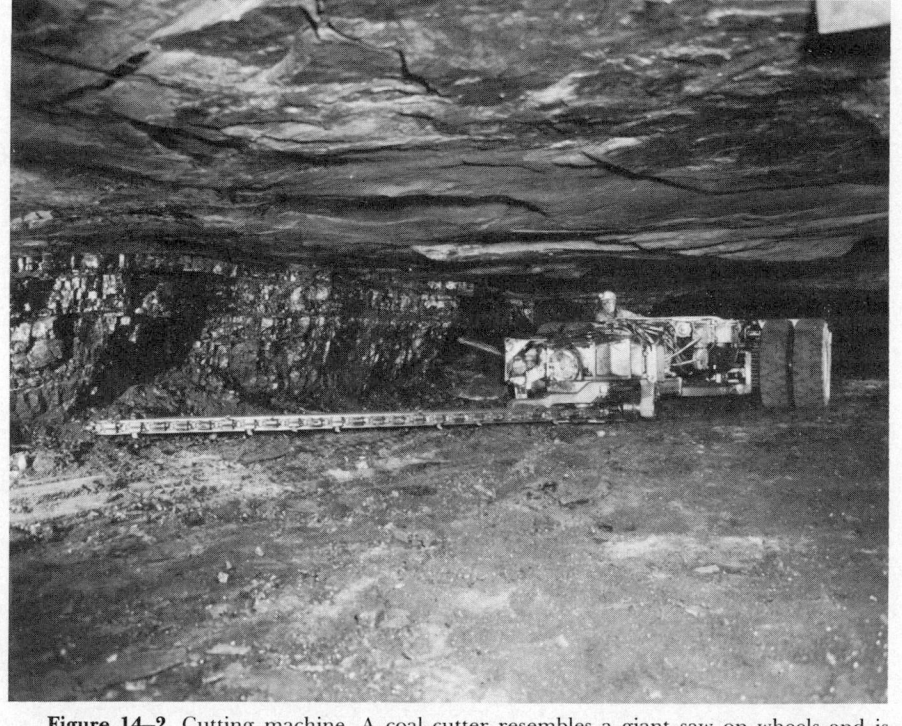

Figure 14–2. Cutting machine. A coal cutter resembles a giant saw on wheels and is used to cut a slot at the base of the seam. The cut is around 6 inches high and may be up to 12 feet deep. When the coal is blasted, the slot allows expansion. (Courtesy of Mining Equipment Division, Westinghouse Air Brake Co.)

conveyor belts are often used. The train is operated by a motorman who often drops sand on the rails in order to provide traction, a practice which, owing to the aerosolization of small particles of silica, occasionally leads to the development of classical silicosis. Motormen, brakemen, drivers, and shuttle car operators are usually regarded as part of "transportation." As such, they are exposed to less dust than those at the face.

Still farther away from the face, and only intermittently working in the dusty areas, are a small group of miners who maintain utilities and act as mechanics and electricians. These workers are exposed to less dust than are those employed in transportation and are classified as maintenance and miscellaneous personnel. Finally, a small proportion of miners work completely on the surface, viz., at the tipple or maintaining the cage and portal equipment. It is pertinent to bear in mind that many miners have held several jobs in the mine, although not infrequently men will be found who have spent all of their working life at the face or on transportation. In both Britain and the United States there is a tendency for older men to move away from the face.

Prior to the advent of mechanization, coal mining was one of the

more arduous jobs. Now this is no longer true, least of all in the United States, where a significant number of women have started working underground, many of whom are employed at the coal face. In this connection, most face operations require little exertion, since they are almost entirely mechanized, and the few underground jobs that are physically more demanding are those concerned with the maintenance of haulage equipment. Workers in these jobs are not exposed to high concentrations of dust, since in general they are at a distance from the face.

HISTORY OF COAL MINERS' LUNG DISEASE

The earliest reports of occupational lung disease occurring in coal miners made their appearance in the early 1800s. Laennec, shortly after the turn of the nineteenth century, separated melanosis of the lungs into four types, (1) melanotic masses enclosed by cysts, (2) melanotic masses lying unencysted, (3) melanosis in which the black matter infiltrates into the lung, and (4) melanosis with deposits on the lung surface. Later he separated malignant melanoma, which he clearly recognized as a form of cancer, from the black coloration of the lungs produced by pigments. Coal miners' lungs were characterized according to him by deposition of "la matière noire pulmonaire."

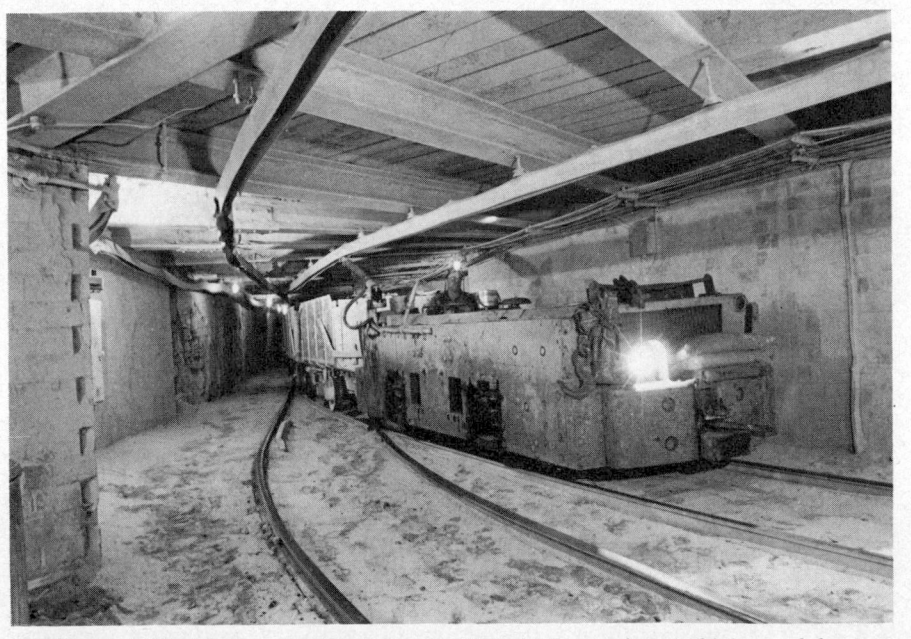

Figure 14–3. Modern transportation in United States mine. A high-speed haulage locomotive pulls a string of loaded cars from the coal fall. Notice sandbags in front, sand being dropped on the rails to obtain traction.

The history of coal workers' lung disease is described in detail by Meiklejohn.[2, 8, 9] In the nineteenth century lung diseases were observed to occur with great frequency in coal miners. The condition from which miners suffered was variously referred to as spurious melanosis, miners' asthma, anthracosis, miners' phthisis, and silicosis. By 1982 Arlidge wrote, "There is a widespread belief at the present day that the serious lesions of the lungs associated with the calling of coal-getters belong to past history, or, at the most, are very uncommon; and no doubt can exist that, compared with the past, they are becoming rarer, thanks to the introduction of efficient ventilation, of shortened hours of labour and of the increased attention given to the hygiene of mines."[10] Subsequent studies have shown that his optimism was misplaced.

For many years, in both Britain and the United States, the inhalation of coal dust was thought to be completely innocuous. That this concept was so widely held can be traced to the profound influence of two men: J. S. Haldane in Britain and Leroy Gardner in the United States. Haldane, a great respiratory physiologist, had catholic interests ranging from industrial hygiene to deep-water diving and parasitology. He first showed that Cornish tin miners suffered from hookworm disease and also conducted some classic studies of the relationship between silicosis and tuberculosis. Because tuberculosis was shown to be uncommon in coal miners, he assumed that silicosis was equally uncommon and that coal dust had little effect on the lungs. Despite Haldane's belief that coal dust was not harmful, his insistence that silicosis, coal workers' pneumoconiosis, and bronchitis were clinically and pathologically distinct disease states has been amply vindicated by time.[9]

For a variety of reasons little attention was given in the United States to the problem of coal miners' respiratory disease until the late 1960s. Such neglect was mainly a consequence of the fact that there was no federal governmental agency with responsibility for health, each state being responsible for its own occupational health activities. Moreover, the Bureau of Mines, the only federal agency involved, had minimal powers in regard to safety only. The investigations conducted by the Trudeau Group directed by Dr. Leroy Gardner indicated that coal dust was nonfibrogenic, and since bituminous coal miners were not exposed to significant quantities of silica, he assumed they were not at risk. Like Haldane, Gardner was a pioneer and had made great contributions to the understanding of silicosis, and as such, his opinion was almost sacrosanct.

Since coal mining was thought not to be associated with any danger to health, only a few epidemiological studies of coal miners were carried out in the United States between 1900 and 1960. Most were conducted in Pennsylvania by the Pennsylvania Department of Industrial Hygiene,[11] but a small study was also conducted in Utah with similar findings.[12] As a result almost no data on the prevalence of coal workers' pneumoconiosis were available until the United States Public Health Service (U.S.P.H.S.) conducted its pilot prevalence study in 1962 and 1963.[13]

Although improved ventilation greatly lessened the dust levels in the late nineteenth century, the introduction of even a minor degree of mechanization restored the status quo, and indeed in South Wales coal miners' lung disease reached almost epidemic proportions in the 1930s. The problem was recognized in Britain many years before it was in the United States, and in 1936 the Medical Research Council of Great Britain started an investigation of the problem of chronic pulmonary disease in coal miners. In 1942 Hart and Aslett published their report on coal miners' respiratory disease,[14] and shortly after this the Pneumoconiosis Research Unit was established at Cardiff in 1945. A comparable facility in the United States was not established until 1966, when the Appalachian Laboratory for Occupational Respiratory Diseases of the U.S.P.H.S. was founded in Morgantown, West Virginia.

THE ROLE OF SILICA IN COAL MINERS' LUNG DISEASE

The discovery of x-rays by Roentgen in 1896 was a great stimulus to the development of an understanding of occupational lung diseases. Although radiographic abnormalities were soon noted in the chest films of coal, gold, and other miners, the appearances were similar no matter to which dust the miner had been exposed. Silicosis, because its effects were more obvious and dramatic, received more attention, and it was soon clearly established that the inhalation of silica dust could lead to the production of radiographic abnormalities. When, at a later date, coal miners were observed to have similar radiographic changes, it was assumed that it was the silica present in the coal dust that was responsible for the abnormal chest film. To date, many Europeans and also some Americans subscribe to this view.

While coal workers' pneumoconiosis is predominantly associated with underground coal mining, it was the occurrence of the disease in Welsh coal trimmers that first called attention to its existence as a separate entity from silicosis. A coal trimmer was a special type of stevedore responsible for the loading and distribution of coal in the holds of ships. Unless the coal was evenly distributed, the ship became unstable and developed a list when it put to sea. Mechanized loading has removed the need for coal trimmers. The coal that used to be exported from Wales had been washed and separated from the rock before it was loaded onto the boat. Its silica content was hence minimal. Collis and Gilchrist[15] and later Gough[16] showed that Cardiff and Swansea trimmers had radiographic abnormalities that were indistinguishable from those seen in classical silicosis. At postmortem the trimmer's lungs were found to contain no more silica than was present in the normal nonmining population of South Wales. Later it was shown that the prevalence of coal workers' pneumoconiosis bore a poor relationship to the silica content of the coal mine dust to which the miners were exposed. In contrast, the relationship between radiographic category and

the coal dust content of the lungs was shown to be excellent.[17] Additional support for the hypothesis that coal dust or carbon alone may produce disease was forthcoming from the demonstration of a type of pneumoconiosis due to exposure to pure carbon. This was pathologically and radiographically similar to coal workers' pneumoconiosis.[18] The development of lung disease in graphite electrotypers has also been described and, similarly, some of these subjects were exposed to carbon only.[19, 20]

The final verdict in the coal versus quartz controversy is still awaited but recently there has been renewed interest in the role of quartz in the development of coal workers' pneumoconiosis. Davis and colleagues have shown that in subjects with progressive massive fibrosis (PMF) there is a preferential retention of quartz in the lungs of those subjects who have the most extensive and rapidly progressive lesions.[21] Subsequently Seaton et al. noted that a minority of coal miners at a Scottish colliery showed rapid radiographic progression of the disease despite generally low exposures to mixed coal mine dust.[22] It was subsequently shown that the mixed dust to which the miners had been exposed had an unusually high quartz content. The subjects who showed the most rapid progression also appeared most prone to develop PMF.[22a] Seaton and colleagues expressed the opinion that in a minority of miners quartz plays an important role in producing rapid radiological progression.

EPIDEMIOLOGY OF RESPIRATORY DISEASE IN COAL MINERS

Reliable data concerning the prevalence of various diseases in the United States coal mining population are scanty; nonetheless, it is widely believed that coal miners have a higher prevalence of lung disease than does the general male population. The cause of the increased respiratory morbidity and mortality is not completely understood, and moreover cannot be attributed to a single respiratory disease or any particular set of circumstances that the coal miner encounters in the performance of his job. Several respiratory diseases have been reported to occur with greater frequency in coal miners. In some instances, viz., in coal workers' pneumoconiosis (CWP), there is a direct relationship between the inhalation of coal dust and the disease that results; however, most of the increased respiratory morbidity and mortality appears to be a consequence of nonspecific airways obstruction. Furthermore, although obstructive airways disease has been reported to occur more frequently in coal miners, coal dust inhalation plays only a minor role in its etiology.[23]

The association between respiratory disease death rates and occupation was noted many years ago in the statistics of the Registrar General of England and Wales. Data published in the United States show similar trends, and the standardized mortality ratio (SMR) for respiratory disease is markedly increased in certain occupations. Thus it can be seen from Table 14-1 that the SMR for bronchitis and emphysema is much higher

for manual laborers than it is for the professional classes. A similar but lesser trend is present for lung cancer. Much of the difference in the incidence of lung cancer and emphysema that exists between different socioeconomic groups is a consequence of the fact that blue-collar workers smoke appreciably more; however, some doubt remains as to whether cigarette smoking is the entire explanation for the disparity.[24]

It is reasonable to assume that some of the deaths included in Table 14–1 under the heading bronchitis, emphysema, and other respiratory diseases are the result of industrial pulmonary disease, viz., silicosis and coal workers' pneumoconiosis. The fact that laborers not exposed to dust have a higher SMR for bronchitis and emphysema than do the operatives and miners indicates that the number of occupationally related respiratory deaths cannot be unduly great.

Enterline, in retrospective analyses, has shown that the standard mortality rates of coal miners in the United States were considerably elevated above those of nonminers.[25] Much of this excess was a consequence of trauma and accidents. If deaths due to these causes were excluded, a relationship between excess mortality and age emerged. This ranged from a 23 per cent excess between the ages of 20 and 24 years to a 122 per cent excess between 60 and 64. This excess at all ages is felt to represent the cumulative effect of environmental factors—some of which may be occupational—on the health of coal miners.

Much of the excess mortality noted by Enterline appeared to be a consequence of respiratory disease.[25] Although deaths due to chronic bronchitis and emphysema were increased, a finding that had been noted also in Britain, so were deaths due to tuberculosis and lung cancer. While it is relatively easy to postulate a relationship between chronic bronchitis and occupation, the same cannot be said for lung cancer and tuberculosis. Until 20 to 30 years ago, United States coal miners constituted a distinctly underprivileged group and as such suffered from overcrowding and poor

Table 14–1. STANDARDIZED MORTALITY RATIOS FOR SELECTED RESPIRATORY DISEASES FOR CERTAIN OCCUPATIONAL GROUPS (MALES 20–64)*

Occupation	Bronchitis, Emphysema, and Other Respiratory Disease	Lung Cancer	Percentage of Smokers (Age Corrected)
Laborers, except farm and mine	168	127	79
Operatives— including miners	158	107	81
Clerical workers	79	95	77
Managers, officials and proprietors	58	94	77

*From Guralick, L.: Mortality by Occupations and Causes of Death: United States, 1950, Vital Statistics, Special Reports, Vol. 53, No. 3. Washington, D.C., Department of Health, Education and Welfare, September, 1963.

economic circumstances, both of which may have contributed significantly to a higher death rate from tuberculosis. The same argument cannot explain the increased death rate due to lung cancer, since this condition is not related to overcrowding, and lung cancer now occurs less often in miners than it does in the general population. The explanation probably lies in the lack of uniformity and reliability in death certification in the United States. This situation is likely to have been compounded by the recent legislation that awards black lung compensation to any miner whose death certificate mentions coal workers' pneumoconiosis or any other respirable disease the effects of which could conceivably have been worsened by exposure to coal dust.

In 1973, Liddell studied the morbidity of a group of over 29,000 British coal miners.[3] He showed that miners lost more time from work than workers in other occupations. This state of affairs prevailed even when mining was compared to other nonmining tasks of an arduous nature. Among underground miners as a whole, those who were paid the least had the greatest amount of time off work. Incapacity varied between coal fields and was related to the worker's financial status, the category of pneumoconiosis, and the depth of the mine. Beat knee, as might be expected, was related to the height of the coal seam.

An additional study published at the same time studied the mortality of British coal miners.[26] In this, Liddell showed that miners generally had high death rates from accidents and pneumoconiosis, but low rates from lung cancer. Face workers, perhaps surprisingly, had lower death rates than expected. The Scottish coal fields had the highest respiratory death rates among British coal fields, a fact which may be explained by the greater number of cigarettes smoked by the average Scotsman.

Although in the past there was little doubt that coal miners had a decreased life expectancy, due mainly to accidents and to a lesser extent respiratory disease, at the present time coal miners live as long as does the general population. This statement is true for the United States, Britain, South Africa, Germany, and Australia. Thus in a randomly selected group of Appalachian coal miners who were followed for a period of 10 years, Ortmeyer and colleagues showed that they had a normal life expectancy.[27] Neither simple CWP nor years underground was associated with an increased SMR. In contrast, both PMF and cigarette smoking were shown to decrease life expectancy. In this connection it might be asked why, if coal miners die more frequently as a result of contracting complicated pneumoconiosis, the effects are not reflected as an increase in the overall SMR. The explanation lies in the fact that the increased death rate from CWP is more than counterbalanced by the decreased death rates from heart disease and lung cancer.[28, 29] Subsequent studies of the same cohort of Appalachian miners clearly demonstrated that both heart disease and lung cancer occurred less frequently than in the general population.[28, 29] The normal life expectancy has subsequently been confirmed in a larger study conducted by Rockette.[30] The cohort selected for this study

was derived from the records of miners who were eligible for medical benefits from the Health and Retirement Funds of the United Mine Workers of America. Unfortunately, the population included in the Rockette study was not randomly chosen and in addition no smoking history was available. This contrasts to the studies conducted by Ortmeyer and co-workers and Costello and colleagues.[27–29] Although the overall SMR for Rockette's group of coal miners was similar to that of the general population, the SMR for lung cancer was marginally increased at 112. The explanation for this probably lies in the fact that miners from Charleston and southern West Virginia were over-represented in the study population. These areas have a significantly increased rate of lung cancer compared with the United States as a whole.

In Britain, Cochrane has likewise demonstrated that simple CWP is not associated with an increased SMR.[31] Subsequently in a 20-year follow-up study of a cohort of miners from the Rhondda Fach, Cochrane and colleagues were again unable to demonstrate an effect of simple CWP on the life expectancy of coal miners; however, the SMR for bronchitis and other respiratory diseases was slightly but significantly increased.[32] Nevertheless, there was no real difference between the SMRs for those with and without pneumoconiosis. Additional long-term follow-up studies in coal miners and foundry workers from Stavely, Derbyshire, have yielded similar results. Unlike the miners from the Rhondda Fach, who showed a slight increase in their SMR, Derbyshire coal miners had a normal life expectancy.[33]

A lengthy and detailed report relating the mortality of British coal miners to a number of factors, including radiographic category, lung function, and dust exposure, was recently published.[34] Older miners, who formed the main population studied, had a lower death rate than expected when compared to recent recruits to coal mining, a finding that may be partially explained by the healthy worker effect. As in other studies, miners with PMF, except for stage A, had an increased SMR. Simple CWP had no effect on life expectancy, except in the 25 to 34 age group. This suggests that those miners who contract the disease while young are unduly prone to progress to PMF. The magnitude of dust exposure was likewise not associated with a general increase in mortality.

Death rates from gastrointestinal cancer were noted to be increased in coal miners, an observation that has also been noted in the United States.[35, 36] In a case control study, Ames and co-workers noted that gastric carcinoma occurs more frequently in coal miners who have prolonged exposure to both coal dust and cigarette smoke; however, CWP per se was not associated with an increased risk of gastric cancer.[36] These data suggest that in coal miners with impaired pulmonary function, coal mine dust in conjunction with long-term cigarette smoking poses an increased risk of stomach cancer. In contrast, in smoking miners with normal pulmonary function, the main risk from cigarette smoking appeared to be lung cancer.

The death rate from lung cancer in coal miners has been shown to be less than expected, and this applies to virtually all of the reliable studies from both Britain and the United States.[23, 26, 29, 34] The decreased incidence of lung cancer is probably related to the fact that the number of cigarette smokers in the mining population tends to be 5 to 10 per cent less than in the general population and that miners, for the most part, smoke fewer cigarettes per person. One assumes that this is a consequence of not being allowed to smoke while underground.

COAL WORKERS' PNEUMOCONIOSIS

Coal workers' pneumoconiosis (CWP) is best defined as the accumulation of coal dust in the lungs and the tissue's reaction to its presence. Necessary for establishing a diagnosis of CWP are a history of exposure to coal dust—usually at least 10 years underground—and certain relatively characteristic abnormalities on the chest radiograph. CWP is separated into simple and complicated forms according to the appearances of the chest film. The pathological basis for the distinction between the two forms of CWP was laid by the pioneer investigations carried out by the Cardiff school.[15, 37–39]

Simple Coal Workers' Pneumoconiosis

Clinical Features

Simple coal workers' pneumoconiosis is a consequence of the inhalation of coal mine dust alone. Clinically, it has almost no symptoms. While almost all miners have a slight cough and some blackish sputum, the symptoms are nonspecific and certainly are of no help in establishing whether or not the disease is present. Shortness of breath is seldom marked in the absence of coincident chronic airways obstruction. There is no evidence to indicate that dyspnea is any more common in miners with simple CWP than it is in those without the condition.

Simple CWP does not progress in the absence of further exposure. This statement must not be taken out of context, since it only applies to the small opacities of simple CWP. Thus, progressive massive fibrosis (PMF) may develop in a lung that has been suitably primed by a heavy dust burden, even though the subject is no longer exposed. The major importance of simple CWP lies in the fact that it is a precursor of complicated disease; nonetheless, it does have certain effects on the function of the lungs. These are described later in the chapter.

Radiological Features

Simple CWP is diagnosed and classified according to the number of small opacities present in the chest film.[40] Such opacities may occur

anywhere in the lung fields, but virtually always make their appearance in the upper zones. As the disease progresses the small opacities often become evident in other regions of the lungs, but the predominant upper lobe involvement persists. Although irregular opacities are seen in a minority of coal miners, they do not have the same connotation as do small rounded opacities. Scanty irregular opacities (0/1, 1/0) occur frequently in smokers who have had no industrial exposure.[41] This is also true for smoking coal miners, and they may be observed in surface workers with little or no exposure to dust. [42] Small irregular opacities are seen with increased frequency in older subjects, in bronchitics, in those exposed to asbestos and manmade mineral fibers, and commonly in subjects with interstitial fibrosis.[43] An association between the presence of irregular opacities, airways obstruction, and overdistension of the lungs has been demonstrated in coal miners.[42] It is important to bear in mind that the presence of scanty irregular opacities in the lower zones only should not be accepted as an indication that the miner has CWP; rather, an alternative explanation should be sought.

As mentioned earlier, simple CWP does not progress in the absence of further exposure, but whether the condition ever regresses is uncertain. Most commonly, the so-called regression results from a change in film technique, such that a later film of a pair is more overpenetrative compared with the earlier film. The development of emphysema, especially of the compensatory variety, may appear to reduce the profusion of nodules in certain regions of the lung. This is not a consequence of an absolute reduction in the number of nodules, but rather a consequence of the concerned lobe becoming overdistended so that the nodules that are present become separated by greater distances. In rare instances, paired radiographs apparently show definite regression, but even so it is difficult to know whether the nodules that were noted previously were not a consequence of some process that spontaneously regresses, e.g., sarcoidosis or welders' siderosis. (For a complete description of the ILO classification, see Chap. 5.)

In simple CWP the profusion of small rounded opacities is related to the weight of retained dust and to its measured constituents.[17, 34] Subjects with p-type opacities show the highest mean dust content regardless of the rank of coal mined. The lung dust contents of subjects with p-type opacities show a higher proportion of coal and a lower proportion of ash.[34] In contrast, the lungs of subjects with r opacities show significantly lower lung dust contents, and relatively greater ash and quartz percentages. The foci of dust in the lungs of subjects with p-type opacities tend to be smaller, less often palpable, and more numerous than those present in the lungs of subjects with q and r opacities. In addition, there appears to be more emphysema present in subjects whose chest film shows p opacities. The presence of r opacities was associated with larger, more easily palpable, but less numerous nodules.[34] Musk et al. found a reduced diffusing capacity, no increase in compliance, and a tendency toward

increased recoil pressure in coal workers with irregular opacities.[44] They postulated that the physiological findings were a consequence of coexisting fibrosis and emphysema. They also suggest that p-type opacities were associated with physiological evidence of emphysema. However, their data showed that subjects with this type of opacity, when compared to subjects with q and r opacities, had a higher FEV_1 and FVC but a lower RV and TLC, along with essentially unchanged recoil pressures.

Small rounded opacities of the p and q type are found most often in CWP, while the nodular or r type of opacity predominates in silicosis. The micronodular type of opacity (q) is found in both conditions; however, p-type opacities are virtually never seen in classical silicosis. Nevertheless, in most instances CWP and silicosis are radiologically indistinguishable unless either calcification of parenchymal opacities or egg-shell calcification is present.

Radiographic Progression

The usual method of determining radiographic progression is to place side by side two radiographs taken at an appropriate interval. Their appearances are then compared by a reader who knows the dates on which both films were taken. There is seldom any point in comparing paired films unless there is at least a five-year interval between them. Even with this five-year gap, progression is often difficult to detect and affects only a minority of miners. Furthermore, changes are generally so slight that it is imperative to use the full-point 12-point scale; indeed, Liddell and May devised the elaboration of the ILO classification for the specific purpose of determining radiographic progression.[45] Similarly, it is rare for a miner to progress more than one subcategory over a five-year period. For a more complete discussion of the methods of assessing progression, the reader is referred to Chapter 5.

Relationship of Radiographic Progression to Dust Levels. There is a definite paucity of long-term studies relating the levels of respirable dust to radiographic progression. Almost the only reliable ones come from the National Coal Board of Great Britain and the Steinkohlenberg-bauverein of West Germany.

The National Coal Board began their Pneumoconiosis Field Research (PFR) in 1952. Twenty-five pits were selected and were visited by mobile x-ray units at intervals of five years. The collieries were representative of the range of environmental conditions prevailing in British coal fields. Later, spirometry was added to the examination, as was a simple respiratory questionnaire.[46]

The British PFR Study was designed to answer the following questions:

1. Can radiographic progression of pneumoconiosis be related to airborne dust measurements?

2. Does the risk of developing pneumoconiosis increase with increasing dust exposure, and if so, does a linear relationship exist?

3. What dust levels produce pneumoconiosis? How does the composition of the dust affect the risk of developing coal workers' pneumoconiosis?

A series of papers have summarized the findings. The earliest was published in 1967 and summarized the first 10 years of the study.[47] A radiographic progression index was related to the mean coal face dust concentrations. The latter were measured using the standard thermal precipitator and were later converted from particle counts into mass concentrations by means of conversion factors that have been established previously in trials conducted by the National Coal Board.[48] The relationship between radiographic progression and particle counts was weak and statistically insignificant. In contrast, progression and mean mass concentrations were significantly related.

At a meeting held in Luxembourg in 1972, Jacobsen analyzed in detail the findings of the study up to 1971.[49] He was able to demonstrate:

1. A significant correlation between radiographic progression and exposure to airborne dust.

2. That miners with early signs of dust retention (categories 0/1 to 1/0) are more likely to have progression than those with category 0/0, or, expressed in a different fashion, in those men in whom the disease develops sooner, it continues to progress more rapidly.

He constructed a series of curves to predict the probability of progression occurring with various dust exposures. Further follow-up has resulted in slight modifications of his original predictions.[50] Thus at the present time the best available evidence suggests that exposure to a dust level of 2 mg/m^3 for eight hours a day for 35 years would result in the development of category 2 or above in between 1 and 2 per cent of those who started work with a clear radiograph and no prior history of exposure. For a dust level of 3.5 mg/m^3, under the same conditions, the probability that a worker would develop category 2 or above was 3.5 per cent.

Since 1960, Reisner has been conducting a similar investigation in Germany which involves 17,000 men at 13 pits.[51] The similarity of Reisner's results to those of the National Coal Board is remarkable when it is borne in mind that a totally different methodology was and is used for measuring dust concentrations. The Germans use a tyndalloscope for measuring respirable dust levels and derive what they term a "k" value. Reisner has also shown that the risks of developing pneumoconiosis at different coal mines cannot be explained solely by the concentrations of dust to which the men are exposed. He maintains that different dusts have different degrees of "injuriousness," and that the harmful qualities of the dust cannot entirely be explained by the quartz or dirt content of the respirable dust.[52] His latest predictions closely resemble those of Jacobsen.[53]

Relationship of Lung Dust Content to Radiographic and Other Changes in the Lung. The relationships between lung dust, work history,

pathological stage of disease, and radiographic category have been studied by a number of workers.[17, 34, 54, 55] Faulds and colleagues observed differences between the composition of lung dust of Welsh, Cumbrian, and Lancastrian miners.[56] Their studies have been continued and extended by the Safety in Mines Research Establishment and the Pneumoconiosis Research Unit at Cardiff.[57, 58] It is now apparent that the dust found in the lungs of coal miners consists mainly of coal and the minerals quartz, mica, and kaolin. Needless to say, quartz represents a definite and distinct threat to the lungs, producing silicosis when its content in the airborne dust is sufficiently high. Although coal is the main constituent of coal mine dust, weight for weight it contributes less to the radiographic category than quartz and other clay minerals. In addition, iron-containing minerals are found in excess in pneumoconiotic lungs. The iron content is too high to be accounted for by exogenous inhaled iron and therefore must partly be derived from endogenous sources.

The significance of the iron, coal, and mineral contents of the lungs and their relationship to radiographic category have been reviewed by Bergman and Casswell.[58] These workers showed that the average lung dust composition varies significantly with the rank of coal. The higher the rank, the higher the coal percentage and the lower the quartz content of the lungs. The iron content is closely related to mineral and coal contents of the lungs and also to years spent underground. A further report of this study was made by Rossiter in New York.[59] From a homogeneous group of 98 miners, the correlation between radiographic evidence of simple CWP and coal and other minerals was 0.9. The ratio of their relative contribution to the radiographic appearances was 1:3.8, which corresponds approximately to their x-ray mass absorption coefficient. The iron content of the lungs did not add much to the correlation despite the fact that by itself it was closely related to the radiographic category. Miners with the r type of opacity had a lower than expected dust content. Recent work suggests that fibrotic palpable nodules have a closer association with the presence of small rounded opacities in the chest film than do smaller nonpalpable macules.[34] This would suggest that tissue reaction has a significant effect in the induction of radiographic changes. Nagelschmidt demonstrated earlier that, rather surprisingly, the lungs of subjects dying of progressive massive fibrosis usually contain only about the same weight of coal dust as do the lungs of subjects with category 2 or 3 simple CWP.[60]

Comparable studies in the United States are lacking; however, the metal and mineral contents of the lungs have been studied in a small sample of West Virginia miners.[61, 62] The lungs of the miners contained an excess of beryllium, cobalt, copper, and other minerals, but the significance, if any, of the increases was and is not apparent. In another study, the lungs of urban dwellers who served as controls were also shown to contain a fairly high concentration of both coal and other dusts; indeed, there was often an overlap between the miners and the controls. The silica content of the lungs of the controls, however, was significantly less than that found in the lungs of coal miners.[63]

It is often suggested that coal dust, or at least the carbon in coal dust, cannot account for the opacities present in the lung. Some persons feel that the radiographic opacities are mainly a consequence of the collagen and fibrous protein content of the lungs, and indeed there is often substantial truth in this assertion. Nevertheless, the one outstanding fact that emerges from these studies is the excellent relationship between the coal dust content of the lungs and radiographic category. Thus the chest film, despite drawbacks in its interpretation, at present remains the only feasible method of determining and quantifying dust exposure in life. Recently, a noninvasive method utilizing magnetopneumography has been used to estimate the dust load present in the lungs. A correlation has been shown between radiographic category and coal dust content as determined by this method. At present this technique remains experimental.[64]

Prevalence

Numerous studies of the prevalence of coal workers' pneumoconiosis have been carried out in all the major coal-producing countries of the world. Unfortunately, the methodology has often differed and comparisons between prevalence rates in different countries are often not possible. In this regard, the increasing acceptance of standard radiological classifications for the pneumoconioses has led to a marked improvement, but much still remains to be done. Furthermore, all prevalence studies suffer from a major drawback in that they only give information about the number of subjects with the condition at any one time, and tell the investigators little or nothing about when or how the disease originated. Thus in many instances the development of coal workers' pneumoconiosis is a consequence of the environmental conditions that prevailed 20 years ago rather than what is happening at the present time.

Prevalence in the United States. From 1963 to 1965 the United States Public Health Service (U.S.P.H.S.) examined 3602 working bituminous coal miners.[65] The percentage of miners showing definite radiographic evidence of either simple or complicated pneumoconiosis ranged from approximately 11 per cent in Appalachia to 6 per cent in the Midwest to approximately 4 per cent in Utah. Face workers had the highest prevalence, followed by transportation, maintenance, and miscellaneous workers with the disease being seen least often in surface workers.

Late in 1969, the Interagency Study was instituted by the Appalachian Laboratory for Occupational Respiratory Diseases of the National Institute of Occupational Safety and Health, and the Bureau of Mines of the Department of the Interior. Thirty-one coal mines were selected for study; of these, 2 were anthracite mines and 29 were bituminous.[66, 67] The mines were chosen to represent different geographical areas, coal seams, and mining methods. Between October 1969 and July 1971, over 9000 miners were examined. Participation in the survey was over 90 per cent. An overall prevalence of nearly 30 per cent was found; however, only 2.5 per cent of the sample had progressive massive fibrosis (PMF). Again, a wide

difference in prevalence was apparent between the various regions. Thus, in eastern Pennsylvania anthracite miners, 46 per cent had simple pneumoconiosis and 14.3 per cent had complicated disease. In contrast, in Colorado miners only 4.6 per cent had simple pneumoconiosis and none had complicated disease. A decreasing prevalence was noted from East to West, and a clear-cut relationship between years spent underground and radiographic category was apparent. Again, there was more disease in face workers than in surface workers.

Inevitably, prevalence data from the Interagency Study will be compared to that of the previous U.S.P.H.S. Prevalence Study of 1963 to 1965.[58] A superficial assessment might suggest that the prevalence of the disease increased and the situation had deteriorated. However, such an interpretation is not warranted because the methodologies of the two studies differed profoundly. First, the panel of interpreters had changed. Second, in the later of the two studies a consensus of two of the three panel members was accepted in regard to the category of the radiographs, whereas in the 1963–1965 study, when there was a difference of opinion between the three readers, a meeting was held and a unanimous decision forced. Third, the radiographs in the earlier study were interpreted according to the 1958 ILO classification; in contrast the 1969–1971 study utilized the UICC/Cincinnati classification.[68] Studies have shown that the substitution of the UICC/Cincinnati classification results in an appreciably greater number of films being placed in category 1. This is related to the fact that many of the radiographs formerly interpreted as either category Z (suspicious) or L (linear) would now be read as category 1.[69] Nonetheless, of those categories not affected by the change in classification, viz., categories 2 and 3 and PMF, there appears to be little difference between the studies, and indeed the prevalence of PMF appeared to have declined. Finally, it is apparent that there was significant over-reading by the panel of readers in the first round of the Interagency study. Rereading with the use of the standard ILO films led to a significant reduction in the prevalence of pneumoconiosis.

The second round of Interagency study showed an overall pneumoconiosis prevalence of 8 per cent. The findings at the third round were just under 5 per cent, with 3.85 per cent having category 1; 0.48 per cent, category 2; 0.04 per cent, category 3; and 0.17 per cent, PMF.[70] There are several reasons for the decline in the prevalence of pneumoconiosis noted between the first and third rounds, including the use of different readers; an exodus of those with radiographic evidence of pneumoconiosis, since this group automatically qualified for compensation; and possibly a minimal effect from the lower dust levels which might tend to lessen progression and the attack rate. As an additional complicating factor, participation fell from 90 per cent in the first round to 60 per cent in the third.

Prevalence in Other Countries. Complete details of the most recent prevalence data from Britain are published in the Medical Service and

Medical Research Annual Report of the National Coal Board (1979–80).[71] The overall prevalence of CWP in 1979 was 4.2 per cent.[71] The marked geographical differences in prevalence that had been noted in previous surveys persisted. Thus the various regional prevalences were 0.6 per cent in Scotland, 5.3 per cent in the Northumberland area, 2.8 per cent in South Yorkshire, and 11.3 per cent in South Wales. Similar variations in the prevalence of PMF were present, ranging from 0.1 per cent in the Midlands to 1.2 per cent in South Wales. Progression rates in the main mirrored prevalence rates, but over the last 10 years there has been a gradual decline in progression rates for pneumoconiosis throughout Britain.

Figures from Germany and France are not really comparable, owing to different x-ray reading systems, but it has been reported that France has a prevalence of around 12 per cent. In Australia in 1963 to 1965 the prevalence for all forms of pneumoconiosis was 3 per cent and is now below 2 per cent. This contrasts with a figure of 16 per cent in 1948.[72] Prevalence in Yugoslavia varies between 4 and 15 per cent according to the location of the mine.[73]

Relationship of Prevalence to Rank of Coal and Other Factors. The marked regional differences in prevalence of pneumoconiosis cannot be explained by differing number of years spent underground, and other factors have to be considered. Obviously, the most important of these is the respirable dust levels that have prevailed over the past 25 years. Unfortunately, in the United States no systematic dust sampling program existed before 1970.

Other factors that may be partly responsible for regional differences in prevalence are the physical and chemical composition of the coal mined. Certain coals may fragment more easily and tend to produce a greater number of harmful particles of around 1 to 2 microns, while others may generate larger and less dangerous particles of about 4 to 5 microns. Alternatively, the chemical composition of the coal mined may account for the higher prevalence of the disease in certain regions, and as has been mentioned earlier, the silica content can influence both the attack and progression rates.[22, 22a] The rank of the coal may also play a role, as may other chemical constituents.[74, 75] It appears that the areas mining the highest-ranked coal have the highest prevalence of the disease.

Pathology

The primary lesion of simple CWP is the coal macule. In general, such macules are widely but fairly evenly distributed throughout the lungs with a predilection for the upper lobes. They may measure up to 5 mm in diameter.[16, 37–39]

Shortly after coal dust is deposited in the alveoli, it is phagocytosed by macrophages and conveyed proximally toward the respiratory bronchioles. With continued prolonged exposure, small aggregations of dust

begin to accumulate in the pulmonary lymphoid tissue and around the pulmonary arterioles and veins. Larger collections occur in the regional lymph nodes. When the dust-laden phagocytes become so numerous that they can no longer pass beyond the respiratory bronchiole, they tend to cluster round its first and second divisions. The aggregations of dust are characteristically situated in or near the center of the secondary lobule, hence the term centrilobular or centriacinar.[16, 37–39] Such macules are seen in whole lung sections as small black dots (Fig. 14–4).

Initially the macule is characterized by a large amount of dust. Later a little reticulin and collagen fibrosis develops (Figs. 14–5 and 14–6). As the macule enlarges, the bronchial smooth muscle atrophies, and as a consequence the bronchiole dilates. Whether the dilation of the bronchiole is a consequence of pressure from inside acting on the weakened wall or a consequence of extraluminal forces applied to the wall is as yet undecided. Either way, the bronchiolar diameter increases; this situation is usually referred to as focal emphysema.[37–39] A complete and recent discussion of the pathology of CWP and its effects on lung function is to be found in a monograph published by the American College of Pathologists.[39] A notable attempt was made to set standards whereby the condition may be recognized and quantitated.

Focal emphysema is situated in the center of the lobule and hence is difficult to distinguish from the centrilobular variety of emphysema that is commonly seen in the cigarette-smoking general population who have chronic airflow obstruction. Although Gough and Heppleston both maintained that focal emphysema can be distinguished from the more common centrilobular form by the absence of an associated bronchiolitis, others do not share their opinion.[76, 77] The end result of simple CWP is shown in Figure 10–6. According to Heppleston, simple CWP has the same features the world over and appears not to be influenced by the rank of coal mined, whether anthracite, bituminous, or carbonaceous, or by the coal field, whether in the United States, Britain, Australia, or South Africa.[37, 38] Recent work, however, suggests that the histological appearances of the macule are affected by the composition and contents of the coal mine dust to which the miner has been exposed.[34, 78]

In coal miners whose lung residue contains 18 per cent or more of quartz, the pathological lesions are those of classical silicosis. A recent study has shown that the histological appearances of the lesions differ according to the composition of the coal mine dust to which the subject has been exposed.[79] In some subjects there is a vigorous cellular response, and the dust particles are widely separated by granulation tissue consisting mainly of macrophages and fibroblasts intermingled with collagen and reticulin fibers. The collagen in the center of such lesions may be laid down haphazardly, but on other occasions suggests the whorling of classical silicotic nodules. In the other type of response or lesion, few cells are present, and the dust masses and dust residue are tightly packed with little reticulin or collagen present in the lesion. Although in the past both

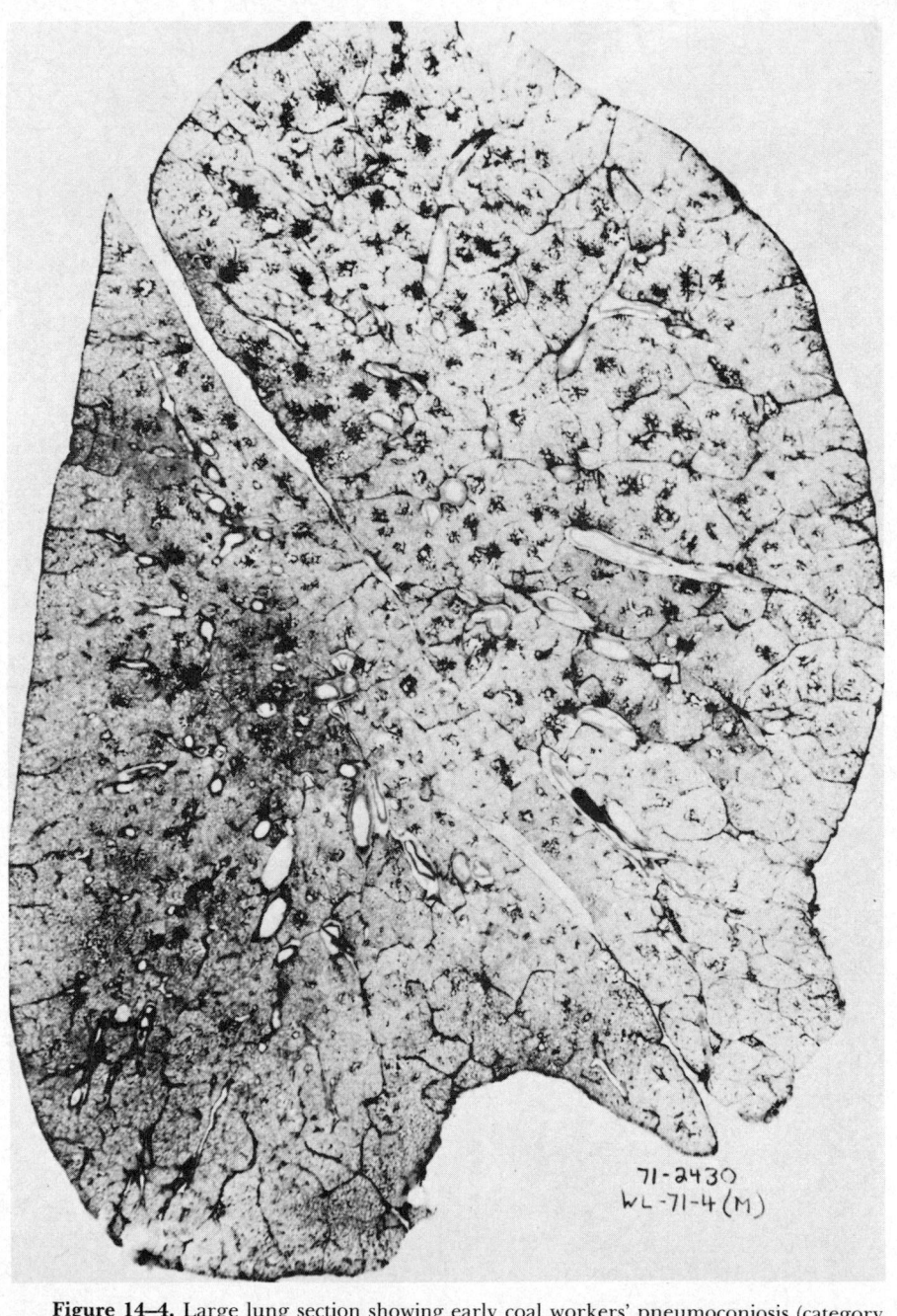

Figure 14–4. Large lung section showing early coal workers' pneumoconiosis (category 1). The black deposits are the coal macules, a few of which show focal emphysema.

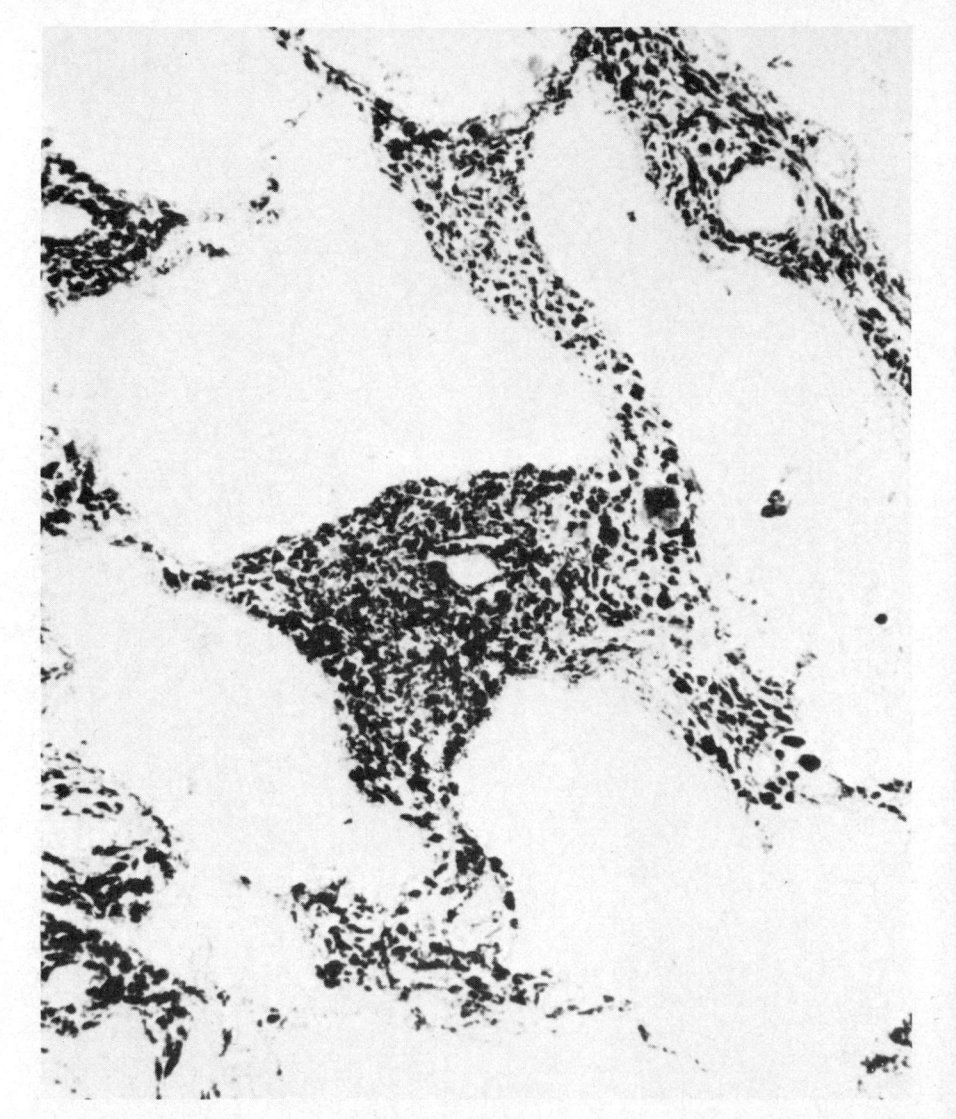

Figure 14–5. Coal macule surrounding distal airway and showing early extension into the pulmonary interstitium.

of these lesions were referred to as macules, some workers are now reserving the term for the second type of lesion. The lungs of subjects who show tightly packed dust macules have a high coal and a low ash content. In contrast, the lungs of subjects who demonstrate palpable nodules with histological evidence of a high collagen and reticulin content have a low coal content but higher ash, quartz, kaolin, and mica contents. In many instances there is a disparity between the percentage composition of retained dust found in the lungs and the lymph nodes, with the latter showing a far greater percentage of quartz.

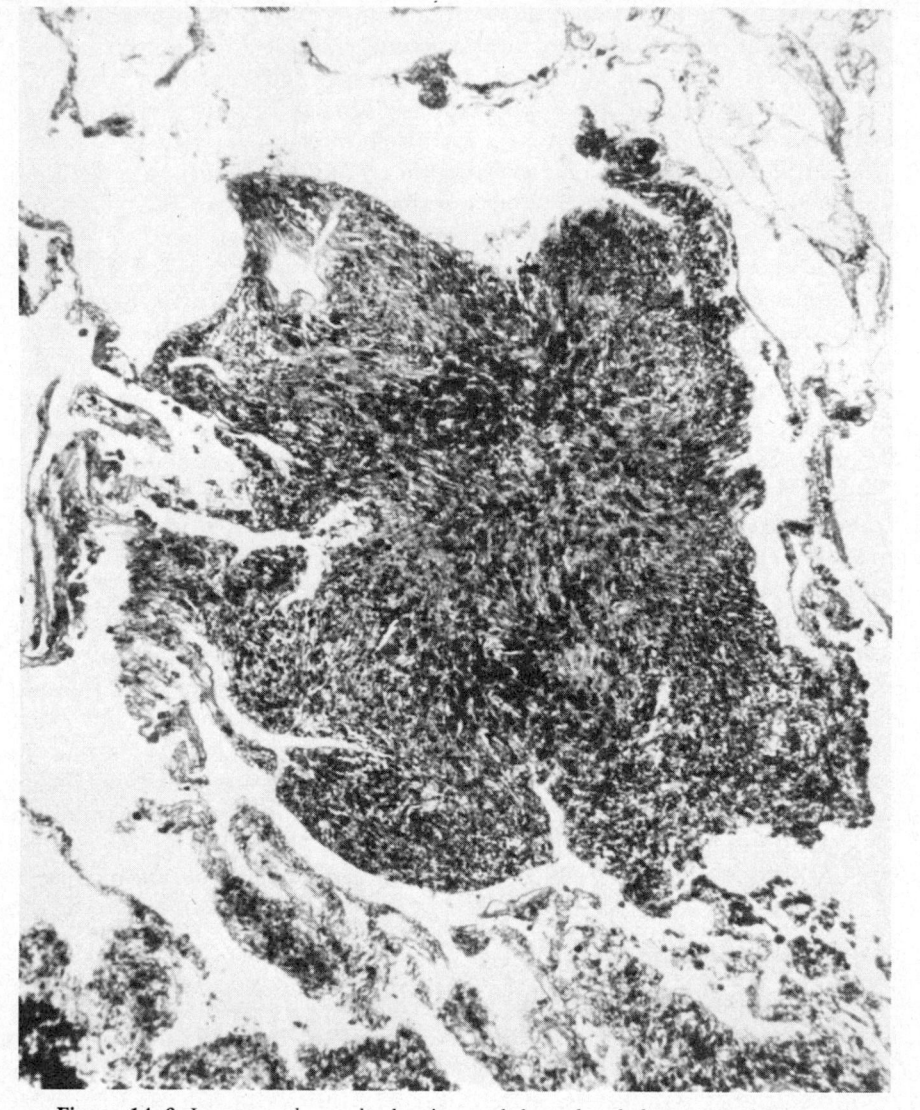

Figure 14–6. Larger coal macule showing coal dust, dust-laden macrophages, reticulin fibers, and minimal collagenous fibrosis.

Two distinct forms of PMF appear to be associated with the different types of simple lesion just described, although in some instances hybrid variants that do not fit readily into either category occur. The first form of PMF presents, as a solitary mass with no evidence to suggest that it originates from aggregation of multiple smaller nodules. The second type of PMF suggests that it is formed by the aggregation and fusion of groups of smaller fibrotic nodules. The latter type of PMF occurs in the cellular type of lesion that shows an absence of heavy dust packing. Simple CWP often occurs concomitantly with chronic bronchitis and emphysema; how-

ever, there is little or no evidence that simple CWP predisposes to the development of chronic bronchitis. In contrast, there is evidence that dust per se, even when it is eliminated by the mucociliary escalator, may play a role in the production of bronchitis. This is discussed in detail in Chapters 4 and 17, and elsewhere in this chapter.

Simple CWP does not affect the heart unless there is a coincident obstructive emphysema.[80, 81] Wells conducted autopsies of the heart and lungs of 388 coal workers from the Rhondda and other Welsh coal valleys.[82] He showed that in simple pneumoconiosis there was a slight loss of capillaries and a variable but usually insignificant effect on the small pulmonary arteries and arterioles. This contrasted with the combined obstructive and restrictive changes seen in progressive massive fibrosis. His study was carefully performed, and the pulmonary vasculature was examined in great detail. His findings were confirmed by James and Thomas,[83] who found that of 546 subjects dying of simple pneumoconiosis, only 8 could be found in which pulmonary heart disease seemed to be a consequence of CWP alone, and even in this small group it was a diagnosis made by exclusion. In seven other subjects who had neither cardiac nor pulmonary disease other than simple CWP, a degree of right ventricular enlargement was present, although this was not the cause of death. Thus it has been accepted for some time that simple CWP seldom leads to right ventricular hypertrophy. Nevertheless, there are those who have claimed that simple CWP may cause cor pulmonale,[85] a claim that has been effectively dismissed by Stanescu.[86] A recent comprehensive postmortem study of the hearts of 215 coal miners settled this issue and showed that right ventricular hypertrophy did not occur except in cigarette smokers with emphysema and in subjects with PMF. The degree of cardiac hypertrophy was closely related to the size of the conglomerate masses.[86a]

Pulmonary Function

The results of many of the early studies of pulmonary function in coal miners were incorrectly interpreted. Most of the early investigations were carried out on coal miners who had both an abnormal radiograph and respiratory symptoms. After carrying out extensive physiological studies, it was concluded that the respiratory impairments that were demonstrated were a consequence of the radiographic abnormalities, an assumption that was subsequently shown to be only partly correct.[87, 88] Since that time the importance of adequately controlled studies has been realized, and the various physiological impairments that occur in simple and complicated pneumoconiosis have been well characterized.[89, 90]

Ventilatory Capacity. Although in their studies Motley and colleagues equated the respiratory impairment they demonstrated with the occupation of coal mining, they were unable to show a relationship between the standard measurements of ventilatory capacity, viz., vital capacity (VC), forced expiratory volume in 1 second (FEV_1), and maximal voluntary

ventilation (MVV), and radiographic category.[87, 88] There was a similar lack of correlation between ventilatory capacity and years worked underground.

Pemberton studied 242 working coal miners by means of simple spirometric tests.[91] He used the FEV_1 as his index of ventilatory capacity and compared the ventilatory capacity of his group of miners to that of the two control groups: one rural and one urban. As a whole, miners had a slightly lower FEV_1 than did either of the control groups, despite the fact that the miners smoked somewhat less. The miners also had more respiratory symptoms, viz., cough, sputum, and shortness of breath; however, there was no relationship between symptoms and radiographic category.

In a well-controlled and excellently designed study, Hyatt and co-workers showed that 39 per cent of their random sample of miners and ex-miners between 45 and 58 years of age had simple pneumoconiosis.[92] A further 7 per cent had progressive massive fibrosis. These workers used the expiratory flow between 25 and 75 per cent of the forced expiratory volume (FEF_{25-75}) as their index of bellows function. They found that there was a relationship between ventilatory function, symptoms of bronchitis, and years worked underground. Only in complicated pneumoconiosis could it be demonstrated that pneumoconiosis led to a reduction of ventilatory capacity. Neither age, smoking habits, nor radiographic category of simple pneumoconiosis explained the small reduction of ventilatory function that occurred with years worked underground.

A random sample of 2432 working miners and 1028 ex-miners was studied in the 1962–63 U.S.P.H.S. prevalence study.[13] The FVC of the miners studied did not differ from predicted values; however, in older miners, the FEV_1 was slightly lower than the predicted figure. In regard to the ratio of FEV_1/FVC, a decline was evident with increasing age, but even so it was not related to radiographic category except in complicated disease. Both bronchitis and smoking history were associated with a decline in FEV_1 and $FEV_1/FVC\%$. Unfortunately, some of the data used in this study were not corrected for age—in particular those relating the decline in FEV_1 to radiographic category—and as a result some of the relationships remain obscure.

For the first round of the Interagency Study, the ventilatory capacity of over 9000 working United States miners was determined.[93] When the observed values for FVC were compared to the predicted figures, there was a minor but statistically significant reduction only in the anthracite miners of Pennsylvania. Indeed, in the Utah and Colorado miners, the observed figure was significantly higher than the predicted. For the FEV_1, there was an appreciable difference between the observed and predicted figures of the anthracite miners. Lesser disparities between observed and predicted values were noted in southern Appalachia and Alabama miners; however, the higher percentage of black miners in Alabama probably accounts for the lower mean FEV_1 in this region[93] (see Chap. 5). This

study shows that there are marked regional variations in ventilatory capacity. Lacking suitable control populations, it is entirely possible, indeed probable, that such differences are the consequence of nonoccupationally related factors. As in other studies, no decline in ventilatory capacity was evident until the advent of progressive massive fibrosis.

Many similar studies have been carried out in Britain and elsewhere.[94-97] Most seem to support the contention that increasing radiographic category has little effect on ventilatory capacity until the miner develops progressive massive fibrosis. Some studies have shown a slight drop in FEV_1 with category 3 pneumoconiosis.[95, 98] Only in anthracite miners does there appear to be a relationship between increasing radiographic category and decline in ventilatory capacity, and even then it is slight.

The problem of chronic respiratory disease in miners has been reviewed by Higgins.[99] This is discussed in detail elsewhere in this chapter (pp. 386–390 and 435–438) and in Chapter 17. The evidence suggests that, in general, miners have more respiratory symptoms (bronchitis) than do nonminers. Ventilatory capacity also tends to be slightly lower in miners, but exceptions exist.[100]

Lung Volumes. Until 1971 no large-scale epidemiological surveys of lung volumes had been carried out in coal miners. Early studies detected no change in lung volumes; however, later studies show that increasing category of simple coal workers' pneumoconiosis is associated with an increase in the residual volume (RV).[101]

Since most techniques that are used for determining total lung capacity are not applicable to field studies, Morgan and colleagues used Barnhard's radiographic method. First, they substantiated that this method could be used in the presence of pneumoconiosis.[102] This they did by comparing the total lung capacity obtained from the radiographic method to that obtained with the body plethysmograph. It was apparent that both methods produced essentially similar results in miners with simple pneumoconiosis; however, in progressive massive fibrosis and in subjects with large conglomerate shadows, the radiographic method was not entirely satisfactory. Residual volume was calculated by subtracting the forced vital capacity from total lung capacity.

Morgan and colleagues reported on the residual volume and total lung capacities of 1455 actively employed Pennsylvania miners.[101, 103] The effect of increasing radiographic category of simple coal workers' pneumoconiosis on lung volumes was investigated. The results were compared to Needham's predicted figures.[104] The subjects were divided into those with and without airways obstruction according to whether their FEV_1/FVC was greater or less than 70 per cent.[90, 101] The population was further divided according to their radiographic category. It was apparent from this study that obstruction and cigarette smoking both had an effect on residual volume (Tables 14–2 and 14–3). Despite a normal FEV_1/FVC, many cigarette-smoking miners had an elevated RV. More importantly,

Table 14–2. RESIDUAL VOLUMES OF MINERS WITH SIMPLE CWP

	Nonobstructed			Obstructed		
	No. of Subjects	Mean $\left[\dfrac{RV\ (obs)}{RV\ (pred)}\right]$ %		No. of Subjects	Mean $\left[\dfrac{RV\ (obs)}{RV\ (pred)}\right]$ %	
Category 0	561	108		214	132	
Category 1	308	119		154	137	
Categories 2 and 3	128	123		55	140	

these investigations also showed that radiographic category of simple pneumoconiosis was associated with an increase in residual volume, and that the increase could not be attributed either to smoking or to large airways obstruction (Figs. 14–7 and 14–8). A later study reporting measurements of the lung volume of all the subjects included in the first round of the Interagency Study[93] showed findings similar to those of the Pennsylvania miners.

Lapp and Seaton carried out an analysis of pressure, volume, and flow relationships of a group of miners.[105] They showed that most miners achieved lower maximal flow rates than their control subjects at comparable lung volumes and pressures. They inferred from their studies that the reduced flow rates were mainly a consequence of an increased upstream airways resistance rather than loss of elastic recoil. Nonetheless, considerable uncertainty exists as to pathogenesis of the increased residual volume. A more recent study of the effect of simple CWP on the lung mechanics of a group of anthracite miners showed no significant alterations either in mechanical properties or in small airways function.[106] In this well-executed study, the authors pointed out that their subjects had a normal coefficient of retraction, normal maximal expiratory flows, and a normal specific compliance, and that these findings made the presence of significant emphysema most unlikely. In this connection it must be remembered that all of their subjects were anthracite miners, and as such, their lungs might well contain a greater percentage of silica than is usually present in the lungs of United States coal miners.

Table 14–3. RESIDUAL VOLUMES OF MINERS ACCORDING TO SMOKING HABITS

	Smoking Habit*	Nonobstructed Mean $\left[\dfrac{RV\ (obs)}{RV\ (pred)}\right]$ %		Obstructed Mean $\left[\dfrac{RV\ (obs)}{RV\ (pred)}\right]$ %	
Category 0	Smokers	111		135	
	Nonsmokers	105		128	
Category 1	Smokers	123		143	
	Nonsmokers	107		122	
Categories 2 and 3	Smokers	125		149	
	Nonsmokers	115		157	

*Ex-smokers omitted.

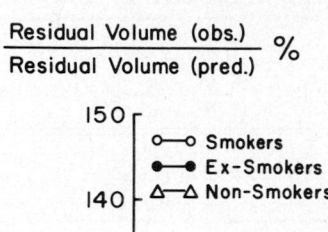

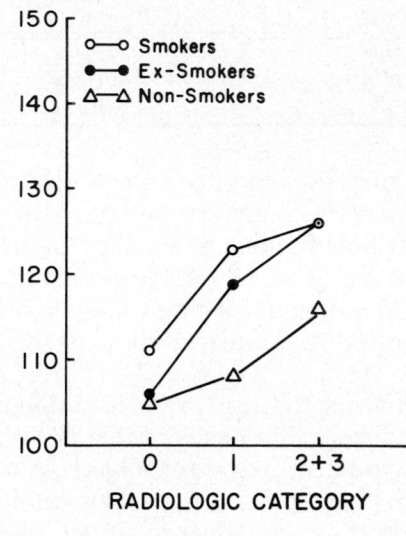

RADIOLOGIC CATEGORY

Figure 14–7. $\dfrac{RV\ (obs)}{RV\ (pred)}$ % in the nonobstructed miners according to smoking habits. (From Morgan, W. K. C., Burgess, D. B., Lapp, N. L., and Seaton, A.: Hyperinflation of the lungs in coal miners. Thorax, 26:585, Sept. 1971. Reproduced by permission.)

Figure 14–8. $\dfrac{RV\ (obs)}{RV\ (pred)}$ % in obstructed miners according to smoking habits. (From Morgan, W. K. C., Burgess, D. B., Lapp, N. L., and Seaton, A.: Hyperinflation of the lungs in coal miners. Thorax, 26:585, Sept. 1971. Reproduced by permission.)

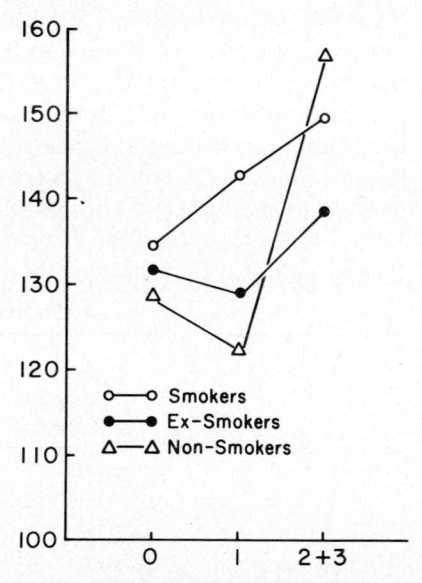

RADIOLOGIC CATEGORY

Diffusing Capacity (Transfer Factor). Until recently relatively few measurements of the diffusing capacity (DL) had been carried out in American and British coal miners. Gilson and Hugh-Jones studied carbon monoxide uptake in a sample of Welsh miners and found it to be slightly reduced in older men and more so in those who had complicated pneumoconiosis.[98]

In contrast, several quite extensive studies are described in the European literature. Sartorelli et al. studied 31 "silicotics" (coal miners) with the steady state method and found the mean DL to be within normal limits, albeit at the lower limit of normality.[107] He observed that miners with the p type of opacity had a lower DL than those with micronodular (q) opacities. Similarly, Billiet et al. measured the DL of 76 miners with "anthracosilicosis" by the single breath technique and found a slight but progressive decrement in DL from categories 0 and 1 through categories 2 and 3.[108] As expected, complicated pneumoconiosis had more severe reductions in DL. Englert and DeCoster studied 41 miners by means of the single breath technique.[109] They showed a minimal reduction in DL with the higher categories of simple coal workers' pneumoconiosis.

Lavenne and colleagues investigated a group of Belgian coal miners to see whether or not they had an abnormality of gas transfer, or alveolocapillary block.[110] In the few subjects they found with a low diffusing capacity, they felt that the reduction was a consequence of ventilation-perfusion abnormalities rather than thickening of the alveolocapillary membrane. Moreover, they pointed out that most of the relatively small number of subjects whose arterial partial pressure for oxygen was low showed improvement with exercise.[111]

Later Lyons and his colleagues studied 17 ex-miners with category 2 or 3 simple coal workers' pneumoconiosis.[112] They subdivided their subjects according to the type of opacity present on the chest radiograph. Using the single breath method, they showed that 10 of 16 with pinpoint (p) lesions had a slight reduction of DL. There were, however, more smokers among the miners who had p-type opacities, and when this was taken into account the data were no longer statistically significant. On the other hand, additional studies by Cotes and Field seem to confirm the lowered DL in miners with the p type of opacity.[113] These workers also claimed that the ratio of physiological dead space to tidal volume was increased in miners with the p type of opacity and that there was an increased ventilation during submaximal exercise.

In a study of 25 United States nonsmoking miners with either category 2 or 3 simple pneumoconiosis, Seaton and colleagues showed that the p type of opacity was associated with a slight reduction in the single breath DL.[114] Lung volumes and pulmonary mechanics of subjects with p opacities did not differ from those of miners with other small regular opacities. In contrast to the findings of the numerous investigators listed above, Rasmussen claimed that "impairment in oxygen transfer is encountered in the majority of symptomatic miners in the absence of airways obstruc-

tion."[115] However, there seems little doubt that his results can be accounted for by what Gaensler so aptly termed the "alarming hyperventilation" that was present in his subjects.[116]

Perhaps the most extensive and complete study of the diffusing capacity in miners was published by Kibelstis.[117] He measured the steady state DL of 133 working, underground bituminous miners at rest and during moderate exercise. He showed that cigarette smoking had a far more potent effect on DL than did years spent underground. Of the nonsmoking miners, the vast majority had a normal DL, and when a reduction was present, it was not of sufficient severity to be associated with disability. The difference in DL between the smoking and nonsmoking miners could not be accounted for by bronchitis, airways obstruction, or radiographic evidence of coal workers' pneumoconiosis.

The diffusing capacity and its components, namely, the capillary blood volume (Vc) and membrane component (DM), were studied in 43 miners and 141 controls by Frans et al.[111] They found the various indices of diffusion to be slightly reduced, and this included both DM and Vc. With exercise the DL_{CO} became normal, and the authors concluded that smoking was apparently more significant than pneumoconiosis in leading to the reduction of DL_{CO}, and as such, a significant loss of the pulmonary vascular bed in coal workers' pneumoconiosis did not occur. They also noted, as have others, that miners with the p type of pneumoconiosis tended to have a lower DL_{CO} than those with q and r opacities.

There would therefore seem to be little doubt that simple coal workers' pneumoconiosis does not lead to respiratory disability through a reduction of the diffusing capacity. Indeed, the diffusing capacity is either within normal limits or slightly reduced; moreover, when there is a reduction, it is seen almost entirely in miners who have the p type of radiographic opacity.

Gas Exchange. Reports of studies of gas exchange in coal miners in the United States are relatively infrequent and have been poorly controlled, with the notable exception of that of Lapp and Seaton.[118] In 1963 Brasseur reported that some miners with simple CWP showed mild hypoxemia at rest.[119] Further studies by Worth and colleagues came up with similar findings.[120] More recently Frans et al. studied a group of 43 coal miners who had no airways obstruction as detected by spirometry. They showed that in older coal miners there may be a slight reduction in PaO_2.[121] With supplemental oxygen administration, it became evident that venous mixture was increased. They also showed that miners with the p type of opacity had a slight increase in the $(A-a)CO_2$ and VD/VT. As a result of these studies, especially those of Brasseur, there remains little doubt that simple pneumoconiosis can lead to an increased alveolo-arterial gradient for oxygen $(A-a)O_2$ and an increased VD/VT ratio.

Rasmussen and co-workers studied the ventilatory function and gas exchange of 192 symptomatic coal miners from southern Appalachia. They demonstrated a tendency for arterial oxygen tension to decrease

and for the (A-a)O_2 gradient to increase with increasing category; however, neither ventilatory capacity nor age was taken into account.[122]

Henschel studied work capacity and gas exchange in five groups of subjects as part of the 1962–1963 U.S.P.H.S. Prevalence Study. He used pulse rate, oxygen consumption, and minute ventilation as his indices of work capacity and gas exchange. He could find no significant difference between miners and nonminers.[13]

In a neglected but most important part of the monograph, Henschel assessed the work capacity of a large group of coal miners and compared it to similar groups of controls.[13] He was unable to show any difference between the coal miners and the nonminers in pulse rate response to four different work levels. Similarly, the maximal aerobic work capacity of miners did not differ significantly from that of the control subjects. The maximal aerobic work capacity was predicted from the recorded pulse rate while the subject was exercising submaximally. Miners as a whole had a higher aerobic working capacity than did nonminers, but it was noted that miners with pneumoconiosis had a slightly but significantly lower capacity than those without the disease.

Most importantly, this study revealed no striking or consistent differences in ventilation for miners and nonminers, and this was apparent at all work levels for each particular age group. Put in more explicit terms, all the miners had more than sufficient respiratory reserve to move air in and out of their lungs for all work levels used in the investigation. In this context, most of these levels exceeded the physical demands made by modern coal mining. Harber, in an elegant study of the work requirements of present-day United States coal miners, has produced some most interesting data.[123] He first determined in a group of coal miners their cardiac response and oxygen consumption at varying work loads. Subsequently, he attached each to a Holter monitor and recorded heart rate throughout the working day. From these data, he calculated total oxygen consumption. He showed the average median estimated oxygen consumption to be 3.3 METS; the average 70th percentile was 4.3 METS and the average 90th percentile was 6.3 METS. The workers studied had a variety of jobs, including operating a continuous miner, operating a shuttle, roof bolting, and track laying and moving. Harber's results make it clear that coal mining is no longer the onerous job that it was and that even peak energy demands are relatively low and short lived.

The most carefully controlled and complete study of gas exchange in United States miners is that reported by Lapp and Seaton.[119] Out of a much larger population, they selected 51 symptomatic coal miners without evidence of large airways obstruction (FEV_1/FVC greater than 70 per cent). Three subjects had category A complicated pneumoconiosis, while the rest ranged from 0 through all the categories of simple pneumoconiosis. Subjects with categories 0 and 1 demonstrated minimal reductions in arterial oxygen tension at rest that returned to normal on exercise (Fig. 14–9). The mean arterial oxygen tension was normal during exercise for

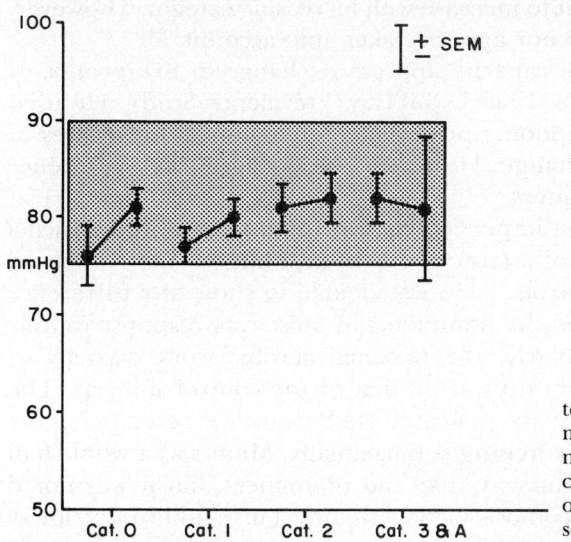

Figure 14–9. Arterial oxygen tensions at rest and exercise of miners with simple pneumoconiosis according to radiographic category (S.E.M. = standard error of the mean). (Shaded area represents normal range.)

all categories, although occasionally subjects did show minor decreases. The mean (A-a)O_2 gradient was abnormally elevated in subjects with category 0, but decreased into the normal range with exercise (Fig. 14–10). The mean value for VD/VT was increased in all categories, but returned to normal with exercise except in those miners with category 3 and in those with complicated pneumoconiosis stage A (Fig. 14–11). The same can be said of minute ventilation.

The results indicate that minor abnormalities of distribution and gas exchange occur in coal miners in the absence of obstruction of the larger airways. They are probably a consequence of focal emphysema, but air flow obstruction in the smaller airways may also play a role. Where there is a general tendency for gas exchange abnormalities to be associated with increasing radiographic evidence of pneumoconiosis, such a relationship is often absent. The occasional presence of minor abnormalities of gas exchange in miners with category 0 pneumoconiosis may be related to the presence of "industrial bronchitis."

Mechanics of Respiration. Leathart studied the respiratory mechanics of 97 British working and former miners, most of whom were disabled or claiming compensation.[124] He noted that compliance tended to decrease with increasing age and with years spent underground, but observed no correlation with radiographic category. Inspiratory airway resistance was normal, but in some of the subjects nonelastic work of breathing was increased, presumably due to airways obstruction.

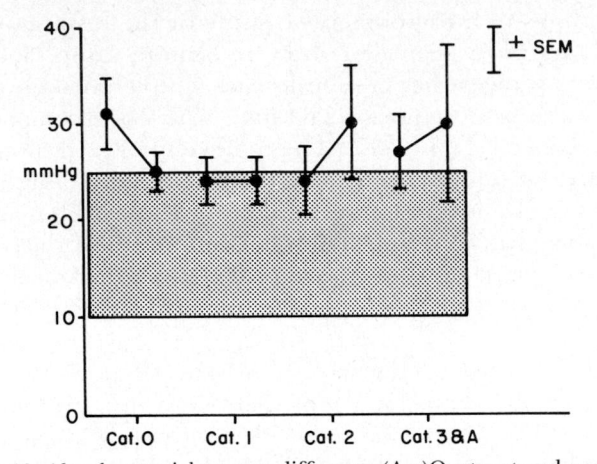

Figure 14–10. Alveolo-arterial oxygen difference (A-a)O$_2$ at rest and exercise of miners with simple pneumoconiosis according to radiographic category (S.E.M. = standard error of the mean). (Shaded area represents normal range.)

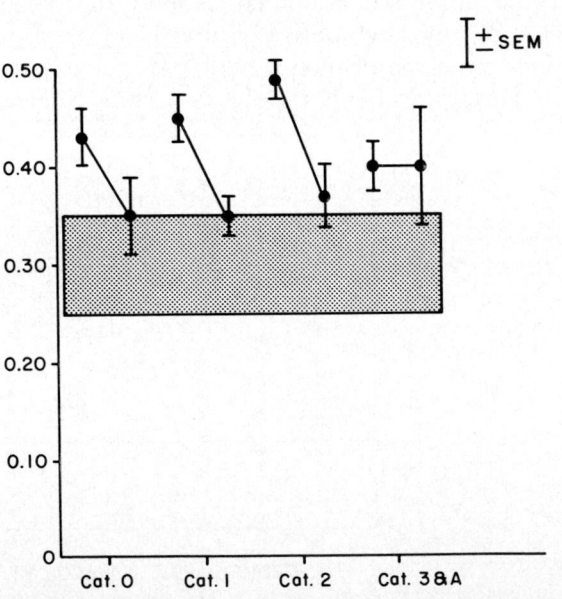

Figure 14–11. Ratio of dead space to tidal volume at rest and exercise of miners with simple pneumoconiosis according to radiographic category (S.E.M. = standard error of the mean). (Shaded area represents normal range.)

The findings of a comprehensive study of the respiratory mechanics in coal workers have been described by Seaton, Lapp, and Morgan.[125] These workers showed that in subjects with simple pneumoconiosis, static compliance was mostly in the normal range, whereas in complicated disease it was often reduced (Fig. 14–12). The coefficient of retraction (pulmonary recoil pressure at total lung capacity divided by total lung capacity) was reduced or normal in most subjects, except those with stages B and C progressive massive fibrosis. Although many of the subjects studied by Seaton and colleagues professed symptoms, none had evidence of large airways obstruction; that is to say, none had an FEV_1/FVC of less than 70 per cent.

They also studied a subgroup of working miners with categories 2 and 3 simple pneumoconiosis. All of this subgroup were nonsmokers, all had an FEV_1/FVC of greater than 70 per cent, and all were actively employed. Their static compliance and pulmonary recoil pressure were likewise relatively normal, although one or two miners had slight reductions in these indices, as did one control (Fig. 14–13).

The same authors also looked at dynamic compliance at different frequencies. They argued that since these men were nonsmokers without evidence of large airways obstruction, it would be legitimate to assume that were any of the subjects to demonstrate a fall in the compliance at more rapid rates of breathing, such a fall could only be a consequence of small airways disease. Such an assumption can be made, however, only if the subjects examined have a normal pressure volume curve and no loss of elastic recoil. The subjects examined fulfilled these requirements (Figs. 14–13 and 14–14). It was demonstrated that 17 of the 25 subjects showed a significant fall in the compliance at higher frequencies (less than 80 per cent of initial compliance). Of the 10 bronchitic subjects, 6 displayed

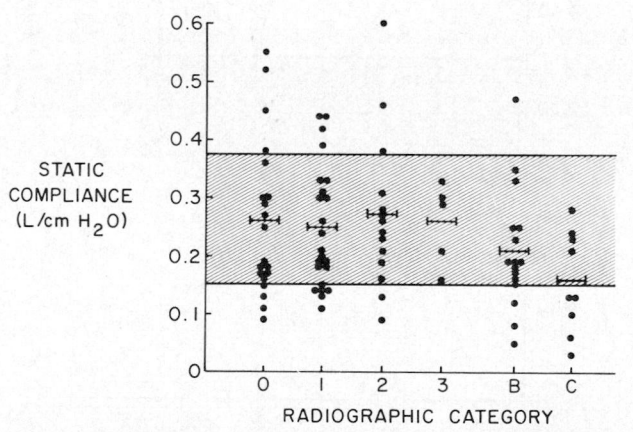

Figure 14–12. Static compliance in miners and ex-miners with different categories of coal workers' pneumoconiosis. (From Seaton, A., et al.: Lung mechanics and frequency dependence of compliance in coal miners. J. Clin. Invest., *51*, 1203, 1972. Reproduced by permission.) (Shaded area represents normal range.)

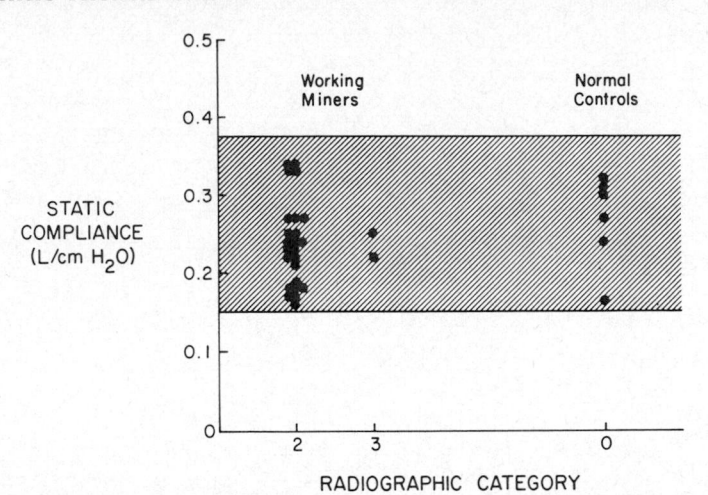

Figure 14–13. Static compliance in 25 working miners with categories 2 and 3 simple coal workers' pneumoconiosis. Comparable controls also shown. (From Seaton, A., et al.: Lung mechanics and frequency dependence of compliance in coal miners. J. Clin. Invest., *51*, 1203, 1972. Reproduced by permission.) (Shaded area represents normal range.)

frequency dependence, while of the 15 nonbronchitic subjects, 11 showed similar findings (Figs. 14–15 and 14–16). Isoproterenol inhalation did not alter the response.

Lapp and Seaton then extended their study and related maximal flow to static recoil pressure and to lung volumes.[105] It appeared that this group of 25 working miners were able to achieve lower flow rates than did

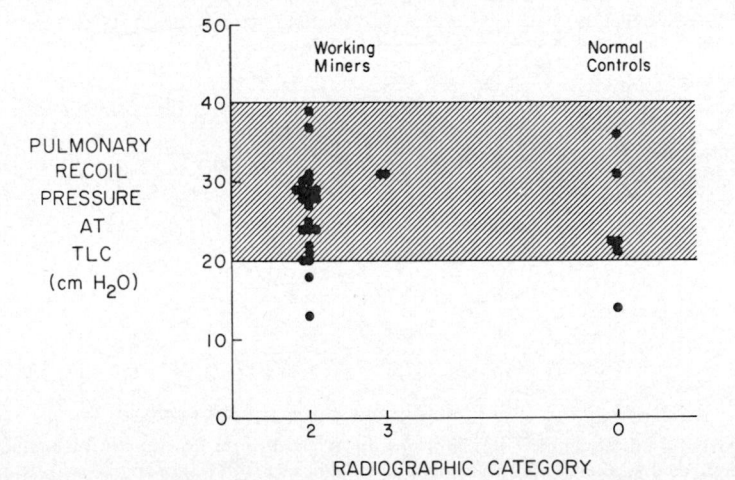

Figure 14–14. Pulmonary recoil pressure at total lung capacity of 25 working miners with simple pneumoconiosis of categories 2 and 3. Controls also shown. (From Seaton, A., et al.: Lung mechanics and frequency dependence of compliance in coal miners. J. Clin. Invest., *51*, 1203, 1972. Reproduced by permission.) (Shaded area represents normal range.)

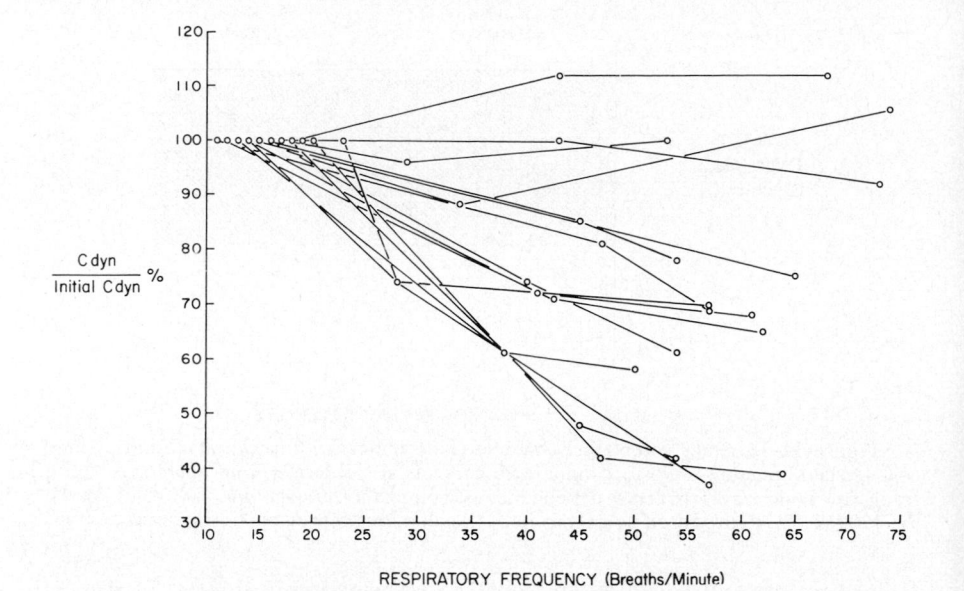

Figure 14–15. Dynamic compliance at different respiratory rates in nonbronchitic miners with simple coal workers' pneumoconiosis of categories 2 and 3 (nonsmokers). (From Seaton, A., et al.: Lung mechanics and frequency dependence of compliance in coal miners. J. Clin. Invest., *51*, 1203, 1972. Reproduced by permission.)

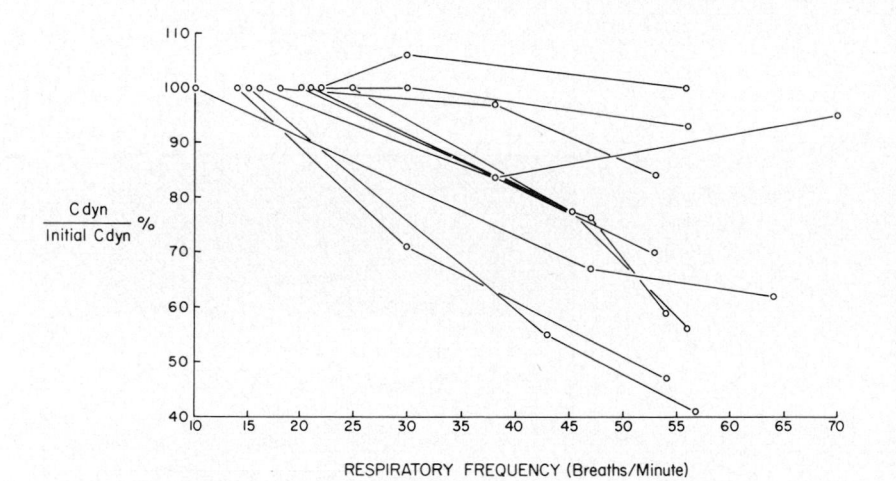

Figure 14–16. Dynamic compliance at different respiratory rates in bronchitic miners with simple coal workers' pneumoconiosis of categories 2 and 3 (nonsmokers). (From Seaton, A., et al.: Lung mechanics and frequency dependence of compliance in coal miners. J. Clin. Invest., *51*, 1203, 1972. Reproduced by permission.)

controls at comparable lung volumes and pressures. The alterations in lung mechanics did not seem to be related to the type of radiographic opacity (p or q) present in the chest film.

Since the publication of the paper of Seaton et al., Morgan and co-workers have investigated miners with categories 0 and 1 simple pneumoconiosis.[126] While a few miners with category 1 showed a slight but significant fall in dynamic compliance at higher rates (Fig. 14–17), this finding was to all intents and purposes absent in miners with category 0 (Fig. 14–18). Unfortunately, one or two of the controls also showed frequency dependence (Fig. 14–19). In some instances, this may have been a result of a resolving viral respiratory tract infection, but in others no obvious explanation was apparent, although age may have been responsible.[127]

As previously mentioned (p. 405), Murphy and co-workers examined most aspects of lung function in a group of anthracite miners with simple pneumoconiosis.[106] They were unable to detect significant changes in either lung mechanics or small airways function. Their findings of normal lung mechanics and an absence of small airways obstruction are in keeping with the results obtained by others.

Although the technique of measuring dynamic compliance at different respiratory frequencies has been hailed as a precise and sensitive means of diagnosing obstruction in the small airways, it has many drawbacks. It can only be applied to subjects who have normal spirometry and a normal pressure volume curve. Until recently it had been assumed that if the

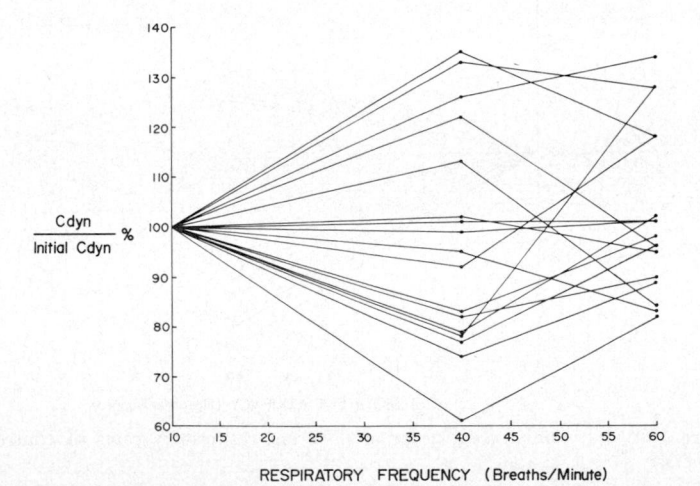

Figure 14–17. Dynamic compliance at different respiratory rates in miners with category 1 simple coal workers' pneumoconiosis (nonsmokers). (From Morgan, W. K. C., et al.: The early detection of occupational lung disease. Brit. J. Dis. Chest, *68*, 75, 1974. Reproduced by permission.)

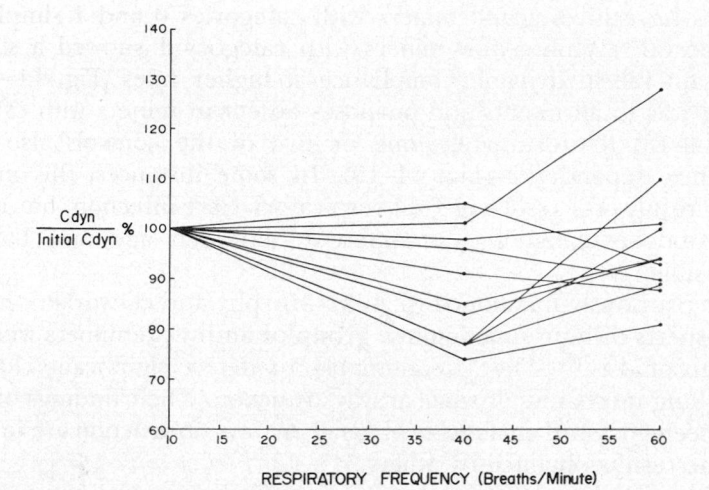

Figure 14–18. Dynamic compliance at different respiratory rates of miners without pneumoconiosis (nonsmokers).

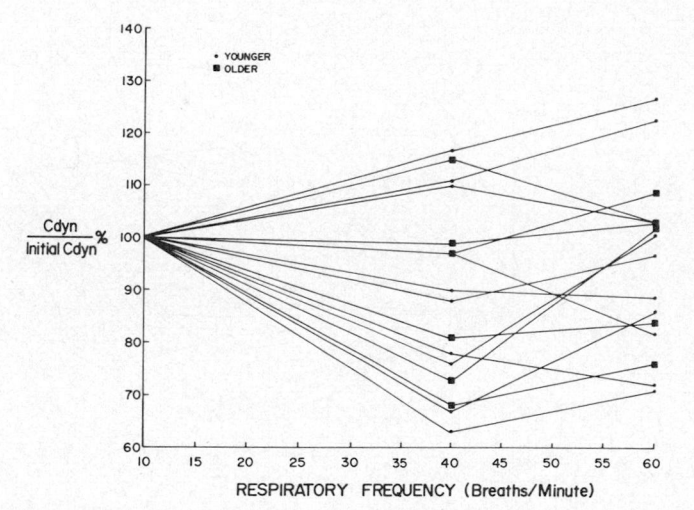

Figure 14–19. Dynamic compliance at different respiratory rates of control subjects (nonsmokers).

latter requirement was met, the elastic properties of the lung were normal—an assumption that may not be justified. Localized areas of emphysema and fibrosis may well be present in the same lung, so that the effects of each process on lung distensibility even out, with the result that the lung as a whole has a normal compliance curve. Such localized areas of emphysema could, however, lead to frequency dependence, and this may well be the case in simple coal workers' pneumoconiosis. Nonuniform involvement of the lungs with focal emphysema could cause frequency dependence and appears to be as likely an explanation for this phenomenon as is an increased resistance to flow in the smaller airways.

Lapp and colleagues have also made measurements of closing volume (CV) and closing capacity (CC) in coal miners with and without CWP. They related these measurements to the presence of bronchitis, whether industrially acquired or due to cigarette smoking.[129] Although CV and CC were often found to be increased in their group of coal miners, the increases were not related to the radiographic presence of CWP or to the presence of industrial bronchitis. While the latter finding may seem unexpected, the evidence suggests that industrial bronchitis predominantly involves the central airways and for the most part spares the peripheral airways.

Hemodynamics. Pathological studies have shown cor pulmonale to be rare in simple pneumoconiosis in the absence of obstructive airways disease.[80-84] Studies of hemodynamics such as those conducted by Bollinelli have in general borne out the above pathological findings. In contrast to simple pneumoconiosis, Bollinelli and co-workers showed that progressive massive fibrosis often leads to pulmonary hypertension through destruction of the pulmonary vascular bed.[130]

Krémer and co-workers in their studies of Belgian miners showed that pulmonary artery pressure was related to the airways resistance, and that obstructed miners differed in no way from obstructed nonmining controls.[131, 132] They demonstrated a statistically significant increase in the pulmonary artery pressure of a group of miners with categories 2 and 3 pneumoconiosis as compared to miners with categories 0 and 1 pneumoconiosis and to normal subjects. None of their unobstructed subjects had a raised pulmonary artery pressure. In a later paper, Krémer described the hemodynamic findings of 100 pneumoconiotic miners and related their pulmonary artery pressure to the presence of obstruction and to the radiographic category of pneumoconiosis.[133] Krémer claimed that categories 2 and 3 lead to slight elevation of the mean pulmonary artery pressure at rest or, more often, on exercise. Although Krémer's data are convincing, he fails to take into account the effect of age on pulmonary artery pressure.

Rasmussen and colleagues suggested on the basis of abnormalities of gas exchange that pulmonary hypertension might be frequent in United States coal miners.[85] They arrived at this conclusion after having demonstrated a high systolic pulmonary artery pressure in certain of the subjects

they were investigating. However, mean pressures were not recorded and the technique of recording systolic pressure rather than mean pressure is generally accepted as unreliable. Moreover, no measurements of pulmonary vascular resistance were made.

Lapp and colleagues selected 47 Appalachian miners, all of whom professed respiratory symptoms and most of whom were claiming compensation.[84] The details of the mean pulmonary artery pressure and oxygen tensions at rest and exercise are shown in Figures 14–20 and 14–21. Seven of the 24 subjects with obstruction of the airways had pulmonary hypertension, the latter being felt to be a consequence of either complicated pneumoconiosis or obstructive airways disease. Of the 23 men without obstruction, many of whom had abnormalities of gas exchange, only 1 had pulmonary hypertension at rest, while 3 others had a slight to moderate elevation on exercise. Two of the group had been exposed to silica rather than coal dust. Again, a significant negative correlation between pulmonary artery pressure and FEV_1 was present. One of the subjects who had an elevation of pulmonary artery pressure on exercise and who had simple pneumoconiosis was markedly obese, and this may have played a role in the genesis of his pulmonary hypertension.

In another paper, Seaton and colleagues describe how they used lung perfusion scans to investigate the pulmonary capillary bed in coal workers' pneumoconiosis.[134] Perfusion in simple pneumoconiosis was to all intents

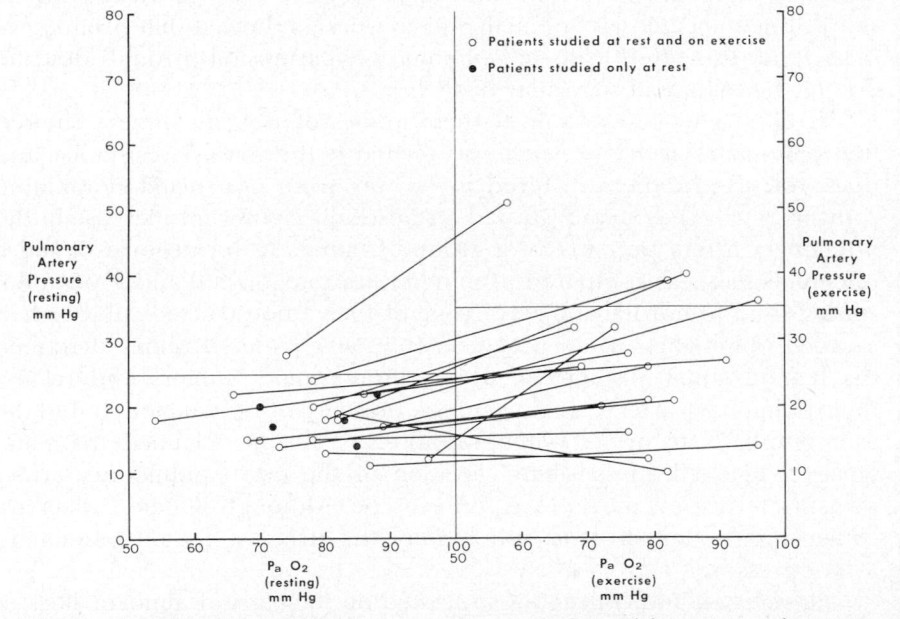

Figure 14–20. Mean pulmonary artery pressures and arterial oxygen tensions at rest and exercise of 23 miners without airways obstruction. (From Lapp, N. L., et al.: Pulmonary haemodynamics in coal workers' pneumoconiosis. *In* Walton, W. A., ed.: Inhaled Particles. Vol. III. London, Unwin Brothers, Ltd., 1971.)

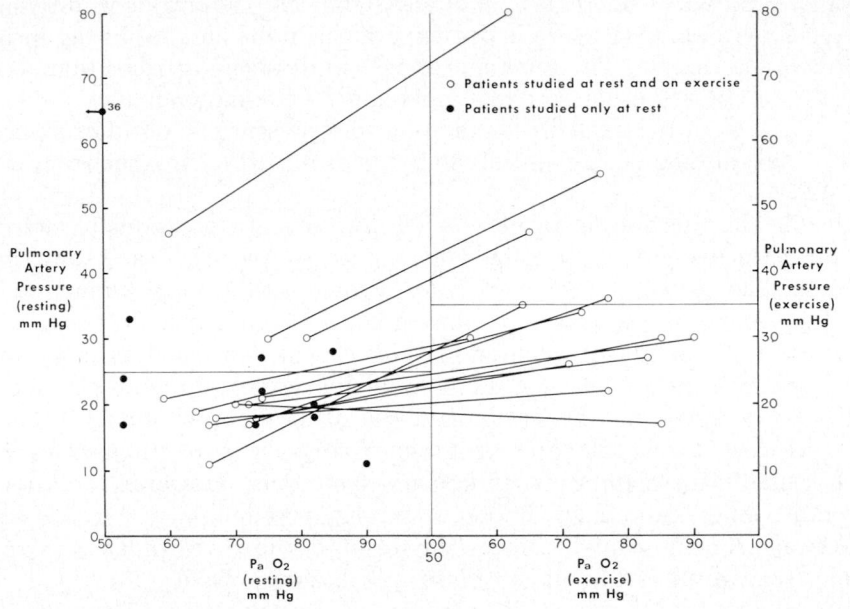

Figure 14–21. Mean pulmonary artery pressures and arterial oxygen tensions at rest and exercise of 24 miners with airways obstruction. (From Lapp, N. L., et al.: Pulmonary haemodynamics in coal workers' pneumoconiosis. *In* Walton, W. A., ed.: Inhaled Particles. Vol. III. London, Unwin Brothers, Ltd., 1971.)

and purposes normal. It is clear that extensive defects in perfusion may be present in the complete absence of symptoms and that perfusion scanning is worthless as a means of detecting impairment and disability in simple CWP. In contrast, gallium scanning is markedly abnormal in CWP and other pneumoconioses.[135] This test is nonspecific and of little practical importance diagnostically.

In summary, it seems that miners with simple pneumoconiosis may suffer from certain minor respiratory impairments, all of which have been reviewed in detail[90]:

1. A minimal reduction of ventilatory capacity may be associated with the higher categories of simple pneumoconiosis, although even this is uncertain.

2. A residual volume (RV) that is often larger than the predicted value is found, the size of the increment being related to the category of simple CWP.

3. Minor abnormalities of gas exchange are sometimes present. Some increase in the physiological dead space and in the ratio of physiological dead space to tidal volume (VD/VT) and other minor ventilation-perfusion abnormalities may be present.

4. Those with the pinhead (or p) type of small opacity tend to have a somewhat lower diffusing capacity than do those with the micronodular

(or q) opacities. Nonetheless, clinically significant reductions in diffusing capacity are extremely rare in our experience in the absence of significant pulmonary disease. The minimal changes in diffusing capacity that occur are felt to be a consequence of ventilation-perfusion inequalities.

5. A slightly elevated pulmonary artery pressure is found exceptionally. This finding is rare and doubt exists in regard to its association with CWP.

6. The mechanical properties of the lung are occasionally altered. The retractive forces in some miners with simple CWP are somewhat diminished, although they more often remain within normal limits.

7. About 50 per cent show that their lung compliance decreases with increased frequency of respiration. This can be construed as suggesting the presence either of some increase in the resistance of the peripheral airways or of irregularly distributed areas of focal emphysema.

It is unlikely that any of these abnormalities by themselves are associated with significant pulmonary symptoms. However, additional abnormalities caused by another unrelated pulmonary disease, e.g., chronic bronchitis, might conceivably result in the development of symptoms that would not occur were only one disease present.

Complicated Pneumoconiosis or Progressive Massive Fibrosis (PMF)

Complicated pneumoconiosis has already been defined in the section dealing with radiographic appearances of the pneumoconioses (Chap. 5). Suffice it to say that any shadow of diameter greater than 1 cm that occurs in a coal miner with simple CWP should be regarded as progressive massive fibrosis (PMF) unless there is definite evidence to suggest another disease, e.g., tuberculosis.

Unlike simple pneumoconiosis, PMF may be associated with severe respiratory disability and premature death.[27, 136, 138] Although PMF may be progressive, this is by no means always the rule, and in some instances the process appears to undergo spontaneous arrest. While numerous theories exist as to its causation, its pathogenesis remains obscure, as do the factors that control its progression.

Etiology

There is excellent evidence that PMF develops most frequently on a background of category 2 or 3 simple pneumoconiosis. While this is not invariable and occasionally it appears in miners with category 1 or even 0, such a state of affairs is unusual.[66] When it does appear in subjects with a lesser background of pneumoconiosis, there may be other factors present that might tend to obscure the number and density of the opacities seen in the chest film, viz., coincident severe emphysema.

Progressive massive fibrosis may appear several years after exposure has ceased and, in addition, may progress in the absence of further dust exposure. Although it is most commonly seen on a background of category 2 or 3 simple pneumoconiosis, only a minority of miners with these categories develop the condition. In a classic study published in 1962, Cochrane first studied the attack rate of progressive massive fibrosis.[139] In this paper, he described how he followed up a population of miners and ex-miners who lived in two Welsh mining communities, the Rhondda Fach and the Aberdare Valley. The populations were x-rayed in 1950–1951 and again in 1958. Cochrane was unable to relate the attack rate of PMF to smoking, energy expenditure, tuberculous infection, or any other obvious factor other than the background of simple pneumoconiosis. He found an attack rate of 0.7 per cent per year in miners with category 1, a rate of 2.6 per cent in category 2, and 4.2 per cent in category 3. Very similar results have been found by the National Coal Board of Great Britain. These are described by McLintock et al., who showed an expected attack rate for the whole of Britain of 1.5 per cent per year in active miners who have category 2 or more simple pneumoconiosis.[140]

The prevalence of PMF varies greatly from one country to another and from one region to another. It is high in eastern Pennsylvania, South Wales, France, and Belgium, but low in Utah, the Midlands of England, and Russia.[58, 90] Cochrane showed that the attack rate declines steeply with age, and thus the prevalence of PMF is obviously influenced by the mean age at which the miner first incurs category 2 simple pneumoconiosis. In South Wales, where the boys used to go down the pit to work at the face at the age of 12 or 14, there was a definite chance of their developing category 2 disease before reaching 30. In Scotland and Northumberland, it was the custom for the boys not to start working at the face until they were 18 or 20, their earlier years being spent on haulage and away from the face. As a result, only rarely was category 2 seen before the age of 30.

In their nationwide study, McLintock et al. showed that not only does the attack rate for PMF rise commensurately with increasing category but it is also influenced by the rate of radiographic progression.[140] Those miners showing the most rapid progression also had the highest attack rates. The attack rates varied greatly according to region, being highest in South Wales and lowest in Scotland. It becomes clear from this work that the earlier category 2 develops in the miner, the longer the period over which he is likely to develop PMF; however, age alone cannot account for the regional differences.

Cochrane, Moore, and Thomas studied the effect of radiographic progression on mortality.[141] They showed that in stage A complicated pneumoconiosis or in those subjects with an opacity less than 20 sq cm, the mortality was little, if any, different from that of the general population or of miners with simple pneumoconiosis. Although continued dust exposure appeared to have no effect on progression, these workers suggested that for the younger miner, at least, it might be worth leaving mining and learning another trade.

Thus it is apparent that aside from dust, some other factor is involved in the etiology of PMF. The nature of this factor has been the subject of debate for many years, and numerous theories exist.

Silica Hypothesis. This theory exists in two forms. The first and simpler advances the point of view that massive fibrosis consists of coalescent silicotic nodules. Such a situation undoubtedly can occur, but classical silicosis is uncommon in coal miners except in brakemen and roof bolters in the United States. The second theory postulates that the coal macule is a silicotic nodule that has been modified by tuberculosis or another infection to produce an atypical response, namely, PMF. This issue has been reviewed earlier (p. 385), and it need be said only that the National Coal Board, despite its extensive dust sampling program, has been able to find only limited support for this theory. Extensive lung dust residue analyses have been carried out in lungs of individuals with PMF, and these have shown a poor correlation between silica content of the lungs and the prevalence of PMF except in a minority of subjects.[22] Nonetheless, the argument continues, and Pratt feels the methodology of the lung analyses has been and still is open to doubt.[142]

Total Dust Hypothesis. This theory proposes that once a certain amount of dust has been deposited in the lungs, a process is started which is self-perpetuating. This theory is unlikely, in that the progression of the disease is not influenced by further dust exposure and often proceeds inexorably in its absence.

Immunological Hypothesis. Recent work has suggested that PMF may be an antigen-antibody reaction. This theory is attractive and will be discussed in more depth later in this chapter, when the immunology of both simple and complicated pneumoconiosis is reviewed.

Nontuberculous Infection Hypothesis. This is a most difficult hypothesis to prove or refute. There is little or no evidence to show that acute pulmonary infections are more common in coal miners than in the general population, and numerous miners are seen who have pneumonia and other acute pulmonary infections without subsequent development of PMF.

Mycobacterium Tuberculosis and Atypical Acid-Fast Bacilli Infection Hypothesis. The observation that silicotics often develop tuberculosis was probably responsible for the formulation of this theory. Additional weight was added to this concept when James found bacteriological or histological evidence of tuberculosis in 40 per cent of massive lesions in an autopsy series of 245 South Wales miners.[143] The occasional finding of tubercle bacilli in the sputum of subjects with what appeared to be radiographic PMF seems to provide additional confirmatory evidence. The subsequent isolation of atypical acid-fast bacilli, viz., *Mycobacterium kansasii* and the scotochromogens, does not argue against the tuberculosis theory.[144] Furthermore, by far the commonest sites in the lung where PMF develops are the posterior segment of the upper lobes or the superior segment (apical lower) of the lower lobes, that is, exactly the same locations that are initially involved by cavitary pulmonary tuberculosis.

Some experimental evidence for this theory came from the work of Zaidi and co-workers.[145] These workers were able to induce massive fibrotic lesions by exposing guinea pigs to a mixture of coal dust and nonpathogenic attenuated tubercle bacilli. Neither the organism by itself nor the dust by itself would induce massive fibrotic lesions.

This work has been extended by Gernez-Rieux and others of the Pasteur Institute in Lille, France, who performed a series of experiments on guinea pigs which had been challenged with coal dust and *M. kansasii*.[146] They showed that dust aggravated experimentally induced infections with *M. Kansasii* and is likely to render pathogenic a host of bacteria which, in its absence, would not induce lesions. There was a linear relationship between the quantity of dust on the lungs and the size of infection due to *M. kansasii*. In animals previously exposed to coal dust for a long time, it was possible by challenging them with *M. kansasii* to induce pulmonary lesions similar to those seen in progressive massive fibrosis.

Despite all the circumstantial evidence, there are many unexplained and contradictory facts that tend to refute the tuberculosis hypothesis. First, a substantial proportion of those with progressive massive fibrosis have negative tuberculin tests, and particularly so in the United States. Second, as the attack rate of tuberculosis declined, a concomitant decline in the attack rate of progressive massive fibrosis should have been observed. However, such decline was absent in the Rhondda Fach.[139] Third, the difference in the attack rates for tuberculosis and PMF are difficult to explain. The higher attack rate of PMF and its progression despite the absence of overt tuberculous infection seem to militate strongly against the theory. Finally, the controlled trial of antituberculosis chemotherapy by Ball and co-workers failed to demonstrate any beneficial effect of antituberculosis treatment.[147] Surprisingly, in view of the other negative findings, progression of PMF was observed to occur more frequently in those with a positive tuberculin test.

Clinical Features

In the early stages of complicated pneumoconiosis there are few if any symptoms or signs. With stages B and C, shortness of breath, cough, and sputum become common. Occasionally the subject will cough up large volumes of black material, so called melanoptysis. As the disease advances, signs of lobar collapse may appear and usually develop in the upper lobes. Tracheal deviation often occurs. Later a right ventricular heave develops with signs of pulmonary hypertension and right ventricular failure. Tricuspid incompetence occurs terminally.

Pathology

As already mentioned, massive lesions are found mainly in the posterior segment of the upper lobes or in the superior segment of the lower lobes. Macroscopically, they consist of a mass of black tissue that is

often adherent to the chest wall. The lesions are of a rubbery consistency and usually are relatively well defined. Unlike conglomerate silicosis, which can be seen to consist of matted aggregates of whorled silicotic nodules, the massive lesion of PMF is amorphous, irregular, and relatively homogeneous (Fig. 14–22). In some instances, its center may contain a cavity filled with a jet-black liquid and whose walls are irregular and thick. Cavitation is virtually always a consequence of ischemic necrosis or secondary infection by tuberculosis.[148] In the United States and Britain the former process is more often responsible; however, there are still areas of the world, e.g., Yugoslavia, where tuberculosis is the usual cause of cavitation.[64] In some cavitated lesions, atypical acid-fast bacilli and rarely other pathogens have been demonstrated.[147, 148]

Macroscopically, the conglomerate masses are composed of dense aggregates of collagenous fibrous tissue. Separating the fibrous bundles are plentiful deposits of coal dust and often a few scattered lymphocytes. The massive lesions encroach on the blood vessels and bronchi of the affected lobe and obliterate them. Traces of their existence still remain on the periphery of the masses, and the persistence of the internal elastic laminae may be evident long after the lumina of the vessels have been occluded and the vessels themselves have been incorporated into the fibrous masses.

In PMF, the arteries and veins and capillaries of the affected region, both large and small, are obliterated. The large arterial vessels of the remainder of the lung not involved by the massive lesion tend to be dilated owing to pulmonary hypertension. In some instances, especially shortly before death, thrombosis of a large pulmonary vessel may take place even when it is not involved by the fibrotic mass. The adventitia and media of muscular arteries are often infiltrated with dust-laden cells, and there is frequent evidence of endarteritis obliterans. Bronchial artery hypertrophy is occasionally seen. These changes are excellently described and beautifully illustrated in a classic paper by Wells.[82]

The descriptions of the morbid anatomy of PMF have been criticized by Wagner.[150] He deplores the artificial separation of the disease into simple and complicated forms on radiological criteria and cogently points out that the process that initiates the massive lesion starts long before the large opacity is 1 cm in diameter. He has incriminated in the pathogenesis of PMF what he chooses to refer to as the perivascular nodule. According to Wagner, the latter varies in size from 1 to 22 mm and may be discrete or consist of several coalescent nodules. It may show evidence of central necrosis and the histological features may suggest the presence of excess silica, tuberculosis, or the rheumatoid diathesis. He advances the thesis that these nodules, with their aggregates of coal dust, act as a nidus on which fibrogenic substances, viz., silica and the macroglobulins of rheumatoid factor, may be deposited. Wagner's theory will be discussed in more detail later, when the immunological factors of coal workers' pneumoconiosis are considered.

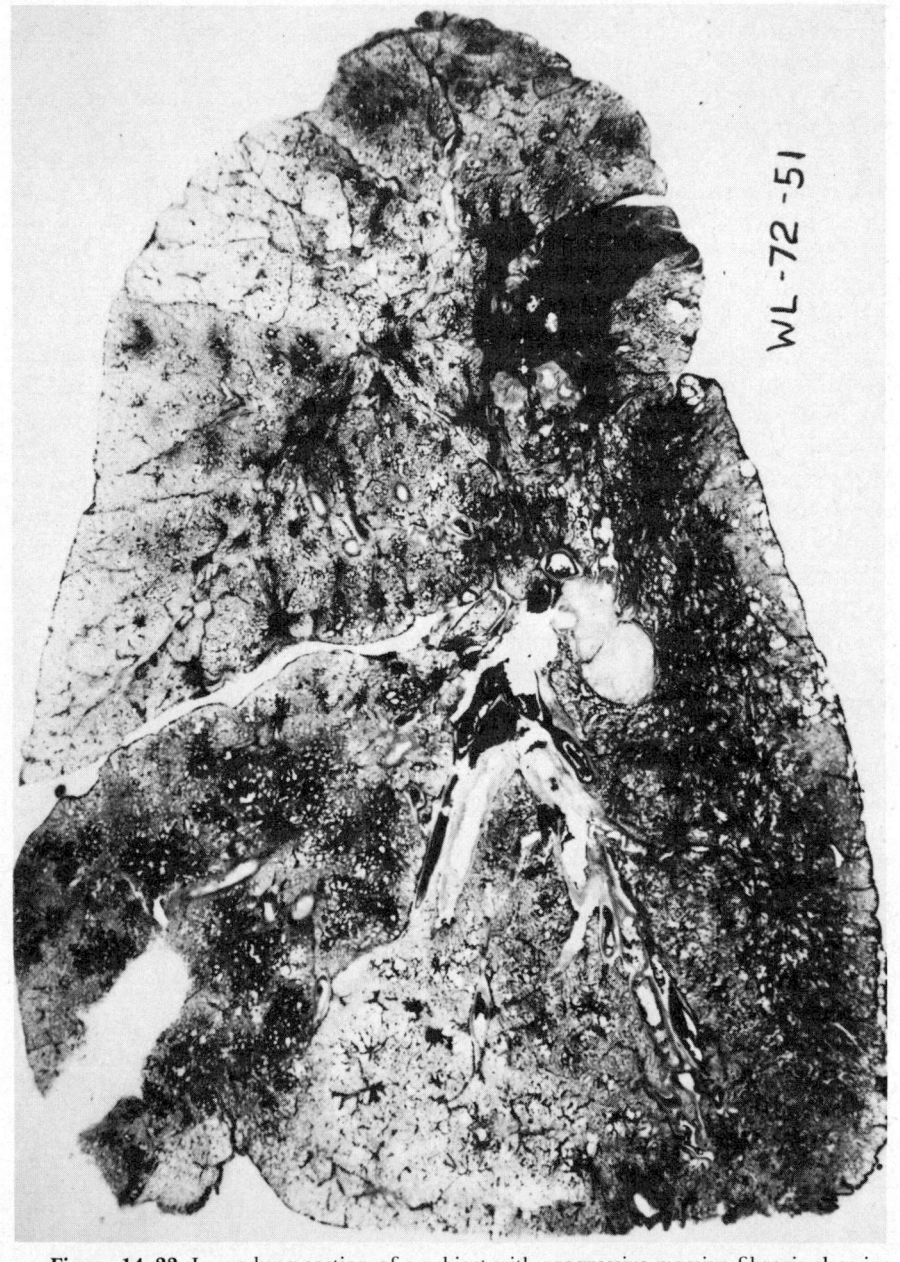

Figure 14–22. Large lung section of a subject with progressive massive fibrosis showing irregular black amorphous conglomerate lesions.

Wagner also reports the results of a series of biochemical studies that tend to cast doubt on previous beliefs concerning the composition of the large masses in complicated pneumoconiosis.[150] He has analyzed fresh tissue from the center of the massive lesions and has demonstrated the following:

1. There is a significant increase in the calcium phosphate content of the lesions as compared to control tissue.

2. The massive lesion contains glycosaminoglycans (hyaluronic acid, chrondroitin sulfate, and so forth) at levels that are consistent with fibrosis.

3. Virtually all the nonmineral content is protein. Hydroxyproline accounts for around 3 to 4 per cent of the protein content and this implies a collagen content of only 25 to 30 per cent. Wagner makes the point that pleural plaques contain up to 90 per cent collagen.

4. The coal dust content varies in different parts of the nodule. Small amounts of coal dust are present in the areas of the lung not affected by the massive lesion, while large quantities are present in the center of the massive lesion. The mucopolysaccharide content falls toward the center of the conglomerate lesion.

It seems that the previously widely accepted belief that the massive lesions of complicated pneumoconiosis consist mainly of collagen is open to question. The studies of Wagner show that although collagen is present at the periphery of the lesion, this is not true of the center, where amorphous material predominates. Wagner's findings are supported by the normal urinary hydroxyproline values found by Resnick and colleagues in both simple and complicated pneumoconiosis.[151, 152]

In a later study Wagner and others showed that fibronectin is an important component of the masses that characterize PMF. This complex extracellular material is also found in the lesions of asbestosis and silicosis.[153]

Pulmonary Function

In general, miners with PMF tend to be older than their co-workers with simple coal workers' pneumoconiosis and as a result often tend to suffer from coincident but unrelated heart and pulmonary disease. In many instances the effects of PMF are difficult to separate from those of the other diseases. Nonetheless, there is ample evidence that in PMF ventilatory capacity is definitely reduced, and the extent of the reduction is related to the size of the large opacity. With stage A, a normal FEV_1 and FVC are the rule, and it is only when stages B and C are reached that the impairment becomes obvious.[89, 90, 93, 98]

Airways obstruction is also common and is nearly always present in stages B and C. The cause of the obstruction is not obvious, but is probably a consequence of the distortion and narrowing of the remaining patent bronchi and bronchioles produced by the conglomerate mass. Similar physiological abnormalities may be observed in long-standing, far ad-

vanced tuberculosis, probably for the same reasons. No matter what the country or who the observer, there seems to be a consensus that stages B and C PMF lead to a reduced ventilatory capacity and to airways obstruction.[154] Increased resistance to air flow, as manifested by the presence of a low $FEV_1/FVC\%$, is related to the size of the pulmonary lesions.[155] While residual volume and RV/TLC ratio are often increased, the changes tend to be less than are usually found in emphysema.[90, 93, 156] In the study of Morgan and colleagues, the RV of miners with complicated pneumoconiosis, although increased, tended to be less than that present in subjects with categories 2 and 3 simple coal workers' pneumoconiosis.[102] There seems little doubt that the increase in RV that is present in PMF is a consequence of the associated obstructive disease. In some instances, the increase in RV may not entirely reflect the degree of obstruction, since in many subjects with PMF large areas of the lung are solid and airless. Recent studies from the Institute of Occupational Medicine have shown an association of PMF with panlobular emphysema.[78]

The diffusing capacity in PMF is reduced in proportion to the size of the lesion or lesions; however, in the absence of obstruction, normal values may be present even in stages B and C.[98, 157] Lapp and Seaton reported on the diffusing capacity of 16 miners and ex-miners with stages B and C complicated pneumoconiosis.[118] The mean D_L expressed as a percentage of predicted normal was 47.1 per cent in those with stage B and 47.2 per cent in those with stage C. These workers showed that substantial reductions in D_L occurred in the presence of only minor degrees of airways obstruction.

In PMF, uneven ventilation and abnormalities of gas exchange are much more frequent than in simple CWP.[158] Lapp and Seaton studied at rest and exercise 14 symptomatic United States coal miners with complicated pneumoconiosis.[118] Their alveolo-arterial gradient for oxygen rose abnormally with exercise, while their arterial oxygen tension generally decreased. The mean values for VD/VT ratio were elevated at rest in stages B and C and did not return to normal on exercise (Table 14–4). Reduction of arterial oxygen tension is common in miners with stages B and C, and this finding may be present at rest.[118] With exercise, the arterial tension usually falls further. In contrast, hypercapnia is not seen until the subject is in the terminal stage of disease, with cor pulmonale.

In a complete and detailed study of the mechanics of coal workers' pneumoconiosis, Seaton and colleagues demonstrated that static compliance is often reduced in PMF.[125] This finding was by no means invariable, and in one instance there was an abnormally high compliance despite the presence of stage B complicated pneumoconiosis. Specific compliance is similarly reduced, and as might be expected, the pulmonary recoil pressure at TLC is often increased. These findings indicate that in complicated pneumoconiosis the lungs tend to be stiffer than normal.

The fibrotic lesions of complicated pneumoconiosis encroach on the pulmonary vascular bed and destroy it. Because pulmonary hypertension

Table 14-4. GAS EXCHANGE IN SUBJECTS WITH COMPLICATED CWP

Radio-graphic Category	Number of Sub-jects		Age	$(A\text{-}a)O_2$ (mm/Hg)		PaO_2 (mm/Hg)		V_D/V_T		Minute Ventilation (L/min/m²)		Oxygen Uptake (L/min/m²)		FEV_1/FVC %
				Rest	Exer.	Rest	Exer.	Rest	Exer.	Rest	Exer.	Rest	Exer.	
B	7	Mean	63	29	31	74	71	0.51	0.40	5.50	16.20	0.148	0.476	57
		S.D.	(8.8)	(14.4)	(12.5)	(6.3)	(14.2)	(0.08)	(0.14)	(1.23)	(5.68)	(0.029)	(0.139)	(19.5)
C	7	Mean	53	25	35	76	64	0.52	0.43	6.42	17.05	0.150	0.476	65
		S.D.	(6.1)	(7.4)	(11.6)	(11.1)	(7.6)	(0.10)	(0.08)	(1.13)	(8.08)	(0.047)	(0.224)	(11.5)

is not seen until more than 50 per cent of the pulmonary capillary bed has been destroyed, pulmonary hypertension and cor pulmonale are late findings in PMF. As such, cor pulmonale is related more to the reduction of the vascular bed than to hypoxemia. They are seen only in late stage B and in stage C, unless there is coincident airways obstruction.[84, 131] The relationship of pulmonary hypertension to coal workers' pneumoconiosis is fully described by Lapp et al. and has been alluded to earlier in the chapter[84] (p. 417). These workers carried out cardiac catheterization in 47 symptomatic coal miners, and concluded that coal workers appear liable to cor pulmonale if their pneumoconiosis is of the complicated type, if they have chronic bronchitis, or if they have classical silicosis rather than coal workers' pneumoconiosis.

The catheterization findings of Lapp et al. have been confirmed by studies conducted by Seaton using lung perfusion scans with macroaggregated human albumin. Areas of absent perfusion were seen both in regions where the masses were located and in areas where bullous changes were present[134] (Figs. 14–23 and 14–24).

Thus it is apparent that complicated pneumoconiosis, at least in stages B and C, leads to a reduction in ventilatory capacity, a low diffusing capacity, abnormalities of gas exchange, a low arterial oxygen tension, and pulmonary hypertension. In addition, the lungs of miners with PMF have a tendency to be stiffer than normal, but this is by no means always true.

Treatment

No effective treatment is known, and antituberculosis drugs have been shown to be ineffective. When *Mycobacterium tuberculosis* is identified in the sputum, standard antituberculosis regimens should be used. These will usually convert the sputum, but, as might be expected, radiographic clearing is far less impressive.[159, 160] The introduction of regimens containing rifampin has been associated with more rapid improvement of concomitant PMF and tuberculosis.[161] There is no evidence to suggest that removal of the miner from further dust exposure is beneficial to him, and such a decision must depend on social and economic factors. Well-meaning advice of this type may deprive an individual of his livelihood and cause severe financial distress to him and his family.

Immunological Aspects of Coal Workers' Pneumoconiosis

Caplan's Syndrome and the Relationship of Rheumatoid Factor to CWP

At a meeting of the Thoracic Society of Great Britain, Caplan first called attention to a syndrome characterized by the presence of certain unusual radiological features in the chest film and by the presence of

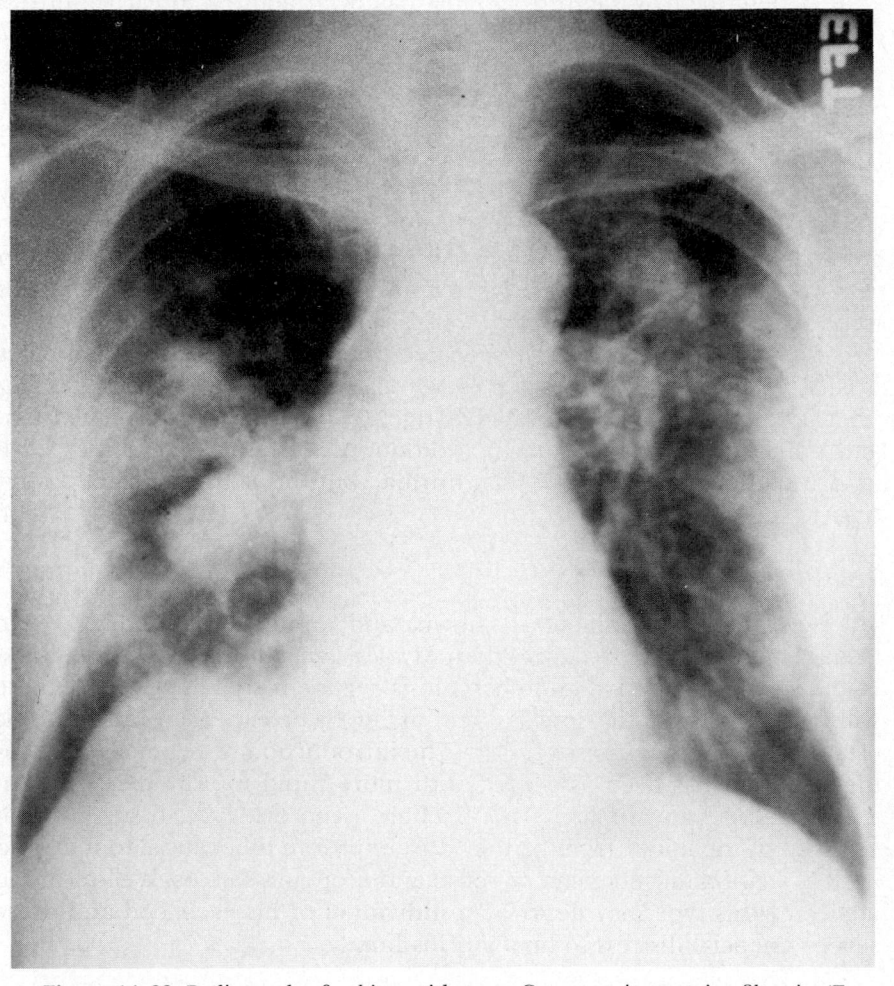

Figure 14–23. Radiograph of subject with stage C progressive massive fibrosis. (From Seaton, A., et al.: Lung perfusion scanning in coal workers' pneumoconiosis. Am. Rev. Resp. Dis., *103*, 338, 1971. Reproduced by permission.)

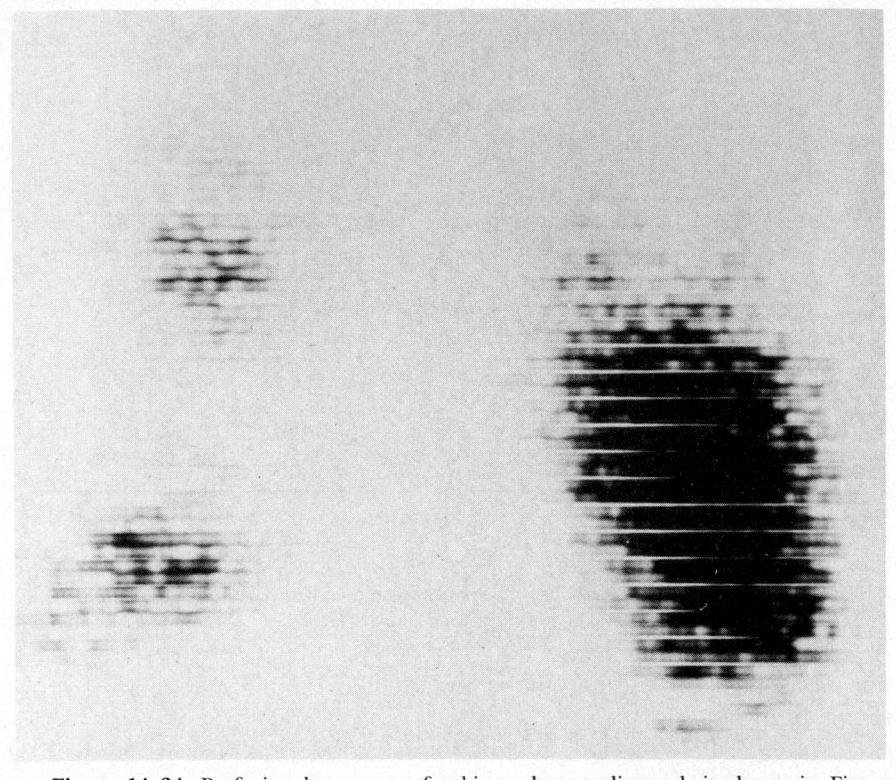

Figure 14–24. Perfusion lung scan of subject whose radiograph is shown in Figure 14–23. Note gross absence of perfusion at sites of large opacities. (From Seaton, A., et al.: Lung perfusion scanning in coal workers' pneumoconiosis. Am. Rev. Resp. Dis., *103*, 338, 1971. Reproduced by permission.)

rheumatoid arthritis.[162] This condition is now referred to as Caplan's syndrome or rheumatoid pneumoconiosis, and while it has some resemblances to progressive massive fibrosis, it has certain distinctive features.

The characteristic radiographic appearances of PMF have been described earlier in the chapter. In contrast to PMF, the opacities which appear in Caplan's syndrome are usually peripherally situated and appear over a short time, e.g., a few weeks.[163, 164,] They usually are seen on a background of category 0 or 1 pneumoconiosis and may undergo cavitation. The pulmonary nodules usually measure between 0.5 and 5 cm and most often develop concomitantly with the joint disease; however, in some instances they may appear either before or after the onset of arthritis (Fig. 14–25). In a few subjects they precede the arthritis by as much as 5 to 10 years. Fresh crops of nodules tend to appear at intervals and they usually portend an exacerbation of the arthritis. Calcification of the lesions is fairly common and pleural effusion may occur. In some instances, the rounded lesions of Caplan's syndrome are present along with the larger opacities typical of PMF. There is a definite association between the

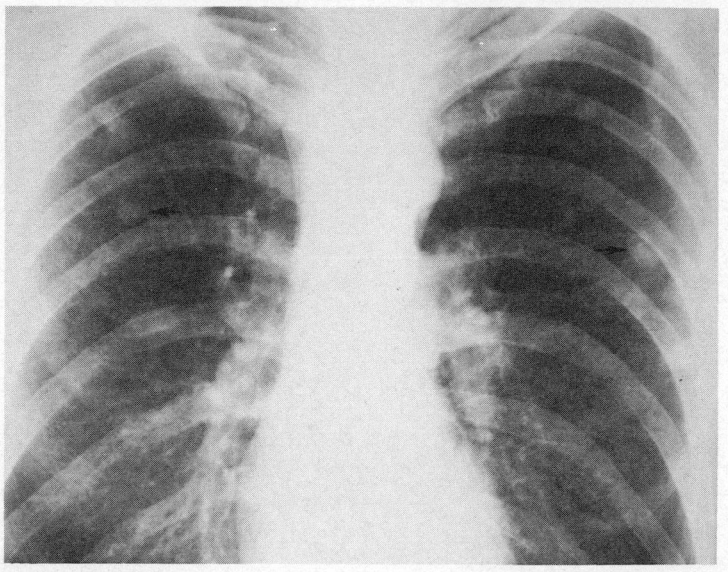

Figure 14–25. Chest radiograph of working miner with Caplan's syndrome.

nodules that occur on the elbows and Achillis tendon and those that are found in the lungs.

The epidemiology of the condition has been intensively studied by Miall et al.[164, 165] These studies have shown that there is an increased prevalence of rheumatoid arthritis in miners with PMF, but Miall was unable to find an increased prevalence of rheumatoid arthritis among miners and ex-miners. He concluded that dust exposure did not predispose to the development of rheumatoid arthritis. The prevalence of PMF and tuberculosis among miners with rheumatoid arthritis was significantly increased,[166] but neither antituberculosis therapy nor steroids influenced the size of the Caplan nodules.

Since Caplan's initial description, the syndrome has been reported in several other mineral pneumoconioses, including silicosis, asbestosis, and the pneumoconiosis of boiler scalers.[167–170]

The pathology of Caplan's syndrome has been well described by Gough, Rivers, and Seal.[171] These workers studied at necropsy 14 subjects who had had rheumatoid pneumoconiosis during life. They found that Caplan nodules and PMF both can occur in the same subject. Cavitation was frequently present and active or "burnt-out" tuberculosis was demonstrated in several instances. Differentiation between the ordinary collagenous nodule of pneumoconiosis, the silicotuberculotic nodule, the lesions of PMF, and the Caplan nodule was occasionally difficult when all four were present in the same subject. In general, to the naked eye, the Caplan nodule resembles a giant silicotic nodule, but histologically it is quite distinct. The Caplan nodule is often found when there is relatively

little dust in the lungs, a finding which contrasts with the massive lesion of typical PMF. Many of the nodules in Caplan's syndrome show a system of concentric layers. Histologically, the center of the nodules is formed of necrotic tissue with varying amounts of collagen and dust present. Outside the necrotic area, there is a cellular zone which is infiltrated with lymphocytes and plasma cells. Endarteritis obliterans is frequently present. In many nodules there is a peripheral zone of active inflammation with polymorphic leukocytic invasion and the presence of a few macrophages. This active inflammation zone is thought by Gough and colleagues to represent the rheumatoid zone.

Since the earlier investigations of Caplan's syndrome, there have been other studies conducted which have suggested that Caplan's original description was too restrictive. Thus Caplan and colleagues have shown that there is an increased prevalence of rheumatoid factors in miners with small nodular and irregular large opacities.[172] Many miners who have no overt arthritis, but who have the classical radiographic appearance of rheumatoid pneumoconiosis, have positive tests for rheumatoid factor.

Since that time Wagner and McCormick have conducted further studies of the immunology of CWP.[173] They correlated the presence of rheumatoid factors with the clinical and radiographic status of several groups of coal miners and also with a control group of nonminers. The coal miners were divided into (1) those with simple pneumoconiosis, (2) those with early PMF (stage A), (3) those with stages B and C PMF, and (4) those with typical Caplan's syndrome.

Wagner and McCormick showed that rheumatoid factor was found most frequently in the serum of subjects with Caplan's syndrome, i.e., in approximately 70 per cent of the group.[173] Around 30 to 40 per cent of the subjects with PMF had a positive titer, and the figure declined further for subjects with simple CWP. The controls had the lowest prevalence of rheumatoid factor, viz., only 2 per cent had a titer of 1:160 or greater. These authors also examined fresh lung tissue by means of immunohistological techniques designed to demonstrate rheumatoid factor in the tissues. As a result of their studies, they suggested that PMF exists in two forms: PMF with vasculitis and nonspecific PMF. The former is associated with marked vasculitis, plasma cell infiltration, and the presence of rheumatoid factor. Nonspecific PMF differs histologically, and is characterized by an irregular deposition of collagen fibers and coal dust but no vasculitis and an absence of rheumatoid factor in the lung. Wagner therefore suggested that many subjects with PMF really had a variant of Caplan's syndrome. He discussed this hypothesis in more detail in a subsequent paper.[150]

Lippmann and co-workers examined the sera of 156 underground United States coal miners for the presence of rheumatoid factor and antinuclear antibody.[174] A relation between humoral autoimmune activity and the radiographic type of nodular opacity was sought. The sera were divided into four groups, according to the miner's chest x-ray: (1) com-

plicated pneumoconiosis (progressive massive fibrosis), (2) simple pneumoconiosis, (3) normal, and (4) features suggestive of Caplan's syndrome.
Group 4 was divided into three subgroups (4a, b, and c): those with
classical features of Caplan's syndrome, those whose films suggested the
syndrome, and those in whom this syndrome was a possibility. Among the
sera from group 4, only 9 per cent showed rheumatoid factor, a rate
which did not differ significantly from those with either simple or complicated pneumoconiosis. None of the sera from the miners with normal
chest films showed rheumatoid factor or antinuclear antibody. In contrast,
antinuclear antibody was present significantly more often in the sera of
anthracite (55 per cent) as opposed to bituminous miners (21 per cent).
In anthracite miners with progressive massive fibrosis the figure was even
higher (74 per cent). There seemed to be a relation between autoimmune
activity and the prevalence of pneumoconiosis in coal workers, those
regions with highest prevalence of pneumoconiosis showing the greatest
number of miners with antinuclear antibody in their serum. With the
exception of serum drawn from subjects whose film had features that
were strongly suggestive of Caplan's syndrome, the type of nodular opacity
(p, q, or r) appears to be unrelated to humoral autoimmune activity.
These findings differ substantially from those of Wagner and would seem
to suggest that while his hypothesis may be valid in Welsh miners with
PMF,[150] it does not apply to PMF as seen in Appalachian coal miners.[175]

The immunoglobulin levels of coal miners with and without CWP
have shown varied results. Hahon and co-workers noted that sera from
anthracite miners with PMF showed greater concentrations of C_3, α_1-
antitrypsin, IgA, and IgG than did comparable sera from bituminous
miners with PMF.[176] In Caplan's syndrome, increases in the same immunoglobulin constituents were noted when compared to the controls without
pneumoconiosis. Few, if any, differences in immunoglobulins and proteins
were observed among miners with simple CWP.

Lung Autoantibodies. In a comprehensive review of the immunological aspects of coal workers' pneumoconiosis, Burrell demonstrated that
lung-reactive antibodies are to be found and that they are distinct from
globulin-reactive materials.[177] His experiments show that connective tissue
components (collagen, elastin, reticulin) are the major antigenic targets of
the immune response. Both types of IgA, viz., secretory and serum, are
involved in the immune response, and such antibodies can be demonstrated in pneumoconiotic nodules and in the alveolar septa after intravenous injection. The antibodies have been shown to enhance the response
to a challenge from *M. tuberculosis;* however, their role in pneumoconiosis
remains conjectural.

It has been suggested that inherited constitutional differences in
response to respirable dust inhalation might explain the different attack
and progression rates for CWP that have been observed in coal miners
with comparable dust exposures. Differing prevalences of histocompatibility antigens have been suggested as a possible explanation, but studies
to confirm this hypothesis have failed to do so.[178]

Chronic Bronchitis in Coal Miners

The relationship of chronic bronchitis to smoking and dust is discussed in detail in Chapter 17. This section will therefore be confined to chronic bronchitis as it occurs in coal miners. Although cigarette smoking is the major cause of cough and sputum in coal miners, it is clear that nonsmoking coal miners are also prone to develop bronchitis and that coal mine dust in itself is responsible.[179, 180] A recent postmortem study of the bronchi of 94 coal miners showed that an increase in the Reid index (viz., mucous gland hypertrophy) was related to both cigarette smoking and coal mine dust exposure.[181] In contrast, no relationship was noted between pneumoconiosis and the gland to wall ratio, as might have been expected.[181]

There has been much argument as to the relative effects of cigarette smoking versus coal dust on ventilatory capacity. In an early paper, Rogan and co-workers suggested that the effects of smoking and dust were approximately equal.[182] In this study, lifetime dust exposure was quantitated and the participating subjects were grouped into those with heavy, medium, and light exposure. Unfortunately, cigarette smoking was not similarly quantitated, and the investigators divided their subjects according to whether they were current smokers or not. No attempt was made to relate the decrement in ventilatory capacity to pack/years, since these data were not available. Moreover, the sample of miners was selected in order to include only those with a long working history. This would ensure that only those who were relatively resistant to the effects of cigarette smoking would be included, since those who had developed disabling emphysema would have already left the work force. In this connection, it must be conceded that the same situation might apply also to those affected by industrial bronchitis, but the currently available evidence suggests that the latter has far less severe effects and would therefore be unlikely to cause disabling impairment.[180, 183]

The currently available evidence indicates that while cigarette smoking affects the ventilatory capacity of about 12 to 13 per cent of those exposed,[184] many quite severely, industrial bronchitis probably affects the majority of those exposed, but to a far lesser extent. This results in a comparison of the effects of a severe affliction that occurs in a substantial minority with those of a minor affliction that occurs in the vast majority. Moreover, although heavy dust exposure leads to a reduction in the FEV_1, airways obstruction associated with dust never leads to the development of right ventricular hypertrophy in the absence of PMF or cigarette smoking.[86a] Industrial bronchitis clearly, then, is of lesser import.

A follow-up study of the subjects included in the original National Coal Board study showed that the effects of coal dust were about one third of those of cigarette smoking; however, here again, the investigators were unable to quantitate cigarette smoking habits.[185] The study gave results more in keeping with studies from the United States in which it has been shown that cigarette smoking has five to six times the effect of

coal dust. Since it is known that cigarette smoking shortens life by approximately 11 years, it can be assumed that the Love and Miller cohort[185] represents a survivor group resistant to the effects of cigarettes. In contrast to the British study, most United States studies have been cross-sectional in type. In one large United States study the relative effects of cigarette smoking and dust exposure were determined by comparing the ventilatory capacity of the least dust-exposed individuals (surface workers) to that of the most dust-exposed individuals (face workers).[179] In order to achieve this comparison, the face and surface workers were subdivided into smokers and nonsmokers, and then the mean FEV_1 of the smoking and nonsmoking face workers and the smoking surface workers was compared to that of the nonsmoking surface workers. The difference between the nonsmoking and smoking surface workers was five to six times greater than the difference between the nonsmoking surface workers and the nonsmoking face workers. For the most part, the effects of dust are apparent only in nonsmokers, mainly because the effects of smoking overwhelm those of dust. Moreover, since the dust-induced changes are relatively small, it is necessary to study a large number of subjects in order to demonstrate a statistically significant difference. As a result, some investigations in which the population base has been limited have failed to show an effect from industrial bronchitis.[183]

An increased annual rate of decline in the FEV_1 in active and retired United States coal miners has been demonstrated by Higgins[186] in a follow-up study of two cohorts of miners who were originally studied by Enterline.[187] The cohorts came from Richwood and Mullins, two separate communities in West Virginia. Higgins showed that coal mining was associated with an increased overall rate of decline of the FEV_1, but there were disparities between the various age groups. Moreover, his results suggested that the Richwood miners were more affected than those from Mullins, results that are diametrically opposed to those obtained by Enterline in his earlier cross-sectional study.[187] In addition, as Higgins pointed out, there was a large drop out between the two studies, and this could have in part accounted for some of the anomalous results. Many miners may have also been reluctant to admit that they were smokers, lest they jeopardize their chance of compensation.

In conclusion, the majority of the evidence suggests that cigarette smoking is far more important than dust exposure as the cause of ventilatory impairment. Over time, and with better dust control, its importance is likely to increase, since cigarette smoking appears to be declining relatively slowly. Widely divergent results obtained by different investigators when comparing the effects of cigarette smoking versus coal dust can be explained partly by different methodologies and partly by differing dust exposures. In this connection the United States coal dust standard is appreciably more stringent than that of Britain, and this might explain to some extent some of the differences noted between the two countries.

Emphysema in Coal Miners

It is generally accepted that coal workers' pneumoconiosis is associated with the presence of focal emphysema.[39] The pathology of CWP and focal emphysema are described earlier in this chapter and also in Chapter 6. While Gough and colleagues have in the past stated they could distinguish focal emphysema of CWP from centrilobular emphysema of cigarette smokers,[76, 77] other workers do not accept this distinction and feel unable to separate the two conditions.[188, 189] Over the past several years a series of papers from South Wales have suggested that emphysema occurs more frequently in coal miners with simple CWP than it does in those without the disease[188-190] These investigators have further suggested that the emphysema of coal workers is associated with a decreased ventilatory capacity and greater proclivity to respiratory disability. Moreover, a recent study of coal miners and nonminers who died of ischemic heart disease compared the postmortem prevalence and degree of emphysema in the two groups.[191] The coal workers were noted to have more emphysema than the control group.

The authors of this and the other previously mentioned studies imply that the focal emphysema that accompanies coal workers' pneumoconiosis is associated with increasing airways obstruction and disability. Although in the study of Cockroft et al.[191] emphysema was quantitated without a knowledge of occupation, the presence of macules and pigment in the coal miners' lungs invariably indicates to the pathologist the individual's prior occupation, and therein lies a possible source of bias, since the black pigment surrounding the focal emphysema may "highlight" it. While the authors tried to take into account the differences in cigarette-smoking habits, in doing so they often relied on a retrospective history of smoking habits rather than on pack/years, a practice which in itself is unsatisfactory. Moreover, it is clear that smoking histories obtained by panels or agencies that are charged with making decisions about compensation are inaccurate. The authors were unable to identify a gradient of emphysema with age; a finding which in itself casts doubt on the appropriateness of the subject selection. They conclude that the findings of the study reflect an excess of emphysema in coal workers as a whole. In doing so they imply that the prevalence of emphysema is increased whether or not the miner has pneumoconiosis, and they also imply that it is emphysema rather than industrial bronchitis that is responsible for the excess obstruction noted in coal miners. They thus ignore the fact that many other dust-exposed populations, including those exposed to silica and asbestos, show an excess of cough and sputum and also a small reduction in ventilatory capacity in the absence of radiological changes. Yet it is well accepted that neither simple silicosis nor asbestosis is associated with emphysema. The South Wales findings differ completely from those of a well-designed epidemiological study of working United States coal miners, which showed that while cigarette smoking led to a loss of lung recoil, no such findings were

present in the nonsmoking coal miners, although many had decreased flow rates at the high lung volumes and symptoms of cough and sputum.[128]

There seems little doubt, however, that simple CWP is associated with some overdistension and that the degree of overdistension is related to the radiographic category.[101] In addition, detailed studies of lung mechanics in nonsmoking miners with simple CWP have shown a trend towards an increased compliance.[90] Similarly, the dimensions of the air spaces in simple CWP have been shown to be increased.[192] Thus it is apparent that simple CWP and its attendant focal emphysema lead to overdistension and a minimal decrease in elastic recoil. However, these changes cannot be equated with airways obstruction, and it has been repeatedly demonstrated that an increasing category of simple CWP, although associated with increasing focal emphysema, does not lead to any concomitant increase in airways obstruction.[90]

The presence of small irregular opacities has been suggested by Cockroft et al. to be associated with a significant reduction in ventilatory and diffusing capacities.[193] Moreover, it is suggested that these effects cannot be accounted for by differences in lung volumes, age, height, and smoking history. It has been postulated that the reduced ventilatory and diffusing capacities are a result of the coincident presence of emphysema and interstitial fibrosis occurring in the same miner. Cockroft and co-workers argue that in those individuals with irregular opacities the absence of an increase in TLC indicates that the predominant lesion present in the lungs cannot be emphysema. However, their results clearly show that an increase in the prevalence of irregular opacities was associated with an increased RV. The latter is a far more sensitive indicator of emphysema and small airways obstruction than is an increase in TLC, and even with severe emphysema it is uncommon to find a TLC of more than 130 per cent of the predicted figure. Their study subjects were not randomly chosen but had been referred to a pneumoconiosis panel, and as such they represent an unusual group. In other studies, a definite increase in the prevalence of irregular opacities has been noted to occur with increasing age.[142, 143]

Musk and co-workers found a reduced diffusing capacity, no increase in compliance, and a tendency towards increased recoil pressure in coal workers with irregular opacities.[44] They postulate that this combination of functional abnormalities is explained by coexisting fibrosis and emphysema. They also suggest that the p type of opacity that occurs in simple coal workers' pneumoconiosis is associated with physiological evidence of emphysema, yet their data shows that subjects with this type of opacity had a higher FEV_1 and FEV_1/FVC ratio but a lower RV and TLC and an essentially unchanged recoil pressure. Were emphysema to be more common in the p type of opacity then one would expect an increased mortality in these subjects. In practice they may have the same life expectancy as do other subjects with simple pneumoconiosis.[194]

Relationship of Pneumoconiosis to Peptic Ulcer

The association between peptic ulcer and chronic airflow limitation has been known for many years, and it has been claimed that peptic ulcer is more common in miners. This thesis is difficult to prove, and it seems that increased incidence of peptic ulcer in coal miners is related to their high prevalence of airways obstruction and emphysema rather than the presence of pneumoconiosis itself.

Phillips studied the influence of surgery for peptic ulcer on pneumoconiosis and tuberculosis.[195] He followed up a group of Welsh miners with simple pneumoconiosis who had had various forms of surgery for peptic ulcer. He showed that active pulmonary tuberculosis occurred more frequently in those who had had a partial gastrectomy than in those who had been treated by vagotomy and gastroenterostomy. PMF also occurred more frequently in those who had had a partial gastrectomy, but Phillips was unable to suggest a cause for the increased incidence.

Association of Scleroderma with Coal Mining

An association between scleroderma and exposure to coal and silica dust has been noted. The great majority of the case reports indicate that it is exposure to coal dust rather than radiographic evidence of pneumoconiosis that seems to be associated with scleroderma.[196]

Factors Influencing Onset of Coal Workers' Pneumoconiosis

It is evident that coal workers' pneumoconiosis is caused by the inhalation of coal dust. Without dust there would be no disease, but other factors play a role in its development. Aside from the quantity, the type and quality of coal mine dust appear to be important. Also influencing the likelihood of the disease developing in a miner is the physical effort necessary to do his job. A high energy expenditure brought on by hard physical work entails a greater minute volume; viz., the worker breathes more air per unit time. This increases the amount of dust reaching the lungs. The effects of smoking on the development of coal workers' pneumoconiosis are probably of no consequence, but smoking might well delay the removal of particles from the ciliated airways. Finally, the problem of individual susceptibility exists. There seems good reason to believe that the same dust exposure in different individuals does not always lead to the same degree of dust retention. This difference is obviously a reflection of the ability of certain individuals to clear their air passages of inhaled particles more effectively. The problem with which we are faced is to lower the dust levels as far as possible and at the same time to allow the industry to remain profitable and productive.

Surface Miners. Surface miners in general are exposed to far lower levels of coal and other dusts.[197] Most surveys have shown that few open-cast coal miners show any radiological evidence of CWP, and that those in whom the condition is present have previously worked underground.[198] Similarly, airways obstruction is uncommon except in smokers. Nevertheless, a particular hazard exists in those few miners who drill the rock prior to placing explosive charges. As such, these drillers are at risk of developing silicosis, and relatively acute forms have been described. Until recently this hazard had not been appreciated in the United States, and few if any precautions had been taken.[199]

Acute Dust-Induced Changes in Ventilatory Function. Measurement of the ventilatory capacity of coal miners before and after a work shift has shown slight but significant decreases.[200] The magnitude of the change was related to the degree and extent of dust exposure. A later study repeated at a time when the dust levels were appreciably less again showed slight but lesser changes.[201] These occurred in the FVC and the FEF_{25-75}, and were limited to smokers. At the time of the second study the mean 8-hour dust level was 1.8 mg/m^3. Measurements of dust had not been made during the first study.

DUST STANDARDS

The present coal mine dust standard in the United States is 2 mg/m^3. The respirable dust is measured with a personal sampler which is worn for an 8-hour shift. The instrument relies on a nylon cyclone to select the respirable fraction.

In Britain the dust is measured in the return airway with a stationary instrument known as the MRE (Mining Research Establishment) gravimetric sampler. The respirable fraction is separated with a horizontal elutriator. The dust concentration in the return airway is higher than that which is present at the coal face, and a return airway measurement of 7 to 8 mg/m^3 corresponds to a face concentration of roughly 4 to 5 mg/m^3. The recommended standard in Britain is currently 7 mg/m^3 measured over the whole shift by the MRE gravimetric sampler at the 70 m control point in the air stream. This is equivalent to an average face concentration of 4.3 mg/m^3. This does not correspond to a United States measurement of 4.3 mg/m^3, since measurements made by the AEC cyclone instrument have to be multiplied by a factor of 1.6 in order to correspond to measurements with the MRE sampler.

References

1. Bremner, D., The Industries of Scotland: Their Rise, Progress, and Present Condition. Edinburgh, 1869.
2. Meiklejohn, A., History of lung disease of coal miners in Great Britain, Part I, 1800–1875. Br. J. Ind. Med., *8*, 127, 1951.

3. Liddell, F. D. K., Morbidity of British coal miners in 1961–1962. Br. J. Ind. Med., *30*, 1, 1973.
4. Lee, H. B., Bloodletting in Appalachia. Morgantown, West Virginia University Press, 1969.
5. Schlick, D. P., and Fannick, N. L., Coal in the United States. *In* Key, M. M., Kerr, L. E., and Bundy M., eds., Pulmonary Reactions to Coal Dust. New York, Academic Press, 1971, Chapter 2.
6. Doyle, H. N., Dust concentration in the mines. Proceedings of the Symposium on Respirable Coal Mine Dust, Washington, D. C., 1970 (Bureau of Mines Information Circular No. 8458).
7. Laennec, R. T. H., Traité de l'Auscultation Médiate, 4th ed. Paris, 1819.
8. Meiklejohn, A., History of lung disease of coal miners in Great Britain, Part II, 1875–1920. Br. J. Ind. Med., *9*, 93, 1952.
9. Meikeljohn A., History of lung disease of coal miners in Great Britain, Part III, 1920–1952. Br. J. Ind. Med., *9*, 208, 1952.
10. Arlidge, J. J., The Hygiene, Diseases and Mortality of Occupations. London, Percival, 1982.
11. Dressen, W. C., and Jones, R. R., Anthracosilicosis. J.A.M.A., *197*, 1179, 1936.
12. Flinn, R. H., Siefert, H. E., Brinton, H. E., et al., Soft Coal Miners' Health and Working Environment. U.S. Public Health Service Bulletin No. 270, Washington, D.C., 1941.
13. Lainhart, W. S., Doyle, H. M., Enterline, P. E., et al., Pneumoconiosis in Appalachian bituminous coal miners. U.S. Department of Health, Education and Welfare. Washington, D. C., U.S. Government Printing Office, 1969.
14. Hart, P. d' A., and Aslett, A. E., Med. Res. Council, Spec. Rep. Ser. No. 243. London, H. M. Stationery Office, 1942.
15. Collis, E. L., and Gilchrist, J. C., Effects of dust upon coal trimmers. J. Ind. Hyg., *10*, 101, 1928.
16. Gough, J., Pneumoconiosis of coal trimmers. J. Pathol. Bact., *51*, 277, 1940.
17. King, E. J., Maguire, B. A., and Nagelschmidt, G., Further studies of dust in lungs of coal miners. Br. J. Ind. Med., *13*, 9, 1956.
18. Watson, A. J., Black, J., Doig, A. T., and Nagelschmidt, G., Pneumoconiosis in carbon electrode makers. Br. J. Ind. Med., *16*, 274, 1959.
19. Gaensler, E. A., Cadigan, J. B., Sasahara, A. A., et al., Graphite pneumoconiosis of electrotypers. Am. J. Med., *41*, 864, 1966.
20: Rüttner, J. R., Bovet, P., and Aufdermaur, M., Graphit, Carborund, Staublunge. Deutsch Med. Wschr., *77*, 1413, 1952.
21. Davis, J. M. G., Ottery, J., and Le Roux, A., The effect of quartz and other non-coal dusts in coal workers' pneumoconiosis. *In* Walton, H. W., ed., Inhaled Particles IV. Oxford, Pergamon Press, 1977, p. 691.
22. Seaton, A., Dick, J. A., Dodgson, J., and Jacobsen, M., Quartz and pneumoconiosis in coal miners. Lancet, *2*, 1272, 1981.
22a. Jacobsen, M., and Maclaren, W. M., Unusual pulmonary observations and exposure to coalmine dust: A case-control study. *In* Walton, H. W., ed., Inhaled Particles V. Oxford, Pergamon Press, 1982.
23. Elmes, P. C., Relative importance of cigarette smoking in occupational lung disease. Br. J. Ind. Med., *38*, 1, 1981.
24. What proportion of cancers are related to occupation. (Editorial) Lancet, *2*, 1238, 1978.
25. Enterline, P. E., Mortality rates among coal miners. Am. J. Pub. Health, *54*, 758, 1964.
26. Liddell, F. D. K., Mortality of British coal miners in 1961. Br. J. Ind. Med., *30*, 15, 1973.
27. Ortmeyer, C. E., Costello, J., Morgan, W. K. C., et al., The mortality of Appalachian coal miners, 1963 to 1971. Arch. Environ. Heath, *29*, 67, 1974.
28. Costello, J., Ortmeyer, C. E., and Morgan, W. K. C., Mortality from heart disease in coal miners. Chest, *67*, 417, 1975.
29. Costello, J., Ortmeyer, C. E., and Morgan, W. K. C., Mortality from lung cancer in U.S. coal miners. Am. J. Pub. Health, *64*, 222, 1974.
30. Rockette, H., Mortality among Coal Miners Covered by the UMWA Health and Retirement Funds. NIOSH Research Report, Publication No. 77–155. Rockville, Maryland, Department of Health, Education and Welfare, 1977.
31. Cochrane, A. L., Relation between radiographic categories of pneumoconiosis and expectation of life. Br. Med. J., *2*, 532, 1973.

32. Cochrane, A. L., Haley, T. J. L., Moore, F., and Hole, D., The mortality of men in the Rhondda Fach, 1950–1970. Br. J. Ind. Med., *36*, 15, 1979.
33. Cochrane, A. L., and Moore, F., A 20-year follow-up of a population sample (aged 25–34) including coal miners and foundry workers in Staveley, Derbyshire. Br. J. Ind. Med., *37*, 230, 1980.
34. Miller, B. G., Jacobsen, M., and Steele R. C., Coal Miners' Mortality in Relation to Radiological Category, Lung Function, and Exposure to Airborne Dust. Final Report of CEC Contract No. 7246, 16/8/001. Edinburgh, Institute of Occupational Medicine, 1981.
35. Ames, R. G., Gastric carcinoma in coal miners: some hypotheses for investigation. J. Soc. Occup. Med., *32*, 73, 1982.
36. Ames, R. G., Gastric carcinoma and coal miner dust exposure: a case control study. cancer, *52*, 1346, 1983.
37. Heppleston, A. G., The essential lesion of pneumokoniosis in Welsh coal workers. J. Pathol. Bact., *59*, 453, 1947.
38. Heppleston, A. G., The pathogenesis of simple pneumokoniosis in coal workers. J. Pathol. Bact., *67*, 51, 1954.
39. Kleinerman, J., Pathology Standards for Coal Workers' Pneumoconiosis. Report of Pneumoconiosis Committee of the College of American Pathologists. Arch. Pathol. Lab. Med., *103*, 375, 1979.
40. Guidelines for the use of ILO International Classification of Radiographs: Occupational Safety and Health Series No. 22, rev. ed. Geneva, International Labour Organization, 1980.
41. Carilli, A. D., Kotzen, L. L., and Fischer, M., The chest roentgenogram in smoking females. Am. Rev. Respir. Dis., *107*, 133, 1973.
42. Amandus, H. H., Lapp, N. L., Jacobson, G., and Reger, R. B., Significance of irregular small opacities in the radiographs of coal miners in the U.S.A. Br. J. Ind. Med., *33*, 13, 1976.
43. Epidemiology Standardization Project. Am. Rev. Respir. Dis., *118* (Suppl), 7, 1978.
44. Musk, A. W., Cotes, J. E., Bevan, C., and Campbell, M. J., Relationship between type of simple coal workers' pneumoconiosis and lung function. Br. J. Ind. Med., *38*, 313, 1981.
45. Liddell, F. D. K., and May, J. D., Assessing the Radiological Progression of Simple Pneumoconiosis. London, National Coal Board Medical Service, 1966.
46. Fay, J. W. J., and Rae, S., The pneumoconiosis field research of the National Coal Board. Ann. Occup. Hyg., *1*, 149, 1959.
47. Rogan, J. M., Rae, S., and Walton, W. H., The National Coal Board's pneumoconiosis field research. *In* Davies, C. N., ed., Inhaled Particles and Vapours II, Oxford, Pergamon Press, 1967, pp. 493–508.
48. Dodgson, J., Hadden, G.G., Jones, C. O., and Walton, W. H., Characteristics of the airborne dust in British coal mines. *In* Walton, W. H., ed., Inhaled Particles III, Vol. 2. London, Unwin Brothers, 1970, p. 757.
49. Jacobsen, M., Progression of coal workers' pneumoconiosis in Britain in relation to environmental conditions underground. *In* Proceedings of Conference on Technical Measures of Dust Prevention and Suppression in Mines, Luxembourg, October 1972.
50. Jacobsen, M., New data on the relationship between simple pneumoconiosis and exposure to coal mine dust. Chest, *78* (Suppl), *408*, 1980.
51. Reisner, M. T. R., Results of epidemiological studies of pneumoconiosis in West German coal mines. *In* Walton, W. H., ed., Inhaled Particles III, Vol 2. London, Unwin Brothers, 1970, p. 921.
52. Reisner, M. T. R., Pneumoconiosis and exposure to dust in coal mines in the German Federal Republic. *In* Proceedings of Conference on Technical Measures of Dust Prevention and Suppression in Mines, Luxembourg, October 1972.
53. Reisner, M. T. R., Results of epidemiological studies on the progress of coal workers' pneumoconiosis. Chest, *78* (Suppl), 406, 1980.
54. Rossiter, C. E., Evidence of a dose-response relationship in pneumoconiosis. Trans. Soc. Occup. Med., *28*, 83, 1972.
55. Rivers, D., Wise, M. E., King, E. J., and Nagelschmidt, G., Dust content, radiology, and pathology in simple pneumoconiosis of coal workers. Br. J. Ind. Med., *17*, 87, 1960.

56. Faulds, J. S., King, E. J., and Nagelschmidt, G., Dust content of lungs of coal workers from Cumberland. Br. J. Ind. Med., *16*, 43, 1959.
57. Casswell, C., Bergman, I., and Rossiter, C. E., The relation of radiological appearance is simple pneumoconiosis of coal workers to the content and composition of the lung. *In* Walton W. H., ed., Inhaled Particles III, Vol. 2. London, Unwin Brothers, 1970, p. 713.
58. Bergman, I., and Casswell, C., Lung dust and lung iron contents of coal workers in different coalfields in Great Britain. Br. J. Ind. Med., *29*, 160, 1972.
59. Rossiter, C. E., Relations of lung dust content to radiological changes in coal workers. Ann. N.Y. Acad. Sci., *200*, 465, 1972.
60. Nagelschmidt, G., The study of lung dust in pneumoconiosis. Am. Ind. Hyg. Assoc. J., *26*, 1, 1965.
61. Crable, J. V., Keenan, R. G., Wolowicz, F. R., et al., The mineral content of bituminous coal miners' lung. Am. Ind. Hyg. Assoc. J., *28*, 8, 1967.
62. Crable, J. V., Keenan, R. G., Kinser, R. E., et al., Metal and mineral concentrations in lungs of bituminous coal miners. Am. Ind. Hyg. Assoc. J., *29*, 106, 1968.
63. Sweet, D. V., Crouse, W. E., Crable, J. V., et al., The relationship of total dust, free silica, and trace metal concentrations to the occupational respiratory disease of bituminous coal miners. Am. Ind. Hyg. Assoc. J., *34*, 479, 1974.
64. Freedman, A. P., Robinson, S. E., and Johnston, R. J., Noninvasive magnetopneumographic estimation of lung dustloads and distribution in bituminous coal workers. J. Occup. Med., *22*, 613, 1980.
65. Lainhart, W. S., and Morgan, W. K. C., Extent and distribution of respiratory effects. *In* Key, M. M., Kerr, L. E., and Bundy, M., eds., Pulmonary Reactions to Coal Dust. New York, Academic Press, 1971, p. 29.
66. Morgan, W. K. C., Reger, R., Burgess, D. B., and Shoub, E., A comparison of the prevalence of coal workers' pneumoconiosis and respiratory impairment in Pennsylvania bituminous and anthracite miners. Ann. N.Y. Acad. Sci., *200*, 252, 1972.
67. Morgan, W. K. C., Burgess, D. B., Jacobson, G., et al., The prevalence of coal workers' pneumoconiosis in U. S. coal miners. Arch. Environ. Health, *27*, 221, 1973.
68. UICC/Cincinnati, Classification of the radiographic appearances of pneumoconioses. Chest, *58*, 57, 1970.
69. Morgan, W. K. C., and Reger, R. B., A comparison of two classifications of coal workers' pneumoconiosis. J.A.M.A., *220*, 1746, 1972.
70. Attfield, M., Radiological Health of Coal Miners. NIOSH Report to Coal Council, Inhouse report, 1982.
71. Medical Service and Medical Research, Annual Report 1979–1980. London, National Coal Board, 1980.
72. Glick, M., Outhred, K. G., and McKenzie, H. I., Pneumoconiosis and respiratory disorders of coal mine workers of New South Wales, Australia. Ann. N.Y. Acad. Sci., *200*, 316, 1972.
73. Saric, M., Prevalence of coal workers' pneumoconiosis in Yugoslavia. Ann. N.Y. Acad. Sci., *200*, 301, 1972.
74. Morgan, W. K. C., Prevalence of coal workers' pneumoconiosis. Am. Rev. Respir. Dis., *98*, 306, 1968.
75. Bennett, J. G., Dick, J. A., and Kaplan, S., The relationship between coal rank and prevalence of pneumoconiosis. Br. J. Ind. Med., *36*, 206, 1979.
76. Gough, J., The pathogenesis of emphysema. *In* Liebow, A., and Smith, D. E., eds., The Lung. Baltimore, Williams & Wilkins, 1968, Chapter 9.
77. Heppleston, A. G., The pathological recognition and pathogenesis of emphysema and fibrocystic disease of the lung with special reference to coal workers. Ann. N. Y. Acad. Sci., *200*, 347, 1972.
78. Ruckley, V. A., Chapman, J. S., Collings, P. L., et al., Autopsy Studies of Coal Miners' Lungs. Final Report on CEC Contract 7246, 15/8/001. Edinburgh, Institute of Occupational Medicine, 1982.
79. Davis, J. M. G., Chapman, J. S., Willings, P., et al., Variations in the histological patterns of the lesions of coal workers' pneumoconiosis in Britain and their relationship to lung dust content. Am. Rev. Respir. Dis., *128*, 118, 1983.
80. Thomas, A. J., The heart in the pneumoconiosis of coalminers. Br. Heart J., *10*, 282, 1948.

81. Thomas, A. J., Right ventricular hypertrophy in the pneumoconiosis of coal miners. Br. Heart J., *13*, 1, 1951.
82. Wells, A. L., Pulmonary vascular changes in coal-workers' pneumoconiosis. J. Pathol. Bact., *68*, 573, 1954.
83. James, W. R. L., Thomas, A. J., Cardiac hypertrophy in coalworkers' pneumoconiosis. Br. J. Ind. Med. *13*, 24, 1956.
84. Lapp, N. L., Seaton, A., Kaplan, K. C., et al., Pulmonary hemodynamics in symptomatic coal miners. Am. Rev. Respir. Dis., *104*, 418, 1971.
85. Rasmussen, D. L., Laquer, W. A., Futterman, P., et al., Pulmonary impairment in Southern West Virginia coal miners. Am. Rev. Respir. Dis., *98*, 658, 1968.
86. Stanescu, D., Pulmonary impairment in coal miners. Am. Rev. Respir. Dis., *100*, 106, 1969.
86a. Fernie, J. M., Douglas, N. A., Lamb, D., and Ruckley, V. A., Right ventricular hypertrophy in a group of coal miners. Thorax, *38*, 436, 1983.
87. Motley, H. L., Lang, L. P., and Gordon, B., Pulmonary emphysema and ventilation measurement in one hundred anthracite coal miners with respiratory complaints. Am. Rev. Tuberc., *59*, 270, 1949.
88. Motley, H. L., Lang, L. P., and Gordon, B., Studies on the respiration gas exchange in one hundred anthracite coal miners with pulmonary complaints. Am. Rev. Tuberc., *61*, 201, 1950.
89. Morgan, W. K. C., Lapp, N. L., and Seaton, A., Respiratory impairment in simple coal workers' pneumoconiosis. J. Occup. Med., *14*, 839, 1972.
90. Morgan, W. K. C., and Lapp, N. L., Respiratory disease in coal miners. State of the art. Am. Rev. Respir. Dis., *113*, 531, 1976.
91. Pemberton, J., Chronic bronchitis, emphysema and bronchial spasm in bituminous coal workers. Arch. Ind. Health, *13*, 529, 1956.
92. Hyatt, R. E., Kistin, A. D., and Mahan, T.K., Respiratory disease in south West Virginia coal miners. Am. Rev. Respir. Dis., *89*, 387, 1964.
93. Morgan, W. K. C., Handelsman, L., Kibelstis, J., et al., Ventilatory capacity and lung volumes of U. S. coal miners. Arch. Environ. Health, *28*, 182, 1974.
94. Cochrane, A. L., Higgins, I. T. T., Pulmonary ventilatory function of coal miners in various areas in relation to the x-ray category of pneumoconiosis. Br. J. Prev. Soc. Med., *15*, 1, 1961.
95. Rogan, J. M., Ashford, J. R., Chapman, P. J., et al., Pneumoconiosis and respiratory symptoms in miners at eight collieries. Br. Med. J., *1*, 1337, 1961.
96. Ashford, J. R., Brown, S., Morgan, D. C., and Rae, S., The pulmonary ventilatory function of coal miners in the United Kingdom. Am. Rev. Respir. Dis., *97*, 810, 1968.
97. Higgins, I. T. T., Oldham, P. D., Ventilatory capacity in miners. Br. J. Ind. Med., *19*, 65, 1962.
98. Gilson, J. C., and Hugh-Jones, P., Lung function in coalworkers' pneumoconiosis. Med. Res. Council, Spec. Rep. Ser. No. 290. London, H. M. Stationery Office, 1955.
99. Higgins, I. T. T., Chronic respiratory disease in mining communities. Ann. N. Y. Acad. Sci., *200*, 197, 1972.
100. Enterline, P., The effects of occupation on chronic respiratory disease. Arch. Envir. Health, *14*, 189, 1967.
101. Morgan, W. K. C., Burgess, D. B., Lapp, N. L., et al., Hyperinflation of the lungs in coal miners. Thorax, *26*, 585, 1971.
102. O'Shea, J., Lapp, N. L., Russakoff, A. D., et al., Determination of lung volumes from chest films. Thorax, *25*, 544, 1970.
103. Morgan, W. K. C., Seaton, A., Burgess, D. B., et al., Lung volumes in working coal miners. Ann. N. Y. Acad. Sci., *200*, 478, 1972.
104. Needham, C. D., Rogan, M. C., and McDonald, I., Normal standards for lung volumes, intrapulmonary gas-mixing and maximum breathing capacity. Thorax, *9*, 313, 1954.
105. Lapp, N. L., and Seaton, A., Lung mechanics in coal workers' pneumoconiosis. Ann. N. Y. Acad. Sci., *200*, 433, 1972.
106. Murphy, D. M. F., Metzger, L.F., Silage, D. A., and Fogarty, M. C., Effect of simple anthracite pneumoconiosis on lung mechanics. Chest, *82*, 744, 1982.
107. Sartorelli, E., Baraldi, V., Grieco, A., and Zedda, S., La capacita di diffusione polmonare

dei gas nei silicotici. Ricerche con un metodo all'ossido di carbonio (1). Med. Lav., *54*, 191, 1963.

108. Billiet, L., van de Woestijne, K. P., Prignot, J., and Gyselin, A., La capacité de diffusion pulmonaire chez le silicotique. Acta Tuberc. Belg., *55*, 255, 1964.

109. Englert, M., and DeCoster, A., La capacité de diffusion pulmonaire dans anthracosilicose micronodulaire. J. Fr. Med. Chir. Thorac., *19*, 159, 1965.

110. Lavenne, F., Meersseman, F., and Brasseur, L., Fibrose interstitielle diffuse et pneumoconiose des houilleurs. Rev. Inst. Hyg. Mines, *20*, 33, 1964.

111. Frans, A., Veriter, C., and Brasseur, L., Pulmonary diffusing capacity for carbon monoxide in simple CWP. Bull. Physiopath. Resp., *11*, 479, 1975.

112. Lyons, J. P., Clarke, W. G., Hall, A. M., and Cotes, J. E., Transfer factor (diffusing capacity) for the lung in simple pneumoconiosis of coal workers. Br. Med. J., *4*, 772, 1967.

113. Cotes, J. E., and Field, G. B., Lung gas exchange in simple pneumoconiosis of coal workers. Br. J. Ind. Med., *29*, 268, 1972.

114. Seaton, A., Lapp, N. L., and Morgan, W. K. C. The relationship of pulmonary impairment in simple coal workers' pneumoconiosis to type of radiographic opacity. Br. J. Ind. Med., *29*, 50, 1972.

115. Rasmussen, D. L., Patterns of physiological impairment in coal workers' pneumoconiosis. Ann. N. Y. Acad. Sci., *200*, 455, 1972.

116. Gaensler, E. A., Discussion. Ann. N. Y. Acad. Sci., *200*, 463, 1972.

117. Kibelstis, J. A., Diffusing capacity in bituminous coal miners. Chest, *63*, 501, 1973.

118. Lapp, N. L., and Seaton, A., Pulmonary function. *In* Key, M. M., Kerr, I. E., and Bundy, M., eds., Pulmonary Reactions to Coal Dust. New York, Academic Press, 1971, p. 153.

119. Brasseur, L., L'exploration fonctionnelle pulmonaire dans la pneumoconiose des houilleurs. Brussels, Editions Arscia, 1963.

120. Worth, G., Muysers, L., and Siehoff, F., Les gradients d'oxygène et de gaz carbonique de fin d'expiration au cours des silicoses du type punctiforme. Poumon. Coeur, *19*, 1377, 1963.

121. Frans, A., Veriter, N., Gerin-Portier, N., and Brasseur, L., Blood gases in simple coal workers' pneumoconiosis. Bull. Physiopath. Resp., *11*, 503, 1975.

122. Rasmussen, D. L., Patterns of physiological impairment in coal workers' pneumoconiosis. Ann. N. Y. Acad. Sci., *200*, 455, 1972.

123. Harber, P., Estimation of the exertion requirements of coal mining work. Chest, *85*, 226, 1982.

124. Leathart, G. L., The mechanical properties of the lung in pneumoconiosis of coal workers. Br. J. Ind. Med., *16*, 153, 1959.

125. Seaton, A., Lapp, N. L., and Morgan, W. K. C., Lung mechanics and frequency dependence of compliance in coal miners. J. Clin. Invest., *51*, 1203, 1972.

126. Morgan, W. K. C., Lapp, N. L., and Morgan, E. J., The early detection of occupational lung disease. Br. J. Dis. Chest, *68*, 75, 1974.

127. Begin, R., Renzetti, A. D., Bigler, A. H., and Watanabe, S., Flow and age dependence of airway closure and dynamic compliance. J. Appl. Physiol., *38*, 199, 1975.

128. Hankinson, J. L., Reger, R. B., and Morgan, W. K. C., Maximal expiratory flow rates in coal miners. Am. Rev. Respir. Dis., *116*, 175, 1977.

129. Lapp, N. L., Block, J., Boehlecke, M., et al., Closing volume in coal miners. Am. Rev. Respir. Dis., *113*, 155, 1976.

130. Bollinelli, R., LeTallee, Y., and Bollinelli, M., Les résultats de l'exploration hémodynamique dans les silicoses pseudotumorales. J. Fr. Med. Chir., Thorac, *11*, 594, 1957.

131. Krémer, R., and Lavenne, F., La circulation pulmonaire dans les pneumoconioses. Poumon. Coeur, *22*, 767, 1966.

132. Krémer, R., Timmerman, G., Baudrez, J., and Lambrecht, P., Hémodynamique pulmonaire dans les pneumoconioses des houilleurs. Rev. Inst. Hyg. Mines, *22*, 3, 1967.

133. Krémer, R., Pulmonary hemodynamics in coal workers' pneumoconiosis. Ann. N. Y. Acad. Sci., *200*, 413, 1972.

134. Seaton, A., Lapp, N. L., and Chang, C. H. J., Lung perfusion scanning in coal workers' pneumoconiosis. Am. Rev. Respir. Dis., *103*, 338, 1971.

135. Siemsen, J. K., Sargent, E. N., Grebe, S. F., et al., Pulmonary concentration of Ga^{67} in pneumoconiosis. Am. J. Roentgen., *120*, 815, 1974.
136. Carpenter, R. G., and Cochrane, A. L., Death rates of miners and ex-miners with and without coalworkers' pneumoconiosis in South Wales. Br. J. Ind. Med., *13*, 102, 1956.
137. Ortmeyer, C. E., Baier, E. J., and Crawford, G. M., Life expectancy of Pennsylvania coal miners compensated for disability as affected by pneumoconiosis and ventilatory impairment. Arch. Environ. Health, *27*, 227, 1973.
138. Oldham, P. D., and Rossiter, C. E., Mortality in coalworkers' pneumoconiosis related to lung function: a prospective study. Br. J. Ind. Med., *22*, 93, 1965.
139. Cochrane, A. L., The attack rate of progressive massive fibrosis. Br. J. Ind. Med., *19*, 52, 1962.
140. McLintock, J. S., Rae, S., and Jacobsen, M., The attack rate of progressive massive fibrosis in British coalminers. *In* Walton, W. H., ed., Inhaled Particles III, Vol 2. London, Unwin Brothers, 1971, p. 933.
141. Cochrane, A. L., Moore, F., and Thomas, J., The radiographic progression of progressive massive fibrosis. Tubercle, *42*, 72, 1961.
142. Pratt, P. C., Role of silica in progressive massive fibrosis. Arch. Environ. Health, *16*, 734, 1968.
143. James, W. R. L., The relationship of tuberculosis to the development of massive pneumokoniosis in coal workers. Br. J. Tuberc., *48*, 89, 1954.
144. Gernez-Rieux, C., and Tacquet, A., Les infections humaines à mycobacteries atypiques au cours des pneumoconioses. Étude clinique et experimentale. 15th International Conference on Tuberculosis, Istanbul, September 1959. Bull. Union Int. Tuberc., *29*, 330, 1959.
145. Zaidi, S. H., Harrison, C. V., King, E. J., and Mitchison, D. A., Experimental infective pneumoconiosis. II. Coal-mine dust with attenuated tubercle bacilli (BCG) in the lung of immunised guinea-pigs. III. Coal-mine dust and isoniazid-resistant tubercle bacilli of moderate virulence. IV. Massive pulmonary fibrosis produced by coal-mine dust and isoniazid-resistant tubercle bacilli of low virulence. Br. J. Exp. Pathol., *36*, 539, 545, 553, 1955.
146. Gernez-Rieux, V., Tacquet, A., Devulder, B., et al., Experimental study of interactions between pneumoconiosis and mycobacterial infections. Ann. N. Y. Acad. Sci., *200*, 106, 1972.
147. Ball, J. D., Berry, G., Clarke, W. G., et al., A controlled trial of anti-tuberculosis chemotherapy in the early complicated pneumoconiosis of coalworkers. Thorax, *24*, 399, 1969.
148. Kilpatrick, G. S., Heppleston, A. G., and Fletcher, C. M., Cavitation in the massive fibrosis of coal workers' pneumoconiosis. Thorax, *9*, 260, 1954.
149. Wagner, J. C., Immunological factors in coal workers' pneumoconiosis. *In* Walton, W. H., ed., Inhaled Particles III, Vol 2. London, Unwin Brothers, 1971, p. 573.
150. Wagner, J. C., Etiological factors in complicated coal workers' pneumoconiosis. Ann. N. Y. Acad. Sci., *200*, 401, 1972.
151. Resnick, H., Lapp, N. L., and Morgan, W. K. C., Urinary hydroxyproline excretion in coal workers' pneumoconiosis. Br. J. Ind. Med., *26*, 135, 1969.
152. Resnick, H., and Morgan, W. K. C., Hydroxyproline excretion in complicated pneumoconiosis. Am. Rev. Respir. Dis., *103*, 849, 1971.
153. Wagner, J. C., Burns, J., Munday, D. E., and McGee, J., Presence of fibronectin in pneumoconiotic lesions. Thorax, *37*, 54, 1982.
154. Ulmer, W. T., and Reichel, G., Functional impairment in coal workers' pneumoconiosis. Ann. N. Y. Acad. Sci., *200*, 405, 1972.
155. Ulmer, W. T., and Reichel, G., Epidemiological problems of coal workers' bronchitis in comparison with the general population. Ann. N. Y. Acad. Sci., *200*, 211, 1972.
156. Lavenne, F., Brasseur, L., Oelbrandt, L., and Belayew, D., Volumes pulmonaires et volume expiratorie maximum par seconde des pneumoconiotiques encore au travail. Rev. Inst. Hyg. Mines, *16*, 3, 1961.
157. Dechoux, J. Pivoteau, C., and Aubertin, X., Analyse des troubles fonctionnels des pneumoconiotiques par le spirographie et le transfert de CO en regime stable et en inspiration unique. Bull. Physiopath. Resp., *5*, 179, 1969.
158. Marek, K., The evaluation of some methods of studying uniform ventilation. Pol. Arch. Med. Wewn., *35*, 1241, 1965.

159. Miall, W. E., Oldham, P. D., and Cochrane, A. L., The treatment of complicated pneumoconiosis with isoniazid. Br. J. Ind. Med., *11*, 186, 1954.
160. Cotes, J. E., and Gilson, J. C., Effects of inactivity, weight gain, and antitubercular chemotherapy upon lung fuction in working coal miners. Ann. Occup. Hyg., *10*, 327, 1967.
161. Jones, F. L., Rifampin-containing chemotherapy for pulmonary tuberculosis associated with coal workers' pneumoconiosis. Am. Rev. Respir. Dis., *125*, 681, 1982.
162. Caplan, A., Certain unusual radiological appearances in the chest of coal-miners suffering from rheumatoid arthritis. Thorax, *8*, 29, 1953.
163. Morgan, W. K. C., Caplan's syndrome. Ann. Intern. Med., *55*, 667, 1961.
164. Miall, W. E., Caplan, A., Cochrane, A. L., et al., An epidemiological study of rheumatoid arthritis associated with characteristic chest x-ray appearances in coal workers. Br. Med. J., *2*, 1231, 1953.
165. Miall, W. E., Rheumatoid arthritis in males. Ann. Rheum. Dis., *14*, 150, 1955.
166. Ball, J., Differential agglutination test in rheumatoid arthritis complicated by pneumoconiosis. Ann. Rheum. Dis., *14*, 159, 1955.
167. Morgan, W. K. C., Rheumatoid pneumoconiosis in association with asbestosis. Thorax, *19*, 433, 1964.
168. Rickards, A. G., and Barrett, G. M., Rheumatoid lung changes associated with asbestosis. Thorax, *13*, 185, 1958.
169. Campbell, J. A., A case of Caplan's syndrome in a boiler-scaler. Thorax, *13*, 177, 1958.
170. Martin, E., and Fallet, G. H., Pneumopathies chroniques et rheumatisme. Schweiz. Med. Woschr., *83*, 776, 1953.
171. Gough, J., Rovers, D., and Seal, R. H. E., Pathologic studies of modified pneumoconiosis in coal-miners with rheumatoid arthritis (Caplan's syndrome). Thorax, *10*, 9, 1955.
172. Caplan, A., Payne, R. B., and Withey, J. L., A broader concept of Caplan's syndrome related to rheumatoid factors. Thorax, *17*, 205, 1962.
173. Wagner, J. C., and McCormick, J. N., Immunological investigations of coal-workers' disease. J. Roy. Coll. Phys., *2*, 49, 1967.
174. Lippman, M., Eckert, H. L., Hahon, N., and Morgan, W. K. C., The prevalence of circulating anti-nuclear and rheumatoid factors in United States coal miners. Ann. Intern. Med., *79*, 807, 1973.
175. Benedek, T. G., Zawadzki, Z. A., and Medsger, T. A., Serum immunoglobulins, rheumatoid factor and pneumoconiosis in coal miners with rheumatoid arthritis. Arth. Rheum., *19*, 731, 1976.
176. Hahon, N., Morgan, W. K. C., and Peterson, M., Serum immunoglobulin levels in coal workers' pneumoconiosis. Ann. Occup. Hyg., *23*, 165, 1980.
177. Burrell, R., Immunological aspects of coal workers' pneumoconiosis. Ann. N. Y. Acad. Sci., *200*, 94, 1974.
178. Heise, M., Mentnech, M. S., Olenchock, S. A., et al., HLA-A1 and coalworkers' pneumoconiosis. Am. Rev. Respir. Dis., *119*, 903, 1979.
179. Kibelstis, J. A., Reger, E. J., Lapp, N. L., et al., Prevalence of bronchitis and airway obstruction in American bituminous coal miners. Am. Rev. Respir. Dis., *108*, 886, 1973.
180. Morgan, W. K. C., Industrial bronchitis. Br. J. Ind. Med., *35*, 285, 1978.
181. Douglas, A. N., Lamb, D., and Ruckley, V. A., Bronchial gland dimensions in coal miners: influence of smoking and dust exposure. Thorax, *37*, 760, 1982.
182. Rogan, J. M., Attfield, M. D., Jacobsen, M., et al., Role of dust in the working environment in development of chronic bronchitis in British coal miners. Br. J. Ind. Med., *30*, 217, 1973.
183. Rom, W. N., Kanner, R. E., Renzetti, A. D., et al., Respiratory disease in Utah coal miners. Am. Rev. Respir. Dis., *123*, 372, 1981.
184. Fletcher, C. M, and Peto, R., The natural history of chronic airflow obstruction. Br. Med. J., *1*, 1645, 1977.
185. Love, R. G., and Miller, B. G., Longitudinal study of lung function in coal miners. Thorax, *37*, 193, 1982.
186. Higgins, I. T. T., and Whittaker, P. E., Chronic respiratory disease in two mining companies in West Virginia. NIOSH Technical Report. Washington, D. C., U. S. Government Printing Office, 1981.
187. Enterline, P. E., The effects of occupation on chronic respiratory disease. Arch. Environ. Health, *14*, 189, 1967.

188. Ryder, R., Lyons, J. P., Campbell, H., and Gough, J., Emphysema in coal workers' pneumoconiosis. Br. Med. J., *3*, 481, 1970.
189. Lyons, J. P., Ryder, R., Campbell, H., and Gough, J., Pulmonary disability in coal workers' pneumoconiosis. Br. Med. J., *1*, 713, 1972.
190. Lyons, J. P., and Campbell, H., Evaluation of disability in coal workers' pneumoconiosis. Thorax, *31*, 527, 1976.
191. Cockroft, A., Seal, R. M. E., Wagner, J. C., et al., Post-mortem study of emphysema in coal workers and noncoal workers. Lancet, *2*, 600, 1982.
192. Hankinson, J. L., Palmes, E. D., and Lapp, N. L., Pulmonary air space size in coal miners. Am. Rev. Respir. Dis., *119*, 391, 1979.
193. Cockroft, A., Berry, G., Cotes, J. E., and Lyons, J. P., Shape of small opacities and lung function in coalworkers. Thorax, *37*, 765, 1982.
194. Waters, W. E., Cochrane, A. L., and Moore, F., Mortality in punctiform type of coalworkers' pneumoconiosis. Br. J. Ind. Med., *31*, 196, 1974.
195. Phillips, T. J. G., Influence of surgery for peptic ulcer on pneumoconiosis and tuberculosis. Br. J. Ind. Med., *27*, 245, 1970.
196. Rodnan, G. P., Benedek, T. G., Medsger, T. A., Jr., and Cammarata, R. J., The association of progressive systemic sclerosis (scleroderma) with coal miners' pneumoconiosis and other forms of silicosis. Ann. Intern. Med., *66*, 323, 1967.
197. Parobeck, P. S., and Tomb, T. F., Respirable dust levels: surface work area of underground coal mines and surface coal mines. Work Environ. Health, *11*, 43, 1974.
198. Fairman, P., O'Brien, R. J., Swecker, S., et al., Respiratory status of surface coal miners in the United States. Arch. Environ. Health, *31*, 1977.
199. Banks, D. E., Bauer, M. A., Castellan, R. M., and Lapp, N. L., Silicosis in surface coal mine drillers. Thorax, *38*, 275, 1983.
200. Lapp, N. L., Hankinson, J. L., Burgess, D. B., et al., Changes in ventilatory function in coal miners after a work shift. Arch. Environ. Health, *24*, 204, 1972.
201. Lapp, N. L., Fairman, P., Hankinson, J. L., et al., Ventilatory function changes in coalminers over a workshift. Paper presented at the International Conference on Occupational Lung Disease, American College of Chest Physicians, San Francisco, 1979.

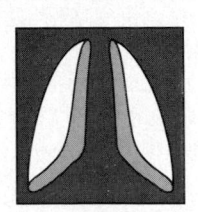

15

OTHER PNEUMOCONIOSES

W. Keith C. Morgan

ALUMINUM

Aluminum is mined as bauxite, and large deposits of this ore are found in Jamaica and, to a lesser extent, in various parts of the southern United States. The ore is also found in Australia, Guyana, France, Hungary, and Surinam. Aluminum is never found in its metallic state, but in combination with oxygen, fluorine, and silica. It also occurs as cryolite, which is sodium aluminum fluoride (Na_2AlF_6), found only in Greenland. Cryolite was at one time a main source of aluminum; however, the deposits have gradually become exhausted. Bauxite is extracted mainly by open-cast mining. It is then crushed and washed to remove clay and silica. The production of aluminum involves two steps. First, alumina (Al_2O_3) is produced from bauxite by what is known as the Bayer process. Bauxite is digested at a high temperature and pressure in a strong solution of caustic soda, and the resultant hydrate is then crystallized and calcined to the oxide in a kiln. Following this, the alumina is reduced by an electrolytic process using carbon electrodes and cryolite flux.

The reduction of Al_2O_3 into metallic aluminum involves electrolytic decomposition in which the Al_2O_3 is first rendered liquid to permit a direct current to flow through it. This is brought about by dissolving the aluminum in cryolite. The electrolytic process then takes place in cells that are known as pots. The latter are steel-coated but have bottoms made of carbon that are connected to a negative polar source. Positive polar carbon electrodes hang above and dip into the cryolite aluminum mixture. When the current flows, the aluminum is split, and the metallic aluminum settles at the bottom of the pot and is removed at intervals. The pot gives off fumes and emissions from the molten cryolite and these contain hydrofluoric acid, fluoride dust, alumina, carbon, and some sulfur dioxide. The carbon electrodes are mostly made from petroleum coke, a waste product

449

of oil refineries. In the manufacture of the carbon electrodes, petroleum coke is first ground in ball mills, so that it becomes a fine powder, and then is made into electrodes.

The National Institute of Occupational Safety and Health (NIOSH) has estimated that there may be 3 million workers in the United States who are exposed to aluminum compounds. Around 1.5 million workers are exposed to alumina, about 100,000 of whom are exposed on a regular basis. Exposure to aluminum may occur during its production or when the finished product is being used for various manufacturing processes.

It is now fairly well accepted that exposure to aluminum may lead to the development of pulmonary fibrosis. The effects of aluminum in the lung tend to differ according to the composition and the amount of inhaled aluminum. Pulmonary fibrosis has been reported in workers involved in the manufacture of aluminum abrasives and in subjects using aluminum powder in the manufacture of explosives.

Pulmonary Fibrosis Due to Inhalation of Bauxite (Shaver's Disease)

This condition is commonly referred to as Shaver's disease and the first detailed report was published in 1947.[1] It occurs in workers who manufacture alumina abrasives, in particular, corundum. The latter, composed of bauxite (aluminum oxide), is of great hardness and is manufactured in special electrical furnaces. The process involves the grinding up of bauxite into a powder that is then intimately mixed with iron and coke. The mixture is placed in large iron pots into which carbon electrodes are lowered. The mixture is fused at over 2000°C., and during the process dense white fumes are given off that contain both aluminum oxide and silica. The fumes contaminate the atmosphere in the furnace rooms, although most escape through openings in the roof.

Shaver and Riddell had each separately encountered a few subjects with what appeared to be idiopathic pulmonary fibrosis associated with pneumothorax before they realized that all of their subjects worked in the same plant manufacturing abrasives.[1] This observation prompted them to survey all the workers employed at the furnaces of four plants that were involved in the manufacture of alumina abrasives. They found 23 subjects with radiographic abnormalities, of whom 8 had had one or more spontaneous pneumothoraces.

Clinical Features

The symptoms of affected subjects are related to the degree of radiographic lung involvement. Shortness of breath is the most common complaint. Paroxysms of shortness of breath occur along with chest pain. Sputum production and cough are common; however, the sputum is

usually mucoid. Tightness in the chest is frequent, as are weakness and fatigue. Pleuritic pain and acute shortness of breath, when they occur together, suggest the presence of pneumothorax. An acute form of the condition occurs when exposure has been intense, and is characterized by cough, low-grade fever, and chest tightness. In many subjects the acute condition progresses to the chronic disease.

Physical findings are nonspecific unless a pneumothorax is present. Tachypnea and cyanosis occur in advanced cases. Dullness to percussion may be present, and basal crackles occur frequently. Finger clubbing is rarely if ever seen.

Radiology

The findings vary according to the severity of involvement, and the less severely affected subject may show little in the way of abnormality. Widening of the mediastinum and elevation of the diaphragm are frequent. Both lungs are usually affected by a diffuse reticulonodular process. As time goes by, numerous blebs appear and regional honeycombing develops. The upper lobes are most affected.[1]

The acute form of the disease is characterized by an acinous filling pattern; however, this often only partially resolves, leaving a reticulonodular pattern. Pneumothorax is common and may be chronic.

Pathology

Macroscopically the lungs appear solid and of a gray-black color, with pleural thickening and adhesions occurring frequently. Emphysematous blebs are usually observed on the pleural surface. The lungs feel fibrotic and are difficult to section. The upper zones are more affected. Dense fibrous masses may extend out from the hila.

Histologically in the acute stage there is often alveolar edema and thickened septa. The damaged alveoli become lined by epithelial cells, and lymphocyte aggregation may be seen in the bronchioles. Interstitial fibrosis occurs later but classical nodular silicotic lesions are absent. Vascular damage is slight.

The respective roles of alumina and silica in the production of the pulmonary changes are still the subject of debate, but there is little doubt that many of the changes were induced by free silica, in particular cristobalite and tridymite. A subsequent analysis of the constituents used in the plants described by Shaver revealed that the mixture that was heated contained 77 to 85 per cent Al_2O_3 and between 4 and 7 per cent of free silica.[2] The concentrations of silica and Al_2O_3 in the fumes were 31 and 62 per cent, respectively. An analysis of the lungs of a number of workers who had died of Shaver's disease showed increases in both the silica and the Al_2O_3 contents. The majority of the evidence suggests that silica was the main agent responsible, perhaps in the form of cristobalite,

which is known to be formed from quartz at high temperatures and is also more fibrogenic than quartz.

Fatal cases occur, and death is usually due to respiratory failure and concomitant pulmonary infection.

Aluminum Lung

The first detailed report of the harmful effects of metallic aluminum came from Goralewski.[3] He drew attention to the fact that German workers engaged in the manufacture of pyro-aluminum powder developed an acute respiratory illness, often within a few months of starting work. The powder was used for making explosives and hence was not coated with stearin, a substance which is often used in the manufacture of aluminum powder. The affected subjects had a cough, low-grade fever, shortness of breath, lethargy, and anorexia. Their radiographs showed pulmonary shadows, and in some a pneumothorax developed. Histological examination of the lungs revealed fibrotic changes. Ten of Goralewski's original 18 patients had died by 1956.[4] Goralewski's material was confiscated during the British advance into Germany in 1945 and sent to the London Hospital, where his findings were subsequently confirmed.

Because of the German experience, epidemiological studies were carried out on British workers involved in the manufacture of incendiary bombs and aluminum airplane propellers.[5] No pulmonary morbidity that could be attributed to aluminum was detected and, moreover, no explanation for the difference between the British and the German findings was forthcoming. In 1959, Mitchell reported a subject with pulmonary fibrosis that appeared to be a consequence of aluminum exposure.[6] In 1961, additional subjects with pulmonary fibrosis were reported by Mitchell et al.[7] and by Jordan.[8]

Aluminum powder is produced in two forms: flake powder, which is formed by stamping cold metal, and granulated powder, which is prepared directly from the molten metal. An unusual form of flake powder known as "pyro" is composed of three-dimensional particles and is used in the manufacture of fireworks. The subjects reported by Mitchell et al. were all exposed to the flake variety of aluminum powder.[7] Their job was to first stamp aluminum into flakes. From the stamped powder, paint and "pyro" were made. To the powder used in the manufacture of paint, large quantities of stearin were added. This was not true of the pyro powder, in which as little stearin as possible was used. A small amount of carbon black was added to the pyro. The mixture was then stamped and ground into a fine blackish powder. During the filling and emptying of the stamping machines, large quantities of dust were liberated. Gravimetric samples of the dust in the room revealed mean concentrations of 95 mg/ m^3, with most particles measuring 1 to 2 microns. Most of the dust consisted of metallic aluminum, but an appreciable concentration of

aluminum oxide and hydroxide was present. Small quantities of copper, magnesium, and carbon were likewise present.

The explanation as to why aluminum induces fibrosis in certain circumstances but not in others remains uncertain. It has been suggested that chloride ions need to be present so that the protein becomes tanned and is then precipitated along with aluminum hydroxide. Since this complex is insoluble and not likely to be phagocytosed, it leaves the metallic aluminum free to cause fibrosis. Koelsch advanced an alternative hypothesis that suggested that high levels of aluminum in the ambient air were necessary for the development of fibrosis.[9] This was certainly true in wartime, when fine plate aluminum was used in the manufacture of explosives, and in working conditions where ventilation was poor.

Aluminum Fibrosis

Clinical Features

These are essentially the same as those in Shaver's disease, namely, cough, sputum, anorexia, and often pneumothorax. Signs are scanty, but basal crackles occur. As in Shaver's disease, clubbing is usually absent. Tachypnea, a small chest expansion, and the characteristic signs of a diffuse fibrosis are present in subjects with advanced disease.

In 1967, McLaughlin and co-workers reported a patient who had developed pulmonary fibrosis and an encephalopathy, which they attributed to the inhalation of aluminum dust.[10] The subject was a 49-year-old man who had worked for 13 years in the ball mill of an aluminum powder factory. His pulmonary symptoms were minor; however, during life he had suffered from epilepsy and had developed a progressive encephalopathy. The lungs and brain were analyzed and found to contain 20 and 122 times the expected aluminum content, respectively.

Pathology

Macroscopically and microscopically the changes are similar if not identical to those seen in Shaver's disease. Interstitial fibrosis and epithelialization of damaged alveoli are common. Analysis of the lungs reveals a grossly increased aluminum content.

Corrin, in a series of experiments, some of which involved animals, demonstrated that stamped aluminum reacts vigorously with water, while the granular powder is unreactive.[11, 12] He showed that the granular particles are inert because they are coated with inert aluminum oxide and thus do not react with water. The formation of aluminum oxide is prevented in the stamping process by the use of stearin. The sudden appearance of aluminum pneumoconiosis in Britain was attributed by Corrin to the substitution of mineral oil for stearin, for, in contrast, to

stearin, mineral oil permits the powder to react with water.[11, 12] He also showed that it was the aluminum and not the stearin that was responsible for the fibrosis, and that granular aluminum was much less fibrogenic than stamped aluminum.

A series of animal experiments conducted by Gross and colleagues has shed some light on the pathogenic effects of inhaled aluminum.[13] The inhalation of fine metallic aluminum dust in rats led to the development of lipoid pneumonitis and alveolar proteinosis. The latter condition was also noted to occur in hamsters and guinea pigs, but there have been no reports of aluminum leading to this condition in humans. In contrast, when intratracheal injection of aluminum dust was substituted for inhalation, powdered aluminum led to the development of areas of focal pulmonary fibrosis. If the dose of aluminum was relatively small, no fibrosis occurred, but with larger doses fibrosis became frequent. The investigators therefore concluded that the development of fibrosis depends largely on the route of entry used to administer the aluminum and hence greatly on the dose administered. Intratracheal injection permits the use of a far greater dose of aluminum, and fibrosis was found to occur only with excessively high doses. In this context, powdered aluminum dust has been used in an effort to prevent silicosis. Ontario metal miners have been exposed at regular intervals to aerosolized aluminum. While there is little evidence of the efficacy of aluminum as a prophylactic, there is even less evidence that this ritual involving the repeated inhalation of aluminum has led to the development of fibrosis. These facts favor the hypothesis that the metal is innocuous unless inhaled in high concentrations.

Other Syndromes Due to Inhalation of Aluminum and Its Compounds

Aside from its association with metallic aluminum, pulmonary fibrosis has been reported in an aluminum arc welder, but a cause-and-effect relationship between exposure to aluminum and the lung condition was not definitely demonstrated.[14] Similarly, a pneumoconiosis has been reported in workers bagging cat litter containing an artificial aluminum silicate (alunite).[15] In these workers there was some suggestion that those exposed showed a reduced diffusing capacity and developed pulmonary fibrosis. Aluminum oxide is also used in the manufacture of abrasives. The two main synthetic abrasives in use are alumina and silicon carbide. In regard to the former, the loose grains of alumina are compacted and then bonded together prior to being made into grinding wheels, stones, or emery cloth. Most grinding wheels are composed of a bonded combination of alumina and silicon carbide. It is of interest to note that it was the recognition of the hazard from grinding with siliceous stones in the Sheffield cutlery industry that stimulated a successful search for less hazardous substitutes.

Natural emery usually is composed of 50 to 70 per cent Al_2O_3, some hematite, occasionally some magnetite, and usually a little free silica. While there have been a few reports of radiographic abnormalities developing in emery workers,[16] it is uncertain whether radiographic changes were a consequence of the inhaled Al_2O_3 or the other constituents, e.g., hematite or other iron ores.

There seems little doubt that potroom workers and aluminum smelters may develop asthma.[17, 18] Both immediate and delayed responses have been shown to occur. The former is precipitated by high exposure to potroom fumes. The delayed response usually occurs 4 to 12 hours following exposure and may develop during the night. Dual responses also occur.[19] The immediate response usually occurs within the first three months of exposure and often within a very short time. It is associated with shortness of breath rather than wheeze, and is likely to be a nonspecific reaction to potroom fumes that occurs in an individual who has either idiopathic asthma or hypersensitive airways. There is some evidence that the delayed response may lead to loss of lung elastic recoil, which suggests that emphysema may develop.[20] This has not, however, been definitely established at the present time.[21]

ANTIMONY PNEUMOCONIOSIS

Antimony is closely related to arsenic and readily forms alloys with lead, tin, zinc, and iron. It occurs normally in several forms: stibnite (SbS_3), valentinite (Sb_2O_3), kermesite (Sb_2S_2O), and senarmontite (Sb_2O_3). It is mined in China, South Africa, Russia, Mexico, and Bolivia.

Antimony has been used in the manufacture and plating of vases since the times of the great Egyptian civilizations. Stibnite has also been used as a cosmetic. At present, the metal is used as a constituent of alloys, in the compounding of rubber, in flame proofing, in safety matches, and in paints and lacquers. Antimony is also used in electronic, semiconductive, and thermoelectric devices because of its low electrical resistance, and in medicine as an emetic (tartar emetic) and in the treatment of schistosomiasis. NIOSH has estimated that 1.4 million workers in the United States are potentially exposed to antimony in their occupational environment. Such ex cathedra pronouncements, although impressive, for the most part appear to be based on extremely tenuous data, and give no indication of the true number of subjects at risk.

The dust that is produced during the mining of antimony often contains some free silica, and the term silicoantimoniosis has been coined to refer to the condition of lungs containing both silica and antimony. The antimony ore, when it is processed, is pulverized into a fine dust. High dust concentrations are thus present during the operations of reduction and scaling. Crushing of the ore generates coarse particles that are not retained by the lungs, and many of the other processes are wet

and relatively dust-free. However, furnacemen who refine the metal prior to its being alloyed with other metals are exposed to appreciable concentrations of antimony dust.

Antimony pneumoconiosis has been described in individuals working with stibnite.[22] The latter is usually emptied from bags through a grill onto a rotating kiln. The metal is volatilized by the heat and forms a fine white powder at the top of the kiln which escapes into the surrounding atmosphere.

Antimony enters the body through the lungs and skin. The metal is absorbed from the lung parenchyma, taken up by the blood and tissues, and excreted in the feces. Some remains in the red blood cells. The inhalation of antimony may produce rhinitis, bronchitis, and nasal septal perforation. Conjunctivitis and dermatitis occur.

Although antimony may produce radiographic changes in the lung (Fig. 15–1), pulmonary function does not appear to be affected.[23] Histological examination of the lungs of workers exposed to antimony has shown alveolar macrophages laden with dust and congregating in and around the alveolar walls and around small vessels.[24, 25] No fibrosis or significant inflammatory action has been observed, and the characteristic radiographic features are those of small rounded opacities similar to those seen in siderosis or stannosis. Massive fibrosis has not been reported.

BARITOSIS

Baritosis was first described by Arrigoni among barytes miners in Italy.[26, 27] Barytes occurs in combination with other minerals such as calcite, fluorite, quartz, and chert. It is found in Mississippi, Nevada, and Georgia, as well as in Italy. Barytes is used in the production of lithopone, a white pigment used in paints; in vulcanization; for x-ray studies; and in glassmaking. During mining, high concentrations of dust are produced. Baritosis has also been described in a few workers in a lithopone plant in Pennsylvania.[28] Those who were affected had markedly abnormal chest radiographs, and it was noted that one of them had features that closely resembled those previously described by Arrigoni in barytes workers. Further inquiries showed that the men in the lithopone plant were exposed to finely dissolved barium sulfate powder. Doig also reported 8 subjects with baritosis in a small factory in which barytes was crushed.[29]

Baritosis is not associated with respiratory symptoms or impairment as far as is known. The radiographic appearances are quite striking (Fig. 15–2). The deposits of barium appear as multiple, extremely dense, small rounded opacities. Some radiographic clearing may occur after exposure ceases. Kerley B lines are sometimes in evidence when silica is present in the inhaled dust, and under such circumstances a mixed-dust pneumoconiosis results. Fibrosis is not a feature of the condition unless inhaled dust has been contaminated by silica or other agents.

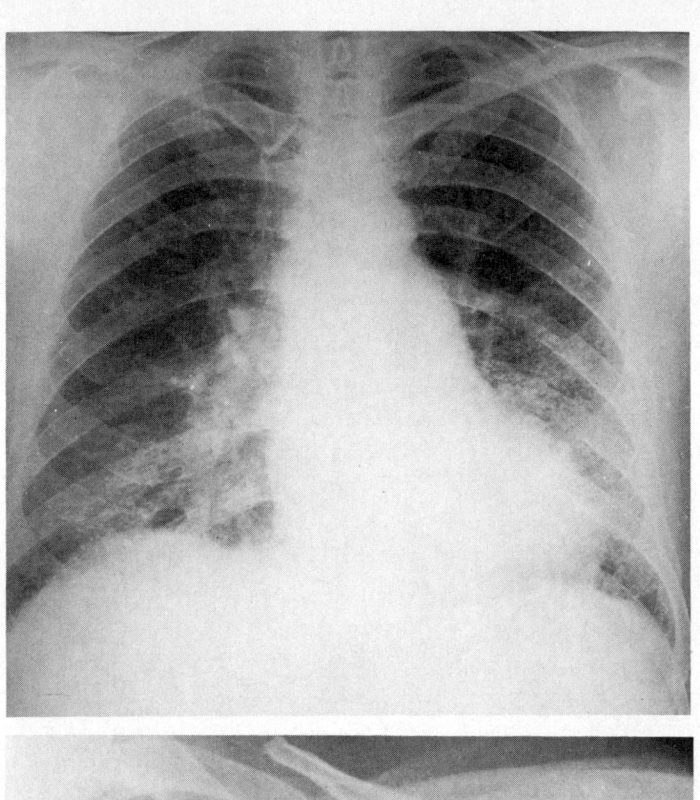

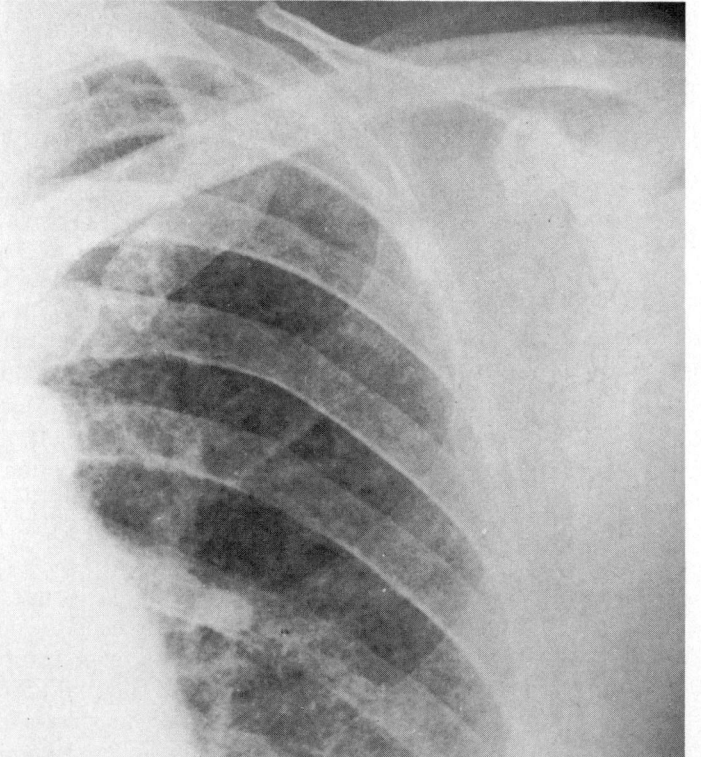

Figure 15–1. Chest radiographs of subject with antimony pneumoconiosis. (Courtesy of Dr. E. P. Pendergrass.)

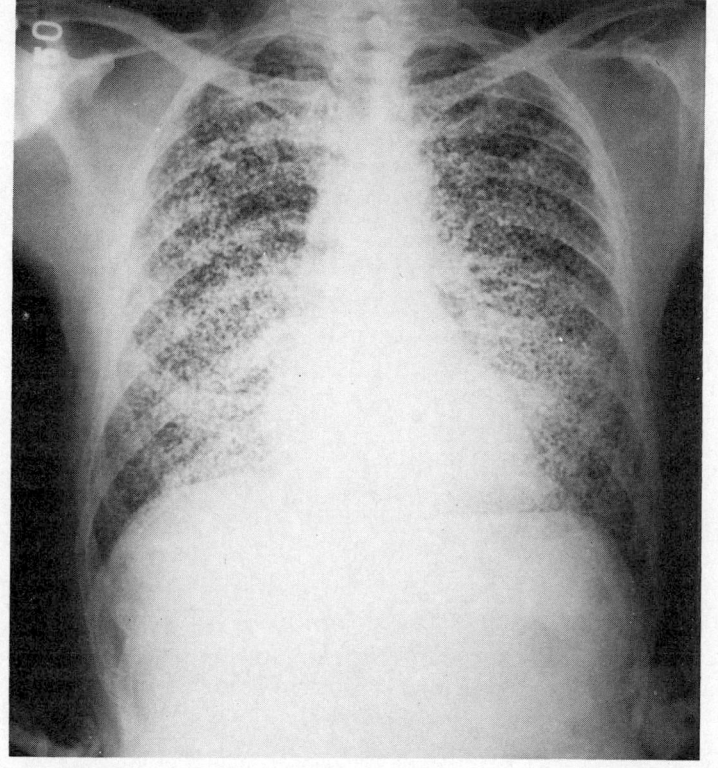

Figure 15–2. Chest radiograph of subject with baritosis. (Courtesy of Dr. E. P. Pendergrass.)

BERYLLIOSIS

Beryllium is a rare element that was discovered by Vanquelin in 1797. About 50 different minerals contain beryllium, but of these beryl is of prime importance. Beryl is beryllium aluminum silicate and yields about 12 per cent of the oxide and around 4 per cent of the metal. Most of the ore comes from South America, and the cost, although fluctuating, is well over 100 dollars per pound. Beryl deposits are found in Argentina, Brazil, India, Zimbabwe, and South Africa. In the United States there are deposits in Colorado, New Mexico, and Utah. Bertrandite is a low-grade ore found in Utah and which is currently being mined.

Beryllium is in demand as a metal because of its lightness and tensile strength. Since it is nonmagnetic and transmits x-rays easily, beryllium is extensively used in x-ray tube manufacture as an alloy in combination with steel, aluminum, and copper. It was also used in the manufacture of fluorescent lighting tubes; however, the recognition of berylliosis led to its replacement in this capacity by other, less toxic substances. Its main uses at the present time are in nuclear physics, since it reduces the speed of

fission reactions, in the space program, in the production of fatigue-resistant alloys and heat-resistant ceramics, and as a "window" in x-ray tubes.

Production of Beryllium

Two processes are used to extract beryllium from the ore. These are known as the sulfate and the fluoride extractions. In the former, crushed beryl is melted in an arc furnace at 1650°C. and poured through a high-velocity water jet to form "frit." Following heat treatment, the frit is pulverized in a ball mill, and then mixed with concentrated sulfuric acid. This mixture, known as slurry, is then sprayed on to a revolving sulfating mill. The beryllium is now in water-soluble form and can be separated or leached from the sludge. Ammonia is added to the leached liquid, which is then transferred to a crystallizer in which ammonium alum is crystallized out. The liquor is next treated with chelating agents to hold iron, nickel, and other metals in solution. Sodium hydroxide is added, and this forms sodium beryllate. The latter is hydrolyzed so that beryllium hydroxide is precipitated, Beryllium hydroxide can be easily converted to metallic beryllium or to beryllium salts.

The fluoride process involves sintering in a rotating furnace a mixture of beryl, sodium, silicofluoride, and soda ash. The sintered residue is pulverized, melted, and separated by leaching. Sodium hydroxide is added to the solution of beryllium fluoride that has been formed by leaching. This leads to the precipitation of beryllium hydroxide which can then be treated as described in the sulfate process.

Several beryllium salts are used industrially. They are (1) beryllium fluoride (BeF_2), (2) beryllium chloride ($BeCl_2$), (3) beryllium nitrate ($Be(NO_3)_23H_2O$), and (4) beryllium sulfate hydrate ($BeSO_44H_2O$).

Aside from health hazards, beryllium is inflammable and its degree of inflammability is related to its particle size.

Effects of Beryllium

Beryllium is highly toxic, and exposure can lead to a condition known as berylliosis. The metal may be absorbed through either the lungs or the skin, especially if the latter is not intact. The metal is not absorbed to any extent by the gastrointestinal canal. Although the metal has local effects, these are relatively unimportant compared with the systemic changes that also may occur. Some beryllium combines with a protein and is deposited in the liver, spleen, and bones. A small residue remains in the lungs. The rate of urinary excretion of the metal depends on how rapidly and in what form the metal has been absorbed. Beryllium persists in bone and liver long after it has been entirely excreted by the lung.

Cutaneous Effects

It is important to bear in mind that aside from the pulmonary effects of beryllium, the skin is also often affected.[30, 31] Erythematous papular or vesicular rashes occur on the exposed parts of the body after an "incubation" period of about two weeks. They are usually itchy. Accidental implantation of the metal in the skin may produce a "beryllium ulcer" or granuloma. Some ulcers are often chronic. Chronic pulmonary berylliosis may undergo an acute exacerbation when the afflicted subject's skin comes into contact with the metal or its salts. Conjunctivitis is also seen and may occur in association with the pulmonary and cutaneous effects. There is some evidence suggesting that the cutaneous manifestations of beryllium exposure are related to hypersensitivity and that sensitization has to occur first. The more soluble the salts are, the more likely is sensitization to occur. The metal itself is thought not to produce sensitization if the skin is intact. Beryllium fluoride is the most potent sensitizing agent, followed by beryllium chloride and sulfate.

Acute Berylliosis

The acute syndrome affects the nasopharynx, trachea, bronchi, and lung parenchyma.[30, 32] The mucous membranes of the nose become hyperemic and swollen. Ulceration may be present and nasal septal perforation occurs. Tracheitis and bronchitis lead to a dry irritative cough. Substernal pain is common. If the exposure to beryllium is severe and intense, a chemical pneumonia develops. The patient complains of the sudden onset of shortness of breath. He rapidly becomes ill, and death is not uncommon. Physical examination reveals cyanosis, tachycardia, and tachypnea. Fever is unusual unless secondary infection occurs. Crackles are often present, especially in the mid and lower regions of the lungs. The chest film may show an appearance that suggests pulmonary edema. In some instances, the radiographic picture resembles that of an acute miliary process, while in others a patchy acinous filling process is present. If the process develops more slowly, weight loss and anorexia are common.

During the acute process, the patient may be severely hypoxic, his lungs are stiff, and he has a low diffusing capacity. The blood count is usually normal.

Treatment consists of giving supplementary oxygen, preferably by mask or nasal catheter. Only if the arterial oxygen cannot be maintained above 50 mm should mechanical ventilation be considered. Antibiotics are useful in preventing secondary infection, and a combination of penicillin and streptomycin is probably the most effective. Steroids should be given in high doses, although there is no conclusive evidence that they are effective. Most of the changes found in acute beryllium pneumonitis resolve completely within one to four weeks, but in around 10 per cent

of affected subjects chronic berylliosis develops. In the subjects who have died of acute berylliosis, the lungs resemble those seen in acute pulmonary edema. The alveoli are filled with fibrin and red cells, while the alveolar walls are infiltrated with lymphocytes and plasma cells. The trachea and bronchi may show acute tracheitis and bronchitis. Epithelialization of the alveolar walls and organization of the exudate may be seen.

Subacute or Reversible Berylliosis

Sprince and colleagues have advanced the concept of a reversible form of berylliosis.[33] Their conclusions were derived from the results of medical and environmental surveys conducted in a beryllium extraction and processing plant. In 1971 they carried out a cross-sectional study and in 1974 they conducted a follow-up study. High concentrations of beryllium were found in the ambient air in 1971, sometimes as much as 50 times the recommended level. They reported that 31 workers showed radiographic evidence of interstitial disease and that a further 20 workers had hypoxemia and an increase in $(A-a)O_2$, with 11 showing both radiographic abnormalities and hypoxemia. The follow-up study indicated that the concentrations of beryllium in the air had declined significantly, and concomitantly that a lesser number of subjects showed hypoxemia and radiographic evidence of berylliosis. The authors attributed the amelioration of the hypoxemia and the improvement in the radiographic changes to the lower levels of beryllium in the air, but the evidence they adduced is less than completely convincing. Thus on the second occasion, although the mean PaO_2 had increased, the $PaCO_2$ had fallen, indicating that the subjects were hyperventilating more, although the hyperventilation may not have accounted entirely for the changes in the PaO_2. In addition, they made no effort to exclude the bias that is introduced by a knowledge of the chronological sequence of the chest x-rays. Similarly, resting $(A-a)O_2$ is a variable test which is not reproducible, and it is unwise to place too much emphasis on it. The improvement in PaO_2 was not accompanied by changes in lung volumes, and the possibility exists that a number of workers had an acute process leading to a physiological shunt and ventilation perfusion inequalities and that as time went by the shunt improved, despite the fact that the mechanical properties of the lung and the diffusing capacity remained unchanged. Similar changes have been observed in sarcoidosis. In the latter condition, an improvement in arterial blood gases due to lessening of the $\dot{V}/\dot{Q}$ mismatching with the passage of time and in the absence of treatment is usual, but is seldom accompanied by an improvement in the DL_{CO} or in the mechanical properties of the lung unless the subject has been treated with steroids. Nevertheless, the authors' recommendation that the concentrations of beryllium in the ambient air should be rigidly controlled has weight.[33]

Chronic Pulmonary Berylliosis

This is a systemic disease which produces granulomata throughout the body but particularly affects the lung. The disease was described by Hardy and Tabershaw in 1946.[34] Most of the early case reports were of workers engaged in the manufacture of fluorescent strip lighting; however, in some instances contact was much less close, and indeed wives of beryllium workers have been reported to incur the disease by inhaling beryllium dust from their husbands' clothes. The ambient air around beryllium refineries may contain enough beryllium to lead to the development of chronic berylliosis.[35, 36] Women seem to be more affected than men. In many instances there is a latent period of 10 to 15 years following exposure before the disease appears.[37] Although beryllium is no longer used in the manufacture of fluorescent tubes, there are still two large beryllium refineries in the United States, and sporadic cases of berylliosis are still occurring and are likely to continue to do so.

Clinical Features. Needless to say, a history of exposure to berylliosis is necessary, but it is important to remember that berylliosis is not limited to workers in beryllium refineries, as previously noted. The onset of symptoms may occur long after exposure has ceased, and it is therefore important to take a complete occupational history.[37] Symptoms of the chronic condition often develop at a time of stress, e.g., during pregnancy or following surgery. At first minimal, dyspnea tends to become progressive and unremitting. A dry unproductive cough is common, and skin lesions may also be present. There may also be a history of previous acute beryllium pneumonitis. In the established cases of chronic berylliosis, there is tachypnea, a small tidal volume, and the typical physical signs found in diffuse fibrosis. Crackles are not common initially. Weight loss and fatigue are also frequent symptoms.

Unfortunately, almost all of the clinical features of berylliosis are also found in sarcoidosis.[38, 39] Thus, lymphadenopathy, especially hilar, occurs in both conditions, although both hilar and generalized lymphadenopathy are less common in berylliosis. Hilar adenopathy in the absence of pulmonary changes is rare in berylliosis but common in sarcoid. Granulomatous skin lesions are likewise common to berylliosis and sarcoidosis. Hepatic and splenic involvement occur in both diseases, and the spleen may be palpable in both. Salivary gland enlargement and cystic bone changes are felt by some to be peculiar to sarcoidosis. Nephrocalcinosis and hypercalcemia occur in both conditions and their presence offers no help in distinguishing them. Meningitis, peripheral neuropathy, and involvement of the myocardium have not been reported in berylliosis, but since they are such rare complications of sarcoidosis, they are usually little help in the differential diagnosis. Ocular involvement such as uveitis is peculiar to sarcoid. Uveoparotid fever is not seen in berylliosis, nor is there a change in tuberculin reactivity. Remission is also much more common in sarcoidosis.

Chronic berylliosis is often accompanied by abnormalities of the serum

proteins and in this, too, resembles sarcoidosis. Gamma globulin production is predominantly affected; however, in chronic berylliosis, unlike sarcoidosis, the IgG fraction is primarily involved, and is found elevated in most subjects.[40] Unfortunately, it is also elevated in beryllium workers who have no clinical evidence of acute or chronic berylliosis. Nor are there blood changes specific to either sarcoidosis or berylliosis.

As the disease progresses the patient becomes increasingly dyspneic. His respiratory rate climbs, his arterial oxygen partial pressure falls, and he becomes cyanosed. Clubbing may develop. As pulmonary scarring and bleb formation develop, the likelihood of pneumothorax increases. A few scattered wheezes may be heard, and there may be some scattered basal crackles. Gradually, cor pulmonale develops and right ventricular hypertrophy becomes evident clinically and electrocardiographically. Progression of the disease is slow, however, and a survival time of 15 to 20 years is relatively frequent.

Radiographic Features. The radiographic features of berylliosis are nonspecific. In some instances, radiographic changes may precede the development of symptoms by several years. Both lungs are commonly affected and there is usually a miliary mottling throughout. Bilateral hilar adenopathy is a rare accompaniment (Fig. 15–3). Larger, blotchy coalescent infiltrates are also seen and closely resemble those seen in sarcoidosis.[41] In long-standing berylliosis, the lungs become small and show widespread reticulonodulation. In some subjects extensive honeycombing occurs.

Pulmonary Function Abnormalities. These too are entirely nonspecific and are identical to those seen in other diffuse fibroses, including sarcoidosis.[42-44] Typically there is an increased respiratory rate and a reduced tidal volume. The vital capacity, total lung capacity, and residual volume are all decreased, but the former is usually most affected. There is arterial desaturation, a slightly low arterial P_{CO_2}, but a relatively normal pH. The lungs are stiff, and the static compliance is reduced. Elastic recoil pressure at total lung capacity is increased. Late in the course of the disease when cor pulmonale supervenes, minor degrees of airways obstruction may develop. The diffusing capacity is reduced, and serial measurement of this function offers the best means of following the course of berylliosis.

Other Diagnostic Tests. A cutaneous test for berylliosis was first discovered by Curtis in 1951.[45] The beryllium patch test is often, but by no means invariably, positive in chronic berylliosis. A positive patch test is probably a consequence of delayed hypersensitivity to beryllium. The test is best done with a piece of gauze or filter paper soaked in 1 or 2 per cent beryllium fluoride, sulfate, or nitrate. Metallic beryllium cannot be used for patch testing. A positive reaction is recognized by the development of an erythematous papule in two to three days. Sneddon biopsied the site of the reaction and showed sarcoid granulomata to be present.[46] There is some evidence that patch testing may lead to an exacerbation of the pulmonary symptoms and to a decrement in pulmonary function.[46, 47] The

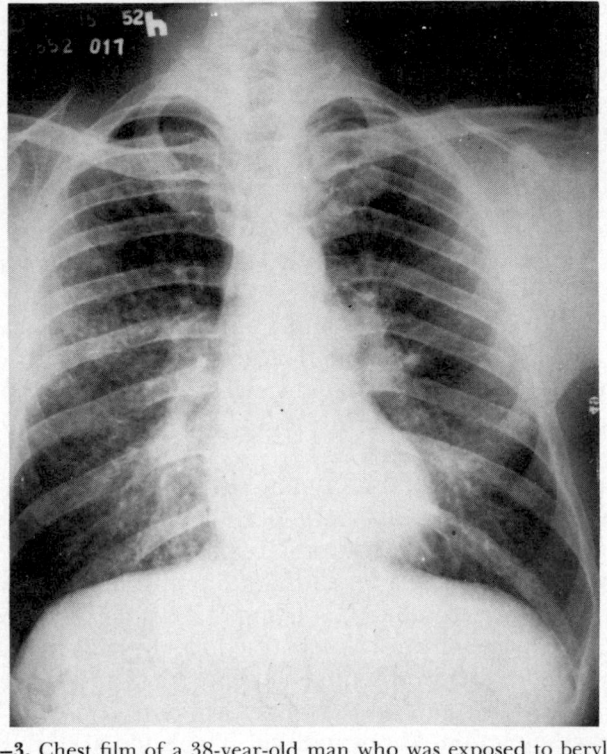

Figure 15–3. Chest film of a 38-year-old man who was exposed to beryllium. There is a fine reticulonodulation present in both lung fields, with bilateral hilar adenopathy. He had no pulmonary function abnormalities other than slight oxygen desaturation on exercise. The question arises as to whether he has berylliosis or has developed sarcoidosis. (Courtesy of Dr. Howard Van Ordstrand.)

test is negative in sarcoidosis, and although often positive in chronic berylliosis, it may be negative. In contrast, the Kveim test, being negative in berylliosis, may be helpful in differentiating the conditions.[48]

Tissue biopsy and spectrographic analysis of the biopsy specimens for beryllium are singularly unhelpful.[49] Most workers who have been exposed to beryllium for any appreciable period will be found to have beryllium present in their bodies. If the exposure is recent, it may be present in the lungs and urine. However, beryllium persists in the bones and liver for many years, and there may be an increased beryllium content in these organs even though the worker has not been exposed for many years. Spectrographic analysis cannot confirm the presence of the disease, since an excess of beryllium in the tissues is found in most subjects who have at some time in their life worked in a beryllium refinery. Moreover, the severity of chronic berylliosis is unrelated to the beryllium content of the tissues. Similarly, a lung biopsy specimen may have a normal beryllium content when there is excellent circumstantial evidence to suggest the presence of berylliosis. The immunological features of the condition are discussed under the section on pathogenesis.

Pathology. Chronic berylliosis is characterized by the presence of noncaseating granulomata,[50] which are indistinguishable from those seen in sarcoidosis. Round cell infiltration is common but necrosis is relatively rare (Fig. 15–4). Asteroid and Schaumann's bodies may be present. Blebs form late in the disease and may rupture, leading to a pneumothorax. Pleural thickening is usual. Right heart hypertrophy occurs late in the course of the disease, as do pulmonary vascular changes. It has also been suggested that beryllium is a carcinogen. In this regard the results of studies have been conflicting, and certainly some of those originating from NIOSH have been both poorly controlled and lacking in credibility.[51, 52] At the present time there is little convincing evidence that beryllium is an occupational carcinogen.

Treatment. Steroids are felt by some to improve the clinical condition of the patient, although there is no evidence that they have ever produced a cure. When starting treatment of a subject with berylliosis, it is probably best to use a large dose for about a week (75 mg prednisone daily). This should be gradually tapered until the subject is taking the smallest possible dose to control the symptoms, viz., around 10 to 20 mg daily. The effects of steroids on the patient's condition are difficult to assess, mainly because of the euphoria they induce. Thus the patient is best followed by serial and objective pulmonary function tests, e.g., diffusing capacity measurements.

Pathogenesis. Despite the most sensitive and extensive diagnostic efforts, a differentiation between berylliosis and sarcoidosis is not always possible. Sarcoidosis can occur in subjects employed in a beryllium refinery, and conversely, berylliosis occurs in those who have never set foot in a refinery. Thus there is little doubt that some patients who were diagnosed as having chronic berylliosis probably had sarcoidosis, and it is equally probable that other cases of so-called sarcoidosis were berylliosis. Studies carried out by Marx and Burrell suggest that differentiation between the two conditions is frequently possible. These workers sensitized guinea pigs by repeated intradermal injection of beryllium sulfate.[53] They were able to produce classical delayed hypersensitivity. They then related the skin hypersensitivity to migration inhibitory factor (MIF) and showed a 74 per cent correlation. The sensitivity to beryllium could be transferred by cells. Lymphocytotoxin was also demonstrated in the cells of the sensitized but not in those of the unsensitized animals. Subjects with chronic pulmonary berylliosis were assessed for sensitivity by *in vitro* inhibition of peripheral blood leukocyte migration and showed MIF production when exposed to beryllium sulfate *in vitro*.

Cellular and immune mechanisms of berylliosis have also been studied by Deodhar and co-workers.[54] They studied blast transformation of lymphocytes, in subjects with berylliosis, in the presence of beryllium sulfate in tissue cultures. Of their 35 patients, approximately three fifths showed blast transformation. The clinical severity of the disease appeared to be related to the degree of blast transformation. In about half of their subjects the serum IgA was reported to be significantly elevated. The

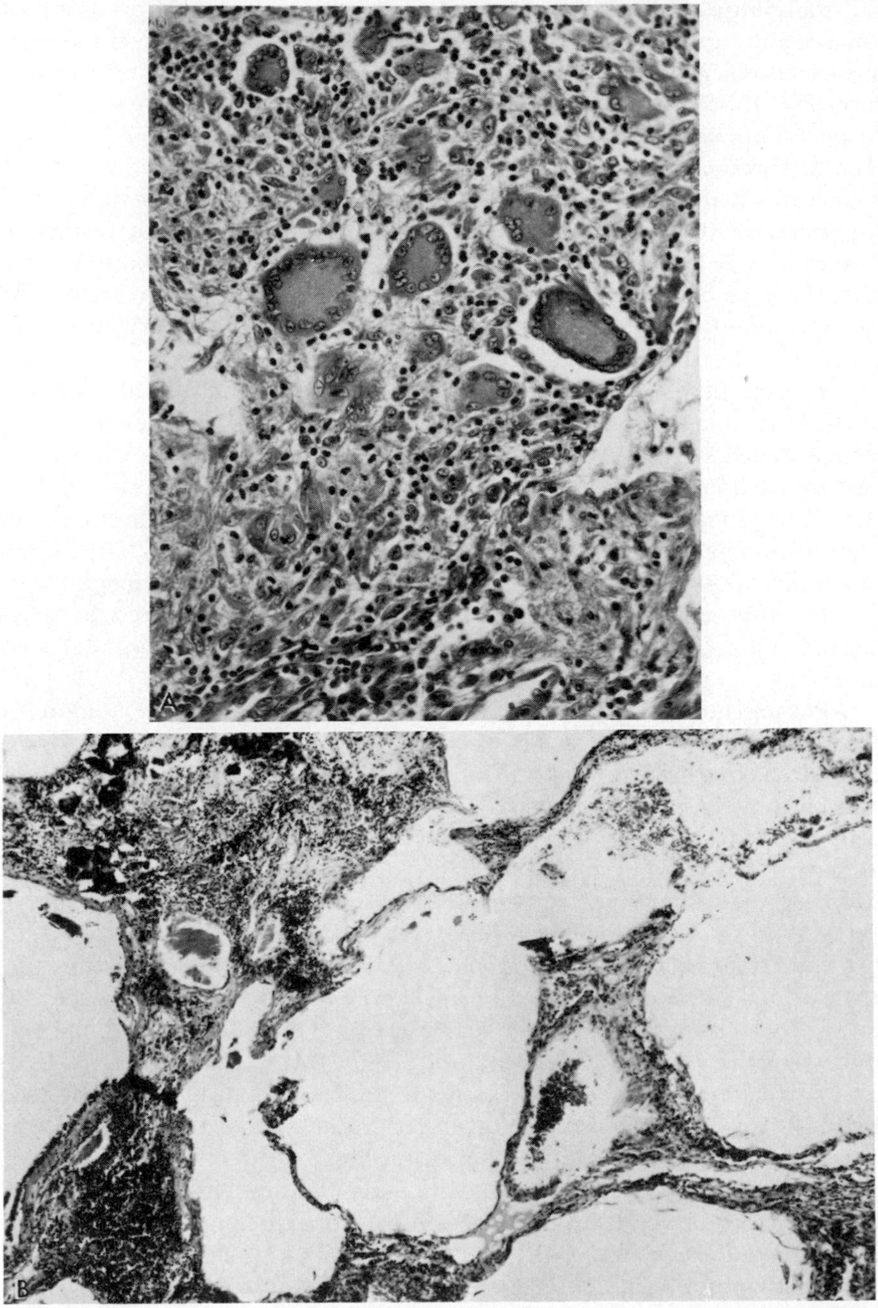

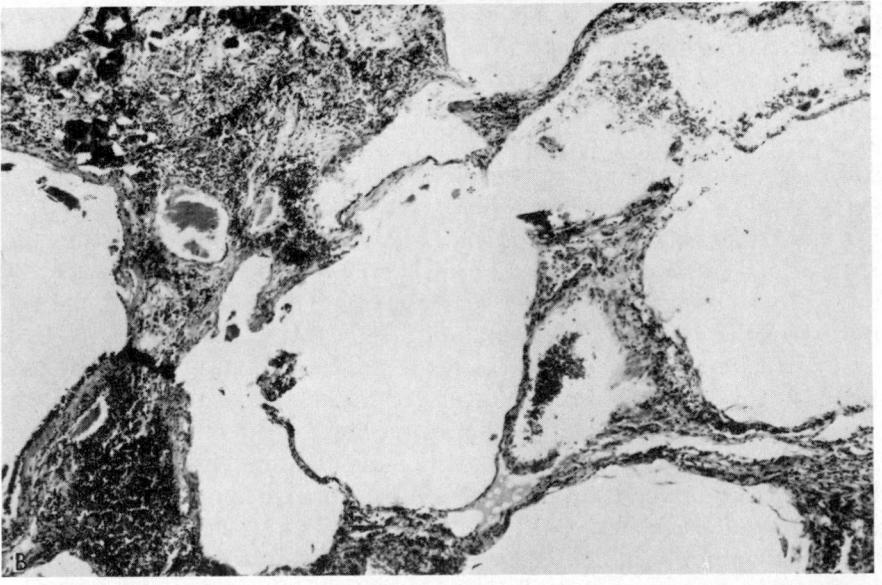

Figure 15–4. *A,* Medium-power photomicrograph of an open lung biopsy specimen. Granulomatous interstitial pneumonitis is present, with obvious giant cells. The beryllium content of the lung was 1.3 micrograms per 100 grams of tissue. (Courtesy of Dr. Howard Van Ordstrand.) *B,* Chronic beryllium disease with interstitial fibrosis, lymphocytic infiltration, an occasional giant cell, and several Schaumann bodies (top left). The patient died of pulmonary fibrosis in 1972, having worked at manufacturing fluorescent lights from 1942 to 1949. This is not the same patient as in *A.*

findings contrast with those of Resnick et al., who found that it was the IgG fraction of the immune globulins that was elevated.[40] Since most of the subjects included in the series of Deodhar and co-workers were taking steroids, and since steroids inhibit blast formation, the authors expressed the opinion that their results provide strong evidence that the etiology of berylliosis is related to immune mechanisms.

Additional support for the hypothesis that the pathogenesis of berylliosis is related to immunological factors came from the studies of Krivanek and Reeves, who demonstrated a delayed type of skin sensitivity in experimental animals.[55] They showed differences in the size of the reactions and in responsiveness according to whether the beryllium was administered to the animal in an ionized or chelated form.

Recently, a beryllium lymphocyte transformation test has been developed, and this has been used with some success in the diagnosis of berylliosis.[56]

The findings in a subject with chronic berylliosis who underwent bronchoalveolar lavage have recently been described.[57] The number and proportion of bronchoalveolar T cells was noted to be increased, and the percentage of activated T cells was five times the control value. Both the peripheral blood and the bronchoalveolar lymphocytes proliferated in response to exposure to $BeSO_4$ and BeF_2, but the bronchoalveolar lymphocytes responded more than did the peripheral lymphocytes. The authors suggest that the findings are consistent with berylliosis being a form of hypersensitivity pneumonitis.

Prevention. All unnecessary beryllium exposure must be avoided. Dust control is of paramount importance so that the generation of fumes and dust is kept to a minimum. Wet processes should be used, and the various work areas of the plant should be self-contained as far as possible. Beryllium-containing preparations should be transported as liquids rather than powders. Masks and protective clothing should be worn when concentrations of beryllium in the ambient air are much above the threshold limit value. Nonetheless, it must be realized that even with optimal care, the concentration of beryllium in the air may be sufficient to induce hypersensitivity in some subjects.

The beryllium content of the ambient air should be measured daily. It is recommended that exposure should not exceed 2 mg/m^3 of air averaged over an 8-hour period. To protect against the acute form of berylliosis it has been recommended that a concentration of 25 $\mu g/m^3$ of beryllium should never be exceeded.[58] Even so, there is good evidence to show that sporadic cases of berylliosis will occur even when exposures remain below the threshold limit value. Such cases are a consequence of the fact that berylliosis is a hypersensitivity disease and that minimal exposures are often sufficient to induce a hypersensitive state.

Pre-employment and periodic medical examinations of all workers in beryllium refineries are desirable. Such examinations should include determination of the vital capacity, the forced expiratory volume, and the

flow rates. If possible, the total lung capacity should be measured. Serial chest radiographs at one-year intervals may conceivably be helpful in controlling the disease.

GRAPHITE AND CARBON PNEUMOCONIOSIS

The term graphite is derived from the Greek word *graphein,* to write. Graphite occurs in three forms: lump, amorphous, and flake. It is also known as plumbago or black lead, and is found almost all over the world; however, it is extracted or mined in Austria, Russia, Sri Lanka (Ceylon), Norway, and Korea. Lump graphite is found in veins that traverse igneous rocks. Quartz, feldspar, mica, and other impurities often occur in the veins. Lump graphite is usually removed by underground mining. Amorphous graphite occurs in underground beds often lying between strata of shale, sandstone, or quartz-containing rocks. It is excavated by blasting, and then is hand-loaded into wagons prior to being brought to the surface. Flake graphite more often occurs near the surface as outcrops from sedimentary rock. This form of graphite is removed by the same methods as are used for open-cast (strip) coal mining.

Small traces of free silica are found in most samples of graphite. After the graphite has been mined, the silica is removed by treating it with hydrofluoric acid and sodium hydroxide. The graphite is then ground, screened, and dried in kilns prior to use. It is used mainly in the manufacture of steel, lubricants, lead pencils, nuclear reactors, and electrodes. Since it conducts electricity, it is often used in generator brushes. Before graphite can be used in any of the above processes, it has to be crushed, ground, and milled to a fine powder. It is also used in electrotyping, a method used in the printing industry for duplicating plates. The exact process is described in detail by Gaensler and colleagues.[59]

It has been known for many years that the inhalation of carbon may induce radiographic changes.[60-62] The changes are usually described as a fine basal reticulation or, in some instances, nodulation. The prevalence of carbon pneumoconiosis varies, but Meiklejohn found it in more than half the workers in two carbon plants.[63] While progressive massive fibrosis was first described in German carbon electrode workers,[64] Watson and colleagues have described similar findings in England.[65] They found both simple and complicated pneumoconiosis occurring in carbon-exposed workers. The complicated form was accompanied by massive fibrosis, cavitation, and right ventricular hypertrophy. Similarly, simple pneumoconiosis in carbon workers was pathologically indistinguishable from coal workers' pneumoconiosis and the condition was characterized by the typical macule and the presence of focal emphysema. Even in subjects with progressive massive fibrosis, the silica content of the lungs was no greater than that found in the lungs of normal subjects. The British and German observations of both simple and complicated pneumoconiosis

occurring in non-silica-exposed carbon electrode workers militate strongly against the silica theory of progressive massive fibrosis. Other case reports have emphasized the low silica content found in both forms of carbon pneumoconiosis.[66, 67]

It is felt by some that graphite modifies the fibrogenic action of silica.[68] Thus, while heavy exposure to pure carbon may induce a slight scattered fibrotic reaction, comparable exposures to a mixture of carbon and silica will induce the formation of nodular foci. In the latter instance, it is thought that the large amounts of carbon dust probably overwhelm the clearing mechanisms so that the silica persists in the lung and thereby has an opportunity to induce a fibrogenic response. Adequately controlled studies of the pulmonary function abnormalities that occur in carbon pneumoconiosis are not available. While individual case reports abound, in many instances it is difficult to demonstrate a cause-and-effect relationship between the physiological impairment and the presence of the pneumoconiosis. In some instances, the respiratory impairment is better explained by the presence of concomitant and coincidental chronic bronchitis and emphysema. Nonetheless, a variety of pulmonary function abnormalities have been reported, including alveolocapillary block (diffuse fibrosis), restrictive disease, and obstructive airways disease. One of Gaensler's subjects had massive fibrosis with severe vascular changes and pulmonary hypertension. Analysis of the lungs in three of his subjects revealed no silica in two instances, and 5 per cent cristobalite in the third. In short, it seems likely that carbon pneumoconiosis produces exactly the same effects on pulmonary function as does coal workers' pneumoconiosis. These are catalogued in detail elsewhere (Chapter 14).

HEMATITE PNEUMOCONIOSIS (SILICOSIDEROSIS) AND OTHER MIXED-DUST FIBROSES

The effects of the inhalation of relatively pure iron are discussed in the section on siderosis; however, many iron miners are exposed not only to iron oxide but also to a fair quantity of free silica. This leads to a condition known as silicosiderosis, or mixed-dust fibrosis. It is seen in the iron miners of Cumbria (England), in the Siegerland miners of Germany, and in the Italian miners of Bergamo. Silicosiderosis seldom occurs without at least 10 years' exposure, and most of the affected subjects have worked in the mines for at least 20 to 30 years.

The first adequate pathological description of the condition was given by Stewart and Faulds.[69] They noted a predominance of diffuse rather than nodular fibrosis, although the latter was present in certain instances. In the diffuse variety of fibrosis, the whole lung is brick red and there is often what appears to be associated focal emphysema. Radiographically, diffuse fibrosis appears as a reticular pattern. The nodular type of silicosiderosis is characterized by the presence of nodules similar to those

seen in silicosis; however, in this instance they are red and are located predominantly in the upper lobes. The remainder of the lung appears brick red.

Massive fibrotic lesions may also be seen. Like progressive massive fibrosis of coal workers, the masses are usually situated in the upper lobes. They encroach on the blood and bronchial supply of the affected region and often undergo cavitation. The presence of massive fibrosis in silicosiderosis appears to be closely related to the silica content of the lung, and tuberculosis is a frequent complication. Microscopically the alveolar walls often show aggregated particles of hematite and silica. Other aggregates occur close to the blood vessels and alveolar septa. Peribronchiolar and periarteriolar fibrosis are frequent findings. Many of the silica and hematite particles are picked up by the macrophages and transported in the lympatics to the regional lymph nodes. Whorled nodules may develop in and along the lymphatic routes. The massive fibrotic areas appear to consist of dense collagenous tissue, heavily impregnated with iron and silica. The adjacent vascular supply is damaged, and endarteritis obliterans is common.

A study of the vasculature of hematite lung showed that the muscular pulmonary arteries between the small fibrotic nodules that characterize the simple form of this condition develop excess longitudinal muscle in the intima, a change that was felt to be a consequence of distortion of these vessels.[70] In some vessels the muscular layer of the intima showed secondary fibrosis. No muscularized pulmonary arteries were observed, and there was an absence of constriction in the terminal region of the pulmonary arterial tree. Vessels adjacent to areas of conglomeration were frequently incorporated into the masses and destroyed by encroachment from fibrous tissue. The occlusive and obliterative changes observed in silicosiderosis were felt to be those of silicosis and not a specific response to hematite. The only peculiar feature of hematite lung is the intense accumulation of iron-containing dust around the pulmonary blood vessels.

There is good evidence that cancer of the lung is found more often in Cumbrian iron miners; however, the cause of the increase is not known.[71] Two theories exist: the first, which seems more probable, relates to the excess radioactivity to which the miners are exposed. In this, it is thought to resemble the radiation-induced lung cancer that occurs in uranium miners. The second theory postulates that the iron ore contains a carcinogenic agent.

The symptoms and signs of silicosiderosis are relatively nonspecific. The miner often complains of shortness of breath, cough, and reddish-brown sputum. The shortness of breath is worse in miners who have massive fibrosis, and many of them develop pulmonary hypertension and cor pulmonale.

Ochre miners also develop silicosiderosis. Ochres are brown-yellow earths that are used in the manufacture of pigments and colors. They are hydrated ferric oxides and are often contaminated with clay, silicates, and

a certain amount of free silica. Ochre miners may have reticular and nodular radiographic changes, but massive fibrosis rarely if ever occurs.[72]

Foundry workers are exposed to both iron and silica, but the proportion of free silica to which they are exposed varies greatly according to their job. While it is undoubtedly true that many foundry workers inhale relatively pure iron and hence are not affected by pulmonary fibrosis or respiratory impairment, in a minority appreciable fibrosis occurs owing to the free silica to which they have been exposed. Mixed-dust fibrosis is commonly seen in foundry welders and burners.[73] The nodule of mixed-dust fibrosis differs macroscopically and microscopically from that seen in classical silicosis. The arrangement of reticulin and collagen fibers is linear or radial rather than concentric, and the outline of the nodule is irregular or stellate.[74] The mixed-dust nodule resembles more closely the coal macule than the typical silicotic nodule. Analysis of the lungs of foundry workers shows that free silica, silicates, and iron are found in varying proportions. The amount of fibrosis is in general related mostly to the free silica content. The radiographic appearances of mixed-dust fibrosis are indistinguishable from those seen in classical silicosis and silicosiderosis. Fettlers and foundry workers show less tendency for their disease to progress radiographically, and there is evidence to indicate that most of the radiological abnormalities are a reflection of iron deposition rather than silica. Iron itself is nonfibrogenic and attenuates the fibrogenicity of the limited amount of silica that is deposited along with the iron.

A recent paper described a cluster of three subjects working in a foundry who developed an uncommon type of pneumonia due to *Acinetobacter pneumoniae*.[75] Two of the men died and were noted to have iron particles in their lungs. The latter finding is hardly surprising, despite the fact that the authors try to attribute the pneumonia to the iron and silica that the workers inhaled in the foundry. There is little evidence to corroborate their hypothesis. While the pneumonia may have been a consequence of the organism being present in dust in the foundry, there is little reason to believe that silica or iron in the concentrations to which the workers were exposed predisposed them to this rare form of pneumonia.

Boiler scalers who clean the water tubes and flues of boilers may also develop pneumoconiosis. This is usually a mixed-dust reaction, since the dust to which they are exposed contains free and combined silica, iron, carbon, and various carbonates. The scale of many marine boilers contains a high proportion of silica, viz., 8 to 10 per cent total silica.[76] Thus, dust exposures in iron and steel workers are usually of the mixed variety and range from pure siderosis at the one extreme to pure silicosis on the other. Most, however, are mixed exposures, and silica, silicates, and numerous other potentially harmful dusts may be inhaled in addition to iron. In some instances, significant exposures to chromium oxide and nickel oxide also occur.[77]

Labrador Lung

An unusual form of mixed-dust pneumoconiosis known as "Labrador lung" has been described in iron miners in West Labrador.[78] The miners were exposed to dust containing iron, silica, and some anthophyllite. Lung biopsies in certain selected subjects have demonstrated large amounts of iron and silica present in the lungs but in addition some subjects have shown a fair number of ferruginous bodies. A granulomatous reaction was seen in a few biopsies of specimens. These latter findings contrast with the typical silicotic reaction observed in most subjects.

The chest symptoms that occurred in the Labrador miners were nonspecific and appeared to be mainly a consequence of bronchitis. Both simple and complicated pneumoconiosis were observed, although the latter was uncommon. Physiological abnormalities were unimpressive even in the complicated form of the disease. Chest films from affected subjects for the most part showed the presence of typical rounded opacities such as are seen in classical silicosis, but a few radiographs also showed the presence of irregular opacities. The latter in general were relatively sparse (0/1 and 1/0), and most could probably be accounted for by cigarette smoking. In a few instances, however, irregular opacities predominated and were relatively profuse. Pleural thickening was also occasionally observed, as was hilar adenopathy.

Labrador lung is thought to be a mixed pneumoconiosis with most of the effects being a consequence of silica. Occasionally the presence of anthophyllite produces atypical features and modifies both the radiographic appearances and the pathological features of the lung.

POLYVINYL CHLORIDE (PVC) PNEUMOCONIOSIS

The manufacture of polyvinyl chloride (PVC) is associated with the generation of a varying number of respirable dust particles. Since the administration of PVC dust to animals is known to lead to bronchiolitis, a minor degree of alveolitis, and the formation of granulomata, the possibility that PVC may be a respiratory hazard in man needs consideration.[79, 80] Over the years there have been isolated case reports of PVC pneumoconiosis, many of them unconvincing, although it is now clear that such a condition exists. A number of epidemiological surveys have also been carried out, but the inferences drawn as a result of such surveys have been suspect, mainly because of a lack of adequate controls and failure to take into account age, cigarette smoking, and other confounding factors.[81, 82]

PVC pneumoconiosis was first described by Szende et al. in 1970.[83] Since then a number of studies have suggested that exposure to PVC dust leads to radiographic changes, respiratory symptoms, and pulmonary impairment. There are few studies of the pathology of PVC pneumoco-

niosis in man. Arnaud et al. describe a subject who had a micronodular infiltrate in his lungs.[84] Histological examination of a drill biopsy specimen revealed infiltration with histiocytes and multinucleated giant cells with some collagenous fibrosis. Macrophage reaction was marked and the macrophages contained many PVC particles (Fig. 15–5).

A well-designed study of a large group of workers exposed to PVC was published in 1980.[85] In this cross-sectional survey involving 818 workers, PVC exposure was found to be associated with a minimal increase

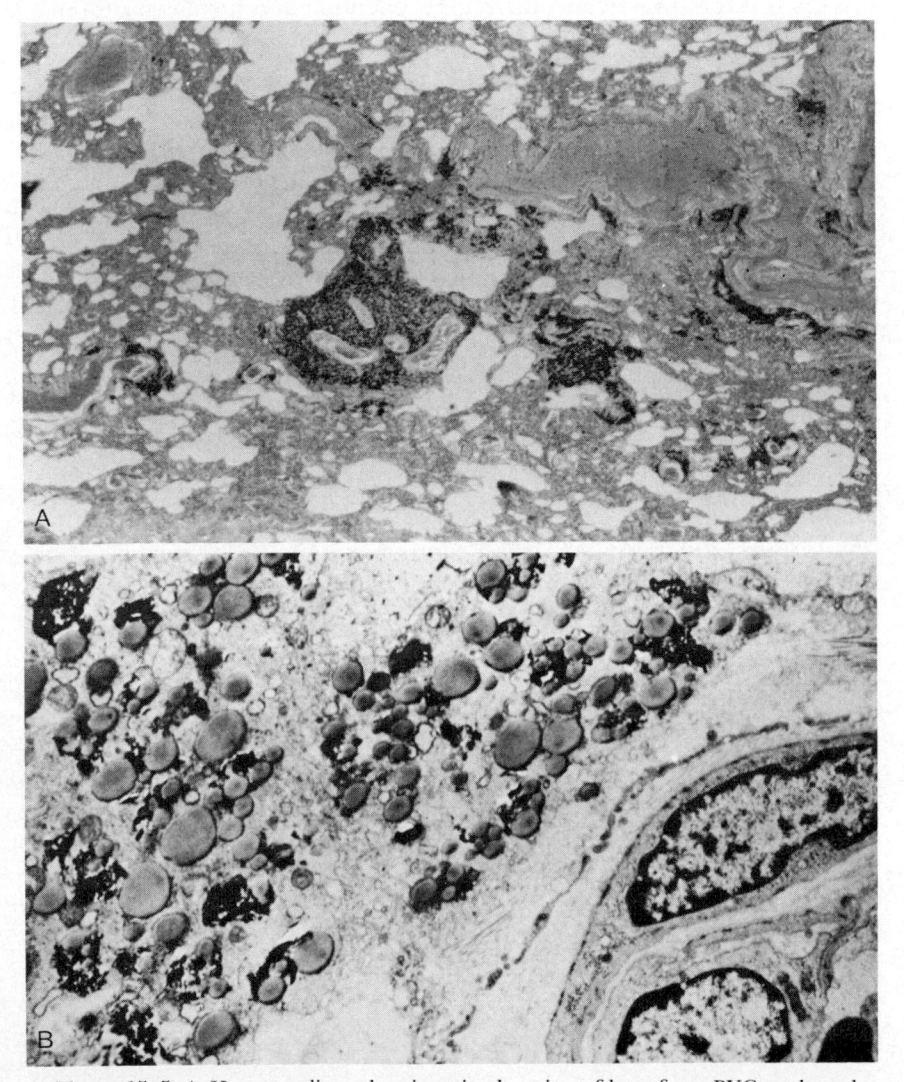

Figure 15–5. *A,* Hematoxylin and eosin stained section of lung from PVC worker whose chest radiograph showed category 1/1 q opacities. A dust macule containing PVC is present. *B,* Electron microscope photomicrograph of PVC particles in lung macrophage. The subject had undergone resection for a tumor. No pneumoconiosis was visible in radiograph.

in respiratory symptoms. After taking into account smoking and age, a slight effect was noted on the FVC and FEV₁. Smoking and PVC dust appeared to have an additive effect. There were minimal radiographic changes, but these were subtle, and higher grades of simple pneumoconiosis were not noted. PVC pneumoconiosis was characterized by the development of scanty small rounded opacities.

Vinyl chloride monomer has effects on other organs, including the liver, where it may produce peripheral fibrosis and lead to the development of angiosarcoma. In addition, a scleroderma-like condition associated with cysts in the fingers and Raynaud's phenomenon has been described.

SHALE PNEUMOCONIOSIS

Shale deposits are a known source of oil and have been commercially mined since the middle of the last century. Production reached a peak in Britain in the early nineteenth century, but with the discovery of oil in the United States and elsewhere the industry declined from lack of demand and an inability to compete. There are extensive deposits of shale in the Colorado Plateau and Alberta, and in recent years consideration has been given to extracting oil from these deposits. Shale consists largely of silicates, including a fair proportion of kaolin and mica, and it might by expected that it would lead to the development of a pneumoconiosis if inhaled in sufficient quantities. Shale mining has not been considered to be a respiratory health hazard, but recent reports have shown that this assumption is incorrect.[86] Shale is mined in both open-cast and underground pits, with the latter being more common. Both scrotal and skin cancer have been reported in workers employed in extraction plants.

It is now evident that simple and complicated shale miners' pneumoconioses occur. The pathology resembles either coal workers' pneumoconiosis (CWP) or kaolin pneumoconiosis, and it is probable that the simple form of the disease has little serious effect on lung function. The complicated form of the disease leads to both restrictive and obstructive impairment such as is seen in CWP. There was a slight but unsubstantiated suggestion that shale pneumoconiosis may predispose to the development of lung cancer.[87] Statistical proof of this is difficult to obtain in view of the rather small number of surviving shale miners. Lung dust studies reveal approximately 70 per cent ash with a high content of kaolin and mica, along with around 5 to 10 per cent free silica.

SIDEROSIS

The condition of siderosis was described by Zenker in the late nineteenth century.[88] The two subjects he reported also had pulmonary tuberculosis, and it can be assumed that the fibrosis which he found in

their lungs was more likely the result of tuberculosis than a response to the dust to which they had been exposed. Iron when inhaled in its pure form does not lead to fibrosis; however, it is often inhaled in conjunction with other fibrogenic dusts such as silica.

Siderosis is seen in its purest form in arc welders, oxyacetylene cutters, and silver finishers. During arc welding and oxyacetylene cutting, iron is melted and boiled by the heat of the arc or torch. The iron is emitted as particles of ferrous oxide which are immediately oxidized to ferric oxide and appear as blue-gray fumes. Prolonged inhalation of these fumes can lead to the development of radiographic changes in the lung that are identical to those seen in silicosis.[89, 90]

Silver finishers use what is known as jeweler's rouge to polish their unfinished wares. The rouge is composed of iron oxide and is often applied with a "buffer" that generates a cloud of small iron and silver particles.[91] The iron miners of Cumbria in Great Britain are subject to silicosiderosis, a condition accompanied by fibrosis and other pathological changes that are not seen in subjects exposed to pure iron. The same is true of the Italian iron miners from Bergamo. Similar changes have been observed in ochre workers.

Welder's siderosis was described by Doig and McLaughlin in 1936.[90] Since its original description, siderosis has generally been assumed to be benign and unassociated with respiratory symptoms. The bases for this assumption have been, first, the published statistics of mortality and morbidity in the United States and Britain,[91, 93] second, the lack of fibrosis in the lungs of welders, [90, 94] and third, the absence of pulmonary function abnormalities in subjects with marked radiographic abnormalities.[94] Over the years there have been several reports of subjects with welders' siderosis who have had both symptoms and impairment of lung function. These reports assumed a cause-and-effect relationship between occupation and respiratory impairment.[95–97] Such inferences have been based on *a posteriori* reasoning. Histological examination of the lungs of these subjects has demonstrated fibrosis and not infrequently emphysema. The presence of these conditions has been attributed to the inhalation of substances other than iron that are often present in the welding fumes. Such substances may be present as impurities in the metal being welded or as constituents of the electrode. Included among them are carbon, manganese, aluminum, silicates, and also some free silica. When emphysema is present, a history of cigarette smoking invariably coexists, unless the welder had been acutely exposed to cadmium fumes. Arc welders, especially those involved in welding aluminum, may also be exposed to ozone in concentrations up to 6 to 9 ppm, and exposures of this magnitude can lead to pulmonary symptoms and bronchitis.

While it must be conceded that other fibrogenic substances may be inhaled during welding, there is usually little reason to assume that any respiratory impairment that may be found in a welder is a consequence of this occupation. Welders are subject to all the diseases that the general

population suffers from, and only by excluding these is it possible to incriminate welding as a cause of chronic respiratory impairment. There is, however, little doubt that welders and oxyacetylene cutters are prone to metal fume fever.[98] In addition, it has been suggested that iron is a carcinogen. An excess risk of lung cancer has been demonstrated in Cumbrian hematite miners, but this is almost certainly a consequence of the inhalation of radon daughters.[99] Other workers have reported an excess of lung cancer among welders.[100] This excess has been noticed in the Registrar General's Decennial Supplement on Occupational Mortality.[101] Although social class and smoking habits may explain part of the excess, they cannot entirely account for the excess death rate from cancer, and another explanation must be sought. Many welders, including those studied by Beaumont and Weiss,[100] have worked either partly or exclusively in shipyards in which the environment frequently contained airborne asbestos. The asbestos exposure is probably responsible for the increased standardized mortality ratio (SMR) for lung cancer. An excess lung cancer rate has likewise been observed in certain foundry workers; this cannot be attributed to iron, but is almost certainly a consequence of exposure to polycyclic aromatic hydrocarbons.[102]

An excellent and relatively complete review of the health effects of welding has been compiled by Challen.[103] It has been suggested that welders are more prone to pneumonia than the general population, but confirmation of this is difficult.[92, 93] It is clear that welders have an increased SMR for pneumonia, but the reason for this is obscure. Moreover, the spouses of welders do not show a comparable increase in morbidity or mortality from this condition. The possibility exists that welders have an increased prevalence of airways obstruction due to smoking and that the presence of preexisting airways obstruction compromises function and increases mortality from pneumonia.

As far as chronic findings are concerned, Challen concludes that while iron is nonfibrogenic, welders are often exposed to other dusts, and a mixed-dust pneumoconiosis can occur.[103] Welders tend to smoke more than the general population, and this explains the high prevalence of bronchitis. Some welders who work in confined spaces are exposed to high concentrations of nitrogen dioxide, and Morley and Silk have suggested that pulmonary edema may occur.[104] Aluminum welders may also be exposed to increased concentrations of ozone, and while these may cause acute nasal and respiratory symptoms, there is little evidence to conclude that such exposures have a permanent effect.

A recent study demonstrated that welders lose more time from work because of respiratory illness than expected (2.3 times higher than expected).[105] Absences due to other diseases were similar to the general population. Smoking welders seem especially prone to absences from respiratory disease, which suggests that they are more susceptible to welding fumes.

Pathology

The first descriptions of the pathological effects of iron were recorded by Harding et al.[90] These workers described the pathological findings in four arc welders and an oxyacetylene cutter who came to autopsy. Some of these subjects had been exposed to silica and in them there was evidence of a mixed-dust fibrosis. The lungs of the cutter showed no fibrosis at all. Harding and his co-workers attributed the fibrosis not to iron oxide but to other constituents of the welding fumes, viz., silica and possibly some of the gases evolved such as the oxides of nitrogen.

Autopsy studies of silver finishers have shown an absence of fibrosis,[91] and chemical inhalation experiments have similarly shown a lack of fibrosis in animals exposed to iron.[106] Morgan and Kerr described seven subjects with welders' siderosis, four of whom had had lung biopsies.[94] The histological appearances of the biopsied lung showed that while some iron lies free in the alveoli and respiratory bronchioles, most is taken up by the macrophages and can be seen in the lymphatic channels (Fig.15–6). Fibrosis was not seen except in subjects with mixed-dust exposures. Analysis of a portion of one subject's lung revealed an iron content of 46

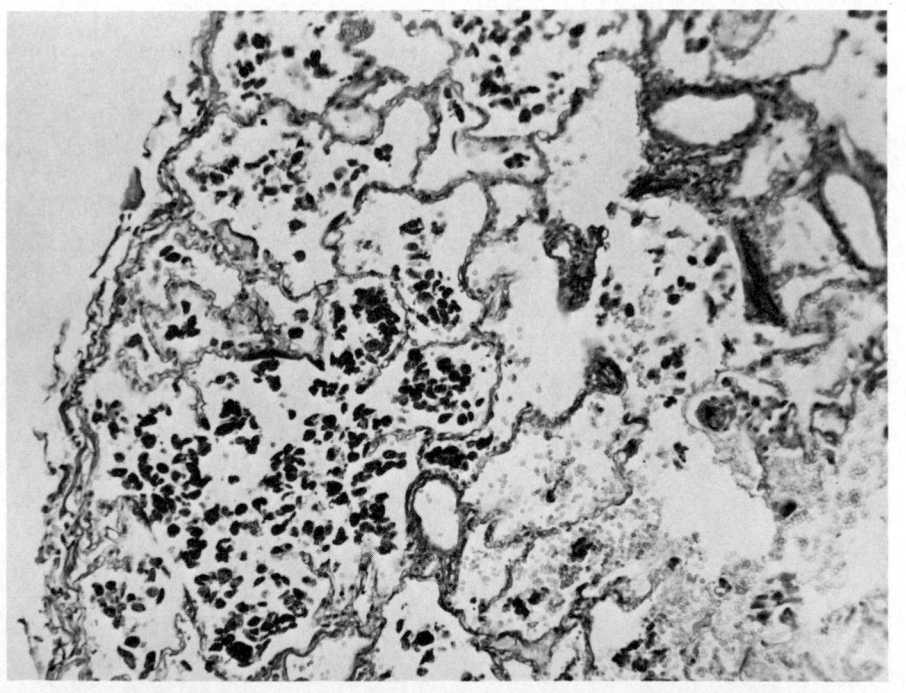

Figure 15–6. Photomicrograph of lung biopsy of subject with welders' siderosis. There is an absence of fibrosis; however, aggregated deposits of iron are much in evidence. Occasional alveolar walls can be seen to be disrupted, but these appearances are due to artifacts introduced in the preparation of the slide. Verhoeff's elastic stain, × 180. (From Morgan, W. K. C., and Kerr, H. D.: Pathologic and physiologic studies of welder's siderosis. Ann. Intern. Med., *58*, 293, 1963. Reproduced by permission.)

mg of iron per gram of dry lung, which is 15 times greater than the normal level. Despite the greatly increased iron content, no fibrosis was present. Another subject whose lung biopsy showed fibrosis was known to have a mixed-dust exposure, and an excess of silica was found in his lung. While the usual radiographic appearances of arc welder's lung are those of simple silicosis, exceptionally a massive shadow appears (Fig. 15–7).[107, 108] It is felt that when conglomeration is seen in a welder, it can be assumed that the worker has been exposed to dusts other than iron, of which by far the most common is silica. Recent postmortem studies of fume contaminants in the lungs of an arc welder, although providing data as to the lungs' constituents, have added little to our understanding of welders' siderosis.[109]

Radiographic Features

Siderosis, whatever its occupational origin, has similar appearances to and cannot be distinguished from simple silicosis. [89, 90, 94] Massive shadows are extremely rare. In some instances the small rounded shadows tend to be "harder" and look more circumscribed than those observed in silicosis.

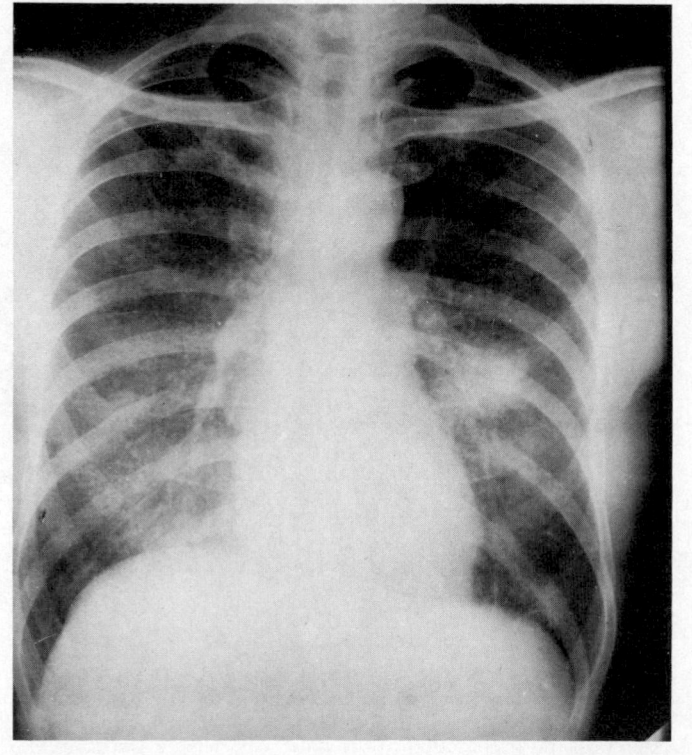

Figure 15–7. Chest radiograph of welder with massive shadow in left lung field. Fine reticulonodulation is present in lower lung fields.

A recent survey of 661 arc welders indicated that about 7 per cent showed radiographic evidence of small rounded opacities of category 0/1 or greater. The authors' observation that there was a correlation between years of exposure and radiological opacities is neither surprising nor original.[110]

Pulmonary Function

There seems little doubt that in its pure form siderosis does not lead to pulmonary impairment. In their study of welders, Morgan and Kerr measured all aspects of pulmonary function with the exception of the diffusing capacity.[94] Despite the fact that the subjects had markedly abnormal chest films and despite the fact that the iron content of their lungs was grossly increased, neither the ventilatory capacity, respiratory mechanics, nor the arterial blood gases were abnormal except in those subjects who had a mixed exposure. At a later date Stanescu and co-workers studied the pulmonary mechanics of a group of 16 working welders with abnormal chest films.[111] They compared the welders to a group of 13 unexposed healthy men and showed that arc welders had a statistically significant reduction in the static and functional compliance of the lungs. However, measurement of elastic recoil at total lung capacity did not separate the welders from the controls. It is difficult to assess the significance of the results of this investigation, and ideally an additional control group of welders without radiographic abnormalities should have been included. Either way, it is difficult to equate slight changes in static compliance with respiratory symptoms, and the effect, if any, that such changes have on the development of respiratory disability can be assumed to be negligible. Additional studies of lung function, including measurement of the diffusing capacity, have been carried out by Teculescu and Albu.[112] Their results agree with those of Morgan and Kerr, and no functional abnormalities to suggest fibrosis were demonstrated.

Well-controlled epidemiological studies of the respiratory status of welders are few. Hunnicutt and colleagues studied the ventilatory capacity of 100 welders and an equal number of controls.[113] Although obstructive airways disease was found in both groups, there was no significant difference between them when the effects of smoking were taken into account. Peters et al. studied 61 welders, using a questionnaire, chest film, and more detailed tests of pulmonary function.[114] During the study, extensive air sampling was also carried out. These workers were unable to show that welders had a significant decrease in pulmonary function when compared to other shipyard workers. Nevertheless, there was some indication that shipyard workers as a whole had a lower ventilatory capacity than did the general population. Like Morgan and Kerr,[94] they concluded that nonsmoking welders do not suffer from a reduction in ventilatory capacity.

Prevention

Although iron in its pure form appears relatively harmless, some welders and oxyacetylene cutters are exposed to various dusts and fumes other than ferric oxide. In some instances these dusts can lead to fibrosis. Such exposures often include the oxides of nitrogen and ozone, and other air pollutants. Siderosis and metal fume fever are seen, and most commonly occur, in welders who work indoors in a poorly ventilated workroom. Both are uncommon when ventilation is adequate and when the men are working outside.

Silver Polishers' Lung

This differs somewhat from the pure siderosis seen in most welders. The jeweler's rouge that is used for polishing formerly consisted of iron oxide mixed with oil; however, with the widespread use of a buffing wheel, also known as a dolly, the powder is now dampened with water only. The dust generated during the polishing process consists of silver and iron oxide particles. As such, the inhaled iron is picked up by the phagocyte, while the silver combines with the protein of the lung, with the result that the elastic tissue is stained black.

Magnetite and Limonite Pneumoconiosis

Radiological abnormalities have also been observed in workers exposed to magnetite dust[115] (Fig. 15–8). Deposits of magnetite (Fe_3O_4) are found in the northeastern United States. Although radiographic abnormalities have been reported in miners and those who process the ore, respiratory impairment has not been observed.[116] The pulverizing of limonite may also be associated with radiographic abnormality.

STANNOSIS

Tin is an important metal because of its pliability and because it readily forms alloys with other metals. After gold and copper, tin was the earliest metal used by man. According to Hoover and Hoover, the smelting of tin took place in the neolithic age, that is to say, about 5000 years ago.[117] Both the Phoenicians and Carthaginians traded with the inhabitants of Cornwall in order to obtain tin.

Deposits of tin are widely distributed throughout the world. Until the industrial revolution most of the world's tin came from Cornwall, Saxony, and Bohemia. Now most comes from Malaysia, Thailand, Bolivia, Nigeria, and to a lesser extent Zaire and Australia. The most important ore is

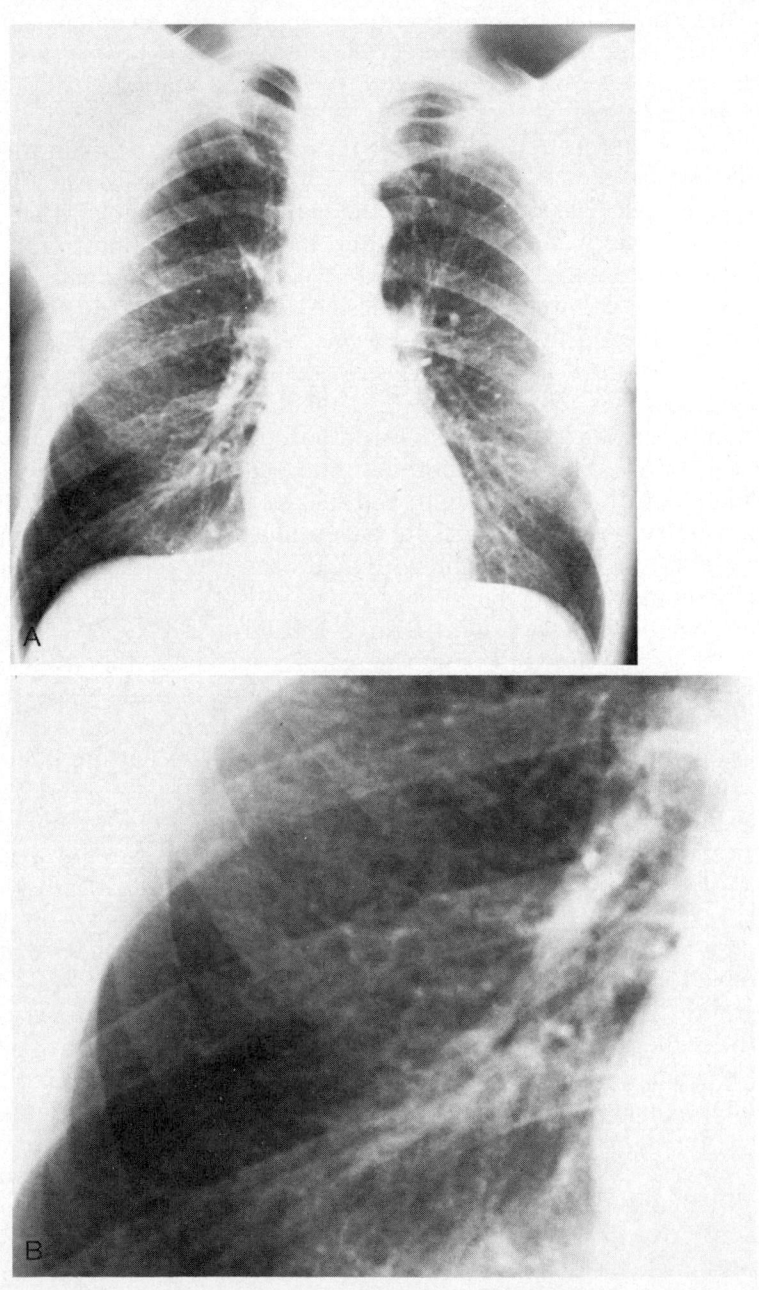

Figure 15–8. *A*, Shows chest radiograph of worker employed pulverizing magnetite. *B*, Magnified view.

known as cassiterite (SnO_2); it occurs in veins that are often intimately related to granite and other rocks with a high silica content. Seventy per cent of the world's total production today comes from secondary alluvial deposits that result from the disintegration of primary deposits. In Bolivia tin is also extracted from various sulfide ores such as stannite (Cu_2FeSnS_2) and tealite ($PbZnSnS_2$).

Lode or underground mining for tin was formerly the main method of extracting the metal. The process involved removing a layer of rock with enough cassiterite in it to make the extraction profitable—that is, at least 1 per cent tin in the rock. However, the concentration of tin in any lode almost never exceeds 10 per cent.[118] A lode mine is usually started as a tunnel that is bored into the hillside and then often is redirected downward. Some Cornish tin mines went down to a depth of 1000 feet, but elsewhere depths of 3000 feet were not uncommon. The cassiterite-containing rock has to be broken up, and this is mainly done by shot-firing. Compressed air drills are used to bore the holes for the insertion of the explosives. The surrounding strata frequently are composed of rock with a high free silica content, and silicosis used to be common in tin miners. Ventilation and wet drilling have reduced the prevalence of the disease greatly. In Cornish tin mines, hookworm infection also used to be relatively common.

The method of extraction of tin is related to the type of deposit. Casserite is usually dredged from the sea or river bed. After it has been dug or excavated, it is washed, and the mud and other superfluous materials are eliminated. In order to achieve this, primary and secondary washing operations are necessary, but even so the concentrate is usually only about 70 per cent pure.

The inhalation of tin leads to a benign pneumoconiosis known as stannosis. Most of the subjects who develop stannosis are involved in bagging of the concentrate or in smelting operations. During the latter process, hot gases containing minute particles of tin are given off from the molten metal as it leaves the furnace, and it is these particles that are responsible for the development of stannosis.

Stannosis is not associated with symptoms, but there is a relatively distinctive radiographic appearance that resembles welders' siderosis (Fig. 15–9). The small opacities present in the radiograph appear extremely radiopaque. The macroscopic appearances of the lung have been described by Robertson and colleagues.[119] Blackish or gray macules ranging between 2 to 5 mm are present in the lungs (Fig. 15–10). These are relatively evenly distributed, and dust pigmentation of the interlobular septa is often evident. Microscopically the dust foci can be seen to be composed of aggregates of dust-laden macrophages that tend to surround the respiratory bronchioles. Occasionally dust-laden cells may be seen in the alveoli, in the interlobular septa, and in the perivascular lymphatics. Focal emphysema occurs but is not as prominent or as frequent as in coal workers'

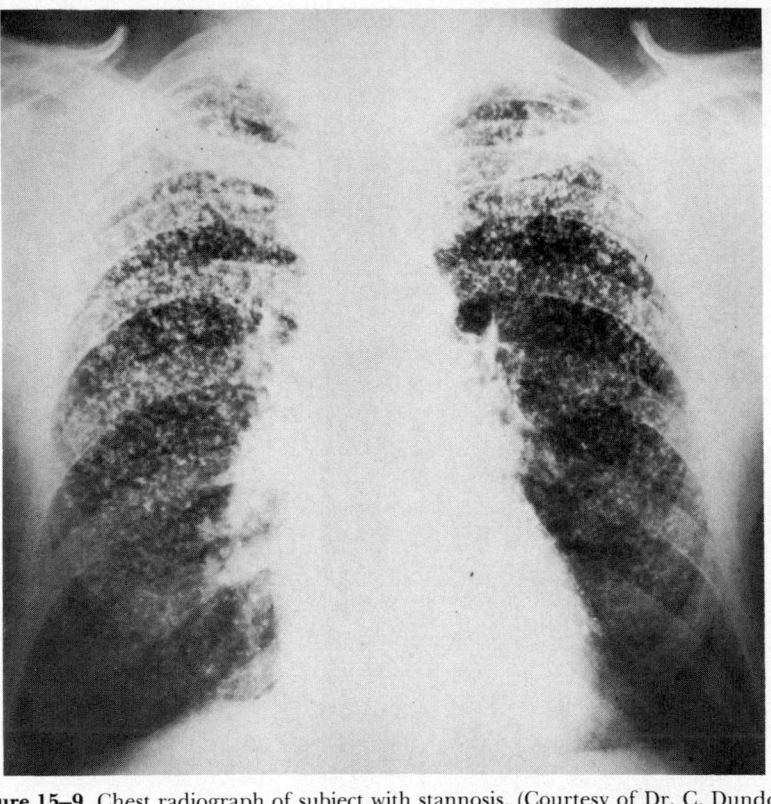

Figure 15–9. Chest radiograph of subject with stannosis. (Courtesy of Dr. C. Dundon.)

pneumoconiosis. Fibrosis is absent, and complicated pneumoconiosis (progressive massive fibrosis) does not occur.

There appears to be no evidence of significant pulmonary impairment in stannosis.[119, 120] Analysis of the lungs of subjects dying with, but not because of, stannosis have yielded between 30 and 40 per cent dry weight of tin oxide. There is a reasonably good relationship between the tin content and the radiographic category of subjects with stannosis. Tin oxide is strongly birefringent. It must, however, be realized that very little tin needs to be retained in the lungs before radiographic abnormalities appear, and indeed 10 times as much coal is required to induce the same radiographic category. This phenomenon is a consequence of the fact that while tin has an atomic number of 50, carbon has an atomic number of 6.

In conclusion, it appears that although the inhalation of tin produces a benign pneumoconiosis generally known as stannosis, the condition is not associated with either morbidity or a decreased life expectancy, and in this context, one wonders whether it is correct to label the condition a pneumoconiosis.

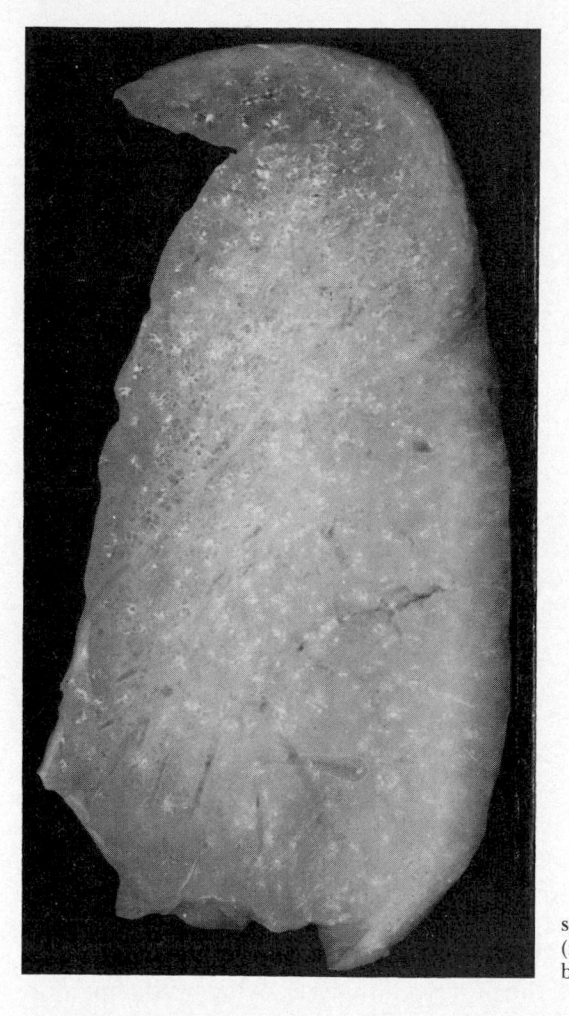

Figure 15–10.   Large lung section showing grayish deposits (macules) of tin. The macules range between 2 and 5 mm in size.

THESAUROSIS

In 1958 Bergmann and colleagues described several subjects with a chronic pulmonary disease that they termed thesaurosis, or storage disease. The condition occurred in young women exposed to hair spray, and was attributed by them to the inhalation of polyvinylpyrrolidone (PVP), the major constituent of hair sprays.[121] The first two patients described were asymptomatic young women with a history of heavy exposure to hair spray. Both had pulmonary infiltrates and hilar adenopathy. A granulomatous reaction was found in an excised scalene lymph node from one subject. In an attempt to develop an animal model for the condition, Bergmann and colleagues injected hair spray residue into the inguinal region of guinea pigs and produced a granulomatous reaction.

In 1962 Bergmann et al. reported 12 new cases, including 3 autopsies.[122] They added a more detailed clinical description, claiming that the condition is characterized radiographically by fluffy, hazy infiltrates and hilar adenopathy. They noted that when the use of hair spray was stopped, the disease resolved. Lymph node biopsy revealed findings that varied from reticuloendothelial hyperplasia to frank sarcoid granulomata. The microscopical lesions in the lung resembled those found in interstitial pneumonitis of the Hamman-Rich type; however, in subjects who had the condition for some time, the appearances were more suggestive of fibrosing alveolitis. Granulomata were sometimes seen in the lung. These workers made much of the presence of PAS-positive granules, which they observed in the lung parenchyma, and at first implied that these were a specific finding in thesaurosis. However, since then, the granules have been described in several other conditions. Following Bergmann and colleagues' description, there have been numerous case reports of one or two subjects with so-called thesaurosis.[123-125]

Unfortunately, good evidence that thesaurosis is an entity in its own right is sadly lacking. The name thesaurosis is presumably derived from the Greek *thēsauros*, which in English becomes "thesaurus" and which is best defined as a treasury or repository. Bergmann et al. regarded the condition as a "storage disease"; however, its relative infrequency in persons exposed to hair spray suggests strongly that it is a manifestation of hypersensitivity, if indeed it exists at all.[121, 122] In many reports of so-called thesaurosis, the clinical picture, x-ray findings, and even pathology were almost pathognomonic of sarcoid. Moreover, most subjects with sarcoidosis, in particular those with hilar adenopathy, improve spontaneously. The subjects described by Bergmann and his colleagues could equally well have had sarcoidosis,[121, 122] and the fact that the condition improved when the subjects stopped using the hair spray is likely to have been entirely fortuitous.

A failure to demonstrate PVP in the lungs of several of the subjects who have been reported as having this condition is further circumstantial evidence against the concept of thesaurosis as a distinct disease entity. The fact that PVP has been shown to be retained in the lymph nodes is to be expected, since as an inert substance, once it is deposited in the lungs it is removed by the macrophage and deposited elsewhere. Animal experiments have likewise failed to give any evidence in favor of the existence of thesaurosis.[126-128] The ultimate acceptance or rejection of thesaurosis must depend on well-controlled epidemiological studies. The study conducted by McLaughlin and Bidstrup best fits this description.[129] These authors were unable to find a single subject with thesaurosis in a survey of 505 hairdressers. A similar study carried out by Sharma and Williams in which the lung volumes and diffusing capacity of 62 exposed cosmetologists were compared to those of 33 controls likewise provided no evidence that thesaurosis exists.[130] Larson also failed to find any evidence of ventilatory impairment in users of hair spray.[131] A large study

purporting to show that hair sprays are harmful was carried out by Palmer.[132] Using matched pairs, he reported that abnormal radiographs and a reduced vital capacity and single breath diffusing capacity were more common in Utah beauticians. The results, however, are not convincing, and the so-called radiological abnormalities were nonspecific and did not conform to a specific pattern. Moreover, beauticians are notoriously heavy cigarette smokers, appreciably more so than the general population in Utah, who for the most part are Mormons and nonsmokers. In a survey of 227 beauticians, Gowdy and Wagstaff claimed to have identified two types of radiographic abnormality, an airways response and a parenchymal response.[125] They noted increased bronchovascular markings in 11 subjects; however, the significance and indeed the very presence of this nonspecific finding are open to doubt. It is difficult to know whether they are describing nonspecific findings in beauticians, an occasional case of sarcoidosis, or what conceivably might be labeled thesaurosis. In a series of circuitous arguments they reviewed the evidence for the existence of thesaurosis, and argued that neither clinically, physiologically, pathologically, nor epidemiologically is there anything that differentiates thesaurosis from sarcoidosis. Then by means of *a posteriori* logic they concluded that thesaurosis could conceivably exist. Suffice it to say that in the absence of epidemiological proof, the existence of thesaurosis cannot be accepted.

It is clear that while brief exposure to hair sprays decreases maximal expiratory flows at low lung volumes, the clinical significance of such a finding is doubtful.[133] A response of this type is likely to be nonspecific and of little import, and shows only that the agent that has been inhaled has reached the small airways. Nevertheless, it is undoubtedly clear that a small minority of subjects react specifically to the fluorochlorohydrocarbons (Freon) that are used as propellants, and a few develop acute symptomatic bronchoconstriction with the characteristic features of asthma.[134]

TUNGSTEN CARBIDE PNEUMOCONIOSIS (HARD METAL DISEASE) AND RELATED SYNDROMES

The currently available evidence suggests that cobalt rather than tungsten is responsible for hard metal disease. The metal is usually recovered as a by-product of gold and silver mining. Cobalt is especially useful in the manufacture of alloys, and is frequently added to other metals such as aluminum, molybdenum, beryllium, chrome, and tungsten carbide. These alloys find their many uses in the production of hard metal and in the manufacture of certain parts of jet engines and large ferromagnets. Cobalt salts have a characteristic blue tint that is frequently useful in coloring glass and for tinting enamel paints and ceramic glazes.

Hard metal is produced by metallurgical blending of tungsten and carbon, with cobalt being used as a binder. Tungsten carbide is a metal

that is extremely hard and resistant to heat, and is therefore used in the cutting of metals and in the manufacture of dental drills and bearings. Tools made of hard metal remain sharp at temperatures up to 3000°F.

Tungsten carbide is prepared by mixing extremely fine particles (0.5 to 15 microns) of tungsten and carbon. The majority of such particles are at the small end of the spectrum and range between 1 and 2 microns. The tungsten carbide is then milled with the addition of between 3 and 25 per cent cobalt. The tiny hard metal crystals are deposited on the cobalt. During this process, nickel, titanium, and other metals may be added according to the desired properties of the hard metal. When the tungsten carbide has been milled, paraffin is added to provide body prior to pressing of the metal into ingots. The carbide is then deparaffinized and sintered into hard metal. In each of these processes, fine dust containing both cobalt and tungsten particles is produced. The manufacturing process is described in detail by Bech, Kipling, and Heather.[135]

Respiratory Disease in Tungsten Carbide Workers[136]

In 1940 Jobs and Ballhausen, following examination of a group of 27 German workers, reported that 8 of them had an abnormal chest radiograph.[137] A fine reticulonodulation was present. In 1959 Moschinski and colleagues examined 696 hard metal workers and found a high prevalence of bronchitis.[138] In a substantial percentage of the sample there also was radiographic evidence of pneumoconiosis. In the United States, Fairhall et al. surveyed almost 2000 tungsten carbide workers.[139] Conjunctivitis, rhinitis, tracheitis, and bronchitis were frequently found. Pruritus and cobalt sensitivity were also common. Some subjects included in this sample had radiographic evidence of a pneumoconiosis. It appears that there are three types of respiratory disease seen in tungsten carbide workers: (1) an interstitial fibrosis which is irreversible, (2) interstital pneumonitis which often disappears when exposure ceases (probably the antecedent disease that leads to the fibrosis), and (3) airways obstruction. The latter may result from simple irritation, but in addition, a distinct form of occupational asthma occurs.

Much experimental work suggests that cobalt is the responsible agent for both the interstitial and the obstructive syndromes. Harding showed powdered cobalt to be toxic when given intratracheally or by inhalation.[140] He also demonstrated that the metal is much more soluble in plasma than in saline. However, tungsten carbide in the absence of cobalt is inert. Delahant produced chronic bronchiolitis and metaplastic changes in the alveoli with pulverized cobalt but not with tungsten carbide, titanium, or tantalum.[141] In animals, the inhalation of metallic cobalt or cobalt salts leads to pulmonary edema. Repeated inhalations over a fairly long period lead to pulmonary fibrosis. Bronchiolitis obliterans, granulomatous pneumonia, and interstitial fibrosis all may occur following the inhalation of metallic cobalt, with the likelihood of fibrosis developing being related to

the dose and duration of inhalation. The administration of cobalt oxide when limited to a few weeks produces a transient pneumonitis.[142] In contrast, continued inhalation of powdered metallic cobalt has been shown to cause permanent changes, stiff lungs, and the laying down of collagen.

Cobalt oxide is less toxic than metallic cobalt. It is felt that the cobalt ions contained in the metal are responsible for most of the deleterious effects.[143] It has been suggested that cobalt impairs oxidative metabolism, and in this regard cysteine has been shown to have an ameliorating influence on lung damage that has been induced by the inhalation of cobalt metal.[144]

Interstitial Fibrosis. A clear and detailed description of hard metal disease is that of Coates and Watson.[145] These workers described 12 subjects with diffuse interstitial lung disease of whom no fewer than 8 died. The early symptoms of hard metal disease are cough and scanty mucoid sputum. Later, the affected subject complains of shortness of breath, which progressively worsens. Tachypnea is frequent, and clubbing of the digits and basal crackles are late features of the condition. Pulmonary function measurements reveal reduced lung volumes, arterial desaturation, and a low diffusing capacity. The pattern is that of classical restrictive disease without significant airways obstruction. Death is usually a consequence of pulmonary hypertension and cor pulmonale.

Chest symptoms usually appear before the film becomes abnormal. Disease is seldom seen without at least 10 years of exposure, but longer and shorter periods of exposure have been reported. Radiographically the disease usually presents as a fine reticulonodular pattern in the mid and lower zones, but the upper zones are occasionally predominantly affected. The heart outline is often blurred, as in asbestosis, and a fine honeycombing may develop, as in other pulmonary fibroses.

Although the lungs in hard metal disease usually appear diffusely involved in the chest film, the fibrosis may be distributed in a patchy fashion. The interstitial tissue is infiltrated with histiocytes and plasma cells, and the alveolar septa are thickened by fibrous tissue. Often present is a granulomatous reaction very similar to that seen in berylliosis.[146] Cystic air spaces lined by cuboidal epithelium are found later on in the disease. The alveoli contain what are assumed to be desquamated mononuclear cells, probably type II alveolar pneumocytes.

Coates and Watson carried out electron microscopy in several of their subjects.[146] They demonstrated excessive deposition of collagen and elastic tissue in the septa and the presence of multifaceted crystals thought to be tungsten carbide. The alveolar lining cells were markedly affected.

A recent study of a series of subjects with hard metal disease describes a nongranulomatous process characterized by intra-alveolar exudate and some interstitial reaction. Mild fibrosis also occurred. Examination of the bronchoalveolar fluid showed bizarre giant forms of the alveolar macrophage. Biopsy specimens revealed a type II pneumocyte response.[146a]

Interstitial Pneumonitis. The recent description of four subjects exposed to cobalt who developed a syndrome similar to extrinsic allergic alveolitis is of considerable clinical significance.[147] All subjects were grinders of hard metal and all developed symptoms and signs compatible with the transient hypersensitivity pneumonitis. After an absence from work, the symptoms improved, the radiographic changes resolved, and the respiratory impairment decreased or resolved. On re-exposure, the symptoms, signs, and radiographic abnormalities reappeared. During the acute pneumonitis, basal crackles could be heard, but these subsequently disappeared. Contact dermatitis occurred in several subjects, and all four subjects described above had positive patch tests for cobalt. The authors pointed out that cobalt, which they believe is responsible for the syndrome, dissolves in the coolant that was used by the workers. As such, it is present in ionic form and probably reacts with the serum protein to form a hapten. The investigators showed quite conclusively that repeated exposure to cobalt coolants may eventually lead to irreversible pulmonary changes and fibrosis. They suggested that all coolants used in the process should not have the ability to dissolve cobalt.

Obstructed Airways Syndrome. This appears most often to be an allergic response and is characterized by wheezing, cough, and shortness of breath while at work. The symptoms often improve when the subject goes home. In this it resembles, to some extent, byssinosis. There is no evidence that this type of disease progresses to interstitial fibrosis. Bech and collagues have shown that in a small proportion of workers who have the obstructive syndrome, the respiratory mechanics deteriorate over the day.[135] Most subjects in whom a severe obstructive response develops leave their job. Coates and colleagues recently described this syndrome in more detail.[148] They described nine subjects with the typical syndrome. Itching was present in three of them. The symptoms cleared up after work and on weekends, and recurred when they returned. The syndrome did not develop until the subjects had had between 6 and 18 months' exposure and sensitization had occurred. They showed that cobalt was toxic to the affected subjects' leukocytes but that tungsten had no effect. Challenge studies with cobalt, but not tungsten, produced an airways response.

The inhalation of cobalt salts or metallic fumes of cobalt, when contained in heavy metal, can lead to conjunctivitis, rhinitis, and tracheitis. These are sometimes associated with a reduction of the ventilatory capacity.

Treatment

No treatment is known for interstitial disease, but steroids may be worth trying, especially when the disease is still reversible, that is to say, when it is a pneumonitis. The obstructive syndrome is best prevented either by limiting exposure to dust or, failing this, by the wearing of a mask.

MISCELLANEOUS PNEUMOCONIOSES

Aside from the well-recognized pneumoconioses, a series of uncommon or esoteric occupationally related conditions have been described.

Bakelite Pneumoconiosis

Two subjects with generalized pulmonary infiltration and exposure to bakelite have been described.[149] Although Pimentel states that the clinical features of bakelite pneumoconiosis resemble those with extrinsic allergic alveolitis, his description is less than convincing. According to him the basic lesion is an epithelial granuloma resembling sarcoid. While Pimentel claims to have developed an animal model, his evidence for the existence of the condition is tenuous, and the existence of bakelite pneumoconiosis must remain sub judice.

Rare Earth Pneumoconioses

A number of elements are referred to as rare earth. These include yttrium, cerium, neodymium, and lanthanum. While intratracheal injection of yttrium and cerium in animals can induce granulomata,[150] there is little evidence that the occupational inhalation of rare earths ever leads to pulmonary fibrosis, although a few reports of radiographic abnormalities induced by cerium have been described. Cerium oxide is used in the optical industry in the manufacture of glassware and in metallurgy. A report from the LaRochelle district of France described two subjects with a miliary process in their lungs which was attributed to the inhalation of cerium oxide.[151]

The subjects had been exposed for 11 and 15 years, respectively. No description of any pulmonary function abnormalities was provided, and there is no evidence that impairment occurs in this condition.

Laundry Workers' Pneumoconiosis

A few subjects who were employed as laundry workers in the pottery district of Britain were reported as developing pneumoconiosis.[152] It is thought that these cases arose from the practice of laundry workers shaking out pottery workers' overalls prior to putting them in the wash. The likelihood is that the radiographic changes were a consequence of exposure to kaolin. No evidence of pulmonary impairment was found in the affected subjects.

Titanium Pneumoconiosis

Titanium oxide is used as a white pigment in the manufacture of paint. The carbide of titanium finds extensive use with tungsten carbide in the manufacture of tools. There is some evidence that titanium oxide may produce radiographic abnormalities similar to those resulting from inhalation of iron and tin; however, there appears to be no associated pulmonary impairment.[152] A recent paper described a number of symp-

toms and changes in pulmonary function in a group of 207 titanium workers.[154] Despite description of a multitude of abnormalities, the authors concluded that the clinically significant disease was infrequent.

Zirconium Pneumoconiosis

Zirconium is a silvery rare metal, and its oxide is used in the manufacture of fused and sintered ceramics and heat-resistant textiles and in the production of furnace bricks. Animal studies for the most part have suggested that zirconium is inert, but it has been shown that the lungs of rats exposed to extremely high concentrations may develop radiographic abnormalities.[155] A slight inflammatory response has been observed.

In man there is doubt as to whether occupational exposure to zirconium ever leads to pulmonary disease. Reed described a granulomatous pulmonary response in a chemical engineer who was involved in the production of the metal[156]; however, this may well have been fortuitous. McCallum has described small round opacities in eight men working in a zirconium processing plant, but here again the men had a mixed exposure.[157] The weight of the evidence is against the association of zirconium with the development of pneumoconiosis in man, except under rare circumstances.

Esoteric Pneumoconioses

A number of truly esoteric conditions have recently been described. These include "dung lung," a pneumonitis caused by the inhalation of liquid manure.[158] The inhalation of hydrogen sulfide from liquid manure caused pulmonary edema. Whether this can be regarded as a true pneumoconiosis is a moot point, but it is included under this term.

A case report of "fly ash lung" described a shipyard worker who developed a nonspecific pulmonary interstitial process.[159] The authors suggested that fly ash, an aluminum silicate, may be the responsible agent.

The development of pulmonary fibrosis in a drug-snorting fire-eater seems to be unique.[160] The affected subject was a drummer in a punk rock band who frequently inhaled powdered drugs, including cocaine, barbiturates, and amphetamines, through a rolled up pound-note. His pièce de résistance involved filling his mouth with paraffin (kerosene), which he would then expel through his lips, at the same time igniting the jet. He was observed to have radiographic changes, and after complete investigation a lung biopsy revealed diffuse pulmonary fibrosis due to the deposition of kerosene and other substances he had been inhaling.

References

1. Shaver, C. G., and Riddell, A. R., Lung changes associated with the manufacture of alumina abrasive. J. Ind. Hyg., 29, 145, 1947.
2. Jephcott, C. M., Fume exposure in the manufacture of aluminum explosives. J. Occup. Med., 5, 701, 1948.

3. Goralewski, G., Die Aluminiumlunge (Arbeithsmedizin No. 26). Leipzig, 1950.
4. Barth, G., Frik, W., and Scheidemandel, H., Die Aluminiumlunge, Verlaufbeobachtungen and neuerkrankungen in der nachkriegszeit. Deutsch Med. Woschr., *81*, 1115, 1956.
5. Hunter, D., Milton, R., Perry, K. M. A., and Thompson, D. R., Effect of aluminium and alumina on the lung in grinders of duralumin aeroplane propellers. Br. J. Ind. Med., *1*, 159, 1944.
6. Mitchell, J., Pulmonary fibrosis in an aluminium worker. Br. J. Ind. Med., *16*, 123, 1959.
7. Mitchell, J., Manning, G. B., Molyneux, M., and Lane, R. E., Pulmonary fibrosis in workers exposed to finely powdered aluminium. Br. J. Ind. Med., *18*, 10, 1961.
8. Jordan, J. W., Pulmonary fibrosis in a worker using an aluminium powder. Br. J. Ind. Med., *18*, 21, 1961.
9. Koelsch, F., Beitr, Klin. Tuber., *97*, 688, 1942. Cited by Hunter, D., et al., Br. J. Ind. Med., *1*, 159, 1944.
10. McLaughlin, A. I. G., Kazantis, G., King, E., et al., Pulmonary fibrosis and encephalopathy associated with the inhalation of aluminium dust. Br. J. Ind. Med., *19*, 253, 1962.
11. Corrin, B., Aluminium pneumoconiosis. I. In vitro comparison of stamped aluminium powders containing different lubricating agents and a granular aluminium powder. Br. J. Ind. Med., *20*, 264, 1963.
12. Corrin, B., Aluminium pneumoconiosis. II. Effect on the rat lung of intratracheal injections of stamped aluminium powders containing different lubricating agents and of a granular aluminium powder. Br. J. Ind. Med., *20*, 268, 1963.
13. Gross, P., Harley, R. A., and De Treville, R. T. P., Pulmonary reaction to metallic aluminum powders. Arch. Environ. Health, *26*, 227, 1973.
14. Vallyathan, V., Bergeron, W. N., Robichaux, P. A., and Craighead, J. E., Pulmonary fibrosis in an aluminum arc welder. Chest, *81*, 372, 1982.
15. Musk, A. W., Greville, H. W., and Tribe, A. E., Pulmonary disease from occupational exposure to an artificial aluminium silicate used for cat litter. Br. J. Ind. Med., *37*, 367, 1980.
16. Bech, A. O., Kipling, M. D., and Zundel, W. E., Emery pneumoconiosis. Trans. Assoc. Ind. Med. Off., *15*, 110, 1965.
17. Kaltreider, N. L., Elder, M. J., and Cralley, L. U., Health survey of aluminum workers with special reference to fluoride exposure. J. Occup. Med., *14*, 1531, 1972.
18. Smith, N. M., The respiratory conditions of potroom workers: Australian experience. *In* Hughes, J. P. (ed.), Health Protection in Primary Aluminium Production. London, New Zealand House, 1977.
19. Dinman, B. D., The respiratory condition of potroom workers. *In* Hughes, J. P. (ed.), Health Protection in Primary Aluminium Production. London, New Zealand House, 1977, p. 95.
20. Field, G. S., Airway function and lung elastic behaviour in potline workers. Second Health Protection Seminar, International Primary Aluminium Institute. Montreal, Sept. 1981.
21. Discher, D., and Breitenstein, B. D., Prevalence of chronic pulmonary disease in aluminum potroom workers. J. Occup. Med., *18*, 379, 1976.
22. Cooper, D. A., Pendergrass, E. P., Vorwald, A. K., et al., Pneumoconiosis in workers in an antimony industry. Am. J. Roent., *103*, 495, 1968.
23. McCallum, R. I., Work on an occupational service in environmental control. Ann. Occup. Hyg., *6*, 60, 1963.
24. Klucik, I., Juck, A., and Gruberova, J., Respiratory and pulmonary lesions caused by antimony trioxide dust. Pracov. Lek., *14*, 363, 1962.
25. McLaughlin, A. I. G., Iron and Other Radio-opaque Dusts. *In* King, E. J., and Fletcher, C. M., eds., Industrial Pulmonary Diseases. Boston, Little Brown & Company, 1960, pp. 146–167.
26. Arrigoni, A., La pneumoconiosis da bario. Clin. Med. Ital., *64*, 299, 1933.
27. Arrigoni, A., La pneumoconiosis da bario, Med. Lav., *24*, 461, 1933.
28. Pendergrass, E., and Greening, R., Baritosis, report of case. A.M.A. Arch. Ind. Hyg., *7*, 44, 1953.
29. Doig, A. T., Baritosis. *In* XV International Congress on Occupational Health. Vienna, Wiener Medizenische Akademie, Verlag, 1966.

30. Van Ordstrand, H. S., Hughes, R., De Nardi, J. M., and Carmody, M. G., Beryllium poisoning. J.A.M.A., *129*, 1084, 1945.
31. Van Ordstrand, H. S., Acute beryllium poisoning. *In* Vorwald, A. J., ed., Sixth Saranac Symposium (1947). Pneumoconiosis; Beryllium, Bauxite Fumes, Compensation. New York, P. B. Hoeber, 1950, p. 65.
32. De Nardi, J. M., Van Ordstrand, H. S., and Carmody, M. G., Acute dermatitis and pneumonitis in beryllium workers: review of 406 cases in 8-year period with follow-up on recoveries. Ohio State Med. J., *45*, 467, 1949.
33. Sprince, N. L., Kanarek, D. J., Weber, A. L., et al., Reversible beryllium disease in beryllium workers. Am. Rev. Respir. Dis., *117*, 1011, 1978.
34. Hardy, H. L., and Tabershaw, I. R., Delayed chemical pneumonitis occurring in workers exposed to beryllium compounds. J. Ind. Hyg. Toxicol., *28*, 197, 1946.
35. Chesner, C., Chronic pulmonary granulomatosis in residents of a community near a beryllium plant: three autopsied cases. Ann. Int. Med., *32*, 1028, 1950.
36. Eisenbud, M., Wanta, R. C., Dunstan, C., et al., Non-occupational berylliosis. J. Ind. Hyg. Toxicol., *31*, 282, 1949.
37. Hardy, H. L., and Stoeckle, J. D., Beryllium disease. J. Chron. Dis., *9*, 152, 1959.
38. Hardy, H. L., Beryllium disease: a continuing diagnostic problem, Am. J. Med. Sci., *142*, 150, 1961.
39. Van Ordstrand, H. S., Diagnosis of beryllium disease. A.M.A. Arch. Ind. Health, *19*, 157, 1959.
40. Resnick, H., Roche, M., and Morgan, W. K. C., Immunoglobulin concentrations in berylliosis. Am. Rev. Respir. Dis., *101*, 504, 1970.
41. Weber, A. L., Stoeckle, J. D., and Hardy, H. L., Roentgenologic patterns in long-standing beryllium disease: report of 8 cases. Am. J. Roentgen, *93*, 879, 1965.
42. Wright, G. W., Chronic pulmonary granulomatosis of beryllium workers. Trans. Am. Clin. Climatol. Assoc., *61*, 161, 1949.
43. Gaensler, E. A., Verstraeten, J. M., Weil, W. B., et al., Respiratory pathophysiology in chronic beryllium disease. A.M.A. Arch. Ind. Health, *19*, 132, 1959.
44. Ferris, B. G., Affeldt, J. E., Kriete, H. A., and Whittenberger, J. L., Pulmonary function in patients with pulmonary disease treated with ACTH. A.M.A. Arch. Ind. Hyg., *3*, 603, 1951.
45. Curtis, G. H., Cutaneous hypersensitivity due to beryllium. A.M.A. Arch. Derm. Syph., *64*, 470, 1951.
46. Sneddon, I. B., Berylliosis, a case report. Br. Med. J., *1*, 1448, 1955.
47. Waksman, B. H., The diagnosis of beryllium disease with special reference to the patch test. A.M.A. Arch. Ind. Health, *19*, 154, 1959.
48. James, D. G., Dermatological aspects of sarcoidosis. Quart. J. Med., *28*, 109, 1959.
49. Dutram, F. R., Cholak, J., and Hubbard, D. M., The value of beryllium determination in the diagnosis of berylliosis. Am. J. Clin. Pathol., *19*, 229, 1949.
50. Williams, W. J., A histological study of the lungs in 52 cases of chronic beryllium disease. Br. J. Ind. Med., *15*, 84, 1958.
51. Shapley, D., Occupational lung cancer. Goverment challenged in beryllium proceedings. Science, *198*, 898, 1977.
52. Round the World column, The beryllium dispute. Lancet, *1*, 202, 1978.
53. Marx, J. J., Jr., and Burrell, R., Delayed hypersensitivity to beryllium compounds. J. Immunol., *111*, 590, 1973.
54. Deodar, S. D., Barna, B., and Van Ordstrand, H. S., A study of the immunologic aspects of chronic berylliosis. Chest, *63*, 309, 1973.
55. Krivanek, N., and Reeves, A. L., The effect of chemical forms of beryllium on the production of the immunologic response. Am. Ind. Hyg. J., *33*, 45, 1972.
56. Williams, W. R., and Williams, W. J., Development of beryllium lymphocyte transformation tests in chronic beryllium disease. Int. Arch. Allergy Appl. Immunol., *67*, 175, 1982.
57. Epstein, P. E., Dauber, J. H., Rossman, M. D., and Daniele, R. P., Bronchoalveolar lavage in a patient with chronic berylliosis. Ann. Intern. Med., *97*, 213, 1982.
58. Schute, H. F., Beryllium, the criteria document. J. Occup. Med., *15*, 663, 1973.
59. Gaensler, E. A., Cadigan, J. B., Sasahara, A. A., et al.: Graphite pneumoconiosis of electrotypers. Am. J. Med., *41*, 864, 1966.
60. Lochtkemper, I., and Teleky, L., Studien uber Staublunge; die in einzelnen besonderen Betrieben und bei besonderen Arbeiten. Arch. Gewerbepath., *3*, 600, 1932.

61. Gartner, K., and Brauss, F. W., Russ pneumoconiosis. Med. Welt, 20, 252, 1951.
62. Gloyne, S. R., Marshall, G., and Hoyle, C., Pneumoconiosis due to graphite dust. Thorax, 4, 31, 1949.
63. Meiklejohn, A., In Reports of the 12th International Congress on Occupational Health, Vol. 3. Helsinki, Helsingfors Publications, 1957, p. 335.
64. Koelsch, F., Zum problem der Graphitpneumoconioses. Zentralbl. Arbeitsmed., 8, 1, 1958.
65. Watson, A. K., Black, J., Doig, A. T., and Nagelschmidt, G., Pneumoconiosis in carbon electrode markers. Br. J. Ind. Med., 16, 274, 1959.
66. Miller, A. A., and Ramsden, F., Carbon pneumoconiosis. Br. J. Ind. Med., 18, 103, 1961.
67. Lister, W. B., Carbon pneumoconiosis in a synthetic graphite worker. Br. J. Ind. Med., 18, 114, 1961.
68. Parmeggiani, L., Graphite pneumoconiosis. Br. J. Ind. Med., 7, 42, 1950.
69. Stewart, M. J., and Faulds, J. S., The pulmonary fibrosis of haematite miners. J. Pathol. Bact., 39, 233, 1934.
70. Heath, D., Mooi, W., and South, P., The pulmonary vasculature in haematite lung. Br. J. Dis. Chest., 72, 88, 1978.
71. Boyd, J. T., Doll, R., Faulds, J. S., and Leiper, J., Cancer of the lung in iron-ore (haematite) miners. Br. J. Ind. Med., 27, 97, 1970.
72. Roche, A. D., Picard, D., and Vernhes, A., Silicosis of ochre workers (a clinical and anatomo-pathologic study). Am. Rev. Tuberc., 77, 839, 1958.
73. McLaughlin, A. I. G., and Harding, H. E., Pneumoconiosis and other causes of death in iron and steel foundry workers. Arch. Ind. Health, 14, 350, 1956.
74. McLaughlin, A. I. G., Pneumoconiosis in foundry workers. Br. J. Tuberc., 51, 297, 1957.
75. Cordes, L. G., Brink, E. W., Checko, P. J., et al., A cluster of Acinetobacter pneumonia in foundry workers. Ann. Intern. Med., 95, 688, 1981.
76. Harding, H. E., and Massie, A. P., Pneumoconiosis in boiler scalers. Br. J. Ind. Med., 8, 256, 1951.
77. Jones, J. G., and Warner, C. G., Chronic exposure to iron oxide, chromium oxide and nickel oxide fumes of metal dressers in a steelworks. Br. J. Ind. Med., 129, 169, 1972.
78. Edstrom, H. W., and Rice, D. M. D., "Labrador lung": an unusual mixed dust pneumoconiosis. Can. Med. Assoc. J., 126, 27, 1982.
79. Agarwal, D. K., Kow, J. L., Srivastava, S. P., and Setth, P. K., Some biochemical and histopathological changes induced by polyvinyl chloride dust in rat lung. Environ. Res., 16, 333, 1978.
80. Richards, R. J., Desai, R., Hext, P. M., and Rose, F. A., Biological reactivity of PVC dust. Nature, 256, 664, 1975.
81. Miller, A., Tiersten, A. S., Chuang, M., et al., Changes in pulmonary function in workers exposed to vinyl chloride and polyvinyl chloride. Ann N.Y. Acad. Sci., 246, 42, 1975.
82. Lilis, R., Anderson, H., Miller, A., and Selikoff, I. J., Pulmonary changes among vinyl chloride polymerization workers. Chest, 69, 299, 1976.
83. Szende, B., Lapis, K., Nemes, A., and Pinter, A., Pneumoconiosis caused by the inhalation of polyvinyl chloride dust. Med. Lav., 61, 433, 1970.
84. Arnaud, A., Pommier De Santi, P., Garbe, L., et al., Polyvinyl chloride pneumoconiosis. Thorax, 33, 19, 1978.
85. Soutar, C. A., Copland, L. H., Thornley, P. E., et al., Epidemiological study of respiratory disease in workers exposed to polyvinyl chloride dust. Thorax, 35, 644, 1980.
86. Costello, J., Morbidity and mortality study of shale oil workers in the United States. Environ. Health Perspect., 30, 205, 1979.
87. Seaton, A., Lamb, D., Rhind Brown, W., Pneumoconiosis of shale miners. Thorax, 36, 412, 1981.
88. Zenker, F. A., Ueber Staublinhalationskrankheiten der Lung. Deutsch. Arch. Klin. Med., 2, 116, 1866.
89. Doig, A. T., and McLaughlin, A. G., X-ray appearances of the lungs of arc-welders. Lancet 1, 771, 1936.

90. Harding, H. E., McLaughlin, A. I. G., and Doig, A. T., Clinical, radiographic, and pathological studies of the lungs of electric arc and oxyacetylene welders. Lancet 2, 394, 1958.

91. Barrie, H. F., and Harding, H. E., Argyro-siderosis of the lungs in silver finishers. Br. J. Ind. Med., 4, 225, 1947.

92. Colleen, M. F., A study of pneumonia in shipyard workers with special reference to welders. J. Ind. Hyg., 29, 113, 1947.

93. Doig, A. T., and Duguid, L. N., The health of welders. Ministry of Labour and National Service, London, H. M. Stationery Office, 1951, p. 68.

94. Morgan, W. K. C., and Kerr, H. D., Pathologic and physiologic studies of welder's siderosis. Ann. Intern. Med., 58, 293, 1963.

95. Charr, R., (a) Respiratory disorders among welders. J.A.M.A., 152, 1520, 1953; (b) Respiratory disorders among welders. Am. Rev. Tuberc., 71, 877, 1955; (c) Pulmonary changes in welders. Ann. Intern. Med., 44, 806, 1956.

96. Mann, B. T., and Lecutier, E. R., Arc welders' lung. Br. Med. J., 2, 921, 1957.

97. Friede, E., and Rachow, D. O., Symptomatic pulmonary disease in arc welders. Ann. Intern. Med., 54, 121, 1961.

98. Schiotz, E. H., Welding regarded from the medical point of view. Acta Med. Scand., 121, 537, 1945.

99. Boyd, J. T., Doll, R., Faulds, J. S., and Leiper, J., Carcinoma of the lung in haematite miners. Br. J. Ind. Med., 27, 106, 1970.

100. Beaumont, J. J., and Weiss, N. S., Lung cancer among welders. J. Occup. Med., 23, 839, 1981.

101. Registrar General's Decennial Supplement, Occupational mortality 1970–72. London, H. M. Stationery Office, 1978.

102. Gibson, F. S., Martin, R. H., and Lockington, J. N., Lung cancer mortality in a steel foundry. J. Occup. Med., 19, 807, 1977.

103. Challen, P. J., R., Some news in welding and welders. J. Soc. Occup. Med., 24, 38, 1974.

104. Morley, R., and Silk, S. J., The industrial hazard from nitrous fumes. Ann. Occup. Hyg., 13, 101, 1970.

105. Fawer, R. F., Gardner, A. W., and Oakes, D., Absences attributed to respiratory diseases in welders. Br. J. Ind. Med., 39, 149, 1982.

106. Harding, H. E., Grout, J. L. A., and Lloyd Davies, T. H., The experimental production of x-ray shadows in the lungs by inhalation of industrial dusts. I. Iron oxide. Br. J. Ind. Med., 4, 223, 1947.

107. Morgan, W. K. C., Arc welders' lung complicated by conglomeration. Am. Rev. Respir. Dis., 85, 570, 1962.

108. Brun, J., Cassan, G., Kofman, J., and Gilly, J., La sidéro-sclérose des soudeurs à l'arc à forme de fibrose interstitielle diffuse et à forme conglomerative pseudo-tumorale. Poumon. Coeur, 28, 3, 1972.

109. Kalliomaki, P. L., Sutinen, S., Kelha, V., et al., Amount and distribution of fume contaminants in the lungs of an arc-welder post mortem. Br. J. Ind. Med., 36, 224, 1979.

110. Attfield, M. D., and Ross, D. S., Radiological abnormalities in electric arc welders. Br. J. Ind. Med., 35, 117, 1978.

111. Stanescu, D. C., Pilat, L., Gavrilescu, N., et al., Aspects of pulmonary mechanics in arc welders' siderosis. Br. J. Ind. Med., 24, 143, 1967.

112. Teculescu, D., and Albu, A., Pulmonary function in workers inhaling iron oxide dust. Int. Arch. Arbeitmed., 31, 163, 1973.

113. Hunnicut, T. N., Cracovaner, D. J., and Myles, J. T., Spirometric measurements in welders. Arch. Environ. Health, 8, 661, 1964.

114. Peters, J. M., Murphy, R. L. H., Ferris, B. G., et al., Pulmonary function in shipyard welders. Arch. Environ. Health, 26, 28, 1973.

115. Morgan, W. K. C., Magnetite pneumoconiosis. J. Occup. Med., 20, 762, 1978.

116. Kleinfeld, M., Messite, J., and Shapiro, J., A clinical, roentgenological and physiological study of magnetite workers. Arch. Environ. Health, 16, 392, 1968.

117. Hoover, H. C., and Hoover, H. L., Footnotes, In Agricola, G., De re metallica, 1556. London, 1912, pp., 283, 354.

118. Robertson, A. J., The romance of tin, Lancet, 1, 1229, 1289, 1964.

119. Robertson, A. J., Rivers, D., Nagelschmidt, G., and Duncumb, P., Stannosis. Lancet, *1*, 1089, 1961.
120. Pendergrass, E. P., and Pryde, A. W., Benign pneumoconiosis due to tin oxide: a case report with experimental investigation of the radiographic density of the tin oxide dust. J. Ind. Hyg., *30*, 119, 1948.
121. Bergmann, M., Flance, I. J., and Blumenthal, H. T., Thesaurosis following inhalation of hair spray: a clinical and experimental study. N. Engl. J. Med., *258*, 471, 1958.
122. Bergmann, M., Flance, I. J., Cruz, P. T., et al., Thesaurosis due to inhalation of hair spray: report of 12 new cases, including three autopsies. N. Engl. J. Med., *266*, 750, 1962.
123. Edelston, B. G., Thesaurosis following inhalation of hair spray. Lancet, *2*, 112, 1959.
124. Nevins, M. A., Stechel, G. H., Fishman, S. I., et al., Pulmonary granulomatoses: two cases associated with inhalation of cosmetic aerosols. J.A.M.A., *193*, 266, 1965.
125. Gowdy, J. M., and Wagstaff, M. J., Pulmonary infiltration due to aerosol thesaurosis. Arch. Environ. Health, *25*, 101, 1972.
126. Draize, H. J., Nelson, A. A., Newburger, S. H., et al., Inhalation toxicity studies of six types of aerosol hair sprays. Proc. Sci. Sec. Toilet Goods Assoc., *31*, 28, 1959.
127. Calandra, J., and Kay, J. A., The effects of aerosol hair sprays on experimental animals. Proc. Sci. Sec. Toilet Goods Assoc., *30*, 41, 1958.
128. Giovacchini, R. P., Becker, G. H., Brunner, M. J., and Dunlap, F. E., Pulmonary disease and hair spray polymers. J.A.M.A., *193*, 298, 1965.
129. McLaughlin, A. I. G., and Bidstrup, P. L., The effects of hair lacquer sprays on the lungs. Fed. Cosmet. Toxicol., *1*, 171, 1963.
130. Sharma, O. P., and Williams, M. H., Thesaurosis. Arch. Environ. Health, *13*, 616, 1966.
131. Larson, R. K., A study of mid-expiratory flow rate in users of hair spray. Am. Rev. Respir. Dis., *91*, 786, 1964.
132. Palmer, A., A morbidity survey of respiratory symptoms and functions among Utah beauticians. Ph.D. dissertation, University of Utah, 1974.
133. Zuskin, E., and Bouhuys, A., Acute airway responses to hair spray preparations. N. Engl. J. Med., *290*, 660, 1974.
134. Frank, R., Are aerosol sprays hazardous? Am. Rev. Respir. Dis., *112*, 485, 1975.
135. Bech, A. O., Kipling, M. D., and Heather, J. C., Hard metal disease. Br. J. Ind. Med., *19*, 239, 1962.
136. Payne, L. R., Hazards of cobalt. J. Soc. Occup. Med., *27*, 20, 1977.
137. Jobs, H., and Ballhausen, C., Powder metallurgy as a source of dust from the medical and technical standpoint. Vertrauensartz u. Krankenkasse, *8*, 142, 1940.
138. Moschinski, G., Jurisch, A., and Reinl, W., Die Lungenveranderungen bei Sinterhart-metallarbeitern. Arch. Gewerbepath, *16*, 697, 1959.
139. Fairhall, L. T., Castberg, H. T., Carrosso, N. J., and Brinton, H. P., Industrial hygiene aspects of the cemented tungsten carbide industry. Occup. Med., *4*, 371, 1947.
140. Harding, H. E., Notes on the toxicology of cobalt metal. Br. J. Ind. Med., *7*, 76, 1950.
141. Delahant, A. B., An experimental study of the affects of rare metals on animal lungs. A.M.A. Arch. Ind. Health, *12*, 116, 1955.
142. Schepers, G. W., The biological action of cobalt metal. A.M.A. Arch. Ind. Health, *12*, 127, 1955.
143. Kerfoot, E. J., Fredrick, W. G., and Domeier, E., Cobalt metal inhalation studies on miniature swine. Am. Ind. Hyg. Assoc. J., *36*, 17, 1975.
144. Griffith, W. H., Paviek, P. L., and Mulford, P. J., The relation of the sulfur amino acids to the toxicity of cobalt and nickel in the rat. J. Nutr., *23*, 603, 1942.
145. Coates, E. O., Jr., and Watson, J. H. L., Diffuse interstitial lung disease in tungsten carbide workers. Ann. Intern. Med., *75*, 709, 1971.
146. Coates, E. O., Jr., and Watson, J. H. L., Pathology of the lung in tungsten carbide workers using light and electron microscopy. J. Occup. Med., *15*, 280, 1973.
146a. Davison, A. G., Haslum, P. L., Corrin, B., et al., Interstitial lung disease and asthma in hard metal workers: bronchoalveolar lavage, ultrastructural and analytical findings and results of bronchial provocation tests. Thorax, *38*, 119, 1983.
147. Sjögren, I., Hillerdal, G., Andersson, A., and Zetterström, O., Hard metal lung disease: the importance of cobalt in coolants. Thorax, *35*, 653, 1980.
148. Coates, E. O., Jr., Sawyer, H. J., Rebuck, J. W., et al., Hypersensitivity bronchitis in tungsten carbide workers. Chest, *64*, 390, 1973.

149. Pimentel, J. C., A granulomatous lung disease produced by bakelite. Am. Rev. Respir. Dis., *108*, 1303, 1973.
150. Haley, T. J., Pharmacology and toxicology of rare earth elements. J. Pharm. Sci., *54*, 663, 1965.
151. Nappée, J., Bobrie, J., and Lambard, D., Pneumoconiose au cérium. Arch. Med. Profess. Med. Travail Sec. Soc., *33*, 13, 1972.
152. Evans, D. J., and Posner, E., Pneumoconiosis in laundry workers. Environ. Res., *4*, 121, 1971.
153. Schmitz-Moorman, P., Horlein, H., and Hanefield, F., Lungenveranderungen bei Titandioxyd staub Exposition. Beitr. Silikose Forschung, *80*, 1, 1964.
154. Daum, S., Anderson, H. A., Lilis, R., et al., Pulmonary changes among titanium workers. (Abstract) Proc. Roy. Soc. Med., *70*, 31, 1977.
155. Harding, H. E., and Lloyd Davies, T. H., The experimental production of industrial dust. Part II. Zirconium. Br. J. Ind. Med., *9*, 70, 1952.
156. Reed, C. E., A study of the effects on the lungs of industrial exposure to zirconium dusts. A.M.A. Arch. Ind. Health, *13*, 578, 1956.
157. McCallum, R. I., The work of an environmental health service in environmental control. Ann. Occup. Hyg., *6*, 55, 1953.
158. Osbern, L. N., and Crapo, R. O., Dung Lung. A report of toxic exposure to liquid manure. Ann. Intern. Med., *95*, 312, 1981.
159. Golden, E. B., Warnock, M. L., Mulett, L. D., and Churg, A., Fly ash lung: a new pneumoconiosis? Am. Rev. Respir. Dis., *125*, 108, 1982.
160. Buchanan, D. R., Lamb, D., and Seaton, A., Punk rocker's lung. Pulmonary fibrosis in a drug-snorting fire-eater. Br. Med. J., *2*, 1661, 1981.

16

OCCUPATIONAL ASTHMA

Anthony Seaton

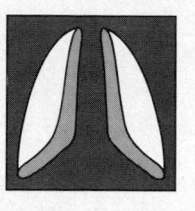

Early in the eighteenth century Ramazzini[1] drew attention to the irritant effect of organic dusts among grain workers in causing both shortness of breath and an urticarial reaction. Since that time it has been recognized that exposure to dusts such as grain, hay, flour, cotton, and sawdust may result in the development of respiratory symptoms in a proportion of workers. An important step in the differentiation of the various mechanisms involved was taken when Coca[2] and Coca and Cooke[3] demonstrated the genetic basis of the development of clinical allergy. These workers described the clinical syndrome of atopy, manifesting itself as asthma and rhinitis and subject to hereditary influence. They demonstrated that first-degree relatives of patients with multiple immediate skin reactions frequently had asthma or hay fever themselves. Such subjects, who may number up to 10 per cent of the population, have been shown to be particularly liable to hypersensitivity to inhaled antigens in the course of occupational exposure.[4] Nevertheless, a proportion of subjects in whom asthma develops in relation to their occupation are not atopic. Such subjects generally develop symptoms only after a more prolonged exposure to the antigen than do those with atopy, or, as in the case of isocyanate asthma, only when the antigen is a very potent sensitizer.

Occupational asthma has in the last few years attracted considerable medical attention. A large number of previously unknown causes have been described, particularly in the plastics, chemicals, and electronic industries, while the development of new, relatively simple investigative techniques has aided the diagnosis of asthma. Occupational asthma is a disease for which industrial disablement benefits can be claimed in West Germany and Finland, and in the former country over 200 claims are lodged each year. It also became a prescribed disease in the United Kingdom in 1982.

MECHANISMS

The different types of immunological responses that may contribute to disease have been classified by Gell and Coombs[5] into Types I to IV

(see Chap. 8). This classification, though useful, is now viewed as an oversimplification, and its uncritical use has led to much confusion when considering the mechanisms of asthma. It would be misleading to claim that these mechanisms are fully understood, but some facts have become clear and these are summarized in the following discussion.

Asthma may present clinically as an attack of wheeze and cough lasting one hour or so and following very shortly after exposure to even minute doses of sensitizer. Alternatively, the attack may start several hours after the exposure and persist for a day or more. Sometimes the two presentations are combined, and the attack, once triggered, recurs for days or weeks.[6, 7] Analogies have been drawn between the immediate and delayed bronchial reactions thus observed and the immediate and delayed responses occurring after antigen challenge testing. For example, inhalation of a small dose of toluene diisocyanate (TDI) may provoke an immediate fall in FEV_1, followed two to three hours later by another, often more severe and always more prolonged fall (Fig. 16–1). It seems

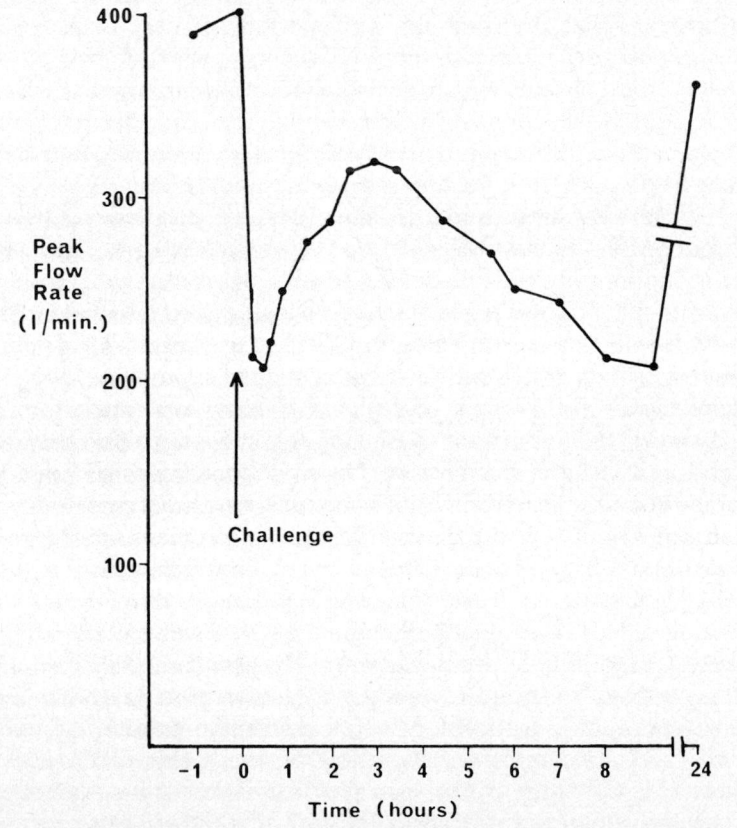

Figure 16–1. Record of peak flow rate of patient before and after a 5-minute challenge with toluene diisocyanate, by using marine varnish. The immediate fall was followed by a later and more prolonged fall.

likely that the mechanisms operating during challenge testing and those that occur as a result of environmental exposure are the same. The further observation that the initial response can often be blocked by cromoglycate and the later one by corticosteroids, but not *vice versa,* gave rise to the concept that the initial fall was a Type I reaction, that is, one mediated by IgE, and the delayed response was a Type III reaction, mediated by IgG. Moreover, this fitted conveniently with what was known of the bronchial responses to *Aspergillus fumigatus,* a ubiquitous mold[8] to the spores of which many asthmatics become sensitized and which causes a curious syndrome known as bronchopulmonary aspergillosis in a proportion of them.[9] Thus the immediate and delayed responses have been labeled Types I and III, respectively.

The classical Types I and III reactions are now quite well understood. Type I hypersensitivity is mediated by a specific immunoglobulin called IgE.[10] Little of this is found in the blood of normal subjects, but larger amounts are present in atopic individuals. It is a glycoprotein with a molecular weight of 190,000 and has remarkable affinity for mast cells and basophils, up to 40,000 molecules being able to bind onto one such cell. It appears that the membrane properties of these cells are altered when pairs of IgE molecules bound by molecules of antigen become attached to the cell surface, resulting in the liberation of mediators of anaphylaxis, slow-reacting substance, histamine, eosinophil chemotactic factor, and other substances. Type III sensitivity, by contrast, is mediated by IgG antibody, which in combination with a moderate excess of antigen forms toxic soluble immune complexes that fix the first component of complement and activate the third, releasing the anaphylatoxin C3a, which in turn causes histamine release. In addition, the reaction attracts poly-morphonuclear leukocytes and mononuclear cells, some of which are destroyed by ingested complexes and liberate their lysosomes, with con-sequent tissue damage. Unfortunately for the concept of Type III asthma, except in bronchopulmonary aspergillosis it is uncommon to find precip-itating antibodies in patients with the delayed response, even though delayed skin reactions may occur. In addition, the histological pattern observed in sputum and bronchial mucosa of all asthmatics, whatever their clinical type, seems to be the same, the predominant cell being the eosinophil. It thus appears that the early and delayed responses are mediated at least through the same final pathway, which seems likely to be the mast cell. However, not all asthmatics have raised levels of IgE, so even if IgE could initiate the delayed response (and there is evidence that it can[11]), it cannot entirely explain the immunology of asthma. A partial explanation has come from the description of a short-term sensitizing IgG molecule,[12] which can cause liberation of mediators from leukocytes. However, the full story is yet to be told and a classification of asthma based on immunological concepts is best avoided at present.

On the assumption that the clinical and pathological features of asthma can be ascribed to liberation of mediators from sensitized mast

cells and basophils, it is possible to proceed a little further in describing the mechanisms of the disease. Once the cell membrane has been activated, as by IgE-antigen complex, there is an intake of calcium into the cell, through channels that may be under the control of cyclic AMP. Secretion of histamine follows immediately, while slow-reacting substance is synthesized. This latter process also appears to be controlled by cyclic AMP. The pathological features, mucosal edema, eosinophilic infiltration, and smooth muscle contraction and hypertrophy, can be explained on the basis of the actions of the mediators released from mast cells.

Two distinct classes of substance seem to provoke occupational asthma. First, materials containing large-molecule proteins, which are often also found in nonoccupational environments. These include grains, dust derived from animals, and wood. The asthma they provoke does not differ from allergic asthma in other environments, in general being more likely to affect the atopic individual and exciting an IgE response. In contrast, an increasing number of substances of low molecular weight have been shown to provoke asthma. IgE responses are less readily detected and atopic and nonatopic subjects often react similarly. These substances, which include isocyanates and components of epoxy resin systems, are often primary irritants. They may act by forming haptens with serum proteins, but the mechanisms are not understood. Moreover, a number of them cause alveolar as well as bronchial reactions, presumably related to their ability to penetrate deep into the lung on account of their small size.

Bronchial hyper-reactivity is present in the majority of subjects with occupational asthma; nevertheless, it needs to be remembered that about one third of those with asthma due to TDI and colophony show no evidence of excessive reactivity of the airways. This would suggest that direct irritation is not the only mechanism involved in these types of asthma.[12a] It has been suggested that increased bronchial reactivity may be genetically determined and as such predisposes to the development of occupational asthma; however, most of the evidence indicates that the hypersensitivity is the result of the asthma rather than the cause.

CLINICAL FEATURES

Occupational asthma is best defined as reversible airways obstruction causally related to agents in the working environment. Characteristically it only affects a proportion of those exposed to the causative agent and develops often after a symptom-free period that varies in length between the individuals, ranging from months to years. Re-exposure to the offending agent almost invariably precipitates an asthmatic response.

The principal complaint is of wheezing related to work. This most typically occurs in an atopic individual who has worked for four or five years in the industry, but nonatopic individuals may become sensitized

and manifest asthma some years later than their atopic co-workers. Asthma may present earlier, even a few weeks after the start of work, especially in industries involving exposure to potent sensitizers such as isocyanates or colophony.

The symptoms vary considerably in their pattern. While most patients notice improvement during weekends and vacations, in some the symptoms start within minutes of exposure, while in others there is a delay of several hours, with symptoms occasionally being most troublesome the following night. It is usual for the symptoms to become gradually worse as the week continues, and sometimes recovery takes several days or even weeks after exposure ceases.[6, 7] Moreover, in some industries exposure is intermittent rather than regular, so that attacks only occur occasionally. Nevertheless, the attacks are almost always episodic, and it is an unusual patient who does not recognize the relationship between his work and his symptoms (though of course patients with other diseases may mistakenly attribute them to their working conditions). Whenever a patient blames the dust or conditions at his workplace for a respiratory illness, he should be taken seriously and appropriate investigations should be undertaken. Only in this way have most of the causes of occupational asthma been described and, in many instances, has the hazard to health been reduced or eliminated.

In addition to dyspnea and rhinitis, most patients will complain of cough and sputum production. These symptoms should always arouse suspicion of allergic disease when they occur in nonsmokers. They are, however, most commonly due to smoking and they may also be produced by a nonspecific irritant effect of dust rather than an allergy. Appropriate investigation of the sputum may be helpful in the differentiation of these causes.

INVESTIGATION OF THE PATIENT

The worker with occupational asthma needs to be distinguished from the subject who has intrinsic asthma but who responds to a variety of irritants, some of which may be encountered at work; therefore, a careful history is essential. The patient will usually be aware of the substances at his work that affect him and some of his co-workers, though in some industries complex chemical and engineering processes may liberate substances that the worker is unaware of. In such instances the factory doctor will usually be able to obtain a list of such chemicals. If these are known to be allergens, management of the situation is relatively easy, but if they are not, a high index of suspicion should be maintained and careful investigation made before incriminating a substance and perhaps eventually forcing an individual to change jobs.

Examination of the patient in the office is generally unhelpful, except in a negative sense, but examination at work during the exposure should

lead to the diagnosis. The patient complains of tightness in the chest, and inspiratory and expiratory wheezes become audible shortly after exposure begins. Often a cough develops, especially on deep expiration, and the forced expiratory time is prolonged to more than 5 seconds. Measurement of peak flow rate will show a fall of greater than 15 per cent of the figure recorded when the patient is without symptoms. This test is of greatest value if repeated measurements are made several times daily over a period including both exposure at work and time spent away from work (Fig. 16–2).

In a patient suspected of having occupational asthma, the implications to his health and future earning power are so important that detailed investigation should be considered. Usually when the patient is not exposed to the allergen his lung function tests are normal, though there may be some residual airways obstruction. A bronchial challenge is therefore a sensible investigation, and a logical and relatively safe one has been introduced by Pepys.[13]

The main indications for inhalational challenges are:

1. When occupational asthma is suspected but when the agent to which the worker is exposed is not recognized as a cause of this condition.

2. When the worker is exposed to more than one recognized cause of occupational asthma.

3. When absolute confirmation of the diagnosis is necessary, i.e., prior to telling a worker to give up a job.

The patient is exposed to the suspected allergen in a manner similar to that in which he comes into contact with it at work, though in a setting where symptoms can be controlled and lung function can be measured (Fig. 16–3). A 15 per cent or greater fall in peak flow or timed vital

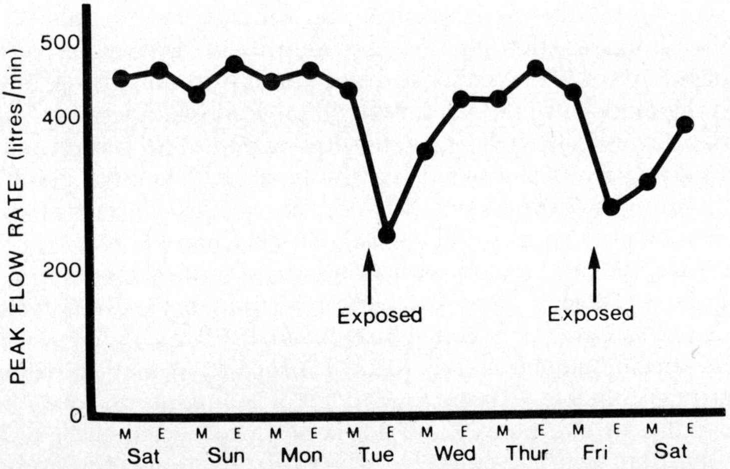

Figure 16–2. Record of peak flow rate kept by patient during a working week. Subsequent investigation revealed the use of isocyanates in the factory on Tuesday and Friday.

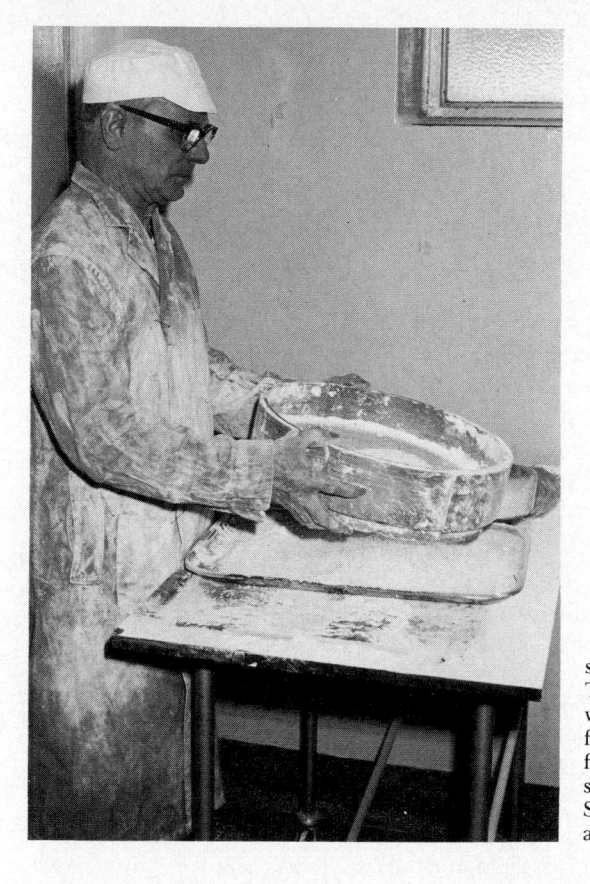

Figure 16–3. Investigation of suspected occupational asthma. The patient, a fitter in a bakery, was suspected of being allergic to flour. Wheezing and a fall in peak flow rates developed after he had spent 15 minutes sieving flour. Similar changes were not recorded after he had sieved sugar.

capacity is sufficient to demonstrate a cause-and-effect relationship, provided no such fall followed a control test using an inert substance.

Other lung function tests are less helpful. Measurements of airways resistance require more expensive apparatus without giving any more useful information, while measurements of lung volumes show only the overinflation associated with airways obstruction. The carbon monoxide diffusing capacity is normal, and this may be a helpful point in the differentiation of occupational asthma from extrinsic allergic alveolitis, in which challenge testing produces a fall (see Chap. 15). A standard 8-minute exercise test, on stairs or a treadmill rather than on a bicycle ergometer, will permit differentiation of occupational asthma from exercise-induced asthma,[14] which may present in an occupational setting.

Less specific but frequently helpful information may be obtained by skin testing. Suitable extracts and control solutions may be obtained commercially, or alternatively, an extract of a suspected allergen may be made. The skin is pricked lightly through drops of allergen and control solutions, with a separate needle for each drop. A wheal and flare occurring within 10 to 20 minutes denotes a positive response. It should

be remembered that a proportion of asymptomatic individuals will show positive immediate reactions to skin tests and that there is not an exact correlation between cutaneous and bronchial hypersensitivity.

The advent of radioallergosorbent tests (RAST) for specific IgE antibody has raised hopes that blood tests may become available for the diagnosis of some forms of occupational asthma. As with precipitating antibody in allergic alveolitis, such tests are likely to detect sensitization rather than bronchial disease, but a combination of clinical and serological evidence should be an aid to the diagnosis. Such tests should prove valuable in allergy to flour and wood dusts, and there is hope that they may become available for some of the chemical sensitizers in the near future.[15]

In situations in which there is doubt as to whether the patient's symptoms are allergic or bronchitic in origin, it may be helpful to examine the blood and sputum for eosinophilia. Sputum expectorated directly into a bottle containing 70 per cent alcohol may be sectioned and stained as a block of tissue and the stigmata of allergic bronchitis looked for.[16] These include eosinophils, desquamated strips of bronchial mucosa, and pink-staining mucus, altogether similar to the casts found in the bronchi of people who have died in status asthmaticus (Fig. 16–4). Such findings are evidence of an allergic mechanism at work, though they do not of course indicate the cause nor do they necessarily exclude the contribution of other mechanisms.

INVESTIGATION OF THE HAZARD

In general, the discovery of a patient with occupational asthma need not lead to detailed investigation of the place of work, as may be the case with allergic alveolitis. Patients with asthma usually consult their physician soon after the onset of their symptoms, and only a relatively small proportion of those exposed are affected. Periodically, however, a new hazard is discovered, as was the case with enzymatic washing powders in 1969.[17] In these circumstances, full investigation of the source of the allergen, its mode of action, and the frequency of sensitization and symptoms among exposed workers should be carried out. This is particularly important in the case of substances such as isocyanates, which are potent sensitizers even in very low concentrations.

MANAGEMENT

The principles of management of occupational asthma are the same as those for other forms of the disease. Ideally, atopic individuals should be advised to avoid entering trades in which there is an obvious risk of provocation of symptoms. Such trades include the production of silk, the

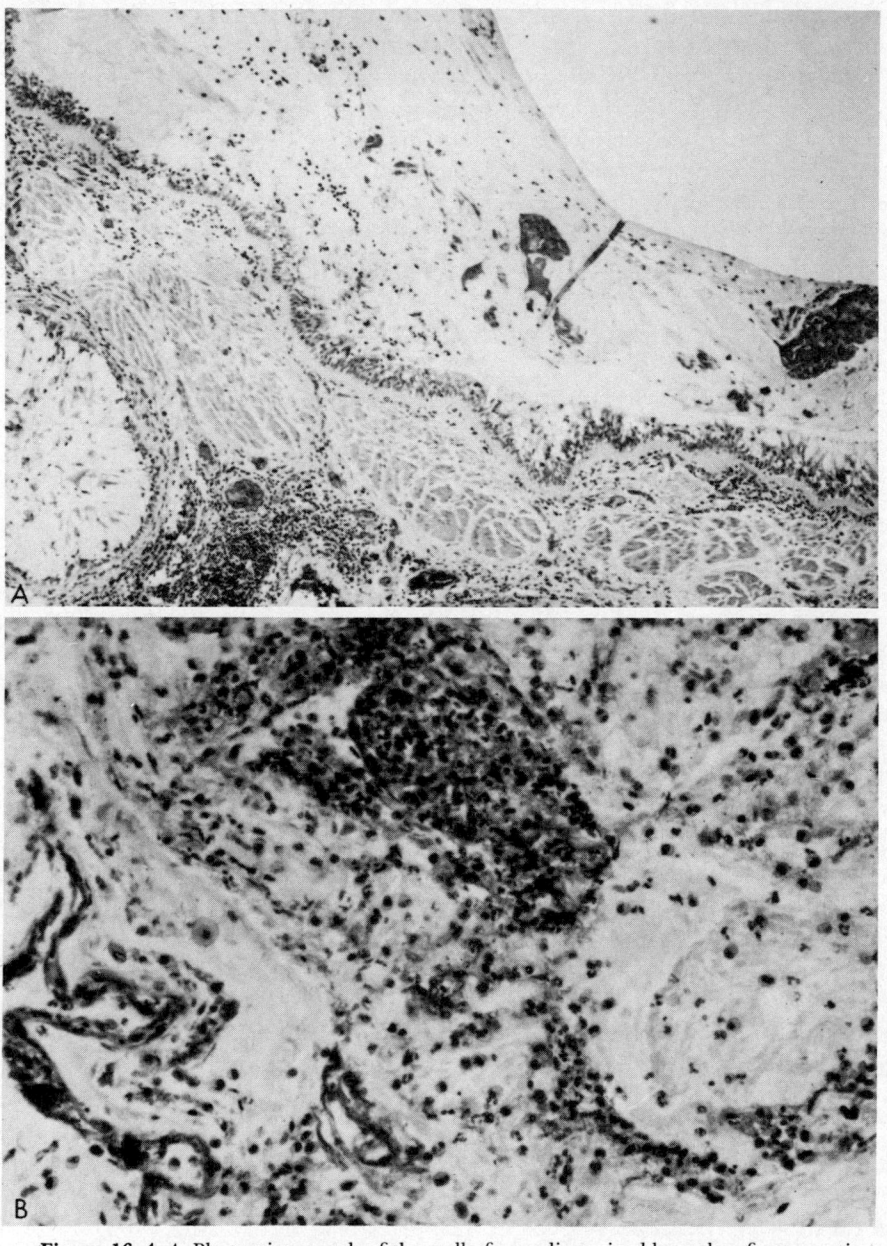

Figure 16–4. *A*, Photomicrograph of the wall of a medium-sized bronchus from a patient who died in severe asthma, illustrating hyperplasia of the mucous glands (bottom left), smooth muscle hyperplasia, and thickening of the basement membrane. The lumen is partly occluded by a characteristic exudate containing desquamated epithelial cells and eosinophils. On the luminal surface these elements have become necrotic and aggregated. *B*, Histologic section of sputum from an asthmatic subject, showing scattered eosinophils, many of which have become necrotic and aggregated (center top), and coiled arrangement of characteristic eosinophilic material (bottom left).

manufacture of enzyme detergents, and in particular those occupations in which workers are exposed to platinum salts. In most causes of occupational asthma there is little evidence to suggest that atopy predisposes to the likelihood that the subject will develop the condition. Moreover, the proportion of atopics in the general population ranges from 10 to 40 per cent, according to the method of detection used. Clearly, for most individuals, economic and social considerations outweigh the theoretical risk of developing occupational asthma. Job satisfaction and adequate remuneration are generally more important than the statistical risk in an individual case.

Trades and industries in which there is known to be a high risk of the provocation of allergy should take steps to exclude atopic individuals at the pre-employment medical examination. When an employee incurs asthma in relation to this work, he should be removed from exposure to the allergen. If this is not possible, the worker should be provided with an effective respirator whenever exposure occurs. It is, of course, axiomatic that the amount of potential allergen in the air should be kept as small as possible by effective ventilation and enclosure of the process whenever this can be done.

Desensitization of affected workers in general proves rather disappointing, though it may be worth a trial in individuals who are unable to be removed entirely from the harmful environment. Apart from this, treatment of attacks should be along standard lines, with the use of bronchodilators, prophylactic treatment with cromolyn sodium, or, in severe cases, corticosteroids.

SPECIFIC TYPES OF OCCUPATIONAL ASTHMA

The number of occupational situations in which asthma has been provoked is large. As new industrial processes are introduced, new chemicals are liberated into the air and bring with them new risks. Some of the most clearly identified agents are described in this section and are listed in Table 16–1.

Cereal Workers

Symptoms of respiratory disease and rhinitis due to grain allergy are found in millers, bakers, and workers exposed to grains on farms, in elevators, and in transportation. The clinical spectrum was described by Ramazzini[1] and its allergic basis was demonstrated by Duke in 1935,[18] when he described four mill workers with asthma caused by an allergen derived from wheat. Studies of bakers[4] have shown that approximately 10 per cent of apprentices may show positive skin reactions to an extract of

Table 16–1. SOME AGENTS CAUSING OCCUPATIONAL ASTHMA

Agent	Occupation
Vegetable Substances	
Grains, flour	Farming, baking, milling
Wood dusts	Mills, joinery, carpentry
Castor bean	Oil, fertilizer production
Coffee bean	Coffee production
Gum acacia	Printing, pharmaceuticals
Tragacanth	Sweet making
Colophony (rosin)	Soldering, electronics
Animals	
Rodents	Laboratories
Horses, dogs, cats	Veterinarians, stable hands
Locusts	Laboratories
Maggots	Anglers
Grain weevil	Millers, laboratories
Grain mites	Farmers
Silkworms	Silkworm culture
Shellfish	Shellfish preparation
Enzymes	
Bacillus subtilis (alcalase)	Detergent production
Trypsin	Plastics
Papain	Food technology, laboratories
Chemicals	
Isocyanates	Foam, paints, varnishes
Epoxy resins	Surface coatings, adhesives
Ethanolamines	Painting, soldering
Platinum salts	Refining
Chromates	Plating, cement
Nickel	Plating
Vanadium	Boiler cleaning
Aluminium	Potroom work
Drugs	
Salbutamol intermediate	
Piperazine	
Spiramycin	
Synthetic penicillins	Production
Tetracycline	
Chloramine-T	

flour within a month of starting work. By the end of the first year, half of these have already become negative, while progressively more apprentices begin to manifest positive skin tests. By the end of three years, approximately 20 per cent of apprentices show a positive skin reaction, and a similar number of trained bakers are also found to have positive reactions after five years of employment. Presumably the amount of allergen in the atmosphere is an important factor in the production of sensitization, but other studies have shown a higher incidence of positive reactors—up to 50 per cent after 10 years.[19] In this latter series 5 to 10

per cent of bakers had symptoms of asthma after 10 years in the trade and an additional 10 per cent had left the baking industry because of their symptoms. Curiously, of those whose asthma is sufficiently mild to allow them to continue at work, symptoms tend to improve or even disappear in almost half, suggesting that spontaneous desensitization may occur. More recent work from Germany has essentially confirmed these findings, showing that about 5 per cent of apprentices and 20 per cent of established bakers have symptoms of allergic disease.[20]

Studies of workers in grain elevators have shown a high prevalence of rhinitis and respiratory symptoms. These symptoms fluctuate with the intensity of exposure to grain dust and are accompanied by evidence of ventilatory impairment.[21-24] Dust levels in grain elevators may be very high, up to several hundred milligrams per cubic meter, of which 40 per cent may be respirable.[25] It seems likely that the respiratory symptoms are related to a combination of asthma and chronic bronchitis, due to chronic irritation as well as allergy. In addition, grain workers commonly complain of malaise, aches, and fever some hours after exposure to dust. The immunological basis of this "grain fever" is not understood, but it does not seem to include a pulmonary component typical of allergic alveolitis.[26] It might be analogous to humidifier fever and is discussed further in Chapter 19.

Respiratory symptoms other than the classic allergic alveolitis have been increasingly described in farmers handling grains and hay. Harvesting grain was shown to produce symptoms in about a quarter of the British farmers exposed in one survey.[27] In this study, fungal spores were shown to be the likely sensitizers, many hundreds of thousands per cubic meter being liberated into the air, with positive skin tests and challenge tests obtained in affected individuals. Asthmatic symptoms also occur in farmers feeding cattle with stored grain and hay, and in these circumstances storage mites have been shown to be potent sensitizers.[28, 29]

It can be seen that many potential allergens are present in grains and flour and that the spectrum of these varies according to the condition and type of the material. This variety of allergens was recognized many years ago[30, 31] and has been re-emphasized recently. The flour itself, wheat hairs, parasitic fungi such as smut and rust, saprophytes such as Aspergillus, Cladosporium, and Aureobasidium, and organisms such as the weevil, *Sitophilus granarius*,[32, 33] and the mites, *Tyrophagus longior* and *Acarus farris*,[29] have all been shown to be responsible for provoking attacks of asthma in exposed workers. It seems that atopic individuals are particularly likely to become sensitized to one or more of these allergens, depending on what is being handled and the density of their liberation into the atmosphere. In addition, in conditions of very heavy exposure, a high proportion of nonatopics become sensitized and acquire hyper-reactive airways that show positive histamine or acetylcholine responses even after exposure has ceased.[20]

Woodworkers

Carpenters, joiners, and papermill and sawmill workers may develop hypersensitivity to wood dust as well as to fungal spores and substances used in the treatment of wood.[34] In particular, hardwoods, such as cedar, oak, and mahogany, and western red cedar *(Thuja plicata),* iroko, cedar of Lebanon, and zebrawood have been described as causes of asthma.[35-39]

Studies of allergy to western red cedar[36, 37] have shown late asthmatic reactions to challenge with both wood dust itself and aqueous extracts. These tend to start about 2 hours after challenge and to last up to 24 hours, being only partly reversible with isoproterenol (Isuprel). Although this reaction has some of the characteristics of a Type III reaction, late Arthus-type skin reactions and serum precipitating antibodies have not invariably been demonstrated, and the sputum contains the eosinophils characteristic of a Type I reaction. Other work has shown immediate, delayed, and combined responses to challenge with extracts of western red cedar, the reactions being probably due to plicatic acid, a low-molecular-weight compound found in the extracts.[40] Follow-up of such patients has shown a gradual improvement in symptoms after exposure ceased, although around 40 per cent of the original group still showed bronchial reactivity over a year later.[41] Those subjects with prolonged exposure in whom the diagnosis was often delayed, and in addition who had a dual response (early and late decrement in ventilatory capacity) and whose ventilatory capacity was most impaired, were the least likely to improve after cessation of exposure.[41a] The same prognostic factors probably apply to occupational asthma as a whole, but in particular it is evident that they are of paramount importance in TDI and western red cedar asthma.

Animals

Allergy to animals is well known in a nonoccupational setting, and those working with animals, such as veterinarians, stable hands, and research workers, are at special risk, especially if they are atopic. The number of animals that have been recognized to cause asthma (and usually also rhinitis) in an occupational setting is large. Laboratory rats and mice are particularly troublesome, and although allergy to their hair may be a factor, it seems that the main allergen is a protein excreted in the urine, especially of older male rats.[42-44] Also in the laboratory, asthma has been described in workers with locusts[45, 46] and the grain weevil, *Sitophilus granarius.*[33] Silkworms, prawn, crabs, maggots, and the Mexican bean weevil have also caused asthma in those engaged in the trades involving exposure to them. In many of these occupations, a high proportion of the individuals exposed developed symptoms, though generally the atopic did so more quickly than the nonatopic.

Other Organic Substances

Coffee and tea workers often develop an excess of respiratory symptoms,[47, 48] and the coffee bean is a known sensitizer.[49] Exposure to soybean, in the manufacture of soybean flour,[50] and to the castor bean and its residue, or pomace, after the oil has been extracted has been shown to provoke asthma.[51] Castor beans are used for their oil and for making fertilizer. Gum acacia, a juice obtained from the bark of a tree, *Acacia senegalis,* was used widely in the printing trade to prevent sheets from sticking together and the print from running. It provoked asthma and rhinitis in those exposed to the spray to such an extent that its use has been superseded.[52–54] It is still used in the preparation of confectioneries and medicaments and could cause asthma in these situations. Tragacanth, another gum, can do the same.

Proteolytic Enzymes

Alcalase, a proteolytic enzyme manufactured by fermentation of *Bacillus subtilis,* was introduced as a component of washing powders in 1966. The product is a fine dusty powder containing 60 per cent sodium sulfate, 5 per cent sodium chloride, and 35 per cent organic material, of which about 5 to 10 per cent is enzyme. It is mixed with water and sprayed onto sodium tripolyphosphate. This complex, containing 4 per cent alcalase, is stored for subsequent mixing with detergent powders, the amount of complex remaining in the commercial preparation being about 5 per cent, and thus the concentration of enzyme is of the order of 60 parts per million.[55]

As the product became more widely used, it became apparent that workers exposed to relatively high concentrations of the dust developed respiratory symptoms, and Flindt[17] reported both immediate asthmatic reactions and more prolonged illnesses suggestive of allergic alveolitis. Immediate skin reactions to extracts of both alcalase and *B. subtilis* were found, and both immediate and late bronchoconstrictor responses were found in some patients on bronchial challenge.[56] Although precipitins were demonstrated in affected subjects, they were also found in the controls and were probably of nonimmunological origin. Subsequent work has failed to confirm the development of allergic alveolitis in exposed workers.

Newhouse and colleagues[55] investigated the epidemiology of the disease. They found 21 per cent of exposed workers to be affected six months after production started. There was a clear relationship between sensitization and level of exposure to the powder. The symptoms of rhinitis, cough, and wheezy breathlessness were suggestive of allergic disease and correlated with skin reactivity, but specific IgE could not be demonstrated, nor was blood eosinophilia found. No radiologic abnormalities were detected.

This study failed to produce evidence of deterioration in lung function over six months, though this was clearly a very short follow-up period. The exposed and sensitized workers showed a reduction in ventilatory capacity compared to those not sensitized, and other studies have confirmed this finding.[57] Though an allergic basis for this reduction seems likely, it is possible that a nonspecific irritant effect of the enzyme may also play a part.

There is some evidence that individuals who use the enzymatic washing powders may become sensitized and may even develop asthma.[58, 59] This problem is probably not very great, and the risks should be reduced further by the change of the enzyme component of washing powders from powder to granule form.

Soon after the condition was recognized, changes were made in production techniques. Dust sources were enclosed, ventilation increased, and vacuum cleaning used instead of sweeping. Effective respirators were also provided for exposed workers, and these measures reduced substantially the frequency of sensitization.[55] A 7-year follow-up of workers exposed to the lower levels of enzyme occurring in the industry since these improvements were made has shown a far lower incidence of skin sensitization and no further evidence of work-related airways disease.[60]

The demonstration of emphysema in individuals with α_1-antitrypsin deficiency in their blood has led to the concept that emphysema in humans may be due to an imbalance, local or general, in the amount of proteolytic and antiproteolytic enzymes in the lungs.[61] Indeed, proteolytic enzymes have been used by tracheal instillation to produce animal models of emphysema. Following the demonstration of protease-provoked airways disease it has been a matter of concern whether workers exposed to such enzymes might be at risk of developing emphysema. Indeed, some work has shown a significant increase in lung volumes and compliance in heavily exposed workers compared with lightly exposed workers.[62] However, these individuals had normal airways function, and it seems unlikely that the usual industrial exposures will lead to appreciable lung damage. There is nevertheless no room for complacency, and all exposure to such materials should be very carefully controlled.

Alcalase is not the only proteolytic enzyme used in industry. Papain is used to tenderize meat and to clarify beer, in tanning and pharmaceuticals and in laboratories, where it has many applications including the production of emphysema in rats. Asthma and rhinitis have been described in workers in most of these situations.[63–65] Again, atopic individuals develop symptoms early. Similar reactions have occurred with the use of extracts of *Aspergillus flavus* in pharmaceuticals,[66] with trypsin,[67] and, in the parents of a cystic fibrotic, with pancreatic extract.[68]

Soldering

Aluminium is widely used as a material for electric cables. When heated in the process of soldering, it forms a film of oxide and the fluxes

normally used in soldering copper wires are not satisfactory. A suitable flux contains aminoethyl ethanolamine mixed with zinc oxide and fluoroborate. In the process of soldering, fumes are liberated which contain particulate fluoride and a mist of the unchanged ethanolamine. McCann[69] described one case of bronchial hypersensitivity in a survey of 3000 cable jointers, and Sterling[70] described two patients in whom there was a late and prolonged bronchoconstrictor reaction after challenge with fumes of both flux and aminoethyl ethanolamine. Skin tests were negative in these patients. Pepys and colleagues[71] described three further cases, all of whom showed a late fall in expiratory flow at about 4 hours, lasting up to 12 hours and not inhibited by cromolyn sodium. One also showed an immediate response, though it was not clear whether this was a primary irritant effect.

The delay in onset and prolonged course of symptoms, the small dose required to precipitate an attack, and the relatively small numbers of those exposed who are affected suggest an allergic basis for the disease. Skin testing is inadvisable, as severe reactions may occur.[69] The allergen is derived from the ethylamino ethanolamine component of the flux, though whether it undergoes chemical changes in the bronchi prior to becoming a sensitizer is not known.

Other mechanisms may provoke asthma in solderers. In particular, colophony has been incriminated in the electronics industry.[72] Colophony, or rosin, is the solid material left after turpentine has been distilled from pine resin and is used as a component of multicore flux and in the production of glue. It is liberated as a fume in the breathing zones of workers soldering electronic circuit boards. A series of studies by Burge and colleagues has shown work-related asthma in about 25 per cent of those exposed to colophony fumes in the electronics industry, with the pattern of development and clinical features similar to those of occupational asthma provoked by other causes.[6, 73, 74] However, these subjects do not seem to have the prick test and IgE response that would be expected, suggesting that a different immunological mechanism may be operating.

Not all asthma in solderers is necessarily due to the flux. Patients have been described in whom the asthma was due to isocyanates liberated from the polyurethane coating of the wires being soldered.[75]

Isocyanates

Isocyanates are used widely in industry in the production of polyurethane, which has applications in the manufacture of plastics, foam, surface coatings including paints and varnishes, synthetic rubber, and fibers. Demand for such materials and, thus, the numbers of workers exposed to isocyanates are steadily increasing.[76] Respiratory symptoms are most likely to occur as a result of exposure to toluene diisocyanate (TDI), which is the most volatile,[77, 78] but asthma has also been described following exposure to hexamethylene diisocyanate (HDI),[79] diphenylmethane diiso-

cyanate (MDI),[80] and 1,5-naphthylamine diisocyanate (NDI).[81] The latter two rarely cause problems unless heated, as they are solids at room temperature.

The acute effects of exposure to TDI, first described by Fuchs and Valade[77] and subsequently by Gandevia,[78] take the form of cough, shortness of breath, and wheezing. Though the substance is an irritant, in some instances demonstration of late bronchial reactions inhibited by cromolyn sodium, sputum eosinophilia,[75] and the finding of circulating antibody[82] suggest that an immunological mechanism is operative.

Apart from asthmatic reactions in sensitized subjects, progressive falls in ventilatory capacity through the week and over periods of up to two years have been shown in workers exposed to levels of TDI below the threshold limit value.[83] There is some evidence that a high prevalence of cough and sputum may occur in workers exposed both acutely to high concentrations and repeatedly to low concentrations.[84] It is not clear whether these symptoms are due to allergy or to nonspecific irritation, though the latter seems more likely in view of the probable relationship to the atmospheric concentrations of TDI.

Asthmatic reactions to TDI have been described not only in workers producing the substance but also in people using the finished products, such as varnishes,[71] do-it-yourself polyurethane foam,[85] and polyurethane-coated wires,[71] foams, and fabrics. In addition, the liberation of isocyanates from furniture in burning buildings may well be a cause of respiratory symptoms in fire fighters.

Industry has a great responsibility for the reduction of levels of isocyanates in the production process. A longitudinal study carried out long after the hazards were recognized has shown frequent excursions of TDI levels above the threshold limit values, with resulting sensitization of a third of those exposed.[86] It is apparent that earlier estimates of toxic levels have been too high and revised lower levels have stretched detection technology to its limits. Aside from this, subjects who have become sensitized may have asthma induced by undetectable concentrations of TDI. Such people should be excluded from contact with the substance.

Metals and Their Salts

Complex salts of platinum are used in the manufacture of catalysts and in electroplating, photography, and the production of fluorescent screens. Subjects may be exposed in these occupations as well as in jewelry and platinum refinery. The salts have been known to be potent sensitizers since their original description in 1929,[87] and the potential hazards of skin and bronchial testing are well recognized. A syndrome of asthma, urticaria, and rhinitis has been described and is known as platinosis.[88] Pepys and colleagues have demonstrated immediate bronchial reactions blocked by cromolyn sodium, using an industrial-type bronchial challenge.[89]

Cutaneous allergy to nickel has been well known for many years, and bronchial reactions to nickel have also been described in metal plating, welding, and work with nickel carbonyl.[90, 91] Chromium,[92, 93] vanadium,[94] and aluminum and their salts, and tungsten carbide are other metals that may provoke asthma. In the latter case it is possible that cobalt in the coolant used when grinding the metal, rather than tungsten carbide itself, is responsible for sensitization,[95] while in the case of aluminium extraction it is not clear whether aluminum itself or fluorides in the potroom fumes are responsible for the bronchoconstriction.[96]

Epoxy Resins

Epoxy resins are widely used in industry and in the home as adhesives, as surface coatings, and in plastics. The resins themselves are long-chain polymers that are converted into hard solids by the addition of a hardener, or curing agent. When the two components are mixed, fumes may be emitted, and these are the cause of bronchial sensitization. The curing agents, which include amines such as ethylene diamine, dimethyl ethanolamine, triethylene tetramine, and aminoethyl ethanolamine, and the phthalic, tetrachlorophthalic, and trimellitic anhydrides, are the usual component responsible.[97] Apart from use of the resins, heating or cutting of material containing them may also release fumes and this is probably the usual cause of meat wrappers' asthma when phthalic anhydride is a component of the label or epoxidized soybean oil is a component of the polyvinyl chloride (PVC) wrapping.[98]

A variety of respiratory syndromes may occur following exposure to trimellitic anhydride (TMA), including rhinitis, TMA flu (a condition characterized by a late onset and associated with cough and muscle aches and pains), asthma, and irritative bronchitis. The asthma may be of the immediate type, mediated by IgE antibodies, or of the delayed type, characterized by IgG and IgA antibodies.[99]

Other Chemicals and Pharmaceuticals

Reactive dyes, used in coloring cotton and synthetic fibers and by hairdressers, may cause bronchial as well as skin sensitization.[100, 101] Formalin is also well known as a skin sensitizer and has been described as a cause of occupational asthma in nurses and laboratory workers.[102] Asthma has also been described in workers involved in the production of a wide range of pharmaceutical preparations, including synthetic penicillins, spiramycin, piperazine, tetracyclines, salbutamol, sulfonamides, and chloramine-T.[13, 103–107]

CONCLUSION

This chapter has described many situations in industry in which workers may become sensitized to powders, fumes, and gases liberated into the air. While in general the atopic individual is likely to develop asthma and rhinitis more readily than the nonatopic person, the latter is far from immune. It is probable that relatively high exposures are usually necessary to sensitize the less susceptible individual, but once sensitized he will respond to minute doses and may frequently have to change jobs on this account.

It is important for industry to be aware that the prevention of occupational asthma requires a somewhat different attitude toward occupational hygiene than that necessary for the prevention of disease due to the cumulative effect of a dust. To prevent occupational asthma, any excursion above statutory levels is a potential threat. Much work remains to be done to learn what doses are required to initiate the disease. Doctors too must become increasingly aware of the possibility that a patient's asthma may be due to the working environment and be prepared to investigate such cases with serial recordings of peak flow rate.

References

1. Ramazzini, B., De morbis artificum diatriba, 1713, Cave, W., trans. Chicago, Wright, 1940.
2. Coca, A. F., Studies in specific hypersensitiveness: preparation of fluid extracts with solutions for use in diagnosis and treatment of allergies, with notes on collection of pollens. J. Immunol., 7, 163, 1922.
3. Coca, A. F., and Cooke, R. A., Classification of phenomena of hypersensitiveness. J. Immunol., 8, 163, 1923.
4. Herxheimer, H., The skin sensitivity to flour of bakers' apprentices. Acta Allerg., 28, 42, 1973.
5. Coombs, P. G. H., and Gell, R. R. A., Classification of allergic reactions responsible for clinical hypersensitivity and disease. In Gell, R. R. A., and Coombs, P. F. H., eds., Clinical Aspects of Immunology. Oxford, Blackwell, 1967.
6. Burge, P. S., O'Brien, I. M., and Harries, M. G., Peak flow records in the diagnosis of occupational asthma due to colophony. Thorax, 34, 308, 1979.
7. Burge, P. S., O'Brien, I. M., and Harries, M. G., Peak flow records in the diagnosis of occupational asthma due to isocyanates. Thorax, 34, 317, 1979.
8. Mullins, J., Harvey, R., and Seaton, A., The sources and incidence of Aspergillus fumigatus (Fres.). Clin. Allergy, 6, 209, 1976.
9. McCarthy, D. S., and Pepys, J., Allergic bronchopulmonary aspergillosis. Clinical immunology (2): skin, nasal and bronchial tests. Clin Allergy, 1, 415, 1971.
10. Ishizaka, M., Function of IgE antibody and regulation of IgE antibody response. In Stein, M., ed., New Directions in Asthma. Park Ridge, Ill., American College of Chest Physicians, 1975.
11. Dolovich, J., Hargreave, F. E., Chalmers, R., et al., Late cutaneous allergic responses in isolated IgE dependent reactions. J. Allergy Clin. Immunol., 52, 38, 1973.
12. Parish, W. E., Short-term anaphylactic IgG antibodies in human sera. Lancet, 2, 591, 1970.
12a. Burge, P. S., Non-specific bronchial hyper-reactivity in workers exposed to toluene di-isocyante, diphenyl methane di-isocyante and colophony. Eur. J. Respir. Dis., 63(Suppl. 123) 91, 1982.

13. Pepys, J., Pickering, C. A. C., and Loudon, H. W. G., Asthma due to inhaled chemical agents—piperazine dihydrochloride. Clin. Allergy, 2, 189, 1972.
14. Seaton, A., Davies, F., Gaziano, D., and Hughes, R. O., Exercise-induced asthma. Br. Med. J., 2, 556, 1969.
15. Newman-Taylor, A. J., Occupational asthma. Thorax, 36, 241, 1980.
16. Sanerkin, N. G., and Evans, D. M. D., The sputum in bronchial asthma: pathognomonic patterns. J. Pathol. Bact., 89, 535, 1965.
17. Flindt, M. L. H., Pulmonary disease due to inhalation of derivatives of Bacillus subtilis containing proteolytic enzyme. Lancet, 1, 1177, 1969.
18. Duke, W. W., Wheat hairs and dust as a common cause of asthma among workers in wheat flour mills. J.A.M.A., 105, 957, 1935.
19. Gadborg, E., Unpublished M.D. thesis. Quoted in Bonnevie, P., Occupational Allergy. Leiden, H. E. Stenfert Kroese, 1956, p. 161.
20. Thiel, H., and Ulmer, W. T., Baker's asthma: development and possibility for treatment. Chest, 78(Suppl), 400, 1980.
21. do Pico, G. A., Reddan, W., Flaherty, D., et al., Respiratory abnormalities among grain handlers. A clinical physiologic and immunologic study. Am. Rev. Respir. Dis., 115, 915, 1977.
22. Broder, I., Mintz, S., Hutcheon, M. A., et al., Comparison of respiratory variables in grain elevator workers and civic outside workers of Thunder Bay, Canada. Am. Rev. Respir. Dis., 119, 193, 1979.
23. Broder, I., Mintz, S., Hutcheon, M. A., et al., Effect of layoff and rehire on respiratory variables of grain elevator workers. Am. Rev. Respir. Dis., 122, 601, 1980.
24. Dosman, J. A., Cotton, D. J., Graham, B. L., et al., Chronic bronchitis and decreased forced expiratory flow rates in lifetime nonsmoking grain workers. Am. Rev. Respir. Dis., 121, 11, 1980.
25. Dosman, J. A., Graham, B. L., and Cotton, D. J., Chronic bronchitis and exposure to cereal grain dust. Am. Rev. Respir. Dis., 120, 477, 1979.
26. Tse, K. S., Warren, P., Janusz, M., McCarthy, D. S., Cherniack, R. M., Respiratory abnormalities in workers exposed to grain dust. Arch. Environ. Health, 27, 74, 1973.
27. Darke, C. S., Knowelden, J., Lacey, J., and Ward, A. M., Respiratory disease of workers harvesting grain. Thorax, 31, 294, 1976.
28. Cuthbert, O. D., Brostoff, J., Wraith, D. G., and Brighton, W. D., "Barn allergy." Asthma and rhinitis due to storage mites. Clin. Allergy, 9, 229, 1979.
29. Ingram, C. G., Jeffrey, I. G., Symington, I. S., and Cuthbert, O. D., Bronchial provocation studies in farmers allergic to storage mites. Lancet, 2, 1330, 1979.
30. Wittich, F. W., Nature of various milldust allergens. J. Lancet, 60, 418, 1940.
31. Jiminez-Diaz, C., Lahoz, C., and Canto, G., The allergens of mill dust. Ann. Allergy., 5, 519, 1947.
32. Lunn, J. A., Millworkers' Asthma. Allergic responses to the grain weevil. Br. J. Ind. Med., 23, 149, 1966.
33. Frankland, A. W., and Lunn, J. A., Asthma caused by the grain weevil. Br. J. Ind. Med., 22, 157, 1965.
34. Fillassier, G., Le bois. Cah. Méd., 28, 205, 1967.
35. Sossman, A. J., Schlueter, D. P., Fink, J. N., and Barboriak, J. J., Hypersensitivity to wood dust. N. Engl. J. Med., 281, 977, 1969.
36. Gandevia, B., and Milne, J., Occupational asthma and rhinitis due to western red cedar. Br. J. Ind. Med., 27, 235, 1970.
37. Pickering, C. A. C., Batten, J. C., and Pepys, J., Asthma due to inhaled wood dusts—western red cedar and iroko. Clin. Allergy, 2, 213, 1972.
38. Greenberg, M., Respiratory symptoms following brief exposure to cedar of Lebanon dust. Clin. Allergy, 2, 219, 1972.
39. Bush, R. K., Junginger, J. W., and Reed, C. E., Asthma due to African zebrawood (Microberlinia) dust. Am. Rev. Respir. Dis., 117, 601, 1978.
40. Chan-Yeung, M., Barton, G., MacLean, L., and Grzybowski, S., Occupational asthma and rhinitis due to Western Red Cedar (Thuja plicata). Am. Rev. Respir. Dis., 108, 1094, 1973.
41. Chan-Yeung, M., Fate of occupational asthma. A follow-up study of patients with occupational asthma due to Western Red Cedar (Thuja plicata). Am. Rev. Resp. Dis., 116, 1023, 1977.

41a. Chan-Yeung, M., Lam, S., and Koener, S., Clinical features and natural history of occupational asthma due to western red cedar *(Thuja plicata).* Am. J. Med., *72,* 411, 1982.

42. Lincoln, T. A., Bolton, N. E., and Garrett, A. S., Occupational allergy to animal dander and sera. J. Occup. Med., *16,* 465, 1974.

43. Carroll, K. B., Pepys, J., Longbottom, J. L., et al., Extrinsic allergic alveolitis due to rat serum proteins. Clin. Allergy, *5,* 443, 1975.

44. Newman-Taylor, A., Longbottom, J. L., and Pepys, J., Respiratory allergy to urine proteins of rats and mice. Lancet, *2.* 847, 1977.

45. Frankland, A. W., Locust sensitivity. Ann. Allergy, *11,* 445, 1953.

46. Burge, P. S., Edge, G., O'Brien, I. M., et al., Occupational asthma in a research centre breeding locusts. Clin. Allergy, *10.* 355, 1980.

47. Bruun, E., Allergy to coffee. Acta Allergy, *1,* 445, 1953.

48. Uragoda, C. G., Respiratory disease in tea workers in Sri Lanka. Thorax, *35,* 114, 1980.

49. Lehrer, S. B., Karr, R. M., and Salvaggio, J. E., Extraction and analysis of coffee bean allergens. Clin. Allergy, *8,* 217, 1978.

50. Bush, R. K., and Cohen, M., Immediate and late onset asthma from occupational exposure to soybean dust. Clin. Allergy, *7,* 369, 1977.

51. Kathren, R. L., Price, H., and Rogers, J. C., Air-borne castor-bean pomace allergy. Arch. Ind. Health, *19,* 487, 1959.

52. Fowler, P. B. S., Printers' asthma. Lancet, *2,* 755, 1952.

53. Bohner, C. B., and Sheldon, J. M., Sensitivity to gum acacia, with a report of ten cases of asthma in printers. J. Allergy, *12.* 290, 1941.

54. Hinaut, G., Blacque-Belair, A., and Buffe, D., L'asthme à la gomme arabique dans un grand atelier de typographie. Franc. Med. Chir. Thorac., *15,* 51, 1961.

55. Newhouse, M. L., Tagg, B., and Pocock, S. J., An epidemiological study of workers producing enzyme washing powders. Lancet, *1,* 689, 1970.

56. Pepys, J., Hargreave, F. E., Longbottom, J. L., and Faux, J., Allergic reactions of the lungs to enzymes of *Bacillus subtilis.* Lancet, *1,* 1181, 1969.

57. Greenberg, M., Milne, J. F., and Watt, A., Survey of workers exposed to dusts containing derivatives of *Bacillus subtilis.* Br. Med. J., *2,* 629, 1970.

58. Belin, L., Falsen, E., Hoborn, J., and André, J., Enzyme sensitization in consumers of enzyme-containing washing powder. Lancet, *2,* 1153, 1970.

59. Falleroni, A. E., and Schwartz, D. P., Immediate hypersensitivity to enzyme detergents. Lancet, *1,* 548, 1971.

60. Juniper, C. P., How, M. J., Goodwin, B. F. J., and Kinshott, A. K., *Bacillus subtilis* enzymes: a 7-year clinical, epidemiological and immunological study of an industrial allergen. J. Soc. Occup. Med., *27,* 3, 1977.

61. Emphysema: beginning of an understanding. Edit., Br. Med. J., *1,* 961, 1980.

62. Musk, A. W., and Gandevia, B., Loss of pulmonary elastic recoil in workers formerly exposed to proteolytic enzyme (alcalase) in the detergent industry. Br. J. Ind. Med., *33,* 158, 1976.

63. Milne, J., and Brand, S., Occupational asthma after inhalation of dust of the proteolytic enzyme papain. Br. J. Ind. Med., *32,* 302, 1975.

64. Tarlo, S. M., Shaikh, W., Bell, B., et al., Papain-induced allergic reactions. Clin. Allergy, *8,* 207, 1978.

65. Novey, H. S., Keenan, W. J., Fairshter, R. D., et al., Pulmonary disease in workers exposed to papain: clinicophysiological and immunological studies. Clin. Allergy, *10,* 721, 1980.

66. Panwells, R., Devos, M., Callens, L., and van der Straeten, M., Respiratory hazards from proteolytic enzymes. Lancet, *1,* 669, 1978.

67. Colten, H. R., Polakoff, P. L., Weinstein, S. E., and Strieder, D. J., Immediate hypersensitivity to hog trypsin resulting from industrial exposure. N. Engl. J. Med., *292,* 1050, 1975.

68. Dolan, T. F., and Meyers, A., Bronchial asthma and allergic rhinitis associated with inhalation of pancreatic extracts. Am. Rev. Respir. Dis., *110,* 812, 1974.

69. McCann, J. K., Health hazard from flux used in joining aluminium electricity cables. Ann. Occup. Hyg., *7,* 261, 1964.

70. Sterling, G. M., Asthma due to aluminium soldering flux. Thorax, *22,* 533, 1967.

71. Pepys, J., Pickering, C. A. C., and Hughes, E. G., Asthma due to inhaled chemical fumes—amino-ethyl ethanolamine in aluminium soldering flux. Clin. Allergy, 2, 197, 1972.
72. Burge, P. S., Harries, M. G., O'Brien, I. M., and Pepys, J., Respiratory disease in workers exposed to solder flux fumes containing colophony (pine resin). Clin. Allergy, 8, 1, 1978.
73. Burge, P. S., Perks, W. H., O'Brien, I. M., et al., Occupational asthma in an electronics factory. Thorax, 34, 13, 1979.
74. Burge, P. S., Perks, W. H., O'Brien, I. M., et al., Occupational asthma in an electronics factory: a case control study to evaluate aetiological factors. Thorax, 34, 300, 1979.
75. Pepys, J., Pickering, C. A. C., Breslin, A. B. X., and Terry, D. J., Asthma due to inhaled chemical agents—tolylene diisocyanate. Clin. Allergy, 2, 225, 1972.
76. Buist, J. M., Isocyanates in industry. Proc. Roy. Soc. Med., 63, 365, 1970.
77. Fuchs, S., and Valade, P., Étude clinique et expérimentale sur quelques cas d'intoxication par de desmondur T. Arch. Mal. Prof., 12, 191, 1951.
78. Gandevia, B., Studies of ventilatory capacity and histamine response during exposure to isocyanate vapour in polyurethane foam manufacture. Br. J. Ind. Med., 20, 204, 1963.
79. Munn, A., Hazards of isocyanates. Ann. Occup. Hyg., 8, 163, 1965.
80. Tanser, A. R., Bourke, M. P., and Blandford, A. G., Isocyanate asthma. Respiratory symptoms caused by diphenylmethane isocyanate. Thorax, 28, 596, 1973.
81. Harries, M. G., Burge, P. S., Samson, M., et al., Isocyanate asthma: respiratory symptoms due to 1:5 naphthylene diisocyanate. Thorax, 34, 762, 1979.
82. Karol, M. H., Ioset, H. H., and Alarie, Y. C., Tolyl-specific IgE antibodies in workers with hypersensitivity to toluene diisocyanate. Am. Ind. Hyg. Assoc. J., 39, 454, 1978.
83. Peters, J. M., Cumulative pulmonary effects in workers exposed to tolylene diisocyanate. Proc. Roy. Soc. Med., 63, 372, 1970.
84. McKerrow, C. B., Davies, H. J., and Jones, A. P., Symptoms and lung function following acute and chronic exposure to tolylene di-isocyanate. Proc. Roy. Soc. Med., 63, 376, 1970.
85. Peters, J. M., and Murphy, R. L. H., Hazards to health—do-it-yourself polyurethane foam. Am. Rev. Respir. Dis., 184, 432, 1971.
86. Butcher, B. T., Jones, R. N., O'Neill, C. E., Longitudinal study of workers employed in the manufacture of toluene-diisocyanate. Am. Rev. Resp. Dis., 116, 411, 1977.
87. Valléry-Radot, L., and Blamoutier, R., Sensibilisation au chloroplatinité de potassium. Accidents graves de choc survenus à la suite d'une cutiréaction avec le cel. Bull. Mem. Soc. Med. Hop. Paris, 45, 222, 1929.
88. Roberts, A. E., Platinosis. A five-year study of soluble platinum salts on employees in a platinum laboratory and refinery. Arch. Ind. Hyg., 4, 549, 1951.
89. Pepys, J., Pickering, C. A. C., and Hughes, E. G., Asthma due to inhaled chemical agents—complex salts of platinum. Clin. Allergy, 2, 391, 1972.
90. McConnell, L. H., Fink, J. N., Schleuter, D. P., and Schmidt, M. G., Asthma caused by nickel sensitivity. Ann. Intern. Med., 78, 888, 1973.
91. Sunderman, F. W., and Sunderman, F. W., Jr., Löffler's syndrome associated with nickel sensitivity. Arch. Intern. Med., 107, 405, 1961.
92. Smith, A. R., Chrome poisoning with manifestations of sensitization: report of a case. J.A.M.A., 97, 95, 1931.
93. Joules, H., Asthma from sensitization to chromium. Lancet, 2, 182, 1932.
94. Williams, N., Vanadium poisoning from cleaning oil-fired boilers. Br. J. Ind. Med., 9, 50, 1952.
95. Sjörgen, I., Hillerdal, G., Anderson, A., and Zetterström, O., Hard metal lung disease: importance of cobalt in coolants. Thorax, 35, 653, 1980.
96. Šarić M., Žuškin, E., Gonzi, M., Bronchoconstriction in potroom workers. Br. J. Ind. Med., 36, 211, 1979.
97. Fawcett, I. W., Taylor, A. J., and Pepys, J., Asthma due to inhaled chemical agents—epoxy resin systems containing phthalic acid anhydride, trimellitic acid anhydride and triethylene tetramine. Clin. Allergy, 7, 1, 1977.
98. Pauli, G., Bessot, J. C., Kopferschmitt, M. C., et al., Meatwrappers' asthma—identification of the causal agent. Clin. Allergy, 10, 263, 1980.

99. Zeiss, C. R., Patterson, R., and Pruzansky, J. J., Trimellitic anhydride–induced airway syndromes. J. Allergy Clin. Immunol., *60*, 96, 1977.

100. Alanko, K., Kerskinen, H., Bjorksten, F., and Ojanen, S., Immediate-type hypersensitivity to reactive dyes. Clin. Allergy, *8*, 25, 1978.

101. Pepys, J., Hutchcroft, B. J., and Breslin, A. B. X., Asthma due to inhaled chemical agents—persulphate salts and henna in hairdressers. Clin. Allergy, *6*, 399, 1976.

102. Hendrick, D. J., and Lane, D. J., Occupational formalin asthma. Br. J. Ind. Med., *34*, 11, 1977.

103. Davies, R. J., Hendrick, D. J., Pepys, J., Asthma due to inhaled chemical agents: ampicillin, benzyl penicillin, 6 amino penicillanic acid and related substances. Clin. Allergy, *4*, 227, 1974.

104. Davies, R. J., and Pepys, J., Asthma due to inhaled chemical agents—the macrolide antibiotic spiramycin. Clin. Allergy, *5*, 99, 1975.

105. Menon, M. P. S., and Das, A. K., Tetracycline asthma. Clin. Allergy, *7*, 285, 1977.

106. Feinberg, S. M., and Watrons, R. M., Atopy to simple chemical compounds—sulphone-chloramides. J. Allergy, *16*, 209, 1945.

107. Fawcett, I. W., Pepys, J., and Erooga, M. A., Asthma due to "glycyl compound" powder—an intermediate in production of salbutamol. Clin. Allergy, *6*, 405, 1976.

17

INDUSTRIAL BRONCHITIS AND OTHER NONSPECIFIC CONDITIONS AFFECTING THE AIRWAYS

W. Keith C. Morgan

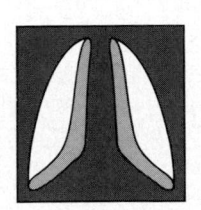

The harmful effects of inhaled dust have been recognized for many years and were alluded to by Agricola and Paracelsus in the sixteenth century. Subsequently Ramazzini in 1700 and Greenhow and Thackrah in the Victorian era emphasized the importance of dust, and in particular textile mill dust, as a cause of bronchitis.[1, 2] In the nineteenth century the term bronchitis was used loosely to indicate a condition characterized by cough and sputum, wheezing, and inanition. It is now obvious that what Thackrah and Greenhow referred to as bronchitis was not a single entity but comprised a large number of different conditions, including tuberculosis, bronchiectasis, byssinosis, asthma, and emphysema. The advent of chest radiography, along with advances in bacteriology, pathology, and epidemiology, made it possible to differentiate these various conditions.

Early in this century Haldane noted that coal miners had a lower mortality from bronchitis than metal miners.[3, 4] His observations were made at a time when cigarette smoking made little contribution to the presence of bronchitis and still less to mortality from this condition. At the turn of the century, the weight of tobacco smoked in the form of cigarettes was less than one fiftieth of that which is now smoked. Subsequently, mechanization greatly increased dust concentrations in British coal mines, and disabling respiratory disease in coal miners became much more prevalent between 1920 and 1940. That this was largely a consequence of coal workers' pneumoconiosis (CWP) became apparent as a result of the studies of the Pneumoconiosis Research Unit (PRU) of the Medical Research Council (MRC) of Great Britain.[5] Nevertheless, the exact role of bronchitis as a cause of increased mortality and morbidity in coal miners and other dust-exposed workers remained uncertain.

In 1961 the Ministry of Pensions and National Insurance in Great Britain conducted a morbidity survey of a 5 per cent sample of the entire working population of Britain. The survey suggested that bronchitis was an important cause of absence from work in the laboring classes, particularly affecting miners and quarrymen. This prompted the Ministry of Pensions to request the MRC to set up a Committee whose charge was to examine the role of occupation in the etiology of bronchitis. The ministry was concerned that while certain dust diseases such as silicosis and coal workers' pneumoconiosis were compensatable, bronchitis, if related to occupation, was not.

The Committee subsequently published a report that to a large extent exonerated dust as a specific cause of disabling bronchitis.[6] The report noted that multiple factors were involved in the etiology of chronic bronchitis, including cigarette smoking, air pollution, and occupationally related dust exposure, and that the symptoms were the same whatever the cause or causes. The Committee expressed the view that it was not going to prove possible to apportion the relative contributions of each etiological factor to the presence of bronchitis in any one individual. They conceded that epidemiological data suggested that dusty occupations had both higher morbidity and higher mortality from bronchitis; however, they pointed out that numerous anomalies existed, and in this context problems with job classification introduced appreciable bias. For example, the Registrar General's statistical surveys were and still are based on the number of workers with a condition among those currently doing a specific job compared with the total number of workers thus employed at the time of the census. Such statistics reflect the individual's job at the time of the census, while death certificates usually reflect the individual's original job or the job he has worked at for most of his life. Thus many coal miners work at the face for a good portion of their life, but as they become older tend to move to less arduous jobs. Problems with selective migration also existed, in that there was evidence to suggest that the fitter workers tended to leave the industry.[7]

Mortality statistics for bronchitis showed a steep gradient according to social class, with the greatest number of deaths occurring in social classes IV and V. However, increased mortality from bronchitis was also observed in the wives of coal miners and steel workers, and the Committee, not without justification, concluded from the epidemiological evidence available that the differences in mortality between the professional and laboring classes owed little to the effects of occupation and more to general socioeconomic and environmental factors. They commented on the role of cigarette smoking in particular. A similar situation prevailed in morbidity statistics for bronchitis. The relationship of coal dust exposure and bronchitis also showed significant variation according to the geographical location of the coal mine. It was suggested that some of these differences might be due to the differing severity of air pollution among regions.

The studies conducted by the PRU showed that coal miners had more

cough and sputum than did nonminers, and that they also occasionally had a lower ventilatory capacity than did a matched control population. While these factors suggested an occupational effect, the observation that miner's wives had an increased prevalence of cough and sputum as compared with nonminers' wives suggested that factors other than occupation might play a role. Based on the evidence then available, the Committee concluded that dust did not appear to be a significant factor in determining the prevalence of bronchitis in coal miners and other dust-exposed groups; however, they recommended that the situation be kept under review. At that time the MRC statement seemed entirely reasonable despite the large number of hostile responses to its publication. The arguments used to refute the Committee's conclusions seemed based on clinical impression and political ideology rather than objective evidence.[8-10] Since the report, additional evidence has become available that permits a reappraisal.

Definition and Pathology of Bronchitis

For many years the term bronchitis implied a condition characterized by cough and sputum, usually either associated with a reduction in ventilatory capacity or likely to lead to one. Subjects with these symptoms and concomitant chronic air flow obstruction were often diagnosed as having chronic bronchitis and emphysema, a practice from which it was inferred that the two diseases were invariably associated and were part and parcel of the same process. At the time the MRC Committee published its statement, it was known that not all subjects with chronic bronchitis demonstrated a decrement in their FEV_1, but nowhere did the Committee define the term bronchitis. However, it was assumed that there was a relationship between the symptoms of cough and sputum and a decreased ventilatory capacity, and that sooner or later most or all subjects with chronic bronchitis would develop chronic air flow obstruction. The attempt of the MRC and Fletcher and colleagues to subdivide bronchitis into simple bronchitis, which is characterized by the presence of cough and sputum in the absence of airways obstruction, and obstructive bronchitis was the first step taken toward a better understanding of the implications of a diagnosis of bronchitis.[11] It was the acceptance and general use of the MRC definition of chronic bronchitis in terms of symptoms without reference to lung function, namely, the presence of cough and sputum for three months of a year for two consecutive years, that facilitated an appreciation of the pathophysiology of this condition.[12]

The characteristic pathological features of bronchitis were first described by Reid and consist of an increase in the mucus-secreting glands of the airways.[13, 14] In the human it is the mucous glands of the large airways that are mostly responsible for mucus secretion and that are predominantly involved in chronic bronchitis. The goblet cells which are found in the smaller airways are also increased in number, but the changes

in them tend to be less impressive. Bronchitis is best quantified by means of the Reid index, which is the ratio of the depth of mucous glands (gland thickness) to the bronchial wall thickness as measured from the surface of the respiratory epithelium to the cartilage.[14] It is now clear that mucous gland hypertrophy occurs as a result of any chronic irritant effect on the airways and that cigarette smoke, dust, and air pollutants, such as sulfur dioxide, ozone, and ammonia, not to mention particulate matter, can all act as the inciting factor.[14a] The heavier and the longer the period of exposure, the greater the likelihood of developing bronchitis. In trying to study the effects and frequency of bronchitis in a working population, it becomes evident that there are two important confounding factors, namely, cigarette smoking and age. In smokers, cigarette smoking completely overshadows the effects of dust and air pollutants. In women, the prevalence of bronchitis does not show the usual clear-cut relationship to smoking and often appears to be better related to educational status. This is a consequence of the fact that middle- and upper-class women are reluctant to admit to coughing up sputum.

Bronchitis, Ventilatory Impairment, and Exposure to Dust. When compared with a comparable control population, workers in many dusty occupations show an increased prevalence of cough and sputum. Such observations have been made in coal miners, steel workers, foundrymen, textile mill workers, gold miners, and cement workers.[15-24] In some instances, a slight reduction in ventilatory capacity has been observed to accompany the increased prevalence of bronchitis.[15, 16, 22] Nevertheless, a reduction in the FEV_1 is not always present and anomalous findings are frequent. The reduced ventilatory capacity observed in coal and gold miners in the absence of progressive massive fibrosis (PMF) can be explained by two hypotheses:

1. That there exists a type of air flow obstruction peculiar to the dusty trades and which affects miners with and without simple pneumoconiosis. This could be either emphysema or bronchitis or both.

2. That differential migration is responsible. Thus, were the fitter and younger men to move out of the industry within a few months or years of starting work, those who remain would have substantially reduced pulmonary function and would be a nonrepresentative sample of the total working population.

The second hypothesis needs consideration, since Cochrane and others have suggested that when unemployment is high, the fittest migrate and seek employment elsewhere.[7] There is, however, little evidence to suggest that this is true at the present time, and a study by McClintock of new entrants into coal mining in Britain indicated that those who are less fit tend to leave the industry first and in addition have more symptoms at the time of entry.[25] The fitter tend to stay in the industry, and perhaps this explains why miners with radiographic evidence of category 3 simple pneumoconiosis often have a higher ventilatory capacity than do those with lower categories.

The Relationship of Obstructive Emphysema to Dust Exposure

A series of papers from South Wales has advanced the hypothesis that coal miners have a higher prevalence of emphysema than do non-miners.[26-28] These studies attempted to relate emphysema demonstrated at postmortem study to measurements of lung function and radiographic category made before death. Emphysema was quantified by point counting. The subjects had all been referred to a pneumoconiosis panel and as a result had radiographic and pulmonary function tests performed for compensation purposes. The authors claimed to have shown a relationship between the presence of simple and complicated CWP and antemortem pulmonary impairment as diagnosed by a reduction in the FEV_1. They further suggested that the p, or punctate, opacity of simple CWP was associated with emphysema more frequently than the larger q and r types of rounded opacities. Their first paper contained the statement that "there is no reason why these deaths should not provide a true sample of the experience of men with this disease." One can only assume that this generalization was meant to imply that their sample was representative of coal miners and ex-miners, not only in Wales, but elsewhere in Britain and in other countries as well. That their group of disability claimants could be regarded as a random and unbiased sample was disputed by Gilson and Oldham, who suggested that miners who had been awarded disability could hardly be regarded as comparable to those who had not.[29] Similarly, in the first paper, Ryder et al. attempted to relate the presence of emphysema to the radiographic category of pneumoconiosis diagnosed from the last chest film prior to death.[26] In doing so they made no distinction between subjects with simple and complicated disease. Since the latter is known to lead to airways obstruction in the absence of smoking, such an assumption can only lead to fallacious results. In the second paper the authors still chose not to separate subjects with simple CWP from those with PMF,[27] and the same criticisms were leveled at them by Oldham and Berry.[30] Numerous other anomalies are present in their results, in particular the fact that miners with category 2 and 3 simple pneumoconiosis had an FEV_1 which was 0.8 L below the predicted value, while those who had a clear chest x-ray had an FEV_1 which was 1.25 L below the predicted value.

Seaton and others compared ventilatory capacity, lung volumes, and diffusing capacity with the various types of small rounded opacity found in the chest film of a group of nonsmoking United States coal miners.[31] Apart from a slight reduction in the diffusing capacity of miners with the punctate opacity (p type), no other differences were noted. Were significant emphysema present in miners with the p type of opacity, the residual volume and total lung capacity might have been expected to be increased when compared to miners with the q and r types of opacity, but no such changes were evident. Nevertheless, an earlier and more extensive study

of the lung volumes of a large group of working coal miners had shown that miners with and without simple CWP had a slight increase in total lung capacity (TLC) and residual volume (RV) and that increasing category of simple CWP was associated with an increment in RV.[32] This finding was thought to suggest either that there was a slight loss of elastic recoil in miners with simple pneumoconiosis or that some small airways obstruction was present. Although increasing category of simple CWP was associated with a concomitant increase in RV, no corresponding increase in obstruction was noted with increasing category of CWP. The study, however, did not separate the subjects according to the type of small rounded opacity, viz., p, q, or r.

Shortly thereafter, Waters et al. considered the possibility that the p type of opacity was associated with decreased longevity, as might be expected were this type of opacity associated with emphysema and a lower ventilatory capacity.[33] They were unable to demonstrate any difference in life expectancy of miners with the various types of small rounded opacity.

It must, however, be conceded that there is evidence that the p type of opacity is associated with certain physiological abnormalities that suggest that there are anatomical changes present in the lungs not seen in those men who have the q and r types of opacity. Thus Hankinson and co-workers observed that miners with the p type of opacity have increased air space size, suggesting that there is a dilatation of either the alveoli or the respiratory bronchioles.[34] However, they were unable to detect any differences in lung function between miners with p, q, and r type opacities. Recent observations made by the Institute of Occupational Medicine have likewise suggested that the radiographic presence of pneumoconiosis is associated with an increased prevalence of centriacinar emphysema.[35] Elsewhere, Musk and colleagues have shown that subjects with the p and r types of opacities have a reduction in their diffusing capacity when compared to miners with the q type of opacity.[36] According to these authors, several subjects with the p type of opacities also demonstrated certain physiological features of emphysema. The elastic recoil at TLC of miners with p type of opacities was minimally reduced as compared to those subjects with q and r type of opacities. However, their mean RV and RV/TLC was smaller than that of subjects with q and r type of opacities. Were the emphysema that is reported to occur in the p type of opacity associated with significant ventilatory impairment, it should be reflected by a significant decrease in ventilatory capacity. As such, any decrement that was present in life was not of a magnitude to be statistically significant. To the disinterested observer, the changes in lung function noted by Musk and colleagues in their sample of miners with the p type of opacity suggested emphysema in some subjects and fibrosis in others. No consistent trend was observed, and the results serve to confuse rather than clarify.

Although focal emphysema occurs more commonly in coal miners with simple CWP and is related to years spent working at the face,[36a] there

is still no evidence that the increased prevalence of emphysema in such subjects leads to increased airways obstruction. In this connection it must be remembered that the postmortem demonstration of emphysema often correlates poorly with antemortem evidence of airways obstruction.[37]

When asymptomatic cigarette smokers assume the supine position, the usual increment in the diffusing capacity (DL_{CO}) that occurs in normal subjects is significantly less. In contrast, in nonsmoking miners with simple CWP, the assumption of the supine position is associated with the normal increase in DL_{CO}. This has important implications, since the failure of asymptomatic cigarette smokers to respond in the usual fashion by increasing their DL_{CO} suggests that this phenomenon is a consequence of early upper-lobe emphysema. Were coal miners with simple CWP to have significant centrilobular emphysema, they should behave in a fashion similar to asymptomatic cigarette smokers. Thus the evidence weighs heavily against dust-induced emphysema being responsible for the lower ventilatory capacity that has been noted to occur in coal miners.

Bronchitis and Dust Exposure

The statement of the Medical Research Council in 1966 implied that bronchitis was a single response to a variety of inhaled agents and that it was impossible to apportion the contribution of each agent to the patient's symptoms and pulmonary impairment.[6] The Committee also included an addendum phrased in the following terms: "Nor is there any reason to believe that it will sometime be possible to determine in any particular individual with chronic bronchitis, how much of his or her illness is attributable to any particular environmental factor."[11] While this statement still retains some element of truth, it is now clear from epidemiological studies that it is possible to assess the role of cigarette smoking versus dust in the etiology of chronic air flow obstruction in those who work in the dusty trades.[16, 39, 40]

As mentioned earlier, for many years the term bronchitis was taken to imply a condition characterized by cough and sputum, which, although not always associated with breathlessness, presaged the onset of ventilatory impairment. This belief has now been shown to be fallacious, and the studies of Fletcher and Peto[41] and of Bates[42] made it clear that, while both bronchitis and airways obstruction are related to smoking, they are separate responses to the same insult. Most subjects who have smoked cigarettes for more than five years develop some cough and sputum. This is a consequence of the hypersecretion of mucus and the mucous gland hypertrophy already described. Aside from cigarette smoking, air pollutants and dust have a similar effect. The main pathological changes seen in bronchitis occur in the large airways. The other response seen in cigarette smokers occurs in the small airways, that is to say, those distal to the 12th generation, and eventually leads to irreversible airways obstruction and emphysema. However, only in 12 to 15 per cent of cigarette

smokers does significant airways obstruction develop.[41] Unlike chronic bronchitis, which tends to clear up when a subject has stopped smoking, emphysema and the irreversible obstruction that are associated with small airways pathology do not improve with the cessation of smoking.

Numerous investigations have shown that the long-continued inhalation of dust leads to the development of bronchitis as manifested by chronic cough and sputum.[16-23, 42] Over the past several years a definite relationship between the prevalence of these symptoms and the level of dust exposure has been demonstrated both in coal miners[16, 44] and in South African gold miners.[22] It is clear that those miners who work in the most dusty conditions, namely, at the coal face, are far more likely to develop bronchitis. It becomes difficult, however, to separate the effects of cigarette smoking and dust in cigarette smokers, since the effects of smoking overwhelm those of dust. For the most part it is possible to detect the consequences of dust exposure only in nonsmokers, although in some studies cigarette smoking and dust appear to have had a synergistic effect.[21]

Bronchitis and Ventilatory Capacity

Although it has been possible to show a relationship between dust exposure and the prevalence of bronchitis, it has been much more difficult to demonstrate a dust-induced reduction of ventilatory capacity. Kibelstis et al. noted a difference in the FEV_1 between nonsmoking face workers and nonsmoking surface workers.[16] The difference, however, was relatively small and, although statistically significant, could hardly be regarded as of great clinical importance. Thus the FEV_1 in the surface workers was 101 per cent of the predicted value, while that of the face workers was 98 per cent. The longitudinal studies that have been conducted in British coal miners over the past 25 years have demonstrated a progressive decrement in the FEV_1 with cumulative dust exposure.[45] These studies have also shown that the presence of simple pneumoconiosis does not lead to an additional decrement above and beyond that attributable to dust exposure. The results were taken to indicate that the dust-induced decrement in the ventilatory capacity was of the same order of magnitude as that due to cigarette smoking. Unfortunately the National Coal Board used current smoking habits rather than pack/years as their index of smoking exposure. This assumes that 20 cigarettes a day for 5 years has the same effect as 20 cigarettes a day for 30 years. In our studies of bronchitis, it became evident that current smoking habits, although correlating well with the prevalence of bronchitis, relate far less well to the presence of ventilatory impairment.[16]

Factors Influencing Ventilatory Capacity. The relative importance of cigarette smoking and dust in inducing airways obstruction has been the subject of considerable discussion recently. Rogan and colleagues showed a progressive decline in ventilatory capacity that was related to

age, with the decline being greater in smokers than in nonsmokers.[45] Although in each age group the men in the dustiest jobs had a slightly lower FEV_1 than men in less dusty jobs, the age-related progression coefficients for low, medium, and high dust-exposed groups were the same. This would suggest that the differences in ventilatory capacity were a consequence of some change in the airways that was a manifestation of current dust exposure but that did not worsen with age.

Were dust to have the same effect on ventilatory capacity as does cigarette smoking, this should be revealed in mortality studies. However, coal miners have a normal life expectancy, and simple pneumoconiosis does not lead to an increased standardized mortality ratio (SMR).[47, 48] Moreover, years spent underground, which, although not a direct measure of dust exposure, correlates well with the prevalence of simple pneumoconiosis, has been shown to have no effect on the SMR, while in contrast, cigarette smoking has been shown to have a profound effect.[48]

Between 1958 and 1969 Brinkman and colleagues carried out a well-planned series of epidemiological investigations in an industrial population that was exposed to various dusts.[40, 49–51] The population studied was composed of four groups:

1. Those with no industrial exposure
2. Those exposed to a variety of inert dusts
3. Those exposed to silica dust but without radiographic evidence of silicosis
4. Those exposed to silica with radiographic evidence of silicosis

Each subject underwent serial tests of ventilatory capacity and had serial chest films taken. The results of these well-conducted investigations have been largely ignored, although it was apparent that the major influences affecting the rate of decline of ventilatory capacity were age and cigarette smoking. Bronchitis and occupational exposure to dust made a relatively small contribution to the annual decrement in FEV_1.[49–51]

An extensive West German study of 6700 workers employed in coal mines, steel works, cement works, asbestos factories, heavy engineering trades, and plants making ceramics and factory ware has recently been published. A questionnaire concerning smoking habits and occupational history was administered to each subject.[52] A clinical examination, chest radiograph, and spirometry were carried out along with measurement of airways resistance and arterial blood gas analysis. In each workplace, dust and other contaminants were measured so that the subjects could be divided into those with high, moderate, and low dust exposure. This study showed that the most important factors relating to the prevalence of bronchitis and airways obstruction were age and smoking habits. In younger workers, there seemed to be an additive effect of smoking, age, and dust; the combined effect of all three equaling the sum of their separate effects. In older workers, smoking appeared to play a relatively greater role, suggesting that while dust may have played a role in the induction of bronchitis and in the development of a minor degree of

ventilatory impairment, the dust-related decrement in ventilatory capacity was not progressive. These studies suggested that by far the most common cause of both bronchitis and airways obstruction was cigarette smoking. Similar findings have been noted in South African gold miners, in whom the contribution of cigarette smoking has been shown to be 14 to 20 times greater than that of mine dust.[53]

Tests of Ventilatory Capacity. The FEV_1 and other commonly used tests of ventilatory capacity mainly reflect the behavior of the large airways during dynamic compression. Much the same can be said for the measurment of the total airways resistance (Raw), which likewise depends mainly on the resistance to flow in the trachea and lobar, segmental, and subsegmental bronchi. Peripheral airways obstruction is difficult to detect with standard tests of ventilatory capacity, in particular the FEV_1 and the FVC. Since 85 to 90 per cent of the total Raw is located in the large airways, it is possible for the resistance in the peripheral airways to double or even quadruple and yet for the FEV_1 and Raw to remain within the predicted normal range.

In the past decade a variety of methods have been used to detect changes in peripheral airways when the FEV_1 and Raw remain normal. These include the use of the flow volume loop, either alone or with helium oxygen mixtures, measurements of closing volume and frequency dependence of dynamic compliance, the determination of alveolo-arterial oxygen gradients, and measurement of residual volume.[54] The flow volume curve can be usefully applied in epidemiological studies. A typical maximal forced expiratory flow volume curve is shown in Figure 17-1. Peak flow and flow at 25 per cent of the vital capacity (FEF_{25}) depend on the state of the large airways. Flow at 50 per cent of the vital capacity (FEF_{50}) is dependent on both small and large airways, while flows at 75 per cent of the vital capacity and 90 per cent of the vital capacity (FEF_{75} and FEF_{90}) reflect the mechanical properties of the lung surrounding the small airways and the resistance to flow in them.

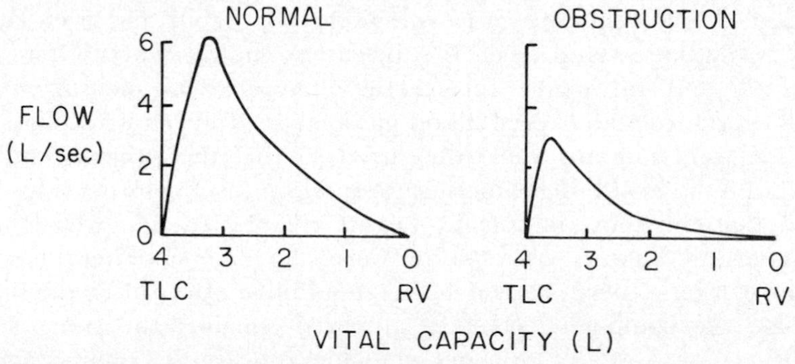

Figure 17-1. A normal expiratory flow volume curve and that of an obstructed subject for comparison. (Reproduced by permission of the editor of the British Journal of Industrial Medicine, *35*, 285, 1978.)

Extensive epidemiological studies of coal miners have been carried out in which the flow volume loop has been used. Flows at various lung volumes have been related to various factors including age, height, radiographic category of pneumoconiosis, cigarette smoking, and years spent underground.[55] Cigarette smoking affects flows at all lung volumes; however, in nonsmoking coal miners with cough and sputum, some effect on ventilatory function was apparent in that peak flow, the FEF_{25}, and FEF_{50} were somewhat reduced (Table 17–1). In contrast the FEF_{75} and FEF_{90} remained relatively unchanged; indeed there was a suggestion that the FEF_{90} of the nonsmoking miners was higher than that of the non-bronchitic nonsmokers. This was explained by an increase in the residual volume of the bronchitic nonsmokers.

While flow rates are customarily expressed as a percentage of the vital capacity, there are problems related to this mode of expression. Thus flows are related to lung volume, and should lung volume change so that the residual volume increases at the expense of the vital capacity, a not uncommon happening, then spuriously high values for the flow rates may be obtained if they are expressed as a percentage of FVC. It is therefore preferable to express flow rates either as a percentage of total lung capacity or ideally at absolute lung volumes.

In a series of studies, Hankinson and colleagues have described the physiological impairments that are associated with the inhalation of dust and cigarette smoke.[55, 56] These studies relied on flow volume curves as a means of assessing ventilatory capacity, but in addition to the standard spirometric measurements, lung volumes were calculated by a radiological method utilizing posteroanterior and left lateral chest films. Since total lung capacity could be measured, it was possible to express the flow rates not only as a percentage of total lung capacity but also at absolute lung volumes.[56] These workers were able to select four age- and height-matched groups based on their smoking history and whether or not they had bronchitis as diagnosed by the presence of daily cough and sputum for three months a year for two consecutive years. Subjects with progressive massive fibrosis were excluded as were ex-smokers. Four groups each containing 428 subjects were selected. These consisted of (1) smokers with bronchitis, (2) smokers without bronchitis, (3) nonsmokers with bronchitis (industrial bronchitis), and (4) nonsmokers without bronchitis.

Figures 17–2 and 17–3 show the mean maximal expiratory flows of the four groups expressed as a percentage of vital capacity and subsequently at absolute lung volumes. It is evident that cigarette smoking affects flows at all lung volumes. The more heavily the subject smoked, the more likely he was to have bronchitis and the greater the effect on ventilatory capacity. It will be noted, however, that those subjects who were nonsmoking bronchitics showed decreased flow rates at high lung volumes. At lower lung volumes the changes were less evident, at least when the flows were expressed as a percentage of vital capacity. When the flows were expressed at absolute lung volumes, several interesting

Table 17–1. FACTORS INFLUENCING EXPIRATORY FLOW RATES IN COAL MINERS

Variable	Multiple Regression Analysis Regression Coefficients for Flow Rates in 1696 Miners (Nonsmokers)				
	Peak Flow	FEF_{25}	FEF_{50}	FEF_{75}	FEF_{90}
Age (years)	−0.0278	−0.0197	−0.0366	−0.0358	−0.0139
Height (cm)	0.0339	0.0193	0.0144	0.0125	0.0085
Weight (kg)	0.0132	0.0132	0.0062	−0.0053	−0.0075
Underground experience (years)	−0.0349	−0.0319	−0.0155	−0.0001*	−0.0012*
Constant (liters/second)	3.2875	4.0725	3.3087	1.4550	0.2052

*Not significant.

features emerged. It is again evident that subjects with industrial bronchitis show a significant reduction in their peak flow and in flows measured from the early portion of their curve. A lesser effect on the small airways is also apparent. What is also clear is that not only do the smokers have an increased residual volume but also that their total lung capacity is likewise increased. This implies that cigarette smoking leads to a loss of elastic recoil, and that these parenchymal changes occur early, are permanent, are a consequence of emphysema, and may occur before the subject has symptoms. Industrial bronchitis, on the other hand, is not associated with an increase in the TLC and therefore is unassociated with the development of emphysema and its associated loss of elastic recoil.

In summary, the present evidence for the existence of industrial bronchitis is overwhelming, and it is equally clear that it is an entity distinct from pneumoconiosis. Industrial bronchitis is a nonspecific response to a variety of agents, including inert dusts and various gases and vapors. The predominant symptoms are those of cough and sputum, and for the most part, these symptoms are of diagnostic import only in nonsmokers. The condition is due to the deposition of particles that are mostly between 3 and 10 microns and are thus larger than the usual

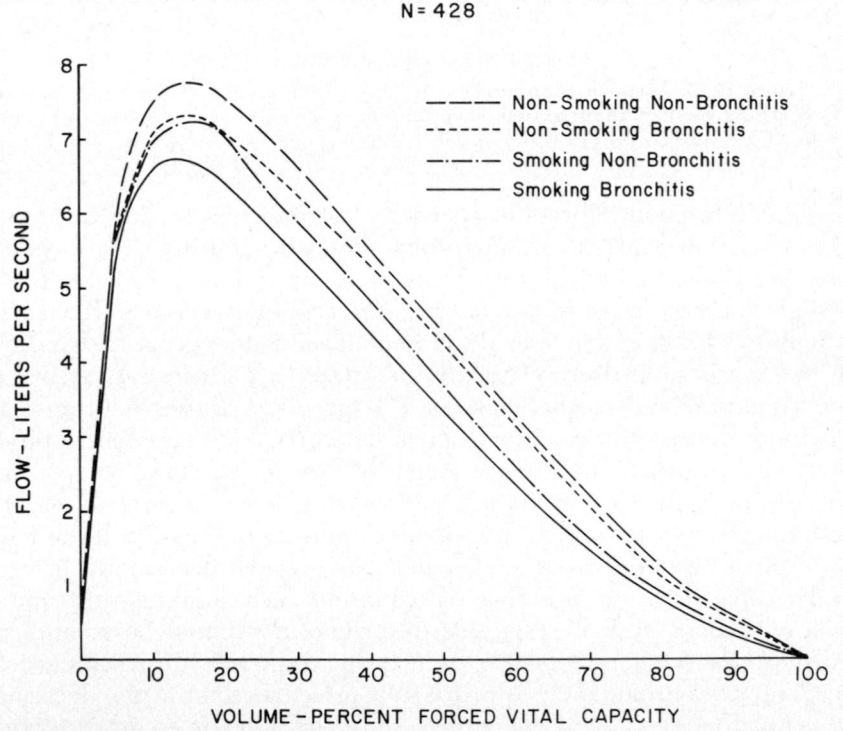

Figure 17–2. Maximal expiratory flows of the four groups of coal miners expressed as a percentage of vital capacity. (Reproduced by permission of the editor of the American Review of Respiratory Disease, *116*, 175, 1977.)

N= 428

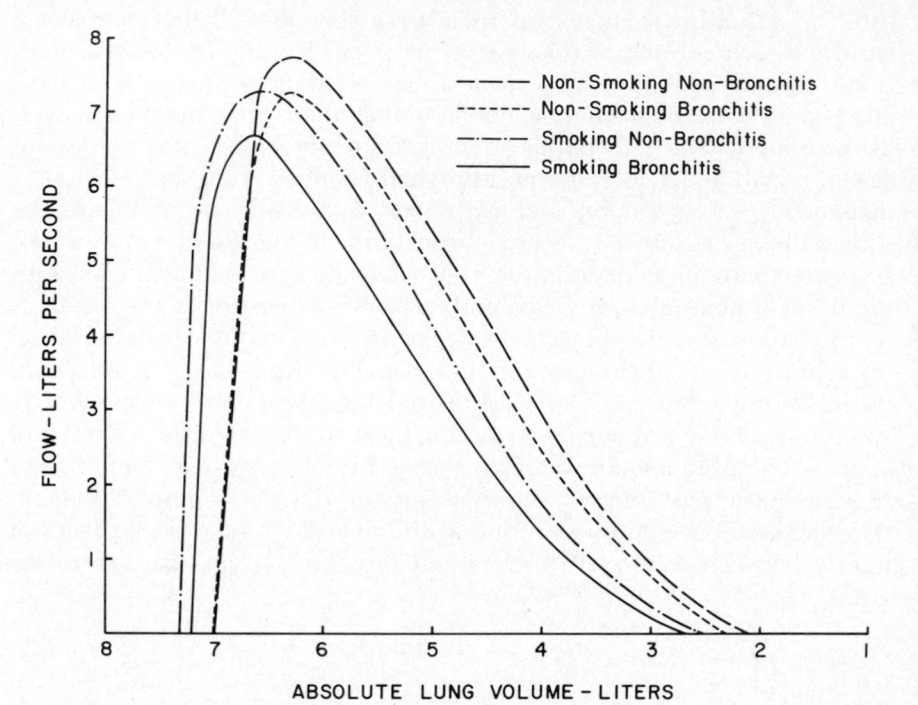

Figure 17–3. Maximal expiratory flows of the four groups of miners expressed as absolute lung volumes. (Reproduced by permission of the editor of the American Review of Respiratory Disease, *116*, 175, 1977.)

respirable fraction. Since such particles are removed by the mucociliary escalator, they leave no radiographic stigmata. Industrial bronchitis is associated with decreased flow in the large airways and occasionally with a slight increase in residual volume. The small airways are affected but usually to a lesser extent. The decrement in ventilatory capacity that occurs in this condition is dose related, but because the particles responsible for the condition are of the most part larger than those that cause the pneumoconioses, there is often only a fair correlation between respirable dust measurements and the prevalence of bronchitis. At the present time, there is no evidence that industrial bronchitis leads to emphysema. The introduction of regulations to control or limit respirable dust levels based on evidence derived from studies that have related decrements in ventilatory capacity or the presence of symptoms such as cough and sputum to a particular level of respirable dust exposure cannot be scientifically justified. Recommendations to reduce the respirable dust standard for coal and silica are unlikely to prove fully effective as far as the decrement in ventilatory capacity is concerned, since the latter is a consequence of industrial bronchitis, not pneumoconiosis. Moreover, monitoring pulmonary function in those exposed to coal dust and silica will yield little or no

useful information concerning CWP or silicosis. The prevalence and incidence of industrial bronchitis are likely to be better related to measurements of total dust or to measurement of those particles that range from 0.5 to 20 microns than to respirable dust. One of the more important questions that remains unanswered is whether the reduction in ventilatory capacity induced by industrial bronchitis is reversible. It is well recognized that the bronchitis of cigarette smokers clears up a few months after the subject stops smoking, but this is not true of the impairment associated with concomitant emphysema. Whether there is an improvement in symptoms and ventilatory capacity in subjects with industrial bronchitis when dust exposure terminates is as yet unknown.

Respiratory Effects of Fire Fighting

The acute effects of smoke inhalation on lung function depend to a large extent on the various fumes and gases that are inhaled. Prolonged exposure to high concentrations is likely to lead to severe acute effects.[57–59] Symptoms of acute exposure include shortness of breath, retrosternal burning pain, burning sensation in the eyes, dry cough, and headache. Upper airway involvement and laryngitis are known to occur.[60] Lung function measurements have been made immediately and at intervals following acute exposure.[59, 61] The consequence of acute exposure to high concentrations of toluene diisocyanate following a fire have been described and include various neurological and physiological sequelae.[62] In certain instances acute exposure has been shown to lead to small reversible changes in the FEV_1, while in others more chronic effects have been reported.[57–59, 61] Hypoxia and carboxyhemoglobinemia immediately following smoke inhalation are known to affect a high proportion of those who have recently been exposed to a fire.[58, 59]

Several cross-sectional studies have demonstrated an association between fire fighting, lung disease, and decrements in lung function.[63–65] In one study of a cohort of Boston fire fighters who were followed for a year, an increased rate of decline for the FVC and FEV_1 was demonstrated.[65] Repeat studies three years later showed no such decline.[66] A longitudinal study of 168 fire fighters and 1476 controls was carried out by Sparrow and colleagues.[67] The authors found that fire fighters had a greater annual loss of pulmonary function than did the reference group and that the occupational effects could not be explained by smoking habits, age, height, or other factors. Fire fighters also tended to have more symptoms than did the reference group. Unfortunately, this study relied on current smoking habits rather than pack/years and, as mentioned previously, while bronchitis correlates well with current smoking habits, ventilatory capacity is far better related to lifelong cigarette consumption as measured by pack/years. A follow-up study of a group of 30 fire fighters over a period of 15 months has recently been published.[61] There was

some suggestion that the FVC and FEV_1 of those exposed were declining at a more rapid rate than the matched control subjects. In reviewing the published evidence it would seem that fire fighters tend to have more respiratory symptoms than do nonexposed reference groups. Acute and usually transient decrements in ventilatory capacity are common following inhalation of smoke and dense fumes, but whether there is an increased annual decline in ventilatory capacity is still unsettled. Although some studies have produced limited circumstantial evidence in favor of this belief, at least in selected groups of fire fighters, the effect on ventilatory capacity is likely to be small, since it is not reflected in the SMR of fire fighters, at least for respiratory disease.[68]

Respiratory Effects of Grain Dust

Ramazzini in 1700 described "diseases of sifters and measurers of grain." He recognized that exposure to grain dust had both acute and chronic effects. Over the past several years there has been a spate of investigations, most of which have taken place in Canada and the United States, designed to look into the hazards of those exposed to grain dust. It is becoming increasingly evident that the effects of grain dust inhalation are far more complex than was originally thought.

Grain dust contains not only the plant matter of the various grains (which range from wheat and rye to rapeseed and sunflower seeds) but also numerous other contaminants. The latter include fungal spores such as Cladosporium and Aspergillus; animal matter including weevils, bird and rodent droppings, and mites; fertilizers; pesticides; and various soils and dust, some of which contains free silica.

The acute effects of exposure to grain dust include conjunctivitis and rhinitis.[70] In addition, some subjects develop grain asthma.[71,72] This latter condition has been described in Chapter 16. The onset of grain asthma may be immediate or delayed for several hours.[72, 73] Recurrent nocturnal asthma has likewise been described, and there is some suggestion that the grain mite Glycyphagus destructor might be an important allergen, although skin and precipitin tests are usually negative.[73, 74] Surveys of grain elevator workers show a lower than normal prevalence of asthma, presumably because most of the susceptible population develop the condition and leave the job early.

Aside from asthma, certain workers develop an acute febrile response characterized by rigors, chills, and sundry aches and pains. This is known as grain fever.[70–72] It occurs after heavy exposure or on return to work. Although the etiology of grain fever is unknown, gram-negative endotoxins must be considered as a likely cause. Extrinsic allergic alveolitis also occasionally occurs in those exposed to grain, usually farmers, and is probably due to a number of fungi, including aspergilli. It is not, as was formerly believed, due to Sitophilus granarius.

The chronic effects of grain dust are less well understood. There seems little doubt that prolonged high exposure can induce both cough and sputum. This may be regarded as a form of industrial bronchitis, since it seems to to be a nonspecific response to dust.[74, 75] Studies of pulmonary function in grain workers have yielded conflicting results, but for the most part seem to suggest that smoking exaggerates the effects of exposure to grain dust. Nonsmokers, for the most part, appear to have normal or near normal pulmonary function.[70, 74–76] Many of the studies of lung function have relied on so-called sensitive tests of ventilatory capacity, such as the FEF_{25-75}, closing volume, and maximal expiratory flow at low lung volumes.[76] The significance of these tests in regard to predicting permanent disability is either dubious or nonexistent. Broder and colleagues have shown that absence from work because of temporary layoffs is associated with a decrease in the symptoms of cough and sputum. Continued exposure, however, usually led to a gradual increase in the prevalence and severity of those symptoms.[77] Those who continued to work also tended to have lower maximal expiratory flow rates. Rehiring of those who were initially laid off was associated with a marked increase in the symptoms and a corresponding fall in the ventilatory capacity. Further studies by the same group have suggested that acute exposure may lead to minor restrictive impairment. The changes induced by exposure are small, but affect both TLC and FVC.[78]

It is becoming increasingly clear that both farmers and those who are exposed to grain may develop a number of diverse respiratory conditions. Since the etiology of some of these conditions remains unknown, prevention is often difficult or impracticable at the present time.[79]

References

1. Greenhow, E. H., Report of the Medical Office of the Privy Council, 1860. Appendix VI, London, H. M. Stationery Office, 1861.
2. Thackrah, C. T., The Effects of Arts, Trades and Professions and of the Civic States and Habits of Living on Health and Longevity, 2nd ed. London, Longman, 1832.
3. Haldane, J. S., The effects of inhaling dust applicable for stone-dusting in coal mines. 7th Report of Explosives in Mines Committee, BMD 8122. London, H. M. Stationery Office, 1915.
4. Haldane, J. S., Quoted in Hunter, D., ed., Diseases of the Occupations, 6th ed. London, Hodder and Stoughton, 1978, pp. 1016–1017.
5. Gilson, J. C., and Hugh-Jones, P., Lung function in coal workers' pneumoconiosis. Medical Research Council's Special Report Series No. 290, London, H. M. Stationery Office, 1955.
6. Medical Research Council, Chronic bronchitis and occupation. Br. Med. J., 1, 101, 1966.
7. Cochrane, A. L., Higgins, I. T. T., and Thomas, J., Pulmonary ventilation functions of coal miners in various areas in relation to x-ray category of pneumoconiosis. Br. J. Prev. Soc. Med.15, 1, 1961.
8. Gough, J., Chronic bronchitis and occupation. Br. Med. J., 1, 480, 1966.
9. Pemberton, J., Occupational lung disease. Br. Med. J., 1, 609, 1966.
10. McLaughlin, A. I. G. Chronic bronchitis and occupation. Br. Med. J., 1, 354, 1966.
11. Fletcher, C. M., Elmes, P. C., Fairbairn, A. S., and Wood, C. H., The significance of respiratory symptoms and the diagnosis of chronic bronchitis in the working population. Br. Med. J., 2, 252, 1969.

12. Medical Research Council, Definition of chronic bronchitis for clinical epidemiological purposes. Lancet, 1, 775, 1965.
13. Reid, L., Pathology of chronic bronchitis. Lancet, 1, 275, 1954.
14. Reid, L., A measurement of the bronchial mucous gland layer: a diagnostic yardstick in chronic bronchitis. Thorax, 15, 132, 1960.
14a. Douglas A. N., Lamb, D., and Ruckley, V. A., Bronchial gland dimensions in coal miners: influence of smoking and dust exposure. Thorax, 37, 760, 1982.
15. Higgins, I. T. T., Chronic respiratory disease in mining communities. Ann. N. Y. Acad. Sci., 200, 197, 1972.
16. Kibelstis, J. A., Morgan, E. J., Reger, R. B., et al., Prevalence of bronchitis and airway obstruction in American bituminous coal miners. Am. Rev. Respir. Dis., 108, 886, 1973.
17. Worth, G. L., Gasthaus, W., Lugning, K., et al., Kritische Bermerkungen zur Diagnostik des Lungenemphysems bei Kohlenbergarbeitern. Arch. Gewerbeoath Gewerbehyg., 17, 442, 1959.
18. Lowe, C. R., Chronic bronchitis and occupation. Proc. R. Soc. Med., 61, 98, 1968.
19. Lowe, C. R., Campbell, H., and Khosla, T., Bronchitis in two integrated steelworks. III. Respiratory signs and ventilatory capacity related to atmospheric pollution. Br. J. Ind. Med., 27, 358, 1970.
20. Merchant, J. A., Kilburn, K. H., O'Fallon, W. M., et al., Byssinosis and chronic bronchitis among cotton textile workers. Ann. Intern. Med., 76, 423, 1972.
21. Sluis-Cremer, G. J., Walters, L. G., and Sichel, H. S., Chronic bronchitis in miners and non-miners: an epidemiological survey of a community in the gold-mining area in the Transvaal. Br. J. Ind. Med., 24, 1, 1967.
22. Irwig, L. M., and Rocks, P., Lung function and respiratory symptoms in silicotic and non-silicotic gold miners. Am. Rev. Respir. Dis., 117, 429, 1978.
23. Kalacic, I., Ventilatory lung function in cement workers. Arch. Environ. Health, 26, 84, 1973.
24. Rom, W. N., Kanner, R. E., Renzetti, A. D., et al., Respiratory disease in Utah coal miners. Am. Rev. Respir. Dis., 123, 372, 1981.
25. McLintock, J. C., The selection of juvenile entrants to mining. Br. J. Ind. Med., 28, 45, 1971.
26. Ryder, R., Lyons, J. P., Campbell, H., and Gough, J., Emphysema in coal workers' pneumoconiosis. Br. Med. J., 3, 481, 1970.
27. Lyons, J. P., Ryder, R., Campbell, H., and Gough, J., Pulmonary disability in coalworkers: pneumoconiosis. Br. Med. J., 1, 713, 1972.
28. Lyons, J. P., and Campbell, H., Evolution of disability in coalworkers' pneumoconiosis. Thorax, 31, 527, 1976.
29. Gilson, J. C., and Oldham, P. D., Coal workers' pneumoconiosis. Br. Med. J., 4, 305, 1970.
30. Oldham, P. D., and Berry, G., Coal miners' pneumoconiosis. Br. Med. J., 2, 292, 1970.
31. Seaton, A., Lapp, N. L., and Morgan, W. K. C., Relationship of pulmonary impairment in simple coalworkers' pneumoconiosis to type of radiographic opacity. Br. J. Ind. Med., 29, 50, 1972.
32. Morgan, W. K. C., Burgess, D. B., Lapp, N. L., et al., Hyperinflation of the lungs in coal miners. Thorax, 26, 585, 1971.
33. Waters, W. E., Cochrane, A. L., and Moore, F., Mortality in punctiform type of coalworkers' pneumoconiosis. Br. J. Ind. Med., 31, 196, 1974.
34. Hankinson, J. L., Palmes, E. D., and Lapp, N. L., Pulmonary air space size in coal miners. Am. Rev. Respir. Dis., 119, 391, 1979.
35. Ruckley, V. A., Chapman, J. S., Collings, P L., et al., Autopsy studies of coal miners' lungs—Phase II. Final Report on CEC Contract 7246–15–8/001. Edinburgh, Institute of Occupational Medicine, 1981.
36. Musk, A. W., Cotes, J. E., Bevan, C., and Campbell, M. J., Relationship between type of simple coal workers' pneumoconiosis and lung function. Br. J. Ind. Med., 38, 313, 1981.
36a. Gough, J., The pathogenesis of emphysema. In Liebow, A. (ed.), The Lung. Baltimore, Williams & Wilkins, 1968.
37. Fletcher, C., Some observations of the bronchial and emphysematous types of patient with severe generalized airways obstruction. In Cumming, G., and Hunt, L. B., eds.,

Form and Function in the Human Lung. Baltimore, Williams & Wilkins, 1968, pp. 231–241.

38. Seaton, D., Lapp, N. L., and Morgan, W. K. C., Measurement of carbon monoxide diffusing capacity in simple coal workers' pneumoconiosis and apical emphysema: the effects of change in body position. Chest, *80*, 350, 1981.

39. Morgan, W. K. C., Industrial bronchitis. Br. J. Ind. Med., *35*, 285, 1978.

40. Brinkman, G. L., and Coates, E. O., Jr., The effect of bronchitis, smoking, and occupation on ventilation. Am. Rev. Respir. Dis., *87*, 684, 1963.

41. Fletcher, C. M., Peto, R., and Tinker, C., The natural history of chronic bronchitis and emphysema. New York, Oxford University Press, 1976.

42. Bates, D. V., The fate of the chronic bronchitic: a report of the ten-year follow-up in the Canadian Department of Veteran's Affairs coordinated study of chronic bronchitics. Am. Rev. Respir. Dis., *108*, 1043, 1973.

43. Minnette, A., Rapport Épidemiologique à l'Étiologie de la Bronchite Chronique des mineurs de Charbon. Hasselt, Belgium, L. and A. Maris, 1976.

44. Rae, S., Walker, D. D., and Attfield, M. D., Chronic bronchitis and dust exposure in British coal miners. *In* Walton, W. H., ed., Inhaled Particles III. London, Unwin Brothers, 1971, pp. 883–894.

45. Rogan, J. M., Attfield, M. D., Jacobsen, M., et al., The role of dust in the working environment in the development of chronic bronchitis in British coal miners. Br. J. Ind. Med., *30*, 217, 1973.

46. Cochrane, A. L., Relationship between radiographic categories of pneumoconiosis and expectation of life. Br. Med. J., *2*, 532, 1973.

47. Cochrane, A. L., Haley, T. J. L., Moore, F., and Hole, D., The mortality of men in the Rhondda Fach, 1950–1970. Br. J. Ind. Med., *36*, 15, 1979.

48. Ortmeyer, C. E., Costello, J., Morgan, W. K. C., et al., The mortality of Appalachian coal miners: 1963 to 1971. Arch. Environ. Health, *29*, 67, 1974.

49. Brinkman, G. L., and Coates, E. L., The prevalence of chronic bronchitis in industrial population. Am. Rev. Respir. Dis., *86*, 47, 1962.

50. Brinkman, G. L., and Block, D. L., The prognosis in chronic bronchitis. J.A.M.A., *197*, 71, 1966.

51. Brinkman, G. L., Block, D. L., and Kress, C., The effects of bronchitis on occupational pulmonary ventilation over an 11-year period. J. Occup. Med., *14*, 615, 1972.

52. Deutsche Forschungsgemeinschaft, Research report on chronic bronchitis and occupational dust exposure. Federal Republic of Germany, Harald Boldt Verlag, 1978.

53. Wiles, F. J., Baskind, E., Irwig, L., and Gonin, R., The comparison of spirometry and plethysmography for measuring airways obstruction in miners. Paper presented at the Symposium on Occupational Lung Disease, Capetown, South Africa, March, 1978.

54. Morgan, W. K. C., Lapp, N. L., and Morgan, E. J., The early detection of occupational lung disease. Br. J. Dis. Chest, *68*, 75, 1974.

55. Hankinson, J. L., Reger, R. B., Fairman, R. P., et al., Factors influencing expiratory flow rates in coal miners. *In* Walton, W. H., Inhaled Particles IV. Oxford, Pergamon Press, 1977, pp. 737–752.

56. Hankinson, J. L., Reger, R. B., and Morgan, W. K. C. Maximal expiratory flows in coal miners. Am. Rev. Respir. Dis., *116*, 175, 1977.

57. Land, A. J., Avery, W., and Sackner, M. A., Some physiologic observations in smoke inhalation. Chest, *61*, 62, 1972.

58. Musk, A. W., Smith, T. J., and McLaughlin, E., Pulmonary function and fire fighters. Acute changes in ventilatory capacity and their correlates. Br. J. Ind. Med., *36*, 29, 1979.

59. Tashkin, D. P., Genovesi, M. G., Chopra, S., et al., Respiratory status of Los Angeles firemen one month after inhalation of dense smoke. Chest, *71*, 445, 1977.

60. Wanner, A., and Cutchavaree, A., Early recognition of upper airways obstruction following smoke inhalation. Am. Rev. Respir. Dis., *108*, 1421, 1973.

61. Unger, K. M., Snow, R. M., Mestas, J. M., and Miller, W. C., Smoke inhalation in firemen. Thorax, *35*, 838, 1980.

62. Le Quesne, P. M., Axford, A. T., McKerrow, C. B., and Jones, A. P., Neurological complications after a single severe exposure to toluene di-isocyanate. Br. J. Ind. Med., *33*, 72, 1976.

63. Sidor, R., and Peters, J. M., Prevalence rates of nonspecific respiratory disease in fire-fighters. Am. Rev. Respir. Dis., *109*, 1421, 1974.
64. Sidor, R., and Peters, J. M., Fire-fighting and pulmonary function. Am. Rev. Respir. Dis., *109*, 249, 1974.
65. Peters, J. M., Theriault, G. P., Fine, L. J., and Wegman, D. H., Chronic effect of fire-fighting on pulmonary function. N. Engl. J. Med., *291*, 1320, 1974.
66. Musk, A. W., Peters, J. M., and Wegmen, D. H., Lung function in fire-fighters: a three-year follow-up of active subjects. Am. J. Public Health, *67*, 626, 1976.
67. Sparrow, D., Bosse, R., Rosner, B., and Weiss, S. T., The effect of occupational exposure on lung function. A longitudinal evaluation of firefighters and non-firefighters. Am. Rev. Respir. Dis., *125*, 319, 1982.
68. Mastromatteo, E., Mortality in city firemen. II. A study of mortality in firemen of a city health department. Arch. Ind. Health, *20*, 227, 1959.
69. Musk, A. W., Monson, R. R., Peters, J. M., and Peters, R. K., Mortality among Boston fire-fighters. Br. J. Ind. Med., *35*, 104, 1978.
70. Becklake, M., Grain dust and health. State of the art. *In* Dosman, J. A., and Cotton, J., eds., Occupational Lung Diseases. New York, Academic Press, 1980, pp. 180–201.
71. Williams, N., Skoulas, A., and Merrimen, J., Exposure to grain dust. I. A survey of health effects. J. Occup. Med., *6*, 319, 1964.
72. DoPico, G., Reddan, W., Flaherty, D., et al., Respiratory abnormalities among grain handlers. Am. Rev. Respir. Dis., *115*, 915, 1977.
73. Davies, R. J., Green, M., and Schofield, N. M., Recurrent nocturnal asthma after exposure to grain dust. Am. Rev. Respir. Dis., *114*, 1011, 1976.
74. Chan-Yeung, M., Wong, R., and MacLean, L., Respiratory abnormalities among grain elevator workers. Chest, *75*, 461, 1979.
75. Dosman, J., Chronic obstructive pulmonary disease and smoking in grain workers. Ann. Intern. Med., *87*, 784, 1977.
76. Broder, I., Mintz, S., Hutcheon, M., et al., Comparison of respiratory variables in grain elevator workers and civic outside workers of Thunder Bay, Canada. Am. Rev. Respir. Dis., *119*, 193, 1970.
77. Broder, I., Mintz, S., Hutcheon, M., et al., Effect of lay-off and rehire on respiratory variables of grain elevator workers. Am. Rev. Respir. Dis., *122*, 601, 1980.
78. Hutcheon, M., Broder, I., Corey, P., et al., Restrictive ventilatory defect in grain elevator workers. *In* Gee, J. B. L., Morgan, W. K. C., and Brooks, S. M. (eds.), Occupational Lung Disease. New York, Raven Press, 1984, pp. 192–193.
79. Warren, C. P. W., Respiratory diseases in Manitoba cattle farmers. Can. Med. Assoc. J., *125*, 41, 1981.

18

BYSSINOSIS AND RELATED CONDITIONS

W. Keith C. Morgan

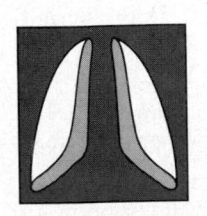

Relatively early in the nineteenth century Kay described a respiratory disease that affected cotton workers.[1] He correctly attributed the symptoms to excessive cotton dust exposure. Because of the onset of chest tightness and fever on Monday morning it became known as Monday morning fever. The condition has been described in cotton, flax, and hemp workers and is known as byssinosis, a term derived from the Greek βύσσοζ, meaning linen or fine flax.

Ramazzini in his treatise *De morbis artificum diatriba* mentioned the chronic cough of combers of flax and hemp. Greenhow described chronic bronchial irritation in a group of about 100 English flax workers.[2] The nineteenth-century cotton famine in England resulted in a great increase in the size and prosperity of the Irish linen industry. Flax spinning, formerly carried out in the crofter homes, was now carried out mainly in Belfast flax mills. Shortly afterward reports of chronic cough and shortness of breath in mill operatives began to make their appearance. The problems of the early Irish flax operatives have been well described by Schilling.[3] Similar problems were later described in hemp workers.[4]

Byssinosis has been described in all countries of the world where cotton, flax, and hemp are spun and processed. Much of the early clinical investigation was carried out in Britain, and for many years byssinosis was assumed to be peculiar to Lancashire and Ulster. Over the past three decades a significant prevalence has been reported from Spain, Egypt, the Netherlands, Sweden, and the United States,[5–9] but no matter where the disease is described, the symptoms are the same. Somewhat similar chest symptoms have been reported in jute, wool, and sisal workers, but doubt exists as to whether these textiles cause byssinosis.

THE MANUFACTURE OF COTTON

A series of processes are involved in the manufacture of cotton yarn. First, the cotton lint has to be separated from the seed. Until Eli Whitney invented the cotton gin this had to be done by hand, and the ginners came into intimate contact with the dust. Since Whitney's time further strides towards mechanization of cotton ginning have taken place, although even now there is evidence that byssinosis may still be occurring in cotton ginners. Seed cotton is first cleaned before being passed to the gin stand, where the lint is separated from the seed. The latter is then transported to the oil mill for separation into linters, oils, and meats. When the lint has been separated by pneumatic suction, it is carried pneumatically into a chamber and there is compressed into bales, which are then transported to cotton mills.

At the mill the cotton bale is first divided up and the cotton cleaned. This is effected by running the cotton through the cotton chamber, blowing room, and card room. The cotton is first broken out of the bales and fed by hand into a machine known as the hopper bale opener. It then passes into the blowing room, where it undergoes a series of processes the purpose of which is to open out and separate the compressed cotton fibers. Treatment of the cotton in the blowing room is designed to ensure that the impurities are removed and that the different qualities of fiber are completely mixed. In general the machines used in the blowing room are protected so that they do not generate much dust. They have to be

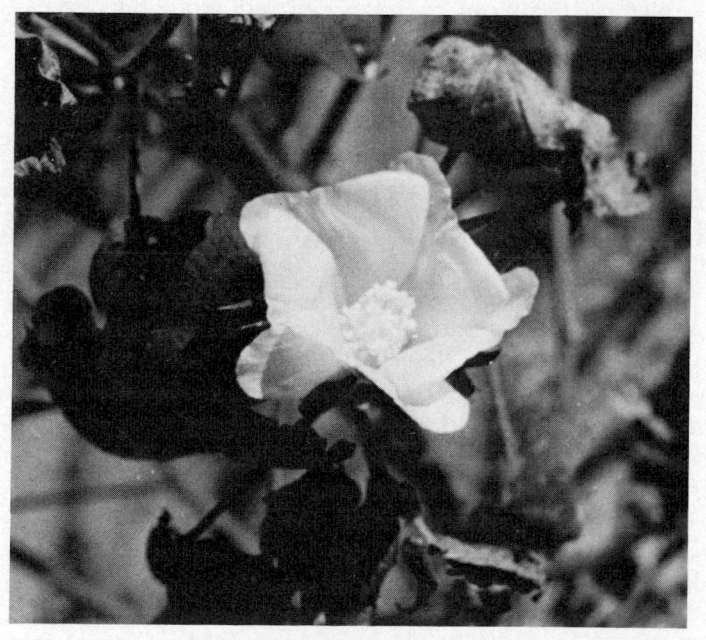

Figure 18–1. Cotton flower.

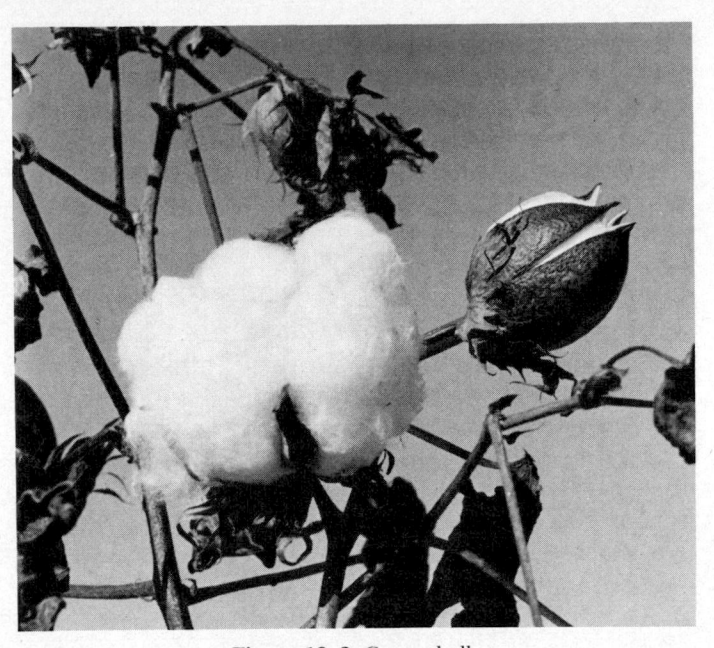

Figure 18–2. Cotton boll.

cleaned, however, and this is a most dusty job and should not be done unless those involved are suitably clad and wearing respirators. Byssinosis is as common in the blowing room as it is in the card room, although fewer workers are at risk.[10]

From the blowing room the cotton is taken to the carding room. Carding involves the final removal of impurities and the aligning of the fibers. The term carding is derived from the Latin *cardus*, meaning thistle. At one time the dried prickly cotton bracts were used for carding, but today the process is done by a carding machine (Fig. 18–3). This consists of a metal cylinder on which are set numerous steel-wire teeth. The cylinder rotates against a separate series of teeth set in the opposite direction, and as a result the cotton is combed into line and the short lengths are removed. Each carding engine has to be cleaned by vacuum several times a day and then later "brush stripped." After prolonged use, the carding cylinder's teeth become dull and deformed and must be reshaped and sharpened. The men who carry out these tasks are known as strippers and grinders, and it is they, rather than the other employees of the card room, who are most affected. Although card room processes and the machines involved tend to differ according to the country in which the cotton is being processed, carding itself is universal. The respiratory symptoms that occur in cardroom workers have long been known as "stripper's asthma."

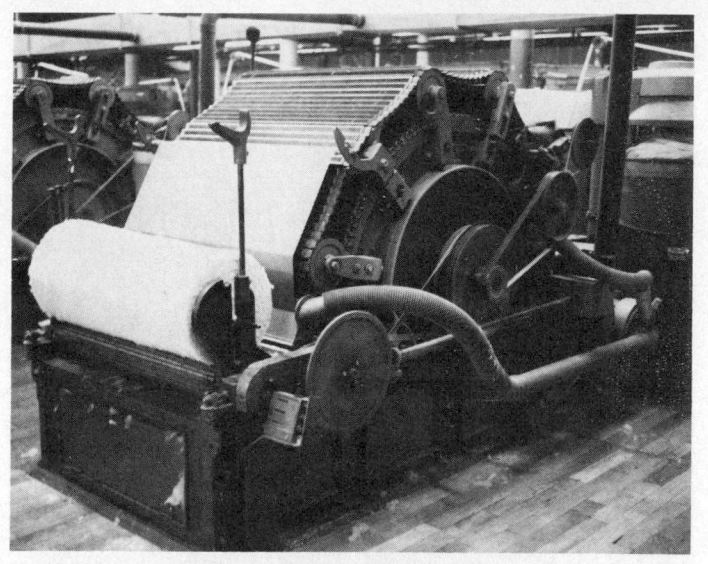

Figure 18–3. Carding machine.

From the carding room the cotton is twisted into threads before being made into the fabric. The final stages, viz., spinning, weaving, and finishing, are relatively free from dust, although byssinosis has been reported in spinners.

THE MANUFACTURE OF FLAX

Certain of the processes involved in the manufacture of yarn from flax differ from those used in the cotton industry. The fibers of the flax plant are 3 to 3.5 cm long and occur in their natural state as compound fibers that have to be separated from the woody part of the stem by a process known as scutching. This involves beating bundles of the plant after they have been softened by allowing bacteria to act on them while they are immersed in water, a process known as retting. Instead of bacteria, molds and fungi can be used to ret the fibers, under which circumstances the fibers are exposed aboveground in a dry state. This is known as dew retting. A third process is also sometimes used in which the fibers are retted in a tank to which chemicals have been added, and this is known as tank retting. After the fibers have been retted they can be separated from the stem by beating. The various procedures and jobs involved in the preparation of flax have been well described by Elwood et al.[11]

Flax fibers are first combed to separate them and to rid them of dirt and other impurities. The separated tow is carded to form a sliver. The slivers are repeatedly drawn through rows of "gills," in contrast to the

cotton fiber, which is drawn through parallel pressure rollers. Spinning of the coarse flax yarn is similar to that of cotton fibers, but when fine linen yarn is needed, the flax slivers have to be softened in hot water, a process known as wet spinning. Byssinosis may be found in all stages of the manufacture of flax, although it is rare in wet spinners. It is most prevalent in flax preparers, namely, those involved in the mixing and carding of the tow.

MORTALITY AND MORBIDITY DATA

Despite the fact that byssinosis has been recognized for many years and is known to occur on every continent, adequate mortality and morbidity data are scarce. Although mortality statistics in textile workers have been available in Britain for some time, many of the data have been contradictory, and to date no one has demonstrated that byssinosis is associated with an increased standardized mortality ratio (SMR) or that cotton textile workers have an increased death rate from occupationally acquired respiratory disease. The Registrar General of Great Britain's report of 1897 showed that cotton, linen, and flax workers had excessive death rates.[12] In 1923, 1927, and 1938, the Registrar General published specific data on the death rates for strippers, grinders, spinners, and weavers for three triennia (1910–12, 1921–23, and 1930–32).[13–15] In each three-year period, strippers and grinders had an excess mortality from respiratory disease, although mortality declined appreciably between the 1921–1923 and the 1930–32 triennia. In the late 1940s it was suggested that cotton workers suffered an excess of cardiovascular disease; however, this claim proved to be largely spurious because cor pulmonale secondary to airways obstruction was being certified as a primary circulatory disease.[16] In addition, it is now apparent that the excess mortality in textile workers in the three triennia arose from a variety of different causes, including tuberculosis, pneumonia and other nonbyssinotic causes of airways obstruction. The Registrar General's Decennial Supplement for 1951 showed an excess mortality for bronchitis and myocardial degeneration in cotton spinners; however, mortality for rheumatic disease was also increased in cotton weavers,[17] an unexpected anomalous finding. In the latest Decennial Supplement (1970–1972) which was published in 1978, no excess death rates from respiratory disease were noted in fiber preparers.[18] Twenty deaths were expected from bronchitis, asthma, and emphysema, whereas 24 occurred, a negligible and statistically insignificant difference.

In the United States, Henderson and Enterline used cotton workers as controls for asbestos workers in a mortality study, and in doing so showed that the cotton workers had no excess deaths from respiratory disease.[19] A more recent study of mortality of textile workers in two North Carolina cotton mills likewise showed no surfeit of respiratory deaths, and indeed for the most part cotton workers had a normal life expectancy.[20]

Berry has also recently described the findings of a mortality study in 16 Lancashire textile mills.[21] He found that in many instances the death rates were lower than expected, and this was equally true for strippers and grinders. He did, however, stress that the number of deaths was relatively few, that the results he described were preliminary, and that before definitive conclusions can be drawn further follow-up is necessary. A comprehensive follow-up study of 2528 flax workers has recently been published. Both male and female deaths were fewer than expected, and the most dust-exposed workers had no increased death rate. These data make it clear that any effect on occupational mortality associated with byssinosis can at the worst be extremely small.[21a] Suffice it to say at the present time there is no evidence to indicate that cotton or flax workers have an increased death rate from respiratory disease.

CLINICAL FEATURES

Byssinosis was originally recognized by a set of characteristic symptoms that occur in cotton workers, namely, chest tightness and shortness of breath that develop on returning to work each Monday. Lee feels that the term tightness does not do justice or fully describe the symptoms experienced by subjects who have byssinosis.[22] He quotes Kay's description of the chest disease that affects cotton spinners: "[The patient] experiences a diffuse and obscure sensation of uneasiness beneath the sternum. On sudden exertion a pectoral oppression occurs as if it were from an inability to dilate the chest fully in ordinary inspiration." Kay's somewhat rococo description is not quite the mode of expression used by patients who have byssinosis and who seem almost invariably to complain of chest tightness. Epidemiological studies in cotton, flax, and hemp workers have made it apparent that those exposed to these textiles may in addition develop a variety of respiratory symptoms that differ from the typical symptoms of chest tightness and shortness of breath. It is now evident that exposure to cotton, hemp, and flax dust may be associated with four responses:

1. The development of chest tightness and shortness of breath on first returning to work.

2. A decline in ventilatory capacity over the first work shift of the week.

3. An increased prevalence of bronchitis as manifested by persistent cough and sputum.

4. A clinical syndrome known as mill fever that usually occurs when a worker first starts working or on returning from a prolonged absence. Mill fever is characterized by the onset of fever and aches and pains, symptoms closely resembling those induced by gram-negative endotoxin.

With the exception of mill fever, all of the above conditions are often loosely referred to as byssinosis. There are, nonetheless, compelling arguments to limit the term byssinosis to the acute response, that is to say,

the chest tightness that develops on first returning to work, and possibly the decrement in ventilatory capacity. While there is some concordance between the symptoms of chest tightness and the acute shift decrement, this relationship is often far from exact. In the case of the more chronic syndrome of bronchitis, this is apparently unrelated to the acute symptoms. Moreover, the previously widely held belief that the acute response, when it occurs over a prolonged period, slowly evolves into chronic irreversible airways obstruction and emphysema is suspect and probably incorrect.[23]

Acute Response

Although some subjects may experience chest tightness on the first occasion they are exposed to cotton dust, more commonly the employee has been working for several years before symptoms develop.[3, 24] Those persons who react on the first day of exposure are likely to leave the job and seek employment elsewhere within a month or two of starting work. To begin with, symptoms usually occur only on the first shift after a subject returns to work, and because this is usually a Monday, the normal history is one of Monday morning chest tightness. Should the subject work over the weekend and have days off in the middle of the week, then he will develop the symptoms the day he resumes work. Initially, the chest tightness and wheeze last for a few hours and then disappear, but with increasing exposure some subjects notice that the symptoms either recur or persist on Tuesdays and occasionally for the rest of the working week.[3-10]

Epidemiological surveys to detect the prevalence of byssinosis in working populations have, to a large extent, relied on the Medical Research Council (MRC) questionnaire on respiratory symptoms.[25] The usefulness of this questionnaire has been greatly enhanced by the addition of some supplementary questions on chest tightness. By means of the responses to the questionnaire, a useful grading system for byssinosis has evolved: Grade ½, occasional tightness on Mondays or the day on which work is resumed; Grade 1, chest tightness and/or difficulty in breathing on Monday or the day on which work is resumed; and Grade 2, chest tightness and difficulty breathing not only on Mondays but on other days of the week. While the questionnaire is a useful approach to quantitating the prevalence of byssinosis, it has to be administered in an objective fashion, and unless the interviewer is careful, bias may result from framing the questions in a tendentious fashion.

The acute symptoms of chest tightness can be duplicated by inhalational challenges with both cotton dust and aqueous extract of cotton bract.[9] Not all workers react, however. Those at risk can be divided into reactors and nonreactors, with the former in the majority and usually constituting up to 65 to 75 per cent of the total. The prevalence of symptoms of byssinosis also appears to be influenced by smoking habits, and in many surveys smokers have been shown to have a greater prevalence of byssinosis.[26, 27] Although it has been suggested that an allergic

diathesis or atopy play a role in the development of byssinosis, evidence in support of this thesis has not accrued, and there is only one study in the literature which suggests that there might be some validity to this hypothesis.[28] The consensus at the present time is that atopy does not predispose to byssinosis. The prevalence of byssinosis also varies from mill to mill, and such differences cannot be explained by a single variable such as dust exposure.[29] There are probably multiple factors that play a role in the so-called mill effect, including the type of cotton that is milled, whether coarse or fine, the degree of bacterial and gram-negative endotoxin contamination of the cotton, and possibly prior exposure of the workers to cotton dust. There is also some suggestion that the risk is greater in men than in women.[27]

In subjects challenged with cotton extract, the acute response may take several hours to develop and in this differs from the typical IgE-mediated asthma and the characteristic timing of the response seen in asthmatics who are challenged with either methacholine or histamine.[30-32] Challenge experiments have been carried out for periods up to four hours, a fact which suggests that factors other than smooth muscle contraction may be playing a role in the development of the acute byssinotic response. The acute response can be attenuated or averted by prior administration of atropine, cromolyn sodium, and chlorphenira-mine, but is enhanced by propranolol.[33-35] It is also known that nonasthmatic responders to cotton bract (byssinotics) do not react to histamine challenge in the same ultrasensitive fashion as asthmatics.[32]

Chronic Effects

For many years it was presumed that the acute response to cotton dust portended the development of irreversible airways obstruction. It was assumed that the acute response gradually became less evident and slowly evolved into a more chronic condition characterized by continuous shortness of breath, cough, and sputum. It was further assumed that chronic exposure eventually led to emphysema and irreversible obstruction, but a number of recent studies have shown that there is either a poor relationship or more commonly no relationship between the acute response and the development of the chronic syndrome. Although certain studies have demonstrated an unusually high decrement in the ventilatory capacity of textile workers,[27, 36] such findings have been inconsistent and are not wholly convincing for a variety of reasons. Moreover, recent studies of the pathology of the condition have shown that while bronchitis and bronchiolitis occur more commonly in the lungs of textile workers, whether smokers or not, emphysema was observed only in the lungs of smokers. Morphological evidence of bronchitis and bronchiolitis was found in the lungs of nonsmoking textile workers. Even in textile workers with dust-associated bronchitis, the relationship between cumulative dust exposure, or the duration of dust exposure, and the presence of bronchitis

is sadly deficient.[23, 37] Much the same situation exists for the annual decrement in FEV_1. A few studies suggest that the annual rate of decline of the FEV_1 is greater in cotton mills than in mills that process synthetic fibers, but the rate of decline was unrelated to symptoms of byssinosis, to past or current dust levels, or to the post-shift decline in the FEV_1.[26, 27, 38] Similar studies of retired mill workers in South Carolina have shown an increased annual decrement in the FEV_1, but it has been impossible to exclude geographical and other selection biases.[39] Moreover, in some studies it seems likely that an unduly high proportion of blacks were included, and no allowance was made for their lower lung volumes.[40] In one widely quoted study, the purpose of which was to detect the effect of steam-treating cotton, the study population was deliberately chosen so as to include a high proportion of byssinotics with heavy exposure to low-grade cotton.[41] The decline in the FEV_1 over an observation period of 10 months was 192 ml, but the observation period in this study was too short. Such an increased annual decrement would profoundly affect mortality and as mentioned earlier no such effect has been observed.

Byssinosis in Hemp and Flax Workers

Exposure to hemp dust is associated with the same effects as exposure to cotton dust. It occurs usually in soft hemp spinners. Carey et al. found that Ulster flax workers who complained of byssinotic symptoms had a lower average FEV_1 than did nonbyssinotic workers.[42] The highest prevalence of symptoms occurred in those exposed to retted flax.[43] The decrease in ventilatory capacity occurs most commonly in preparers, while spinners and polishers are much less likely to be affected. Bronchitis is a common finding in flax mill operatives.

Byssinosis is also found in cottonseed mills in which the raw cottonseed is separated into short cotton fibers or linters, hulls, and meats, the latter being the source of cottonseed oil. The process of separation is often dusty, and there is some evidence that byssinosis occurs in around 2 to 3 per cent of the workers.[44]

PULMONARY FUNCTION

Although certain of the changes in lung function tests have been mentioned in the previous section, further elaboration is necessary.

Acute Response

A degree of biological variability is inherent in all tests, and this is particularly true of tests of ventilatory capacity. Part of the variability is related to the diurnal variation in ventilatory capacity that occurs in both

normal persons and those with respiratory disease. It therefore becomes difficult to establish definite criteria for what constitutes an acute response. Faute de mieux it is suggested that any shift decrement in the FEV_1 of between 5 and 10 per cent should be regarded as strongly suggestive of byssinosis, while any change of greater than 10 per cent should be regarded as diagnostic. Alternatively, should there be a fall in the FEV_1 of greater than 200 ml, the shift decrement should be regarded as strongly suggestive of the presence of byssinosis. The highest of three acceptable FEV_1's, all of which should be within 5 per cent of each other, should be accepted as the subject's value. Although other tests of ventilatory capacity, e.g., maximal flows, FEF_{25-75}, and closing volume, have been suggested as being more sensitive in the detection of byssinosis, these tests are less reproducible and are affected by changes in lung volume, and for this reason the FEV_1 is to be preferred[45] (Fig. 18–4). The FVC also often shows a change over a shift, but as a test it is less sensitive than the FEV_1 in the diagnosis of byssinosis. In testing subjects it is important to remember that the pre- and post-shift ventilatory studies should always be done on the first morning the subject returns to work, whether that be a Monday or any other day, since the back-to-work decrement is usually appreciably larger on that day than on subsequent days of the week.

The National Institute of Occupational Safety and Health (NIOSH) recommended standard for cotton dust contains an Appendix that describes the requirements and criteria that should, and now have to, be met when carrying out serial pulmonary function tests in textile workers.[46] In general, the regulations seem appropriate, with the exception that they permit a 10 per cent difference between the two larger FEV_1's and FVC's. Such a large difference is too lax and can only lead to dubious results and will detract from the medical surveillance program.

A number of other indices of lung function have been used to study the acute effects of cotton dust exposure. These include measurement of

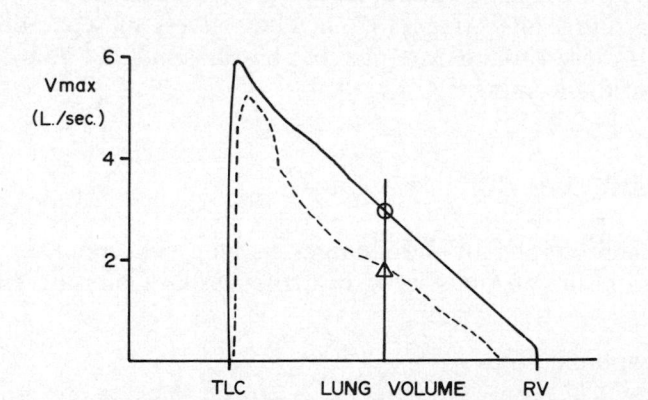

Figure 18–4. Flow volume loops before and after exposure to cotton dust. Vertical lines with circle and triangle represent flow at 50 per cent of vital capacity, assuming that total lung capacity (TLC) is not significantly changed. The FEV_1 fell 14 per cent.

lung volumes, diffusing capacity, and arterial blood gases.[47, 48] Small increases in residual volume may occur following acute exposure, but the total lung capacity is for the most part unaffected. The diffusing capacity remains unchanged over a work shift. Significant falls in PaO_2 and oxygen saturation have also been reported in active and retired hemp workers following challenges with hemp fibers.[47] The decrement in the PaO_2 is the consequence of worsening of ventilation perfusion mismatching. Guyatt and co-workers have also made a study of lung mechanics in subjects with byssinosis.[49] They concluded that there was a loss of elastic recoil in affected subjects, and this in part contributed to the decreased flows observed in cotton workers with chronic airways obstruction. Unfortunately the subject selection in the study was less than optimal, and there may have been appreciable bias. Moreover, the results for smokers and nonsmokers were considered together, thereby to a large extent making it difficult to separate the effects of dust exposure from those of smoking. Furthermore, only 6 of the 23 subjects included in the study were nonsmokers. Bouhuys and Van de Woestijne carried out detailed studies of lung mechanics in hemp workers and suggested that two responses to the offending agent are seen.[50] They termed the first a flow rate response and suggested that this is seen in subjects with typical byssinotic symptoms, i.e., chest tightness. In these subjects there is a decrement in the FEV_1 and flow rates. While the FVC may also decrease to a limited extent, the subjects' airways conductance remains unchanged. Bouhuys attributed the decline in the flow rates to pharmacologically induced bronchoconstriction taking place in the small airways. The second type of response was seen in those subjects who, following challenge, developed no symptoms. These subjects showed no decrement in the FEV_1, vital capacity, or maximal flows, but did show a decrease in their airways conductance. The latter response was attributed to a reflex or a mechanical effect on the large airways. It was noted that both types of response could be abolished by the prior administration of bronchodilators.

Chronic Effects

Although the ventilatory capacity of flax, hemp, and cotton workers has repeatedly been demonstrated to be lower than that of comparable controls, it is often difficult separating the effects of the acute response from the more chronic effects. The decreased ventilatory capacity that characterizes the acute response is seen for the most part in carders, pickers, and those involved in early processing of cotton. It has also been observed that workers with symptoms of byssinosis—in this instance, chest tightness and wheeze—have significantly lower spirometric values than do asymptomatic workers,[27, 36] but again it is not known whether the lower FEV_1 is permanent and irreversible or simply a delayed manifestation of acute exposure that is likely to completely resolve when exposure ceases. Other studies have shown that cough and sputum are more common in

textile workers than in nonexposed workers, but the exact implications of these symptoms are not clear.[26, 27] The clinical significance of the increased prevalence of cough and sputum is debatable, but there is excellent evidence to indicate that these symptoms do not necessarily portend the onset of irreversible obstruction.[51] Indeed, such symptoms are present in numerous dust-exposed populations, and the majority of the evidence points to the fact that the symptoms are of little moment. When it comes to comparing ventilatory capacity in exposed and nonexposed populations there have been problems in the selection of the control or reference population. Differing smoking habits; differing types of fibers, whether coarse or fine; different ethnic origins of the workers surveyed—all may play a role in introducing bias. Moreover, the results of many of these studies have been conflicting. There is ample morphological and epidemiological evidence to indicate that bronchitis and bronchiolitis occur more frequently in those exposed to cotton dust. The same cannot be said for emphysema, which appears to be limited to smoking textile workers.[23, 37]

There are a few studies that have suggested that cotton textile workers have a greater than normal annual decrement in ventilatory capacity.[38, 39] One such study reported a decrement of "54 ml/year (expected 25 ml/year)" in a group of Lancashire mill workers.[38] Those processing synthetic fibers had a decrement of 32 ml/year. However, only two synthetic mills were included in the study, one of which seemed to be mainly responsible for the overall relatively normal rate of decline observed in the noncotton textile workers. Whether these two mills represent the general population of noncotton-exposed textile workers is doubtful. Furthermore, dust sampling was carried out only at the time of the survey and not over a longer period. The annual decline in ventilatory capacity noted in the cotton workers was not related to the current dust levels, to the symptoms of byssinosis, to the acute shift decline in FEV_1, or to the symptoms of bronchitis.[38]

In another study, a survivor population of active and retired cotton workers in South Carolina was shown to have a lower mean FEV_1 and FVC than did the reference population, who came from Connecticut.[39] Whether the latter group can be regarded as comparable to the study group is a moot point because of the geographical difference. Elsewhere, studies have shown that the FEV_1 of nonbyssinotic cotton workers was below the predicted value for all durations of employment beyond two years.[40] Incongruously, however, the nonsmoking byssinotic workers with the longest employment had the best ventilatory capacity, making it difficult to reconcile dust exposure with any chronic decline in lung function. This study probably had a greater than normal percentage of black subjects included in it, and no obvious effort was made to correct for the smaller lung volumes of the black subjects.

Other studies have also shown an excess annual decrement in lung

function.[26, 41] As previously mentioned, in one of these studies the mean 10-month decrease in FEV_1 was 192 ml.[41] Were this the usual rate of decline in the FEV_1, it would be difficult to explain why such a rapid deterioration in lung function is not reflected in increased mortality figures. Moreover, the cohort chosen had the heaviest exposure and was unrepresentative of the cotton industry as a whole. Both these studies relied on only two measurements of FEV_1 over a period of less than a year, and it is inaccurate to try and predict the rate of decline from such a limited period of observation. Similar but lesser effects on lung function have been observed in workers in wool mills,[52] and the whole concept of the specificity of cotton dust as the agent responsible for the so-called chronic syndrome observed in textile workers must remain sub judice. There is a dire need for a longer prospective study relating any decline in ventilatory capacity to cotton dust levels and other variables including smoking and type of cotton fiber.

PATHOLOGY

Until recently there have been few descriptions of the morphological changes found in the lungs of textile workers, and the few observations that have been made have generally been nonspecific or suggested the presence of emphysema. Moreover, little attempt was made to relate postmortem findings to premortem dust exposure, smoking habits, and pulmonary function tests.

A recent study by Edwards and co-workers examined the heart and lungs of 43 subjects who in life had been diagnosed as having byssinosis and subsequently were awarded compensation.[53] Although some emphysema was found at post mortem, there appeared to be no relationship between the presence of this condition and prior cotton dust exposure. In contrast, bronchitis and bronchiolitis were found more frequently in the textile workers than in the general population. Neither right ventricular hypertrophy nor pulmonary vascular abnormalities were noted. In addition, a recent study found that emphysema is not associated with exposure to cotton dust per se, and when observed in a cotton worker at post mortem it is almost certainly a consequence of the individual's smoking habits.[23] Additional careful studies carried out by Rooke have demonstrated similar findings. He was completely unable to show any evidence of interstitial fibrosis or emphysema in the lungs of textile workers and likewise could not demonstrate emphysema unless the subjects were cigarette smokers.[37] He also made the observation that so-called byssinotic bodies are uncommon in the lungs of textile workers. Byssinotic bodies are rounded aggregates of debris with a central black core that is surrounded by yellowish material and are composed for the most part of degenerated alveolar macrophages.

ETIOLOGY

Before the late 1940s little attention had been given to the investigation of the etiology of byssinosis; however, the situation has changed radically. Many theories have been put forward to explain the airway changes seen in byssinosis, but none is entirely satisfactory. There is little doubt that the agent or agents responsible for the bronchoconstriction are located in the cotton bract; however, their identity remains unknown.

Early observers noted the similarity between the symptoms of byssinosis and those of asthma, and for years byssinosis was believed to be a form of asthma. Nevertheless, there are features of byssinosis that are completely different from those of asthma. Extrinsic asthma is associated with an immediate response that develops in 10 to 30 minutes. Such a reaction is brought on by exposure to antigenic proteins. In contrast, the symptoms of byssinosis develop slowly over several hours and improve as the week goes by, despite continued exposure. Subjects with byssinotic symptoms do not demonstrate the acute response to histamine or methacholine challenge. Furthermore, some subjects with byssinosis have undergone repeated challenges with antigen for periods up to four hours, a procedure that would be quite intolerable in asthmatics. Another difference is that, in contrast to asthma, byssinosis affects a large proportion of those exposed to the offending agent, usually well over 50 per cent. Likewise, asthmatic attacks occur unpredictably and may remit in an equally unpredictable fashion. The absence of both a family history and the allergic diathesis in byssinosis serves to distinguish the two conditions. Such differences seem a most telling argument against considering byssinosis to be a form of asthma.

A variety of pathophysiological mechanisms have been put forward to explain the symptoms and decrement in ventilatory capacity that are seen in byssinotics. At least three of these can be dismissed fairly summarily. At one time the symptoms and ventilatory decrement were felt to be a consequence of an inert dust reaction; however, cotton dust produces a response at much lower concentrations (roughly one thirtieth to one fiftieth) of coal and other inert dusts. Moreover, washed cotton dust and other fibers such as polyesters do not have the same effect on the FEV_1. Other persons have suggested that cotton dust contains agents that act directly on the airways and induce bronchoconstriction. Included in this category are histamine and serotonin, which are present, albeit in minute quantities insufficient to induce bronchoconstriction. The third hypothesis is that byssinosis is an immediate asthmatic reaction to an allergen. Reasons have already been stated for rejecting this theory.

Several other more likely theories of the pathogenesis of byssinosis exist,[54] including the following hypotheses.

1. *Pharmacologic release of histamine or other mediators.* There is no doubt that cotton dust can cause liberation of histamine.[55] Similar observations have been made with cotton extracts. Inhalation experiments with cotton

dust and aqueous extracts of cotton bract have been shown to induce a fall in the FEV_1 which can be prevented by the prior administration of antihistamines. Extracts of cotton dust will liberate histamine from platelets.[58] An increase of histamine metabolites has been shown to occur in the urine of subjects exposed to cotton dust, but the site of histamine release has not been established.[30] Although the histamine hypothesis has a certain meretricious appeal, there are certain weaknesses to it. First, the time course of the reaction with reference to the changes in ventilatory capacity is inappropriate and cannot be explained by histamine alone. Second, the evidence from the use of histamine antagonists is nonspecific and questionable.

The possibility that mediators other than histamine are important in the pathogenesis of byssinosis needs further study. It is known that slow-reactive substance (SRS–A) induces not only bronchoconstriction but is also an eosinophil chemotaxin. SRS–A is released from several cells that are commonly found in the lung, including polymorphonuclear leukocytes. In addition, it has been shown that aqueous extract of cotton dust will mobilize polymorphonuclear leukocytes in lung tissue. Leukotrienes C and E are derivatives of arachidonic acid and are released by the cell surfaces of polymorphonuclear leukocytes, mononuclear phagocytes, and basophils, and as such are 200 to 2000 times more powerful than histamine in inducing smooth muscle contraction.[59] Other potential mediators include platelet activating factors, which also may be released in the lung under certain circumstances and are capable of inducing bronchoconstriction.[60]

2. *Chemotactic mechanisms.* It has been suggested that the induction of chemotaxis by cotton dust may play a role in the pathogenesis of byssinosis. Certain polyphenolic extracts of cotton trash and quercetin have been shown to recruit polymorphonuclear leukocytes into hamsters' airways, Lancinilene C and lancinilene E-7 methyl ether have been isolated from water extracts of the cotton bract and have been demonstrated to be chemotactic.[61] Even so, the mechanism whereby chemotaxis might induce acute bronchoconstriction is unclear and the exact role of chemotaxis, if any, in the induction of the acute byssinotic reaction is not known.

3. *Endotoxin activity.* A group of Italian workers showed that the inhalation of purified *Escherichia coli* endotoxin will induce a fall in the ventilatory capacity and that an associated febrile response was frequently absent.[62, 63] The levels of endotoxin were roughly equal to those that are found in exposed cotton mill workers. Rylander and colleagues have extended these observations and have shown that symptoms of byssinosis correlate better with endotoxin levels that occur in cotton dust than they do with measurements of respirable dust. It is also abundantly clear that cotton plants are invariably contaminated with gram-negative organisms, and the same can be said for the air of most cotton mills. Gram-negative bacilli contain a particularly toxic substance that is known as lipopolysaccharide (LPS). This consists of hydrophilic and lipid-rich fractions. The

hydrophilic fraction consists of a polysaccharide chain with repeating units, constituting the somatic O antigens and a core polysaccharide. The lipid-rich fraction consists of phosphate groups, diglucosamine, and fatty acids and is probably the active fraction.[65] It seems that the lower the LPS content of cotton dust, the less likely are exposed subjects to react. While the role of endotoxin in the etiology of byssinosis is by no means certain, further investigations, including human challenges with LPS, would seem desirable in investigating the role of endotoxin in the etiology of byssinosis.

4. *Antigen-antibody reaction.* Various workers have put forward the hypothesis that byssinosis is a Type III hypersensitivity reaction, but there is little scientific evidence in support of this notion. Massoud and Taylor reported that cotton bract extracts produce lines of precipitation in sera from byssinotic patients, but the presence of antibody was subsequently shown to be nonspecific precipitation of IgG.[66] In later work, Taylor and collagues isolated a polyphenyl, 5,7,3,4,tetrahydroxy-flavan 3,4 diol (THF), that they suggested was the agent responsible. In a double blind trial, although challenges with THF induced symptoms of byssinosis, it failed to induce a drop in the FEV_1.[67] Firm evidence that THF has a role in the etiology of byssinosis is lacking, and the Type III hypothesis has been examined in more detail by Kutz et al. and found unconvincing.[68] They are of the opinion that true precipitating antibodies do not exist.

It is thus apparent that there is a great divergence of opinion as to the causative agent of byssinosis. Various groups of workers with a vested interest in a particular agent have become unduly preoccupied with that agent to the extent that they tend to dismiss other hypotheses too summarily. At the present time it seems probable that several agents may play a role or that there may be a multicomponent etiology, with various agents enhancing the effects of one another. The majority of the evidence suggests that cotton dust contains an agent or agents that will induce both chest tightness and an associated decrement in ventilatory capacity. Such a response appears to involve the liberation of mediators that will contract bronchial smooth muscle. For reasons previously stated, this seems unlikely to be related to any specific immunological reaction. Such a nonspecific response might originate first, as a result of an inhaled component of cotton dust activating complement components that have been synthesized by activated macrophages with the formation of C3a and C5a anaphyla-toxins, or second, as a result of two or more constituents of the inhaled dust activating lymphocytes, macrophages, mast cells, or basophils in a polyclonal and nonimmune fashion. The second hypothesis appears to be more likely.

A recent review of byssinosis and related conditions summarizes the present state of knowledge and emphasizes areas of uncertainty.[68a]

Host Factors

A variety of host factors have been suggested as possibly predisposing to the development of byssinosis. These include atopy, aspirin sensitivity,

and airways hyperreactivity. Most such suggestions do not bear close examination. HLA antigen frequency has been investigated in flax workers with byssinosis, with the finding that HLA-B27 predisposes to the development of byssinosis, but this observation has little importance, since byssinosis occurs so frequently with other HLA types.[69]

PREVENTION

Dust Measurement

A number of different instruments have been used in the measurement of cotton dust[43] (see also Chap. 9). These include the cascade impactor, the high-volume total dust sampler, the vertical elutriator, and the horizontal elutriator. The vertical elutriator excludes all particles with an aerodynamic diameter greater than 14.5 microns, while the horizontal elutriator of Roach segregates particles into coarse, medium, and fine. In the United States the recommended instrument is the vertical elutriator, and dust concentration is expressed as mg/m^3.

Cotton Dust Standard. The current United States Cotton Dust Standard, which takes effect in 1984, is 0.2 mg/m^3. The standard is to be introduced gradually, with a progressive decline in the allowable concentration. The 0.2 mg/m^3 limit applies only to the picking, carding, and spinning areas, whereas in the slashing and weaving stages the allowable concentration is 0.750 mg/m^3. The standard does not apply to cotton ginners.

Several problems exist with the recommended standard other than those relating to its financial impact on industry. The standard is based largely on the results of one or two United States cross-sectional studies,[71] the conclusions of which have repeatedly been questioned. Nowhere is it apparent which of the features of byssinosis the standard has been designed to control, the impression being that the standard will be equally effective in controlling both the acute and chronic effects of cotton dust.

Other recommendations included in the United States Cotton Dust Standard are as follows:

1. A preplacement examination to include a history, FVC, and FEV_1. The history is to include a respiratory questionnaire and is based on Schilling's modification of the British MRC questionnaire.[25]

2. Each newly employed cotton mill worker will have a repeat FVC and FEV_1 within six months of starting employment.

3. Periodic testing of ventilatory capacity will take place on the first day after return to work and shall be performed both before and following an exposure for at least six hours. These tests will be repeated at varying intervals, and specific criteria are laid down for those persons who showed a ventilatory decrement. The OSHA standard also suggests that the FEV_1 variation should not exceed 10 per cent; however, this would seem unduly generous, since a 5 per cent drop in FEV_1 strongly suggests the presence of byssinosis.

Treatment of Cotton to Remove Bronchoconstrictor Agents

A variety of approaches have been used in the attempt to reduce the prevalence of byssinosis,[41, 72] including cotton steaming to reduce the biological effects of cotton dust. Another approach relies on washing the cotton prior to carding and processing. An ingenious process was recently devised in which a small quantity of cotton was harvested before the opening of the boll. This was compared with standard cotton collected when the boll had already opened.[73] Cotton dust from the closed boll had a lesser effect on ventilatory capacity than the dust derived from the open boll.

These modifications have resulted in a lesser decrement in expiratory flow per mg of dust exposure. The effects on the FEV_1 for the most part occurred in those subjects working in areas where dust levels were highest.

ACUTE NONBYSSINOTIC RESPIRATORY ILLNESS IN COTTON AND OTHER TEXTILE WORKERS

There have been frequent reports of outbreaks of acute respiratory illness among cotton workers. The symptoms and signs of these illnesses suggest that they are distinct from those of byssinosis; however, the clear-cut distinction that was formerly made between byssinosis and mill fever may not be as justifiable as was believed in the recent past. No single factor appears to be concerned in their pathogeneses, and a variety of agents have been implicated. Molds and vegetable allergens are amongst those incriminated, and in particular, the dust of the tamarind seed (Tamarindis indica) has been thought to be responsible for some outbreaks. In 1913, an outbreak of cough and respiratory illness among Lancashire weavers was described by Collis.[74] The condition was characterized by bronchoconstriction, cough, purulent sputum, and shortness of breath. The material woven was cotton that had been sized with a mixture of flour, tallow, and china clay. At the time of the outbreak the warp threads were observed to be mildewed, and furthermore, the outbreak disappeared when dry threads were substituted. The recurrence of mildew in the threads led to a further outbreak of the illness. The air over the looms was found to contain many mycelia and conidia. Penicillium, Aspergillus, and Mucor were identified in the loom dust.

In 1954 Vigliani and associates reported an epidemic of bronchoconstriction among cotton weavers.[75] The cotton yarn had been sized with locust bean gum and potato starch. About half the weavers were affected by wheezing, breathlessness, and a dry irritative cough. The symptoms were worse on Mondays, and the illness lasted between two and six months. Skin tests with molds of Aerobacter aerogenes produced positive results in many of the affected subjects, but the organism was never definitely incriminated.

An outbreak of similar respiratory symptoms was reported in a group of Indian workers involved in the sizing of jute and cotton.[76] The weavers had started using tamarind seed a short time previously. No effect occurred with the first exposure, but with repeated exposure sensitization seemed to take place. In some of the affected workers, but not in controls, inhalational challenges using tamarind powder produced acute symptoms of the syndrome.

A few cotton and hemp workers suffer from chills, fever, nausea, and vomiting when they first return to work after a prolonged absence. This complaint is known as mill fever or hemp fever and usually disappears in a few days. Although the term mill fever is often used as if it were a distinct entity and separate from byssinosis, some doubt remains as to whether this distinction is justifiable. In practice, while mill fever is uncommon in cotton workers, this is less true in mattress workers. Most subjects with byssinosis have characteristic symptoms, in particular, chest tightness. This is much less marked in subjects who complain of mill fever. There is evidence to indicate that *Aerobacter cloacae* is one of the responsible agents. This bacterium is found as a normal soil inhabitant and as a contaminant of cotton in cold and wet seasons. More recent studies by Rylander and Lundholm have shown that cotton products are contaminated by many gram-negative bacteria, particularly Enterobacter, Pseudomonas, and Agrobacterium species.[64] These bacteria are also present in the cotton plant itself. Exposure to inhaled endotoxins may lead to the development of fever, chills, and malaise, and also to a decrement in the FEV_1. Gram-negative bacteria are frequently found in the air of cotton mills, and the concentration of endotoxin dust from cotton mills has been shown to range from 0.2 to 1.6 mg/gram of dust—with the higher level being greatly in excess of that at which symptoms will develop in exposed workers.[65] Endotoxins are also capable of activating complement and liberating anaphylatoxins and chemotaxins. Tolerance to endotoxin follows prolonged exposure.[77] Thus the possibility still exists that mill fever and byssinosis are just variants of the same condition, with both being due to endotoxins.

RESPIRATORY DISEASE IN SISAL AND JUTE WORKERS

Sisal is a hard fiber produced from the leaves of *Agave sisalana*, a species of amaryllis. First found in Yucatan, Mexico, it is now grown in the United States, Europe, and Africa. It is used in the manufacture of ropes, coarse textiles, carpets, and twine. The leaves are first removed from the sisal plant. After the fibers have been extracted, they are combed and carded in a fashion similar to cotton fibers.

A byssinosis-like condition has been described in sisal workers,[78] reportedly affecting the combers more often than the drawers and spinners. Significant mean reductions in ventilatory capacity over a work

shift have been recorded. This has been attributed to sisal dust causing histamine release, with its associated bronchoconstriction.[79] More recently, lung function was measured in 66 workers in a sisal rope-making factory and in a matched control population.[80] A major contaminant found in the air was a lubricant used to soften the fiber. At the start of the work shift, comparison of lung function in the control and exposed groups showed no significant difference between them. However, those exposed to sisal did not change their lung function over the shift, while the control group showed the usual and expected increase in FEV_1. Baker and colleagues suggested that perhaps the lubricant and softeners used were responsible for the effect on ventilatory capacity.[80] A further study involved 77 sisal spinners and 83 sisal brushers working in 6 Tanzanian sisal factories.[81] Symptoms of byssinosis were low in the spinners, but relatively high in those workers employed in the brushing departments. As has been observed with other textile workers, sisal workers who smoked were more prone to develop symptoms of byssinosis.[26, 27] Acute changes in the FVC and FEV_1 occurred over the work shift, but in some instances acute falls in the FEV_1 were not accompanied by symptoms. Unfortunately, no dust measurements were available at the time of the survey, although prior measurements showed that brushers were exposed to higher levels than spinners.

The prevalence of symptoms of byssinosis in two groups who were exposed simultaneously to jute or hemp has been compared. Classical symptoms of byssinosis did not occur in those exposed to jute.[82] Although most studies have shown no effect from jute processing,[83, 84] Popa and co-workers suggested that byssinosis could result from exposure to jute.[85] A study of the ventilatory capacity of 46 workers exposed to jute dust likewise showed a significant decrease in the FEV_1 on the first day of work.[86] A subsequent study carried out by Valic and Zuskin compared the effects of cotton and jute dust on respiratory symptoms and respiratory function in 60 cotton and 91 jute nonsmoking female workers of similar age and similar length of dust exposure.[87] They showed that cotton workers had a significantly higher prevalence of byssinosis and of dyspnea than did jute workers. None of the jute workers had the characteristic symptoms of byssinosis. Both cotton and jute caused a significant reduction in ventilatory capacity on the first working shift in the week; however, cotton dust had a significantly greater effect. Thus it would seem that jute probably does lead to a shift decrement in the FEV_1, but its effect is much less than that of cotton and flax and may be nonspecific.

References

1. Kay, J. P., Trades producing phthisis. New Eng. Med. Surg., *1*, 357, 1831.
2. Greenhow, E. H., Report of the Medical Officer of the Privy Council, 1860, Appendix VI. London, H. M. Stationery Office, 1861.
3. Schilling, R. S. F., Byssinosis in cotton and other textile workers. Lancet, *2*, 319, 1956.
4. Jimenez Diaz, C., and Lahoz, C., La cannobosis (enfermedad de los trabajadores del canamo). Rev. Clin. Esp., *14*, 366, 1944.

5. Bouhuys, A., Barbero, A., Lindell, S.-E., et al., Byssinosis in hemp workers. Arch. Environ. Health, *14*, 533, 1967.
6. El Batawi, M. A., Byssinosis in cotton industry in Egypt. Br. J. Ind. Med., *19*, 126, 1962.
7. Lammers, B., Schilling, R. S. F., and Walford, J., A study of byssinosis, chronic respiratory symptoms and ventilatory capacity in English and Dutch cotton workers, with special reference to atmospheric pollution. Br. J. Ind. Med., *21*, 124, 1964.
8. Belin, L., Bouhuys, A., Hoekstra, W., et al., Byssinosis in cardroom workers in Swedish cotton mills. Br. J. Ind. Med., *22*, 101, 1965.
9. Bouhuys, A., Heaphy, L. J., Jr., Schilling, R. S. F., and Welborn, J. W., Byssinosis in the United States. N. Engl. J. Med., *277*, 170, 1967.
10. Schilling, R. S. F., Hughes, J. P. W., Dingwall-Fordyce, I., and Gilson, J. C., Epidemiological study of byssinosis among Lancashire cotton workers. Br. J. Ind. Med., *12*, 217, 1955.
11. Elwood, P. C., Pemberton, J., Merrett, J. D., et al., Byssinosis and other respiratory symptoms in flax workers in Northern Ireland. Br. J. Ind. Med., *22*, 27, 1965.
12. Registrar General Supplement to 55th Annual Report for England and Wales 1891. London, H. M. Stationery Office, 1897.
13. Registrar General Supplement to 75th Annual Report for England and Wales 1910–12. London, H. M. Stationery Office, 1923.
14. Registrar General Decennial Supplement, England and Wales for 1921. London, H. M. Stationery Office, 1927.
15. Registrar General Decennial Supplement, England and Wales for 1931. London, H. M. Stationery Office, 1938.
16. Schilling, R. S. F., and Goodman, N., Cardiovascular disease in cotton workers: Part I. Br. J. Ind. Med., *8*, 77, 1951.
17. Registrar General Decennial Supplement, England and Wales 1951. Occupational Mortality Part II, Vol 1. London, H. M. Stationery Office, 1958.
18. Registrar General Decennial Supplement (1970–1972). Occupational Mortality. London, H. M. Stationery Office, 1978, pp. 87–88.
19. Henderson, V. L., and Enterline, P. E., An unusual mortality experience in cotton textile workers. J. Occup. Med., *15*, 717, 1973.
20. Merchant, J. A., and Ortmeyer, C. E., Mortality of employees of two cotton mills in North Carolina. Chest, *79* (Suppl), 6, 1981.
21. Berry, G., and Molyneux, M. K. B., A mortality study of workers in Lancashire cotton mills. Chest, *79* (Suppl), 11, 1981.
21a. Elwood, P. C., Thomas, H. F., Sweetman, P. M., and Elwood, J. H., Mortality of flax workers. Br. J. Ind. Med., *39*, 18, 1982.
22. Lee, W. R., Clinical diagnosis of byssinosis. Thorax, *34*:287, 1979.
23. Pratt, P. C., Vollmer, R. T., and Miller, J. A., Epidemiology of pulmonary lesions in non-textile and cotton workers. Arch. Environ. Health, *35*, 133, 1980.
24. Schilling, R. S. F., Byssinosis in the British cotton textile industry. Br. Med. Bull., *7*, 52, 1950.
25. Roach, S. A., and Schilling, R. S. F., A clinical and environmental study of byssinosis in the Lancashire cotton industry. Br. J. Med., *17*, 1, 1960.
26. Fox, A. J., Tombleson, J. B. L., Watt, A., and Wilkie, A. G., A survey of respiratory disease in cotton operatives. Part II. Symptoms, dust estimations and the effect of smoking habit. Br. J. Ind. Med., *30*, 48, 1973.
27. Berry, G., Molyneux, M. K. B., and Tombleson, J. B. L., Relationship between dust level and byssinosis and bronchitis in Lancashire cotton mills. Br. J. Ind. Med., *31*, 18, 1974.
28. Jones, R. N., Butcher, B. T., Hammad, Y. Y., et al., Interaction of atopy and exposure to cotton dust in the bronchoconstrictor response. Br. J. Ind. Med., *37*, 141, 1980.
29. Jones, R. N., Diem, J. E., Glindmeyer, H., et al., Mill effect and dose-response relationship in byssinosis. Br. J. Ind. Med., *36*, 305, 1979.
30. Edwards, J., McCarthy, P., McDermott, M., et al., The acute physiological pharmacological effects of inhaled cotton dust in normal subjects. J. Physiol., *298*, 63, 1970.
31. Bouhuys, A., Lindell, S.-E., and Lundin, G., Experimental studies on byssinosis. Br. Med. J., *1*, 32, 1960.
32. Massoud, A. A. E., Altounyan, R. C., Howell, J. B. L., and Lane, R. E., Effect of histamine aerosol in byssinotic subjects. Br. J. Ind. Med., *24*, 38, 1967.
33. Valić, F., and Zuškin, E., Pharmacological prevention of acute ventilatory capacity reduction in flax dust exposure. Br. J. Ind. Med., *30*, 381, 1973.

34. Schacter, E. N., Brown, S., Zuškin, E., et al., The effect of mediator modifying drugs in cotton bract–induced bronchospasm. Chest, 79 (Suppl), 73, 1981.
35. Zuškin, E., and Bouhuys, A., Protective effect of disodium cromoglycate against airway constriction induced by hemp dust extract. J. Allergy Clin. Immunol., 57, 473, 1976.
36. Bouhuys, A., Schoenberg, J. B., Beck, G. J., and Schilling, R. S. F., Epidemiology of chronic lung disease in a cotton mill community. Lung, 154, 167, 1977.
37. Rooke, G. B., The pathology of byssinosis. Chest, 79 (Suppl), 67, 1981.
38. Berry, G., McKerrow, C. W., Molyneux, M. K. B., et al., A study of the acute and chronic changes in ventilatory capacity in Lancashire cotton mills. Br. J. Ind. Med., 30, 25, 1973.
39. Beck, G. J., Schacter, E. N., Maunder, L. R., and Bouhuys, A., The relation of lung function to subsequent employment status and mortality in cotton textile workers. Chest, 79 (Suppl), 26, 1981.
40. Imbus, H. R., and Suh, M. W., Byssinosis: a study of 10,133 textile workers. Arch. Environ. Health, 26, 183, 1973.
41. Merchant, J. A., Lumsden, J. C., Kilburn, K. H., et al., Intervention studies of cotton steaming to reduce biological effects of cotton dust. Br. J. Ind. Med., 31, 261, 1974.
42. Carey, G. G. R., and Merrett, J. C., Changes in ventilatory capacity in a group of flax workers in Northern Ireland. Br. J. Ind. Med., 22, 121, 1965.
43. Zuškin, E., and Valić, F., Respiratory changes in two groups of flax workers with different exposure patterns. Thorax, 28, 579, 1973.
44. Jones, R. N., Carr, J., Glindmeyer, H., et al., Respiratory health and dust levels in cotton seed mills. Thorax, 32, 281, 1977.
45. Fairman, P., Hankinson, J. L., Lapp, N. L., and Morgan, W. K. C., A pilot study of closing volume in byssinosis. Br. J. Ind. Med., 32, 235, 1974.
46. Occupational Exposure to Cotton Dust. HEW Publication (NIOSH) 75–118, U.S. Department of Health, Education & Welfare. Washington, D.C., Government Printing Office, 1974.
47. Merino, V. L., Lombart, R. L., Marco, R. F., et al., Arterial blood gas tension and lung function during acute responses to hemp dust. Am. Rev. Respir. Dis., 107, 809, 1973.
48. Zuškin, E., Valić, F., Butkovic, D., and Bouhuys, A., Lung function in textile workers. Br. J. Ind. Med., 32, 283, 1975.
49. Guyatt, A. R., Douglas, J. S., Zuškin, E., and Bouhuys, A., Lung static recoil and airway obstruction in hemp workers with byssinosis. Am. Rev. Respir. Dis., 108, 1111, 1973.
50. Bouhuys, A., and Van de Woestijne, K. P., Respiratory mechanics in dust exposure in byssinosis. J. Clin. Invest., 49, 106, 1970.
51. Morgan, W. K. C., Industrial bronchitis. Br. J. Ind. Med., 35:285, 1978.
52. Zuškin, E., Valić, F., and Bouhuys, A., Effect of wool dust on respiratory function. Am. Rev. Respir. Dis., 114, 705, 1976.
53. Edwards, C., Macartney, J., Rooke, G., and Ward, F., The pathology of the lung in byssinosis. Thorax, 30, 612, 1975.
54. Edwards, J., Mechanisms of disease induction. Chest, 79 (Suppl), 38, 1981.
55. Antweiler, H., Histamine liberation by cotton dust extract. Br. J. Ind. Med., 18, 130, 1961.
56. Davenport, A., and Paton, W. D. M., The pharmacological activity of extracts of cotton dust. Br. J. Ind. Med., 19, 19, 1962.
57. Hitchcock, M., In vitro histamine release from human lungs as a model for the acute response to cotton dust. Ann. N.Y. Acad. Sci., 221, 124, 1974.
58. Ainsworth, S. K., Neuman, R. E., and Harley, R. A., Histamine releases from platelets for assay of byssinogenic substances in cotton mill dust and related materials. Br. J. Ind. Med., 36, 35, 1979.
59. Murphy, R. C., Hammarström, S., and Samuelsson, B., Leukotriene C: a slow-reacting substance from murine mastocytoma cells. Proc. Natl. Acad. Sci. U.S.A., 76, 4275, 1979.
60. Knauer, K. A., Lichtenstein, L. M., Adkinson, N. F., and Fish, J. E., Platelet activation during antigen induced airway reactions in asthmatic subjects. N. Engl. J. Med., 304, 1404, 1981.

61. Lynn, W. S., Munoz, S., Campbell, J. A., and Jeffs, P. M., Chemotaxis and cotton extracts. Ann. N.Y. Acad. Sci., *221*, 163, 1974.
62. Pernis, B., Vigliani, E. C., Cavagna, C., and Finulli, M., The role of bacterial endotoxins in occupational disease caused by inhaling vegetable dust. Br. J. Ind. Med., *18*, 120, 1967.
63. Cavagna, C., Foa, V., and Vigliani, E. C., Effects in men and rabbits of inhalation of cotton dust or extracts and purified endotoxins. Br. J. Ind. Med., *26*, 314, 1969.
64. Rylander, R., and Lundholm, M., Bacterial contamination of cotton and cotton dust and effects on the lung. Br. J. Ind. Med., *35*, 204, 1978.
65. Rylander, R., Bacterial toxins and the etiology of byssinosis. Chest, *79* (Suppl), 34, 1981.
66. Massoud, A. A. E., and Taylor, G., Byssinosis: antibodies to cotton antigens in normal subjects and in cotton cardroom workers. Lancet, *2*, 607, 1966.
67. Taylor, G., Massoud, A. A. E., and Lucas, F., Studies in the aetiology of byssinosis. Br. J. Ind. Med., *28*, 143, 1971.
68. Kutz, S. A., Mentnech, S., Olenchock, S., and Major, P. C., Immune mechanisms in byssinosis. Chest, *79* (Suppl), 53, 1981.
68a. Morgan, W. K. C., Vesterlund, J., Burrell, R., et al., Byssinosis: some unanswered questions. Am. Rev. Respir. Dis., *126*, 354, 1982.
69. Middleton, D., Logan, J. S., Magennis, B. P., and Nelson, S. D., HLA antigen frequencies in flax byssinosis patients. Br. J. Ind. Med., *36*, 123, 1979.
70. Cotton Dust Standard. Federal Register, Vol. 43, No. 122, June 23, 1978, pp. 27394–27399. Washington, D.C., Government Printing Office.
71. Merchant, J. A., Lumsden, J. C., Kilburn, K. H., et al., I, An industrial study of the biological effects of cotton dust and cigarette smoke exposure. II, Dose-response studies in cotton textile workers. J. Occup. Med., *15*, 212 and 222, 1973.
72. Imbus, H. R., and Suh, M. W., Steaming of cotton to prevent byssinosis. Br. J. Ind. Med., *31*, 209, 1974.
73. Boehlecke, B., Cocke, J., Bragge, K., et al., Pulmonary function response to dust from standard and closed boll harvested cotton. Chest, *79* (Suppl), 77, 1981.
74. Collis, E. L., Annual Report of Chief Inspector of Factories, 1953, p. 150. Reprinted in Pub. Health, *28*, 252, 1915.
75. Vigliani, E. C., Parmeggiani, L., and Sassi, C., Studio di un'epidemia di una tessiture di cotone. Med. Lavoro, *45*, 349, 1954.
76. Murray, R., Dingwall-Fordyce, I., and Lane, R. E., An outbreak of weaver's cough associated with tamarind seed powder. Br. J. Ind. Med., *14*, 105, 1957.
77. Woolf, S. M., Biological effects of bacterial endotoxins in man. *In* Kass, E. H., and Woolf, S. M., eds., Bacterial Lipopolysaccharides. Chicago, University of Chicago Press, 1973, p. 251.
78. Munt, D. F., Gauvain, S., Walford, J., Schilling, R. S. F., Study of respiratory symptoms and ventilatory capacities among rope workers. Br. J. Ind. Med., *22*, 196, 1965.
79. Nicholls, P. J., Evans, E., Valić, F., and Zuškin, E., Histamine-releasing activity and bronchoconstricting effects of sisal. Br. J. Ind. Med., *30*, 142, 1973.
80. Baker, M. D., Irwig, L. M., Johnston, J. R., et al., Lung function in sisal ropemakers. Br. J. Ind. Med., *36*, 216, 1979.
81. Mustafa, K. Y., Lakha, A. S., Milla, M. H., and Dahoma, U., Byssinosis, respiratory symptoms and spirometric lung function tests in Tanzanian sisal workers. Br. J. Ind. Med., *35*, 123, 1978.
82. El Ghawabi, S. H., Respiratory function and symptoms in workers exposed simultaneously to jute and hemp. Br. J. Ind. Med., *35*, 16, 1978.
83. Mair, A., Smith, D. H., Wilson, W. A., and Lockhart, W., Dust diseases in Dundee textile workers. Br. J. Ind. Med., *17*, 272, 1960.
84. Siddhu, C. M. S., Nath, J., and Mehotra, R. K., Byssinosis amongst cotton and jute workers in Kanpur. Ind. J. Med. Res., *54*, 980, 1966.
85. Popa, V., Gavrilescu, N., Preda, N., et al., An investigation of allergy in byssinosis: sensitization to cotton, hemp, flax and jute antigens. Br. J. Ind. Med., *26*, 101, 1968.
86. Gandevia, B., and Milne, J., Ventilatory capacity on exposure to jute dust and the relevance of productive cough and smoking to the response. Br. J. Ind. Med., *22*, 187, 1965.
87. Valić, F., and Zuškin, E., A comparative study of respiratory function in female nonsmoking cotton and jute workers. Br. J. Ind. Med., *28*, 364, 1971.

19

HYPERSENSITIVITY PNEUMONITIS

Anthony Seaton and W. Keith C. Morgan

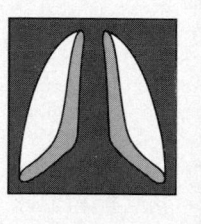

The inhalation of organic particles or gases may lead to a number of different pulmonary responses. The best understood of these is asthma, characterized by increased resistance to flow in the airways and usually mediated by reaginic antibody (see Chap. 16). Less common is a reaction involving the lung acinus, including the bronchioles, and known as allergic alveolitis or allergic bronchiolo-alveolitis.[1] There is still considerable debate about the immunological mechanisms involved in this disease, and indeed the different clinical patterns seen in various manifestations of allergic alveolitis suggest that several mechanisms may be involved. In addition to these diseases, there are also several even less well-understood conditions in which the lung may be involved as part of a response to organic antigen. Humidifier fever, sewage worker's disease and grain fever are examples. Finally, an occasional patient may present with a dual reaction at both bronchial and acinar level. This may occur with exposure to gases or fumes, such as isocyanates and cobalt, as well as to particulate organic matter. In view of the variety of pulmonary responses to inhaled organic material and the uncertainties surrounding their pathogenesis, this chapter has been given the rather general heading of hypersensitivity pneumonitis. Under this rubric, the classical syndromes recognized as allergic alveolitis, as well as the other less well-defined syndromes, are discussed.

ALLERGIC ALVEOLITIS

Clinical Features

The classical acute episode of allergic alveolitis starts with fever, muscular aches, and general malaise some four to eight hours after exposure to an antigen. Occasionally this is preceded or accompanied by wheeze or tightness in the chest and a dry cough. Shortness of breath is

564

a feature of more severe attacks and may occasionally be dramatic and disabling or even fatal. The symptoms typically reach a peak at about 8 to 12 hours after exposure and then improve over another 12 to 24 hours, in the absence of further exposure. The physical signs during such an attack are fever, tachycardia, and tachypnea. The latter sign may only be detected in mild cases if the patient is exercised. Auscultation of the lungs invariably reveals repetitive mid- and end-inspiratory crackles. Wheeze may occasionally be heard also and should not put one off the diagnosis. Acute attacks are associated with leukocytosis and a relative lymphopenia in the peripheral blood.

Such an acute attack usually resolves rapidly, but occasionally it may persist much longer and require the patient's admission to a hospital (Fig. 19–1). These episodes may cause diagnostic difficulties if the physician is unaware of this presentation; the most frequent condition with which it may be confused is a mycoplasmal or another atypical pneumonia, which it mimics closely, and this confusion may be compounded by the anamnestic rise in viral antibody titers that may occur in acute allergic alveolitis.[2] Even more confusing is that spurious false-positive precipitins to farmer's lung antigen may occur in mycoplasmal pneumonia.[3] In such difficult cases, the diagnosis initially depends on a careful record of the patient's exposure history.

A third way in which allergic alveolitis may manifest itself is as a recurrent, subacute illness. In this case, patients complain of general malaise, cough, wheeze or shortness of breath, laryngitis, and other symptoms, none of which is specific or dramatic. They will commonly have consulted doctors repeatedly for what both patient and doctor believe to be upper respiratory tract infections and in some cases there may even have been thoughts of involving a psychiatrist. Such patients usually respond promptly to removal of the antigen. This type of presentation is found most frequently among people exposed to relatively low doses of an antigen on a regular basis, such as keepers of parakeets or canaries.

It should be pointed out that though age may modify the body's immune response to antigen, allergic alveolitis may occur at any age. Children who help their parents on farms and with racing pigeons are at risk, and it is important that pediatricians be aware of this, since permanent lung damage may well occur. Besides age, another factor that may modify the response to inhaled antigen is cigarette smoking, and there is now good evidence that smokers are less susceptible to allergic alveolitis than non-smokers.[4, 5] This should not, of course, be used as an argument in favor of smoking!

It is likely that any acute attack of allergic alveolitis causes some scarring of acinar structures pathologically. However, the patients who are most likely to develop irreversible pulmonary fibrosis are those with the recurrent subacute type of presentation and, to a lesser extent, those with recurrent episodes of the persistent acute attacks. Such patients may develop clinical evidence of pulmonary fibrosis, with retraction of upper

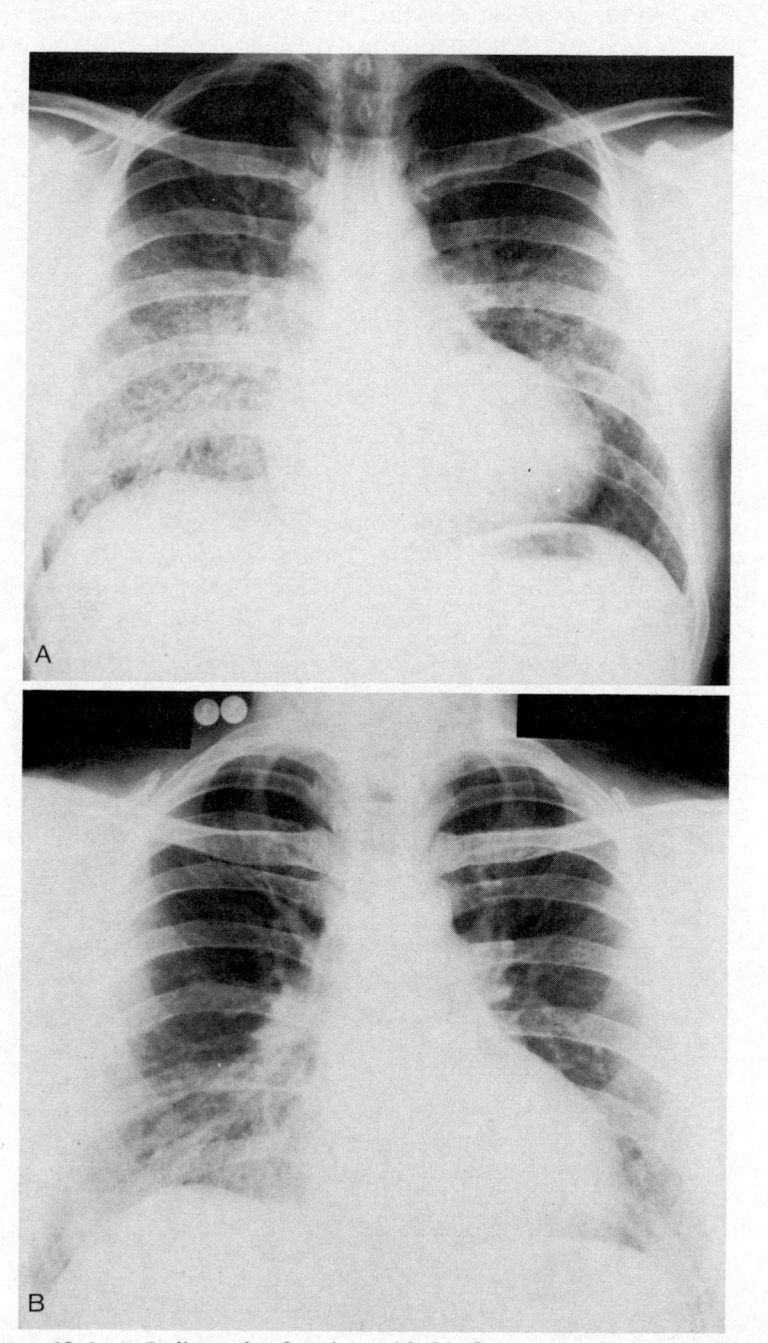

Figure 19–1. *A,* Radiograph of patient with his first attack of acute farmer's lung, showing diffuse ground glass opacification. *B,* Same patient 5 weeks later. Slow resolution has taken place, but some residual shadowing remains.

lobes and basal crackles, but not usually finger clubbing. A proportion of patients with chronic allergic alveolitis develop a syndrome of airways obstruction clinically indistinguishable from emphysema.[6] Any nonsmoker who presents with emphysema should be carefully questioned about possible exposure to organic antigen. Ultimately, patients with chronic allergic alveolitis may develop respiratory failure and cor pulmonale.

Radiographic Features

The radiographic appearances of allergic alveolitis are very variable.[6] In the acute episode there may be a dramatic bilateral acinar filling process indistinguishable from pulmonary edema (Fig. 19–2) or a diffuse miliary mottling (Fig. 19–3). There is often an irregular linear component to the

Text continued on page 571.

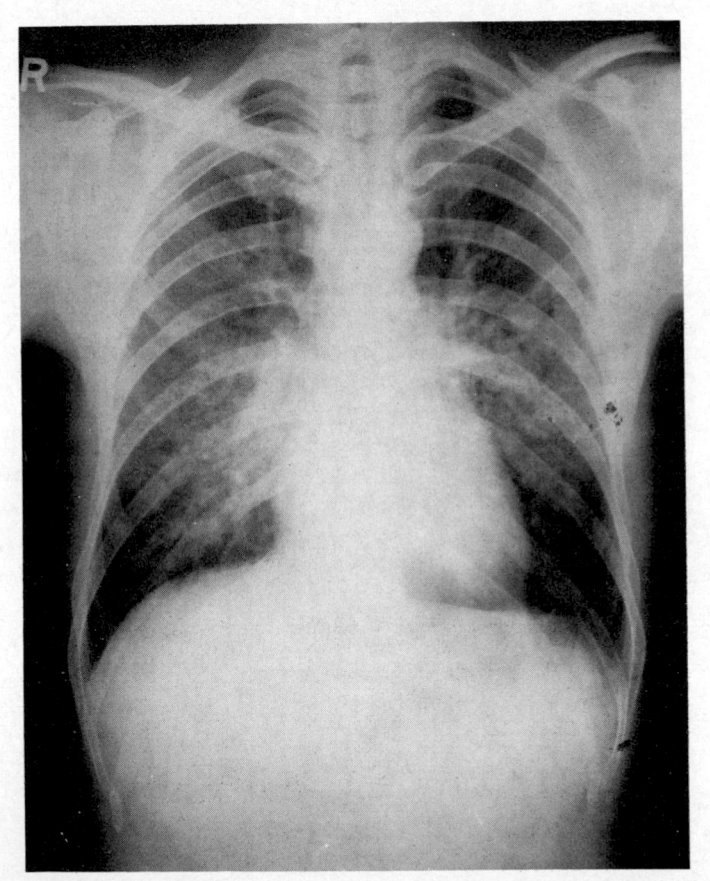

Figure 19–2. Farmer's lung. Acute episode of fever and dyspnea occurring 4 hours after the patient had forked moldy hay for feeding cattle. Radiograph shows a fine nodular infiltrate, confluent toward the hila and sparing the peripheries. Patient recovered rapidly with steroid treatment. (Courtesy of Dr. J. Meek.)

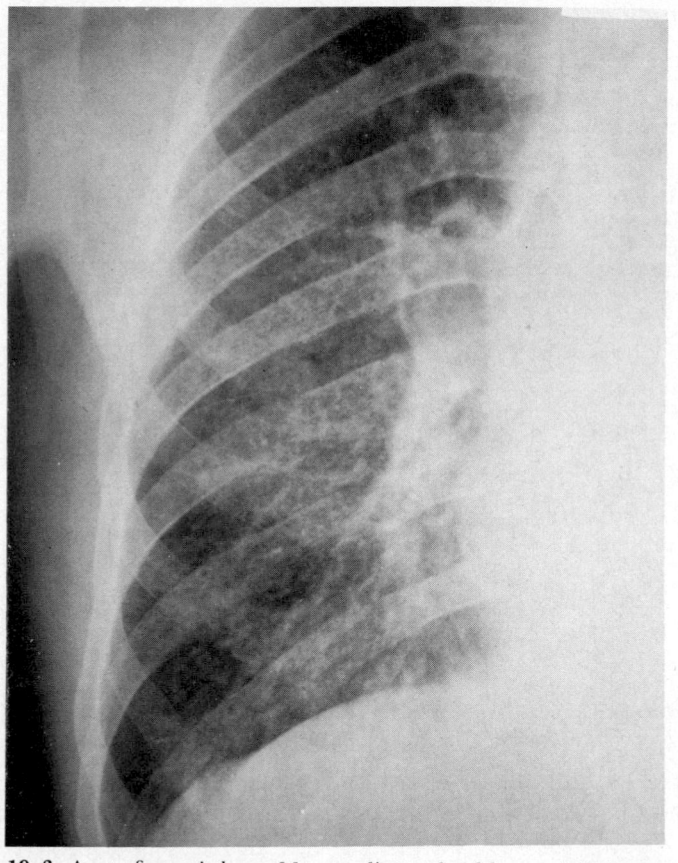

Figure 19–3. Acute farmer's lung. Macroradiograph of lower right lung to show the typical pattern of fine miliary mottling. (Courtesy of Dr. J. Meek.)

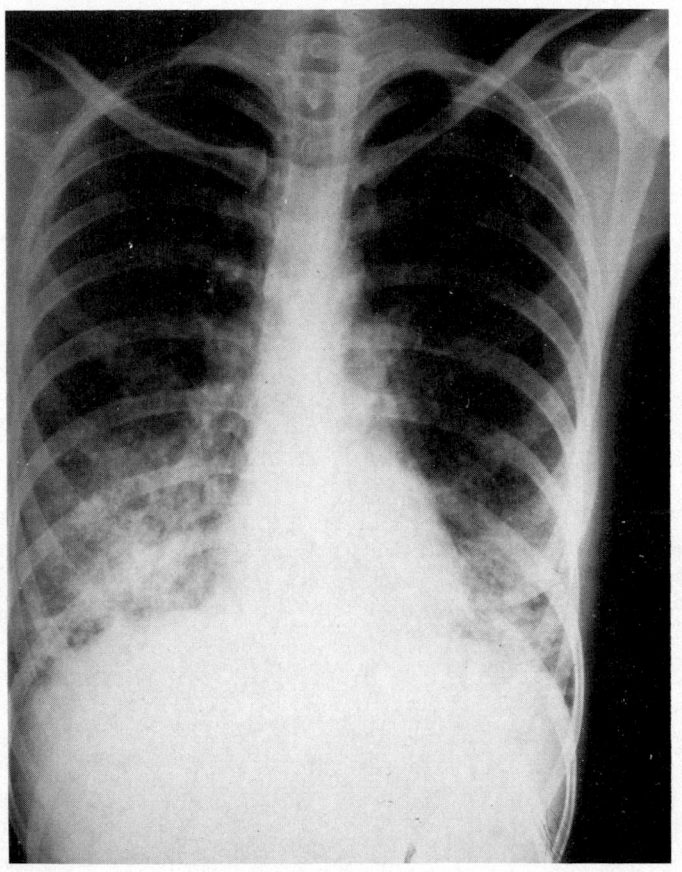

Figure 19–4. Acute farmer's lung in farmer's wife following feeding cattle with hay. Radiograph shows a pattern of miliary mottling with a linear component at the bases. (Courtesy of Dr. J. Meek.)

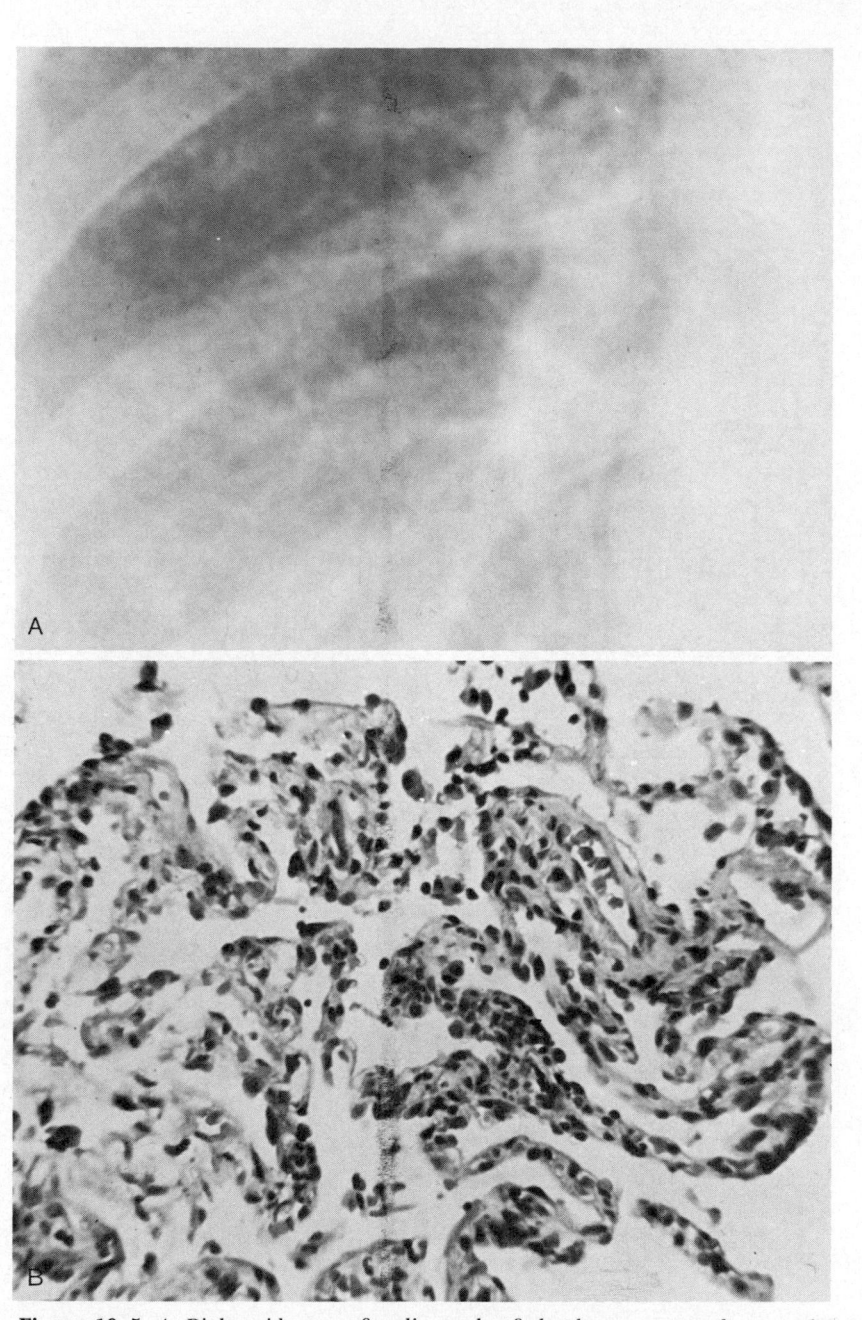

Figure 19–5. *A*, Right mid zone of radiograph of shopkeeper exposed to parakeets, showing possible diffuse nodularity. *B*, Needle lung biopsy specimen from same patient, showing nonspecific alveolitis.

Illustration continued on opposite page.

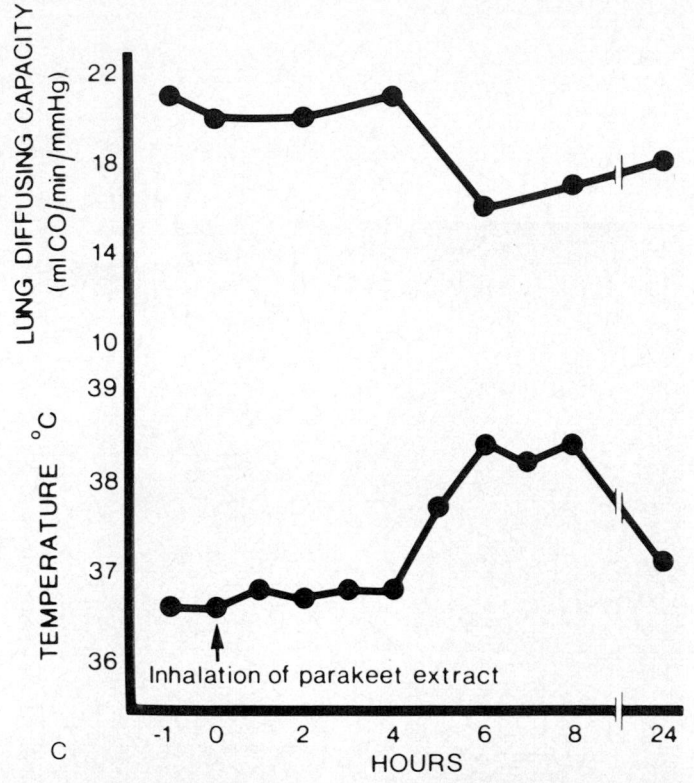

Figure 19–5 (*Continued*). *C,* Challenge test with parakeet serum showed delayed rise in temperature and fall in diffusing capacity, diagnostic of allergic alveolitis.

shadowing in the lower zones (Fig. 19–4), and Kerley B lines may be seen. The shadowing is usually diffuse and shows no preference for any parts of the lung.

In the subacute type of allergic alveolitis, radiographic changes may be minimal or absent, even in the presence of profuse inspiratory crackles on auscultation (Fig. 19–5). As the disease becomes chronic, irregular linear and cystic shadows of fibrosis occur, predominantly in the upper zones. The upper zones become contracted with traction upwards of the pulmonary arteries (Fig. 19–6), and the final appearance may be indistinguishable from that in tuberculosis, sarcoidosis, ankylosing spondylitis, or histiocytosis X, all of which figure in the differential diagnosis of upper zone fibrosis.

Pulmonary Function

During the acute attack, the subject's lung volumes and in particular vital capacity are reduced. Although there are regional changes in the distribution of ventilation and perfusion, airways resistance remains nor-

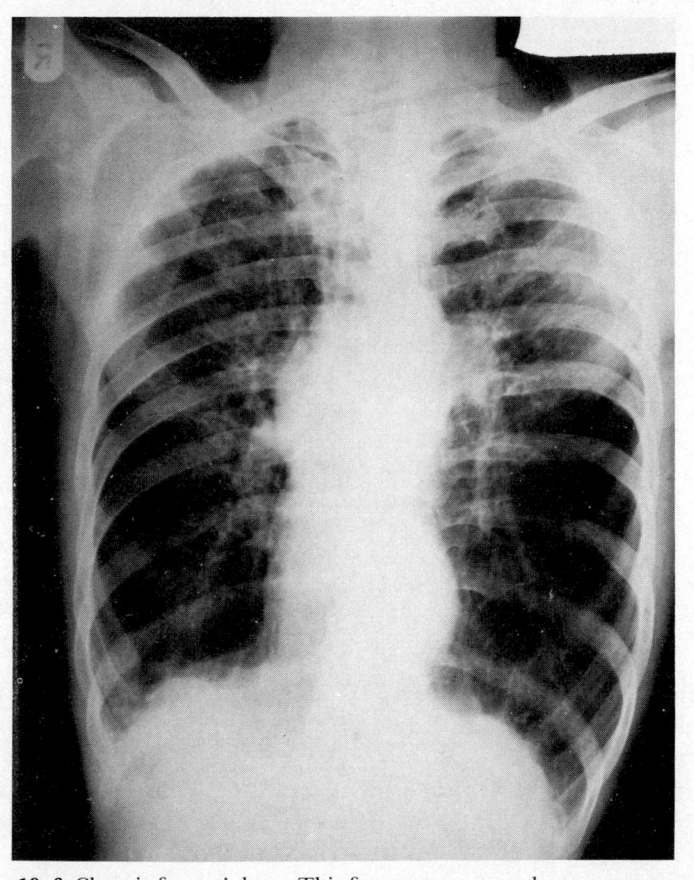

Figure 19–6. Chronic farmer's lung. This farmer was exposed over many years to moldy hay dust, and had several previous episodes of shivering and dyspnea following exposure. Now he is persistently short of breath on moderate exertion with lung function tests showing a mixed pattern of restriction and obstruction. Radiograph shows linear shadows extending into contracted upper lobes and compensatory emphysematous changes in lower zones. (Courtesy of Dr. J. Meek.)

mal. The diffusing capacity (transfer factor) is reduced and the lungs have a reduced compliance.[6, 7] Blood gases at this stage show arterial oxygen desaturation, which may be profound. The arterial carbon dioxide tension is usually slightly reduced due to alveolar hyperventilation, though renal compensation for this respiratory alkalosis tends to keep the pH normal (Table 19–1). In the acute attack, exercise testing is usually impracticable, but when it becomes possible it usually causes a further fall in arterial oxygen tension. Neither does diffusing capacity rise as expected on exercise at this stage. The administration of 100 per cent oxygen produces complete saturation, and the arterial oxygen tension rises to a level sufficient to indicate that the basic defect responsible for desaturation is an inequality in ventilation-perfusion ratios. Concomitant with the hyperventilation and desaturation is an increase in the ratio of physiological dead space to tidal volume. Some studies have suggested that the reduction in diffusing capacity is related to a fall in the membrane component rather than the pulmonary capillary blood volume.[6, 7] Pulmonary artery pressure and vascular resistance may, however, be slightly elevated in the acute stages, an increase possibly related to the fall in arterial oxygen tension.

In the typical acute attack, these abnormalities resolve over a few days. Prolonged attacks may, however, be associated with severe impairment of volumes and diffusing capacity for several weeks, and in some cases these abnormalities may persist indefinitely as the chronic disease. In the subacute cases, reduced diffusing capacity and compliance may be

Table 19–1. PULMONARY FUNCTION CHANGES IN A SUBJECT WITH ACUTE FARMER'S LUNG

	Predicted	Observed	3 Weeks Later	6 Months Later
Lung Volumes				
VC (L)	5.10	3.80	4.20	5.30
RV (L)	1.50	1.90	1.80	1.80
TLC (L)	6.60	5.70	6.00	7.10
Mechanics				
FEV$_1$ (l)	4.08	3.04	3.21	4.20
MVV (l/m)	145	95	107	144
Static Compliance				
(l/cm H$_2$O)	0.20	0.045	0.10	0.21
Gas Diffusion				
Carbon monoxide diffusing capacity (steady state) (ml/min/ mm Hg)	37.00	18.00	22.00	34.00
Arterial Po$_2$ (mm Hg)	95.00	52.00	75.00	92.00
Arterial Pco$_2$ (mm Hg)	38.0–42.0	34.00	38.00	39.00
pH	7.38–7.42	7.44	7.40	7.40

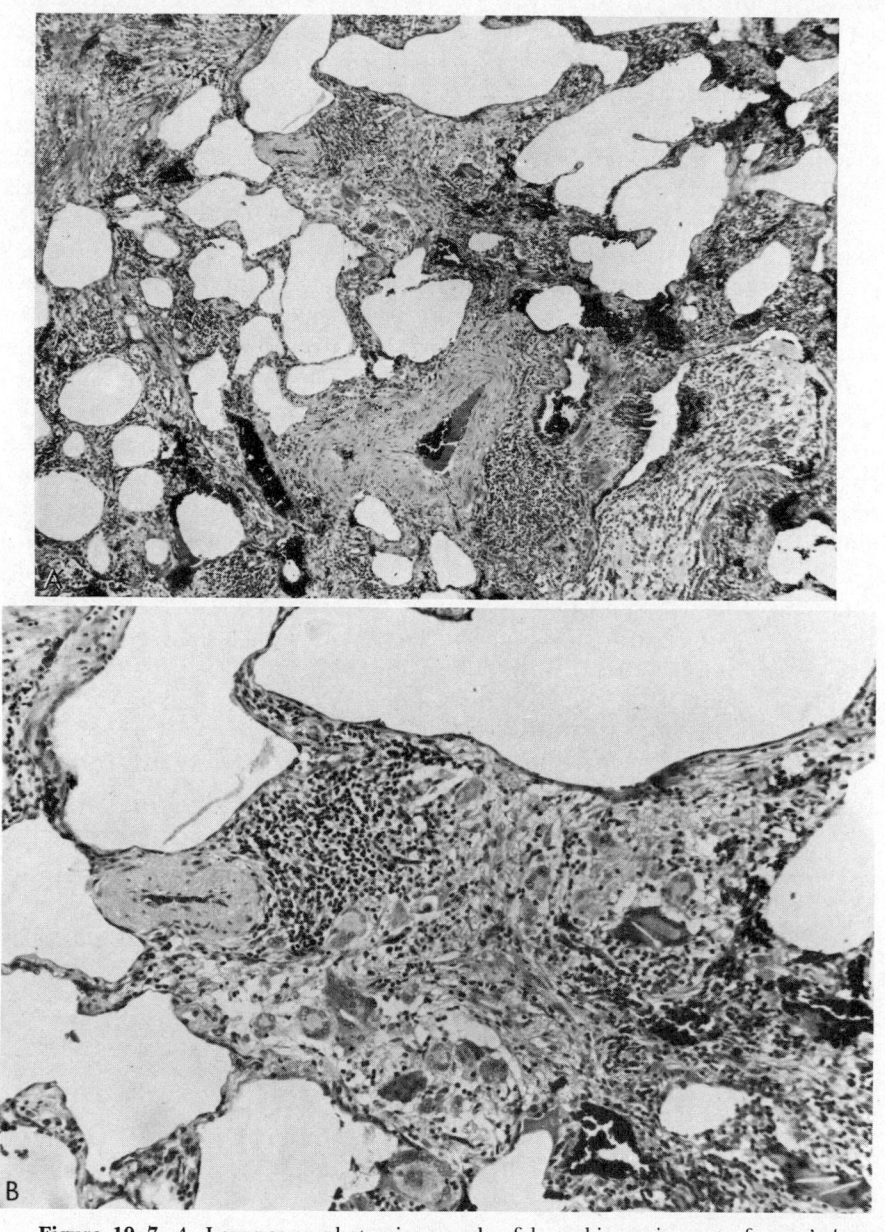

Figure 19–7. *A,* Low-power photomicrograph of lung biopsy in acute farmer's lung, showing extensive inflammatory changes in centrilobular areas, bronchiolitis (bottom right), and thickening of related pulmonary arteries. There is an interstitial mononuclear inflammatory infiltrate (alveolitis), and a perivascular giant cell granuloma is present (top center), The disease in this patient progressed to chronic fibrosis in spite of treatment with steroids. *B,* Higher-power photomicrograph of the perivascular granuloma in *A,* showing epithelioid cells, giant cells of both Langhans and foreign body type (with inclusions in the latter), and focal collections of lymphocytes.

the only abnormalities found. It should also be remembered that up to one third of chronic cases present an obstructive pattern, sometimes with raised residual volume and low diffusing capacity mimicking emphysema.[6]

Pathology

Often the most characteristic feature of the pathology of allergic alveolitis is its distribution maximally around the respiratory bronchiole at the center of the acinus (Fig. 19–7). There is frequently an inflammatory reaction in the bronchiolar wall and this may be intense. Occasionally, the alveolar wall is also involved (Fig. 19–8). Another conspicuous feature of the pathology of the acute disease is the presence of numerous noncaseating sarcoid-like granulomata, usually associated with giant cells, and again predominantly in the center of the acinus. The giant cells may be of both Langhans' and foreign-body types (Fig. 19–7). The alveolar walls are typically thickened by edema and infiltration with monocytes, predominantly lymphocytes, plasma cells, and histiocytes.[8, 9] Alveolar macrophages may be profuse and, especially in bird breeder's lung, have a foamy appearance. In very acute severe cases, alveolar edema may be present with some macrophages within alveoli.[10] If biopsies are performed months after an acute attack, the granulomata have usually resolved, unlike sarcoidosis, in which they typically become hyalinized.

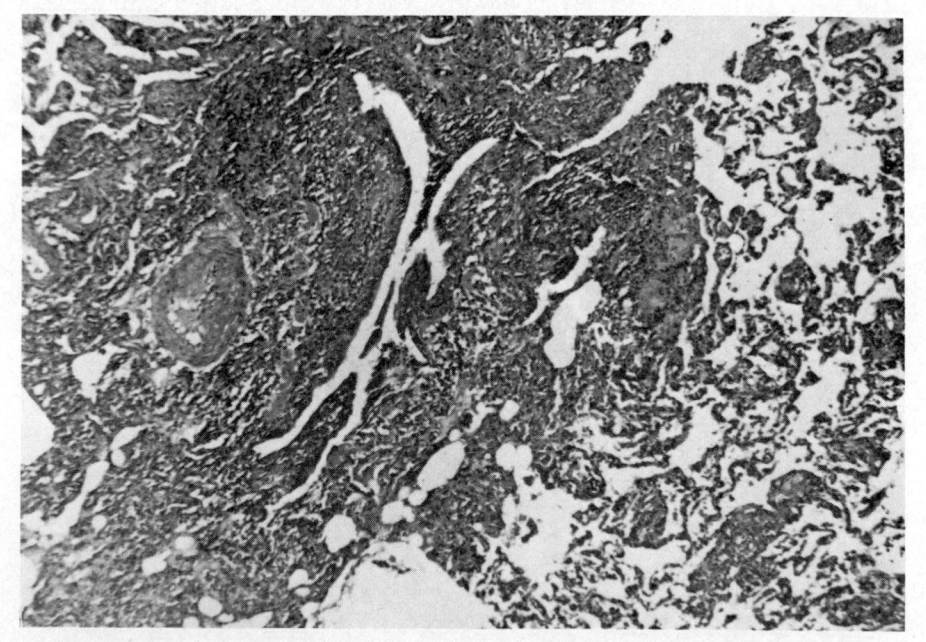

Figure 19–8. Low-power photomicrograph of biopsy from patient with acute farmer's lung, showing proliferative bronchiolar changes, ballooning of arteriolar endothelial cells, and mononuclear infiltration maximal in the center of the lobule, the peripheral alveolar septa being less involved.

While some alveolar wall fibrin may be seen in acute cases (Fig. 19–9), collagenous fibrosis is an important feature in chronic cases.[8] Macroscopically, irregular fibrosis and honeycombing is present, predominantly in the upper zones (Figs. 19–10 and 19–11). Microscopically, focal fibrosis is found around bronchioles and small bronchi (Fig. 19–12). Alveolar septa are thickened with collagen and around the bronchioles the alveolar architecture may be totally destroyed. Pulmonary hypertensive changes may be seen in the vessels, and in such cases right ventricular hypertrophy will be evident. Occasionally, chronic cases may be seen in which emphysema is the main pathological finding but in which microscopy reveals this to be associated with a fine interstitial fibrosis (Fig. 19–13). It is probable that such cases,. as well as those with extensive peribronchiolar fibrosis, are responsible for the syndrome of airways obstruction occurring in a proportion of patients with chronic allergic alveolitis.

Pathogenesis

The first step in the pathogenesis of allergic alveolitis is the inhalation of particulate organic matter sufficiently small in aerodynamic diameter to reach the lung acinus. In many instances this means the inhalation of fungal spores. These particles are present in the normal atmosphere throughout the year,[11] often in large numbers, and may sometimes provoke asthma in atopic subjects. However, the much larger numbers of

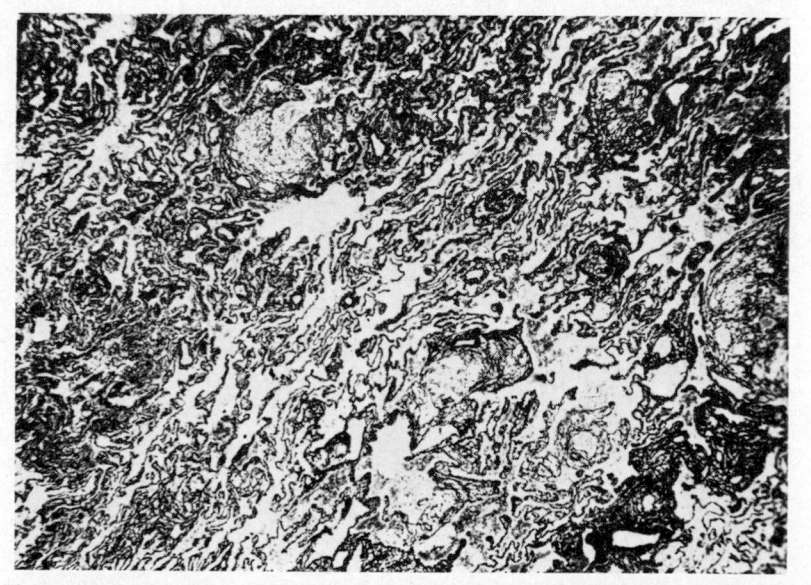

Figure 19–9. Low-power photomicrograph (reticulin stain) showing generalized increase in reticulin and three epithelioid tubercles. This biopsy was taken from a 20-year-old farmer following his second attack of farmer's lung. He has made a complete recovery and has normal lung function tests 20 years later.

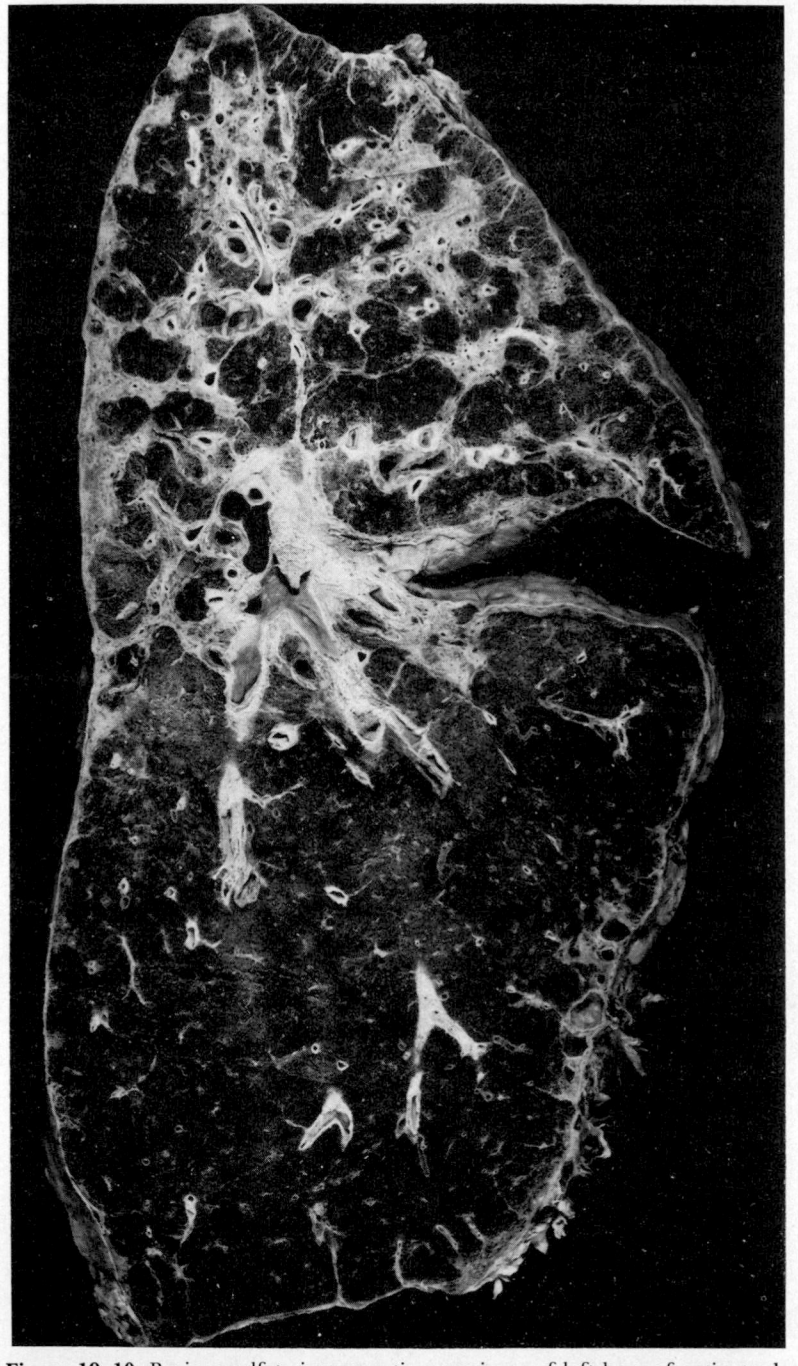

Figure 19–10. Barium sulfate impregnation specimen of left lung of patient who died in the chronic stage of farmer's lung, illustrating the more extensive involvement of the upper lobe with areas of focal fibrosis and interlacing communications. (From Seal, R. M. E., et al.: The pathology of the acute and chronic stages of farmer's lung, Thorax, *23*, 469, 1968.)

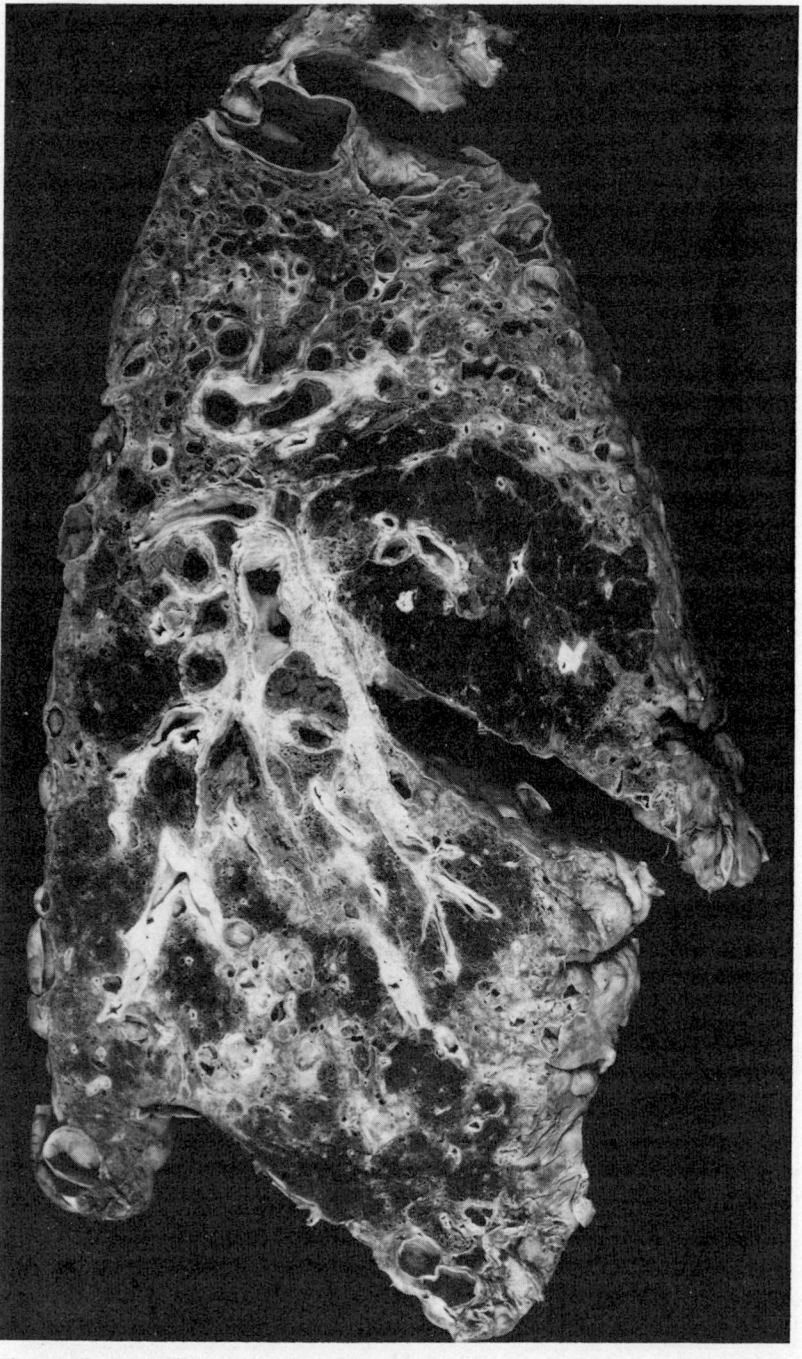

Figure 19–11. Barium sulfate impregnation specimen of left lung of patient who died of chronic farmer's lung, showing generalized disease, accentuation in the upper lobe and extensive honeycomb change. (From Seal, R. M. E., et al.: The pathology of the acute and chronic stages of farmer's lung, Thorax *23*:469, 1968.)

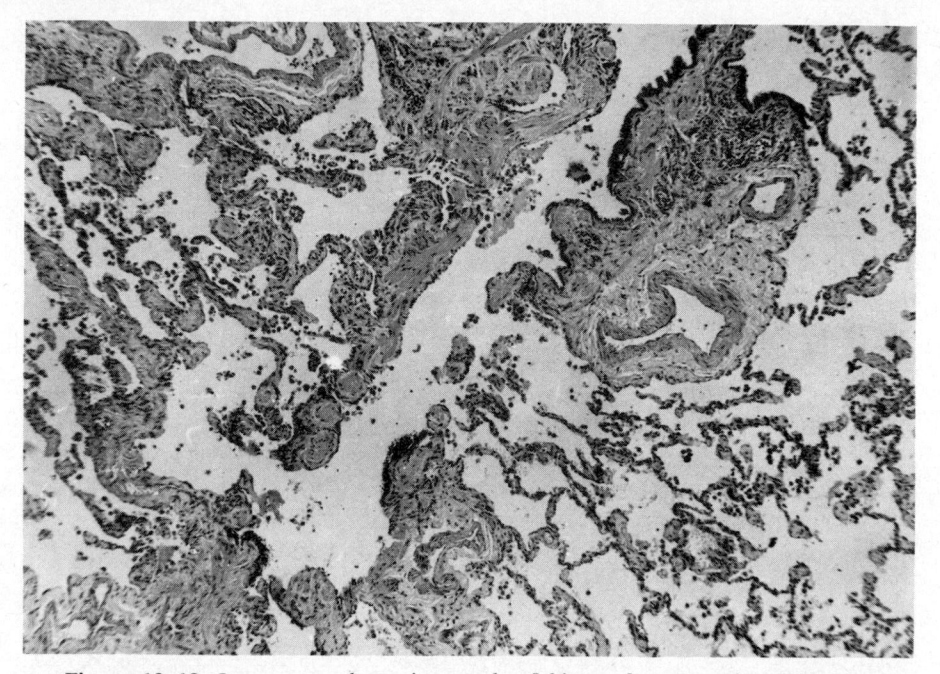

Figure 19–12. Low-power photomicrograph of biopsy from a patient with chronic farmer's lung, showing fibrosis maximal around the respiratory bronchiole but occurring also in peripheral alveolar walls.

particles associated with profuse growth on dead organic matter at appropriate conditions of temperature and humidity[12] are necessary in most cases for sensitization of the allergic alveolitis type to occur. Other organic particles that may be sufficiently small to cause acinar disease may be derived from feathers and animal dander or excreta. In a few instances a similar reaction has also been recorded following inhalation of organic vapor or even inorganic fumes, presumably on the basis of hapten formation with protein within the lung.

The original concept of pathogenesis was that the inhalation of relatively large amounts of antigenic material stimulated an IgG antibody response and that immune complexes were formed with this precipitating antibody that in the presence of excess antigen cause local activation of complement, recruitment of neutrophils, and consequent tissue damage; that is, a pulmonary Arthus reaction.[13] Central to this concept was the observation that precipitins were frequently observed in the blood of patients with allergic alveolitis. However, subsequent work has shown that the story is not quite so simple. Many patients have now been shown to have allergic alveolitis and yet have no precipitins[14] and, conversely, exposed individuals have been shown to have precipitins and no disease.[15] Moreover, the pathology of the lung is not wholly consistent with that of a typical Arthus reaction, the predominant cell reaction being infiltration

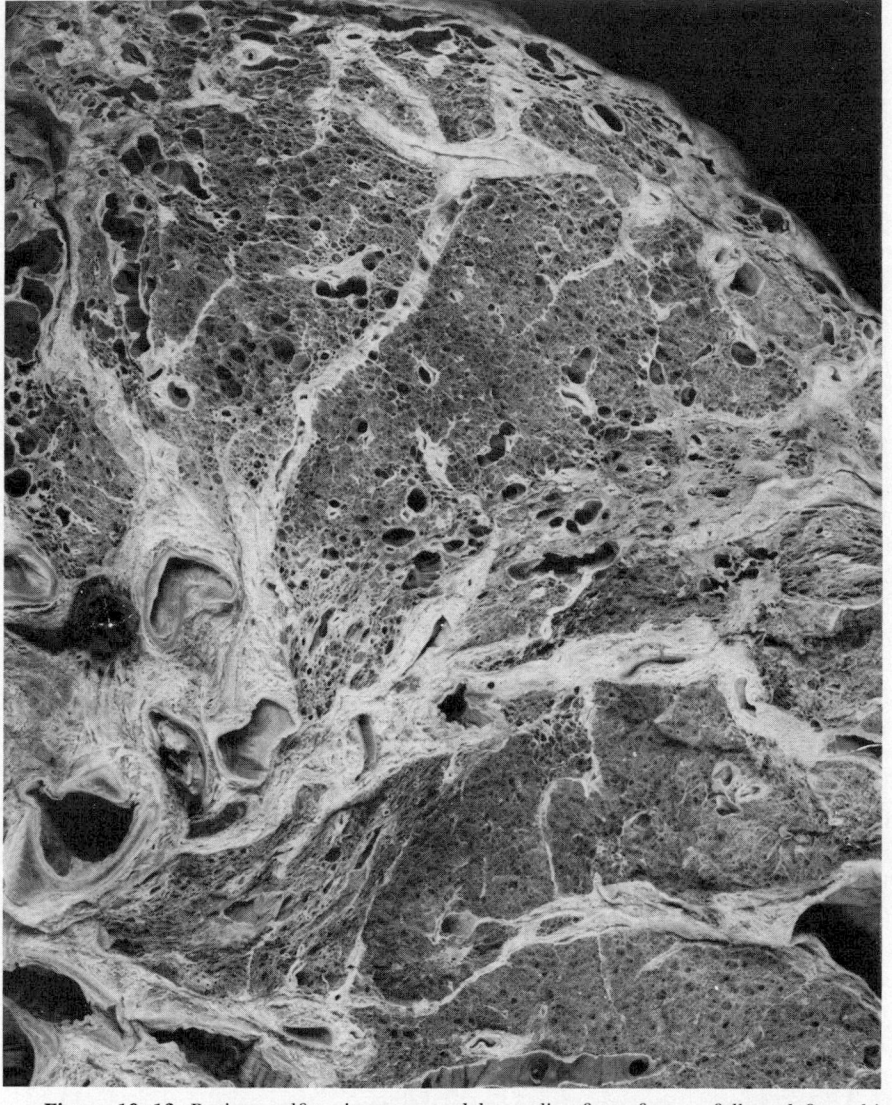

Figure 19–13. Barium sulfate–impregnated lung slice from farmer followed from his second acute attack of farmer's lung 18 years previously. He had minimal radiographic changes but a severely obstructed pattern of lung function and died in respiratory failure. The appearances illustrate fine interstitial fibrosis and dilated airspaces that many might interpret as emphysema. (Courtesy of Dr. R. M. E. Seal.)

with lymphocytes and plasma cells, with granulomata and giant cells forming a prominent feature. Animal studies have also failed to produce a model of the typical histological features of allergic alveolitis by simple aerosol challenge without prior treatment with Freund's adjuvant.[16]

Although an immune complex mechanism probably plays a part in many cases of allergic alveolitis,[17] recent research has pointed towards a role for complement activation by other mechanisms. In particular, insoluble organic particulates can activate complement by the alternative pathway, cleaving C3 and resulting in tissue damage and chemotaxis of macrophages.[18] Perhaps even more pertinently, macrophages that have ingested organic particles may liberate hydrolytic enzymes that are also capable of activating complement. However, the presence of granulomata and mononuclear cell infiltrates in allergic alveolitis suggests strongly that a cell-mediated immune mechanism also plays a part in the pathogenesis, and there is evidence that lymphocytes may be sensitized by organic antigen, particularly cell-wall components, producing lymphokines. This, together with the effect on macrophages mentioned previously, provides a hypothetical explanation for most of the histological appearances seen in allergic alveolitis as well as for the fibrosis found in chronic cases.[16]

Clearly, in spite of much research, the pathogenesis of allergic alveolitis is not yet completely understood.[19] It should be remembered that the clinical spectrum of the disease is very wide, ranging from the acute, possibly fatal, attack to the chronic fibrosing type, and that the histological appearances are variable. In clinical practice, atypical cases are seen. It seems likely that a number of different mechanisms are at work, and it may be unwise to attempt at this stage to fit all clinical and experimental cases into one theory of pathogenesis.

Diagnosis

This diagnosis of allergic alveolitis often presents an interesting challenge to the physician. For example, while the typical acute case of farmer's lung poses no particular problems, many patients seen clinically present with rather nonspecific symptoms and may easily be thought to have other diseases such as bronchitis, asthma, idiopathic pulmonary fibrosis, sarcoidosis, drug-induced lung disease, or even a psychogenic illness. As suggested in Chapter 2, when investigating lung disease it is useful to start from the premise that the cause comes from the external environment. Beginning with that presupposition, the steps to the diagnosis of allergic alveolitis are as follows:

History
A careful note should be made of the patient's occupation and of any organic or chemical aerosols to which the individual may be exposed. In acute attacks, a history of what the patient was doing some hours prior to falling ill is essential. The relationship of symptoms to periods at work

and on vacation is less clear in allergic alveolitis than in occupational asthma, and in subacute and chronic cases may be frankly misleading. In addition, the patient's recreational pursuits should be investigated, and the presence of birds, damp, mold, or air conditioners in the home or place of work noted. In obscure cases, a visit to the patient's home or workplace may be necessary. Any drugs the patient may be taking should be recorded, since drug-induced lung disease is an important cause of diagnostic confusion. Other occupational lung diseases which may cause diagnostic difficulties are silo filler's disease, which may mimic farmer's lung; legionnaires' disease, which may also be spread by aerosol in workplaces; and occupational asthma of the chronic type. Further investigation will usually allow these to be differentiated.

Examination

The only sign on examination of most patients is the presence of bilateral, gravity-dependent, repetitive mid- and end-inspiratory crackles, though tachypnea may be present in acute cases. The absence of other abnormalities such as finger clubbing or signs of left ventricular disease should raise the suspicion of an extrinsic alveolitis, whether due to inhaled or ingested antigen. The signs often do not help distinguish allergic alveolitis from atypical pneumonias or toxic pneumonitis.

Radiography

The chest radiograph shows nonspecific features but, combined with clinical examination and other tests, may be of considerable help. For example, an apparently normal radiograph in someone with basal crackles and low diffusing capacity is more likely to be a sign of allergic alveolitis than anything else. A change in this radiograph after a challenge test is strong evidence of the disease, though challenge testing should normally avoid producing this extreme reaction (see below).

Immunology

The most useful diagnostic test is that for detecting precipitating antibody in the patient's serum to the suspected antigen. As noted previously, this may be misleading, precipitins being absent in some patients with the disease and present in some exposed but well individuals. Nevertheless, when present in someone with appropriate clinical findings it is usually the only test necessary. The simple test by Ouchterlony gel diffusion is sufficient in many cases, but a more sensitive radioimmunoassay based on a modification of the radioallergosorbent test (RAST) is available for quantitation of antibody, and some authorities find this more valuable as a diagnostic test.[20] It is certainly advisable to use such a test if the simple one shows no precipitin lines in the serum of a patient with a consistent clinical picture.

In some cases it will be necessary to make extracts of suspected antigens collected from home or work in order to carry out testing for

antibody. The same extracts, in suitable concentration, can be used also for skin testing intradermally, to look for an Arthus reaction (an indurated tender swelling at 4 hours, lasting about 24 hours) and challenge testing.

Lung Function Testing

In the typical acute case, lung function testing simply confirms the expected reduction in lung volumes, diffusing capacity, and arterial oxygen tension. In obscure cases, its main value lies in demonstrating that a restrictive and diffusion abnormality is present. While this is of no help in itself in the differential diagnosis, it is useful when taken with other findings such as basal crackles or dubious radiographic changes in deciding on further investigation. Lung function testing, however, has its greatest value in monitoring the progress of the disease and its response to treatment.

Challenge Testing

A challenge test is only necessary in obscure cases of allergic alveolitis in which the clinical and immunological findings are equivocal. Thus it has proved useful in the investigation of previously undescribed causes of the disease and in confirming the diagnosis in patients with suggestive clinical findings but absent serum precipitins. The simplest such test is to expose the patient to the suspectedly harmful environment for a limited period of time and observe changes in temperature, white blood cell count, and lung volumes and diffusing capacity. The period of time may vary from a few minutes to a work shift, and a decision on this should be guided by the patient's history. Alternatively, the patient may be asked to bring the suspected agent to the laboratory and be exposed to it there. A third, and widely used, method for investigating soluble organic antigens is to make an extract of the suspected antigen and expose the patient to it via a nebulizer. Again, the strength of solution and length of exposure must be judged from the patient's history. Generally, a relatively light exposure should be used initially, proceeding to increasingly stronger ones if no reaction occurs. The responses are characteristic and include fever, dyspnea, basal crackles, a rise in exercise minute ventilation and neutrophil count, and a fall in lymphocytes, vital capacity, and transfer factor. Hendrick and colleagues[21] have investigated these responses to challenge, finding a specificity of 95 per cent and sensitivity of 85–48 per cent for a combination of six, namely, an increase of $\geq$ 15 per cent in exercise ventilation, a rise in temperature > 37.2°C, of neutrophils $\geq$ 2500/cu mm, and of exercise respiratory rate $\geq$ 25 per cent with a fall in lymphocytes $\geq$ −500/cu mm and vital capacity $\geq$ 15 per cent. These authors have also pointed out that measurements of lung volumes, diffusing capacity, crackles, and radiographic changes proved too insensitive to be useful, though it would seem likely that such changes when provoked are highly specific. It is probably wise, if possible, to challenge

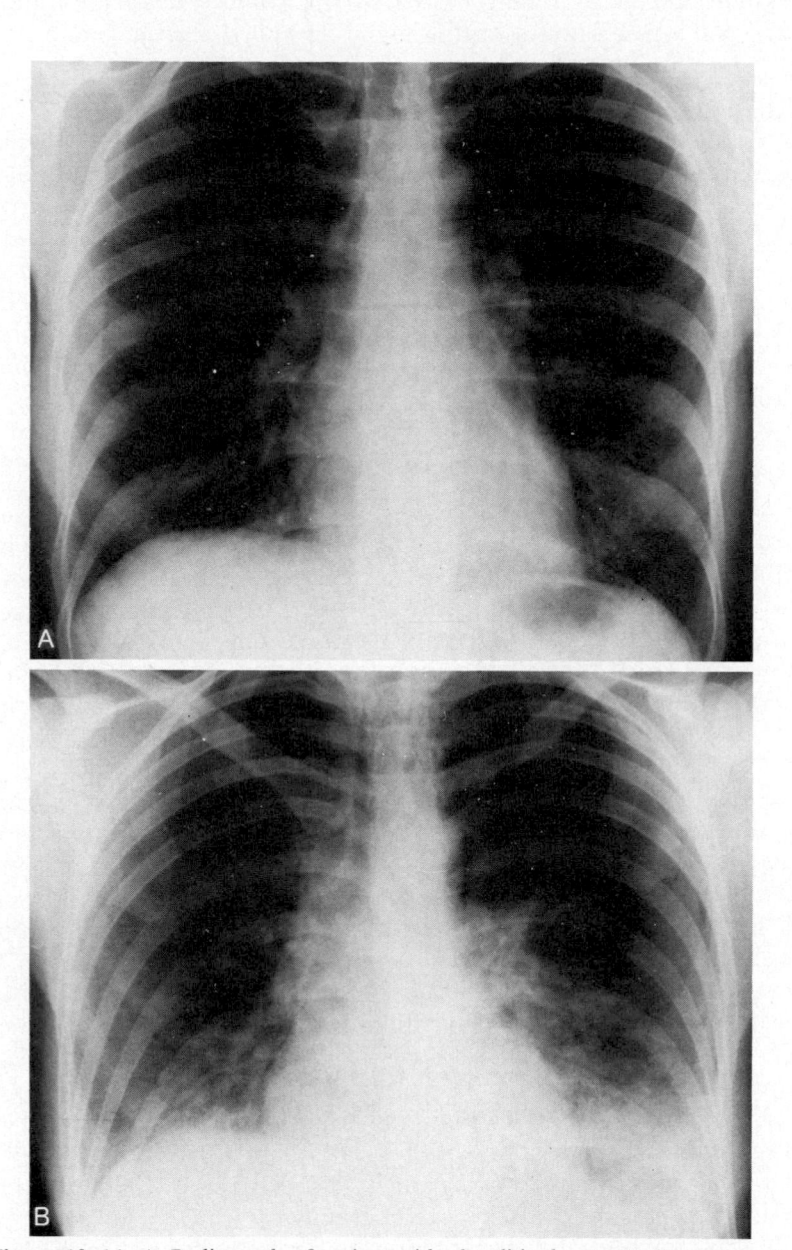

Figure 19–14. *A,* Radiograph of patient with alveolitis due to Pauli's reagent before challenge. *B,* Same patient after challenge test mixing reagents in laboratory.

Illustration continued on opposite page.

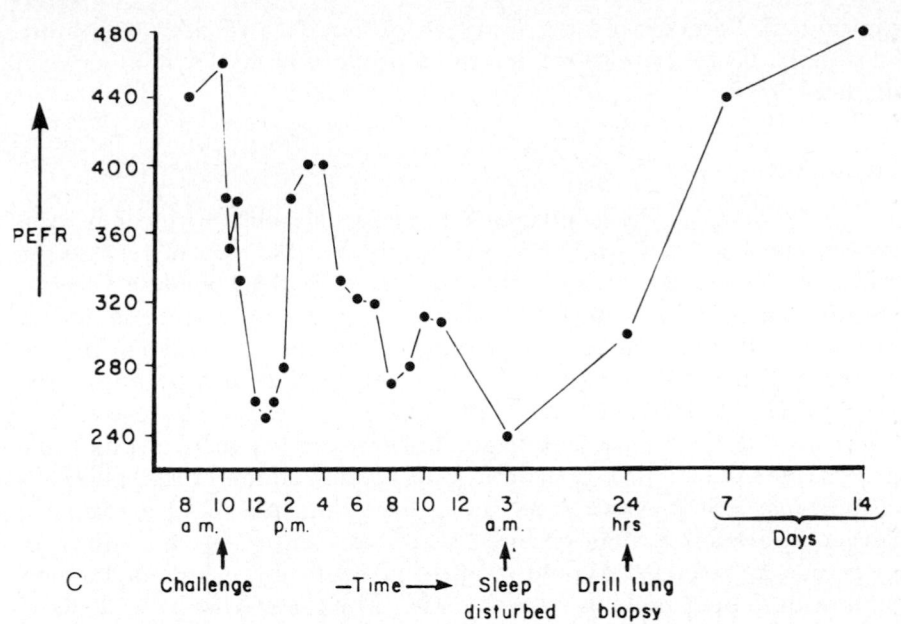

Figure 19–14 (*Continued*). *C*, Recording of peak flow rate during challenge test, showing both immediate and delayed obstructive patterns in addition to interstitial disease apparent on radiograph and also seen on biopsy. (From Evans, W. V., and Seaton, A., Hypersensitivity pneumonitis in a technician using Paul's reagent. Thorax, *34*, 767, 1979.)

with a dose that produces the earlier, less distressing changes in order to avoid an attack that may be harmful to the patient.

It should be pointed out that a challenge test may often provoke a dual obstructive and alveolar response,[22] and the obstructive one may even have immediate and delayed components[23] (Fig. 19–14). Such immunologically mixed cases should be managed with an eye on the potentially more serious alveolar component.

Lung Biopsy

Lung biopsy is neither necessary nor justifiable in most cases of allergic alveolitis. However, the disease may occasionally be suspected but no allergen identified, and in such cases biopsy may be necessary to prove the diagnosis or to exclude other possible diseases. Open biopsy produces the best specimens from the pathologist's point of view, but is a major procedure for the patient. Transbronchial biopsies often provide pieces too small for confident diagnosis. Percutaneous drill biopsy is probably the best compromise, though the relatively nontraumatic transbronchial procedure is now often tried first. It has the additional marginal advantage that it can be preceded by bronchoalveolar lavage, a procedure that holds some hope as a means of monitoring the course of the disease, though in the authors' view it is really only valuable as a means of understanding the immune and other processes involved and is more a research than a

clinical tool.[24] Studies of animal models of allergic alveolitis using bron-choalveolar lavage have shown increased proportions of T lymphocytes in the fluid.[25, 26]

Treatment

While death in the acute attack of allergic alveolitis is uncommon, it is by no means unknown.[10] As corticosteroids are known to reverse the effect of the inhaled antigen, their use in all but the mildest attack is justified. During the acute attack, arterial oxygen desaturation should be relieved by the use of oxygen, which may be given by any convenient means sufficient to raise the arterial oxygen tension to between 60 and 100 mm Hg. There is no risk of provoking carbon dioxide retention in the acute attack, since alveolar hypoventilation is not a feature, unless the patient already has chronic airways obstruction in addition. Exceptionally, if the lungs are very stiff and the patient cannot achieve a sufficient oxygen saturation without excessive respiratory effort, mechanical ventilation may be required. Should this become necessary, nasal endotracheal intubation is preferable to tracheostomy, since the disease almost always responds rapidly to treatment with corticosteroids.

In a proportion of acute attacks, response is not rapid even when adequate doses of prednisone (40 mg daily) are given, and occasionally it may be several weeks before recovery is complete. In such cases the slow response may cause diagnostic uncertainty, and this constitutes one situation in which lung biopsy may be helpful.

The chronic form of the disease responds less well to treatment, especially if the obstructive element predominates. It is, of course, essential that the patient be removed from the allergenic stimulus, and it should always be assumed that at least a part of the disease is potentially reversible. If the patient is unable to be removed from possible exposure, respirators are available that will reduce the exposure to a level that is relatively safe in most cases.[27, 28] Steroids should be given and their efficacy monitored by serial measurements of vital capacity and diffusing capacity. The collagenous component of chronic allergic alveolitis will not respond to any therapy, and once this has become the predominant feature of the disease, therapy should be symptomatic. This includes oxygen when necessary, antibiotics for acute infections, and a cardiac regimen for cor pulmonale.

SPECIFIC TYPES OF ALLERGIC ALVEOLITIS

Any account of the causes of allergic alveolitis must be incomplete, since new ones are being described quite regularly and no doubt many remain to be discovered. However, the causes may be grouped under general headings, in the assumption that other potential antigens in these

Table 19–2. RECOGNIZED TYPES OF ALLERGIC ALVEOLITIS

	Condition	Antigen
Fungal causes	Farmer's lung	Thermophilic actinomycetes
	Air conditioner lung	" "
	Bagassosis	" "
	Mushroom worker's lung	" "
	Maltworker's lung	*Aspergillus clavatus*
	Cheesewasher's lung	*Penicillium casei*
	Maple bark stripper's disease	*Cryptostroma corticale*
	Sequoiosis	*Aureobasidium pullulans*
	Woodworker's disease	*Cryptostroma corticale*
	Suberosis	*Penicillium frequentans*
	Paprika splitter's lung	Mucor
	Dry rot lung	*Merulius lacrymans*
	"Dog house disease"	*Aspergillus versicolor*
	Lycoperdonosis	Lycoperdon
Animal causes	Bird breeder's lung	Avian protein, bloom
	Rat handler's lung	Rat protein
	Wheat weevil disease	Wheat weevil
	Furrier's lung	Animal fur
	Pituitary snuff taker's lung	Ox and pork protein
Chemical causes	Isocyanate lung	TDI, MDI, HDT
	Pauli's reagent lung	Pauli's reagent
	Vineyard sprayer's lung	Bordeaux mixture
	Hard metal disease	Cobalt
	Cromolyn sodium lung	Cromolyn sodium
Bacterial causes	Washing powder lung	*Bacillus subtilis* enzymes
	B. subtilis alveolitis	*Bacillus subtilis*
	B. sereus alveolitis	*Bacillus sereus*
Uncertain causes	Sauna lung	Lake water (?)
	New Guinea lung	Hut thatch (?)
	Ramin lung	Ramin wood (?)
	Insecticide lung	Pyrethrum (?)

categories will in due course be shown to cause disease. Thus it is convenient to consider allergic alveolitis as caused by fungi, animal materials, small-molecular-weight chemicals, and bacteria. In addition, a number of outbreaks have occurred in which the cause has not been clearly defined (Table 19–2).

Diseases of Fungal Etiology

Farmer's Lung

The first detailed description of farmer's lung was published in 1932, and the relationship of the condition to inhalation of hay dust was recognized.[29] The disease was initially thought to be due to fungal infection of the lung. Further and more complete descriptions were given by Fawcitt

in 1936[30] and Fuller in 1953.[31] A similar condition occurs in cattle and is known as fog fever.

In the early case reports it was apparent that farmer's lung occurred mostly in wet summers, and in many instances there was an obvious relationship between exposure to moldy hay and the onset of symptoms. In some outbreaks, barley or oats that had stood in wet weather and been threshed before they were completely dry were incriminated. It is now appreciated that if hay is stored in a damp state, that is, with a moisture content of greater than 30 per cent, heat is generated and this encourages the growth of thermophilic microorganisms. Of these, the most important from the point of view of farmer's lung are *Micropolyspora faeni* and *Thermoactinomyces vulgaris*. These organisms produce vast numbers of spores that are liberated into the air when the hay is raked or turned over (Fig. 19–15). The farm worker inhales these spores and an attack usually

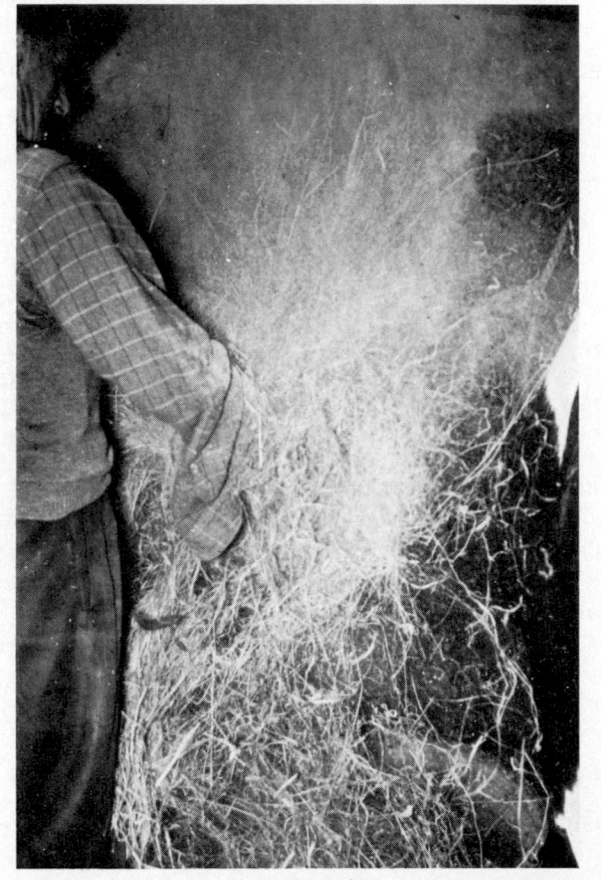

Figure 19–15. Farmer shaking bale of moldy hay. The haze in the upper part of the picutue is a cloud of dust containing respirable spores of thermophilic actinomycetes.

develops a few hours later. Attacks are now seen most commonly in winter, as baled hay is often stored in barns for winter fodder, and during winter the bales are broken and the hay is forked into appropriate portions for the cattle. This is usually done inside the barn, and mild attacks may occur every time the worker handles the hay.

Outbreaks of a disease similar to farmer's lung have also been described in association with exposure to air conditioners and heating systems contaminated by thermophilic actinomycetes.[32-34] This emphasizes the fact that these organisms are widely distributed and may grow and sporulate wherever temperature and humidity are appropriate. The relationship of this condition to humidifier fever is discussed later in this chapter.

The clinical features of farmer's lung may range from the most acute attack to a slowly progressive pulmonary fibrosis, probably depending on the individual's pattern of exposure and natural susceptibility. Though acute attacks have been recognized most frequently, it is likely that more insidious disease without all the classical symptoms develops in a high proportion of exposed subjects.

The immunology of the disease has been studied in great detail. Originally, Williams showed that aerosols of aqueous extracts of mouldy hay would produce the clinical picture of farmer's lung.[35] Subsequently Pepys and Jenkins showed that extracts of *Micropolyspora faeni* had a similar effect.[36] No such reactions were produced by extracts prepared from Aspergillus or Penicillium species, nor by Mucor or other fungi found in hay and grass dust. Adequately dried hay was likewise ineffective. The reactions developed several hours after the challenge and were associated with a fall in vital capacity and diffusing capacity and a rise in temperature. There was also hyperventilation, but no evidence of airways obstruction.

The antigens were extracted in various ways from moldy hay or grain,[37, 38] and Barbee and co-workers showed that they were soluble in trichloroacetic acid.[39] Scratch tests with the antigen rarely produced a reaction, but intradermal injections of extracts may produce a typical late Type III response.

The first demonstration of precipitating antibodies in the sera of subjects with farmer's lung was made by Pepys and his colleagues in the early 1960s.[38, 40, 41] Simple carbol-saline extracts were prepared and tested against the sera of farmers with and without the clinical condition. These workers employed a double diffusion technique. They showed first that the titer of antibodies in different sera varied, and second that not all hay extracts were equally antigenic. A number of other fungal extracts were also shown to produce precipitin lines: challenge of the subject with these extracts failed to produce a clinical response, with the exception of *Thermoactinomyces vulgaris*, which occasionally produced a reaction similar to that of *Micropolyspora faeni*.[41]

Studies of the prevalence of farmer's lung are confounded by the difficulty of deciding on diagnostic criteria. The presence of precipitins

in the sera of farm workers, a test that does not correlate very well with clinical disease but is at least an indication of exposure, varies greatly. In the United States prevalence is highest in Wisconsin and Pennsylvania; in Canada, in Manitoba[42]; and in Britain, in Scotland[14] and the southeast.[5] Studies of the prevalence of clinical disease have indicated figures of about 3 to 5 per cent in both the United States and Britain.[43] These represent between one half and one sixth of those with positive precipitin tests. There is no evidence that patients are genetically predisposed to the disease,[44] though cigarette smoking clearly has a protective effect.[5]

The management of farmer's lung often requires the use of steroids for an acute attack. The disease may largely be prevented by care in the making and use of hay, especially in reducing its water content and allowing free ventilation. Subjects who have had an attack should attempt to avoid exposure completely, if necessary by changing jobs, since the risk of further attacks and production of chronic disease is high.[45] The number of spores inhaled may be reduced by wearing an appropiate respirator.[27] This, together with expert advice on proper haymaking (which can be provided by agricultural scientists in many farming communities), is the form of management most commonly used, as farmers are rarely in a position to change jobs.

In Britain, farmer's lung has been compensable as an industrial disease since 1964. In many Western countries and in most states in the United States, subjects affected by the disease are still not covered by workmen's compensation acts, a situation that is very far from satisfactory.

Bagassosis

This condition bears many resemblances to farmer's lung. Bagasse is a fiber, derived from dried sugar cane, that is used in the manufacture of paper, cardboard, and building materials. The disease is a result of exposure to moldy stored bagasse and is seen in the southern United States, the West Indies, India, Italy, Peru, and even Britain.[46] The outbreak that occurred in Britain was related to exposure to bales of bagasse that had been imported from Louisiana.[47]

The disease develops in approximately 50 per cent of subjects exposed to moldly bagasse. The available evidence suggests that thermophilic actinomycetes are responsible and precipitins are frequently present in the subjects' serum in the acute stages of the disease. Systemic and pulmonary reactions have been produced by inhalation challenges of moldy bagasse.[48] The response usually appears three to six hours after the challenge. The same subjects when challenged with extracts of *Micropolyspora faeni* failed to respond, and it seems likely that the main antigens are from *Thermoactinomyces vulgaris* and *T. sacchari*.

The clinical features, radiology, and pathology of bagassosis are essentially the same as those of farmer's lung. Thus, the presenting symptoms are shortness of breath, fever, chest discomfort, anorexia, and

sweating. While complete recovery is the rule, repeated lesser exposures can lead to a chronic form of the disease. The acute stage is characterized by pulmonary function evidence of interstitial lung involvement, while in the chronic form of the disease airways obstruction is also seen.[49] Though cessation of exposure to bagasse results in remission of symptoms, a restrictive lung function lesion lasting up to 10 years after the acute attack has been described.[50]

Mushroom Worker's Lung

This condition, like bagassosis, is a variant of farmer's lung. It was first described by Bringhurst and colleagues.[51] The common mushroom, *Agaricus hortensis*, is grown on compost whose main constituents are usually straw and horse droppings. The compost is usually allowed to "ferment" in the open for two to three weeks. It is then exposed to a moist heat of no more than 60°C for several days in special chambers. This process eliminates many of the organisms that interfere with the growth of the mushrooms and also provides an ideal medium for the growth of *Micropolyspora faeni* and thermophilic actinomycetes. The compost is later dried and seeded with mushroom mycelia. The latter process involves mechanical mixing of the mushroom spawn with the compost. The compost is then spread on trays, which are placed in mushroom houses where the temperature is kept at 15°C and the humidity at 90 per cent. The first crop of mushrooms usually appears in three to four weeks.

Subjects in whom mushroom worker's lung develops have usually worked in the sheds in which spawning is effected and where the compost and spawn are mechanically mixed. Occasionally the condition occurs following emptying and cleaning of the mushroom sheds. Precipitins against *Micropolyspora faeni* and *Thermoactinomyces vulgaris* have been reported in the serum of the subjects with this condition.[52]

Maltworker's Lung

A further cause of allergic alveolitis was described in 1968 by Riddle and colleagues.[53] The subject was a maltworker who had developed a farmer's lung–like respiratory illness. The illness was associated with low-grade fever, dyspnea, and cough. All the symptoms cleared while he was away from work, only to recur when he returned. When seen after the recurrence of symptoms, he was found to have basal crackles and impairment of his diffusing capacity along with a restrictive ventilatory defect. He was treated with steroids, with a good response.

In the malting process, fresh farm barley is first dried in kilns and then stored for two months in a silo. It is next rehydrated over 36 hours and is then treated with hypochlorite to rid the barley of fungi. It is then allowed to germinate in a hot and humid atmosphere, where both the heat and humidity are controlled. The malt is turned regularly to release

carbon dioxide. It is then dried once again in kilns, and afterwards the rootlets are removed. Lastly, the malt is taken to the distillery.

The subject in whom allergic alveolitis developed had as his main job the turning of the malt on open floors, which produced a spore-laden dusty atmosphere. The patient's sputum grew a mixed fungal flora, as did samples of the maltings. However, *Aspergillus clavatus* was grown both from the patient's sputum and from nearly every sample of the maltings. Moreover, this was the only fungus that could be repeatedly isolated from both sputum and the maltings.

Precipitating and complement-fixing antibodies against *A. clavatus* were demonstrated in the subject's serum. An intradermal injection of an extract of the antigen produced an Arthus-type skin reaction, and an inhalational challenge duplicated the respiratory symptoms of the naturally occurring disease. Subsequent studies showed that approximately 5 per cent of workers in the malting industry had symptoms of the disease, though in most cases it was relatively mild.[54] Modern methods of malting, especially in which a closed drum rather than an open floor process is used, are associated with a much lower prevalence of disease.

Cheesewasher's Disease

This condition was described in Switzerland in 1969.[55] In the process of making some cheeses, aging is carried out in damp cellars. A mold forms on the surface of the cheese, and cheeseworkers are required to wash this off periodically. Some of these subjects developed a disease similar to farmer's lung and were found to have serum precipitins against *Penicillium casei*. Subsequent investigation of the epidemiology of the disease revealed precipitins in 21 per cent of exposed workers, while 55 per cent of those with a past history of symptoms had precipitins. Lung function studies, not usually performed in acute attacks, were mostly normal in this study, suggesting that the disease is usually mild and reversible. It is thought that most cheese producers in the United States avoid the risk of causing this disease by wrapping the cheese in foil during aging.[56]

Maple Bark Stripper's Disease

Maple bark disease was first described by Tower, Sweaney, and Huron in 1932.[57] The condition affected lumber workers whose job it was to strip the bark from maple logs. Further outbreaks of maple bark stripper's disease have been reported by Emanuel et al.[58, 59] The fungus that is responsible is known as *Cryptostroma corticale* and grows beneath the bark of the tree, affecting both the hard maple and the sycamore.

The processes and operations that are involved in the lumber mill have been thoroughly described by Wenzel and Emanuel.[60] The maple

logs are brought into the woodroom on a continuous chain and are first cut in half. The logs then are debarked on a series of drums. The drums have a tumbling action and are sprayed with water. After the bark has been removed, the log is carried to a chipper, which cuts it into small chips. The latter are shaken on a screen and the remnants of the bark removed. The chips are then taken on a conveyor belt to a silo in which they are stored.

Cryptostroma corticale produces ovoid spores of 4 to 5 microns in length. They are brownish red in color but when present in large numbers appear black. Maple logs that are affected by the fungus show large blackened areas underneath the bark. Removal of the bark during the stripping process liberates the spores into the air, and high spore counts were observed in the woodroom, especially in winter, when the doors of the room were kept closed because of the cold.

The clinical features of this condition are very similar to those of farmer's lung. Cough, fever, and shortness of breath are common. Rigors and marked cyanosis with severe arterial oxygen desaturation occur. Subacute forms of the disease are also seen in which the fever is low grade and in which symptoms of chronic shortness of breath and loss of weight predominate. Eosinophilia is unusual. The radiographic findings vary according to the stage of the disease. The subject with acute disease usually shows an extensive confluent acinous filling process; however, reticulonodulation and stringy infiltrates are seen in the more chronic forms of the disease and during the convalescent stage.

Emanuel and colleagues carried out lung biopsies in some of their subjects.[59] The appearances resembled those of farmer's lung in that an extensive granulomatous pneumonitis was present with frequent foreign body giant cells. With silver methenamine fungal stains, in a few instances the spores could be recognized in the lung parenchyma and indeed were initially mistaken for *Histoplasma capsulatum*. Cultures of resected lung tissue are often successful and the organism appears as a white mycelial growth. Despite the presence of the spores in the lung, there is no real evidence that the disease is infectious in origin. Precipitins against extracts of the spores can be demonstrated not only in affected subjects but in some exposed workers who have no overt disease. Intracutaneous tests with an extract of the antigen cause an immediate wheal that persists for up to eight hours.

Most subjects with the condition improve rapidly when exposure to the spores ceases. As they become convalescent, their antibody titers decline. Since the complete description of the disease by Emanuel et al.,[59] the lumber mill in which the subjects worked has introduced preventive measures to lessen the spore counts in the saw area and woodroom by continuous spraying of the logs as they are debarked, by isolation of the chipperman, and by improved ventilation. Immediately after these measures were introduced there was a decline in the incidence of the condition.

Sequoiosis

A subject with granulomatous pneumonitis associated with redwood dust inhalation has been described by Cohen et al.[61] The man had worked for 17 years as a sawyer in a redwood lumber mill. The patient was first seen with dyspnea and a chest radiograph showing a "ground glass" pattern. The symptoms and radiographic findings disappeared spontaneously when he was in the hospital. With further exposures to redwood dust the symptoms returned, and he developed dyspnea and was found to have crackles in his chest. Pulmonary function testing revealed evidence of interstitial disease. Biopsy of the lung showed septal thickening, lymphocytic and plasma cell infiltration, and a granulomatous pneumonitis. He was given steroids, which produced marked improvement.

Skin tests with redwood extracts produced no immediate reaction, though precipitins against redwood sawdust extract were present in the patient's serum. Precipitins were present only rarely in other workers exposed to the redwood dust and not at all in controls. Culture of the sawdust grew several species of fungi, but only Graphium and *Aureobasidium pullulans* showed antigens with immunological identity to the redwood antigen. It was therefore concluded that the latter were probably responsible for the condition.

Woodworker's Disease

Hypersensitivity to wood dust has been described on several occasions.[62, 63] A respiratory illness resembling hypersensitivity pneumonitis has been described in two subjects who worked at a paper mill.[64] Although the clinical and occupational history suggested maple bark disease, inhalation challenge tests with extracts of *Cryptostroma corticale* failed to confirm the diagnosis. The first subject presented with recurrent episodes of dyspnea, chills, and fever. He developed persistent radiographic abnormalities, and a lung biopsy was interpreted as showing chronic interstitial pneumonitis and fibrosis. He was subsequently challenged with an extract of Alternaria, with the development of all the acute symptoms and signs of extrinsic alveolitis. Steroids had to be given because of the severity of the reaction, but within 24 hours the patient's signs and symptoms had ceased. The other patient had a similar but shorter history and he likewise had a positive inhalation test when challenged with an extract of Alternaria. In both of these subjects, a Type I reaction with an immediate reduction in ventilatory capacity occurred following the challenge, in addition to the Type III response. Moreover, the serum of one of the subjects contained rheumatoid factor. Precipitins which reacted against an extract of Alternaria were present in the sera of both subjects.

A similar illness, called suberosis, has been described in workers producing bottle stoppers and discs from cork.[65] Although initially it was thought that this condition, which may have asthmatic features or may be

typical of allergic alveolitis, was due to hypersensitivity to cork itself, the evidence now suggests that it results from exposure to moldy cork bark. The mold that is probably responsible is *Penicillium frequentans*.[66] Finally, allergic alveolitis has been described in a woodworker exposed to Ramin *(Gonystylus bancanus)* dust. In this case the wood itself rather than fungi appeared to be responsible for the disease.[67]

Paprika Splitter's Lung

Capsicum annuum longum, red pepper or paprika, has long been cultivated for medical purposes. It is grown mainly in Hungary and Yugoslavia. The fruit of the plant is about four to five inches long, and was usually split open by women workers in order to remove the "ribs" of the plant. The latter were then thrown away, since they contain an excess of capsaicine. Late in the year, paprika fruits are often parasitized by Mucor species, and the air of the workroom in which the women worked was grossly contaminated with spores. Respiratory complaints were common in the paprika splitters, but not in the workers who handled the finished product.[68]

The clinical features of the disease are cough and loss of weight. Fever and "bronchiectasis" may develop. The development of bronchiectasis must be doubted and is probably explained by the fact that bronchography when performed in subjects with established interstitial fibrosis often shows shortening and a tuberose appearance in the segmental bronchi.[69] The chest film shows consolidation and stringy infiltrates. Death may occur from right heart failure. It is probable that this disease is an allergic alveolitis, but it is now seldom if ever seen. Selective breeding has evolved a plant in which the ribs contain little capsaicine, and hence workers are no longer employed to split the paprika fruit.

Dry Rot Lung

A typical case of allergic alveolitis has been described in a patient exposed to the dry rot fungus, *Merulius lacrymans*, in a house.[70]

"Dog House Disease"

The development of acute, very severe interstitial lung disease in a woman who was exposed to moldy straw has been described by Rhudy et al.[71] She was admitted to hospital in extremis with a history of having been well until a few hours before admission. At the time of her admission she was cyanotic, with gross hypoxia, and was semicomatose. Despite oxygen supplements she required mechanical ventilation. Her chest radiograph showed a diffuse acinous filling process throughout both lungs. She was treated with oxygen, assisted ventilation, and steroids, and in spite of the development of other complications, made a recovery.

She kept two dogs which slept on straw in her basement. The bale of straw that she had been using for their bedding in the week prior to admission had been damp and moldy. It was her custom to spread fresh straw out every day. Culture of the moldy straw grew a mixed fungal flora, but *Micropolyspora faeni* and *Thermoactinomyces vulgaris* could not be isolated despite several attempts to do so. Among the several fungi present was *Aspergillus versicolor*. It was later shown that the patient's serum contained precipitins against an extract prepared from this fungus. As the patient improved and became convalescent, her antibody titer fell, and three months following the illness precipitins were no longer demonstrable. An inhalation challenge was thought inadvisable because of the severity of the patient's illness and because of the difficulty in titrating the dose.

Lycoperdonosis

A respiratory disease caused by the inhalation of large numbers of puffball spores was described by Strand and co-workers in 1967.[72] Lycoperdon is the genus of fungi to which most puffballs belong. They grow in woods and forests on decaying logs and stumps and sometimes in fields. Within the puffball wall vast numbers of clavate spores are contained. Because of their styptic action, these have been used to stop nosebleeds. With the inhalation of large numbers of spores, nausea, fever, dyspnea, and lung crackles appear, and the chest film shows miliary mottling. No attempt has been made to see whether the serum of such patients contains precipitins.

Diseases of Animal Etiology

Allergic Alveolitis due to Birds

The first reports of allergic alveolitis due to birds were published in 1960 and recorded the disease in duck pluckers and people exposed to parakeets.[73, 74] Soon afterwards, the disease was reported in pigeon breeders[75-78] and more recently in people farming chickens[79] and turkeys.[80] The spectrum of symptoms and signs in these patients is the same as in other types of allergic alveolitis, though with a tendency for fewer of the acute cases to occur, most falling into the category of recurrent, nonacute disease. This is especially true of those who keep parakeets in their homes. Children with the disease may present with nonspecific symptoms and failure to thrive. The lung function findings are of a restrictive type with low diffusing capacity,[81, 82] though raised residual volume and obstructive findings may predominate.[22] In the acute recurrent cases, lung function may be normal between attacks. Studies of the prevalence of the condition are again confused by the difficulty of defining a case and by unsatisfactory population sampling. However, studies among pigeon fanciers suggest

that the prevalence of clinical disease may be between 10 and 20 per cent of those regularly exposed in the lofts.[83]

Affected individuals often have serum precipitins to bird serum, feathers, egg white, and droppings,[84] and it is likely that sensitization has occurred to the birds' serum globulin. In pigeons at least, IgA seems to be the predominant antigen, though patients probably become sensitized to one or more of a range of antigens.[17] The route of sensitization is presumably inhalational, and challenge testing uses bird serum administered by this route. Bird droppings, which contain protein, have been considered a likely source of aerosol, but tend to be hygroscopic and do not dry out easily. Exposure to feathers may be a more important source of antigen, and recent work has confirmed that bloom, a waxy material composed of fine 1-micron particles of keratin coated with IgA, is a potential source of antigen.[85] Bloom is produced in large amounts by flying birds, especially pigeons in peak condition, and this may explain why such birds as pigeons and parakeets seem more potent sensitizers than chickens and turkeys.

The diagnosis of allergic alveolitis in people exposed to birds is made more difficult by the relatively high proportion of subjects who have no precipitins when tested by standard gel diffusion. However, the use of more sensitive tests increases the possibility of diagnosing more cases without the need for challenge testing.[17] The disease should be managed by prevention of exposure, generally by avoiding contact with birds or, if this is not possible, by wearing an efficient respirator.[28] Cross reactivity between species occurs, and the authors have seen patients who, having got rid of their pigeons, became ill on exposure to friends' or relatives' parakeets. We have also seen a patient who developed typical disease, proved by challenge test, simply from exposure to feathers in the cushions of her three-piece suite!

A comment should be made on two possible diagnostic pitfalls with respect to bird breeder's lung. First, false-positive viral complement fixation tests may be found in pigeon fanciers with allergic alveolitis, due either to a polyclonal stimulation of antibody formation[86] or to reaction with antigens in the hen's egg on which the virus was grown.[87] Confusion with influenzal or other viral pneumonias may therefore become a real problem. Second, patients with celiac disease frequently have precipitins in their blood to avian antigens, probably derived from egg protein in their food.[88] Since celiac disease is occasionally accompanied by a diffuse pulmonary fibrosis unrelated to bird exposure,[89] diagnostic confusion may occur, especially when the patient keeps a parakeet.[90] Such problems may require a challenge test to resolve.[91]

Allergic Alveolitis due to Small Mammals

Laboratory rats are well described as a cause of occupational asthma and rhinitis, and there is strong evidence that protein excreted in their urine is an important antigen. One case of typical allergic alveolitis due to

exposure to rats has been described in a research assistant.[92] This patient had typical symptoms and signs, precipitating antibody, and responses to work and laboratory challenges. A similar case has been described following exposure to gerbils.[93]

Wheat Weevil Disease

Asthmatic reactions to the wheat weevil, *Sitophilus granarius*, were first described by Jiminez-Diaz et al. in 1947.[94] Subsequent studies showed that the wheat weevil produced asthma in subjects exposed to it in the laboratory and that the affected subjects had positive skin and inhalation tests. Control subjects did not react when similarly challenged.[95, 96]

In a few of the challenged workers, the immediate response was followed by a delayed reaction several hours later. Associated with the latter was a fall in the gas diffusing capacity. Precipitins against an extract of the weevil were present in the subjects' sera.

Furrier's Lung

The antigenic properties of animal hairs were recognized in 1928 by Valléry-Radot and Giroud.[97] It has also been claimed that animal hairs can produce interstitial pulmonary disease.[98] Biopsy showed the process was a granulomatous interstitial pneumonia, though the patient's serum was not examined for precipitating antibodies.

Pituitary Snuff Taker's Lung

The development of pulmonary infiltrates as a result of the inhalation of bovine and porcine pituitary snuff was first reported in the British literature.[99] Since that time there have been further reports from Europe[100] and the United States.[101] Pituitary snuff is used in the treatment of diabetes insipidus, and the method of administration avoids the need for repeated injections. The snuff is prepared from finely ground mixtures of dried bovine and porcine posterior pituitary, the particles usually being below 50 microns, some in the respirable range. Although most are deposited in the nasal passages, some reach the respiratory bronchioles and alveoli. A less finely ground preparation is available in which the particles are around 150 to 180 microns, but it is much more expensive. These preparations have been superseded by synthetic vasopressin.

Two types of pulmonary response have been described following the inhalation of snuff. The first is an immediate reaction and is characterized by asthma and hay fever–like symptoms and occurs within minutes of exposure. It commonly affects the atopic subject. The second type is an allergic alveolitis similar to farmer's lung and maple bark stripper's disease.

In the subjects described by Mahon et al., a generalized reticulonod-ulation of the lungs developed.[99] Bronchospasm and eosinophilia oc-

curred. However, pituitary snuff taker's lung does not seem to be associated with the sharp systemic reactions and fever that have been reported in acute farmer's lung and many of the other allergic alveolitides. The more insidious onset may be related to the repeated small insults that result from nasal administration of the preparation. Nevertheless, the compliance of the lungs falls and the diffusing capacity drops in a fashion similar to that seen in subjects with the other types of allergic alveolitis.

Immunological studies have demonstrated the presence of precipitins in the serum of affected subjects. The precipitins develop not only against hog and ox serum proteins but also against pituitary antigens themselves. The offending antigen in the patient described by Harper and colleagues was identified as a hormone constituent of the pituitary rather than the specific antigens of the animals from which the snuff was prepared.[101] The serum of this patient also failed to react with synthetic lysine 8-vasopressin, probably because the low molecular weight of this substance would make it a hapten and it would not be large enough to form a lattice with homologous antibody. Because this patient continued to have troublesome polyuria, she was challenged with lysine vasopressin. Measurement of her ventilatory and diffusing capacities before and after the challenge showed no change. She was therefore returned to a regimen of the synthetic preparation and has suffered neither symptomatic, physiological, nor radiographic impairment since.

Steroids seem to be beneficial in the treatment of pituitary snuff pneumonitis. A few subjects with this condition go on to develop a chronic form of the disease that cannot be distinguished from the ordinary form of chronic interstitial fibrosis.[99] With the widespread use of synthetic vasopressin, this condition is probably a thing of the past.

Disease due to Low-Molecular-Weight Chemicals

Isocyanate Alveolitis

The uses of isocyanates are described in Chapter 16, as these chemicals are potent causes of occupational asthma. Several subjects, however, have been reported as having developed pulmonary shadowing and a restrictive type of lung function abnormality following exposure. The initial report described four toluene diisocyanate (TDI) workers with radiographic changes.[102] Three of these patients had asthma as well. Subsequently, four patients with restrictive lung function—one of whom had signs of consolidation on chest radiography, biopsy changes of diffuse alveolitis, and an Arthus skin reaction to TDI—were reported.[103] Three of these subjects had been exposed to TDI and one to hexamethylene diisocyanate (HDI). The patients responded to treatment with corticosteroids. Challenge tests with TDI-albumin in sensitized rabbits produced changes of allergic alveolitis, whereas controls challenged with albumin showed no such changes.[103] Since then there have been reports of three further cases of

alveolitis following exposure to isocyanates,[104-106] two in workers exposed to diphenyl methane diisocyanate (MDI) and one in a man exposed to TDI.

Disease due to Pauli's Reagent

Pauli's reagent, sodium diazobenzenesulfonate, is widely used in laboratories for identifying aryl amines and phenols. A laboratory technician working in a medical school developed symptoms and signs of allergic alveolitis following her work in making and using this reagent in a defective fume cupboard. An occupational-type challenge produced immediate and delayed asthmatic reactions and also signs and biopsy evidence of allergic alveolitis. Skin tests showed evidence of atopy and also an immediate response to Pauli's reagent[23] (see Fig. 19–14).

Vineyard Sprayer's Lung

A granulomatous alveolitis has been described in workers spraying vines with Bordeaux mixture, a 1 to 2 per cent solution of copper sulfate neutralized with lime.[107] The histological changes seem typical of a hypersensitivity pneumonitis, with lymphocytes, plasma cells, and histiocytic granulomata that tend to fibrose. The lesions contain copper and tend to regress radiologically when exposure ceases. A somewhat atypical feature is the occasional development of massive fibrosis similar to that seen in silicosis. It has been suggested that these patients have an increased risk of lung cancer, though the evidence for this is flimsy, the patients having been selected partly on the basis of having lung tumors.[108]

Other Chemical Causes

Many drugs taken orally may cause a hypersensitivity pneumonitis, the best known of these probably being sulfasalazine[109] and nitrofurantoin.[110] Discussion of these is outside the scope of this book, but it is possible that workers producing these drugs may become sensitized. Drugs taken by inhalation may, like pituitary snuff, cause an alveolitis, and hypersensitivity to cromolyn sodium, which must be exceedingly rare, has been described.[111] Cobalt, used as a coolant in the grinding of tungsten carbide, presumably binds with protein to act as a hapten and has been shown to cause allergic alveolitis in three patients.[112]

Other Causes of Allergic Alveolitis

There have been occasional reports of allergic alveolitis following exposure to bacteria or the proteolytic enzymes derived from them. Early reports of respiratory disease in detergent workers exposed to *Bacillus subtilis* enzyme stressed the occurrence of asthma and rhinitis but also

hinted that an alveolitis might also develop.[113, 114] Certainly, precipitins were found in exposed workers, though their significance was dubious. More recently, *B. subtilis* has been clearly implicated as the cause of allergic alveolitis in six members of a family who were exposed to dust from decaying wood.[115] *Bacillus sereus* has also been implicated as a cause of allergic alveolitis due to a humidifier.[116]

In other outbreaks of allergic alveolitis, the precise cause has not been identified. One community outbreak in Finland was spread by tap water in baths and saunas, the water coming from a local lake.[117] A subject who had worked for 20 years in a coffee roasting factory was described as having chronic allergic alveolitis, with precipitins to coffee bean dust and compatible biopsy findings. However, long-term follow-up revealed that the patient in fact had pulmonary fibrosis in association with rheumatoid disease.[118] A chronic lung disease in Papuans, termed New Guinea lung, has been ascribed to a hypersensitivity reaction to the thatch roofing of their huts, and precipitins have been found to extracts of the thatch.[119] Prolonged and heavy exposure to pyrethrum in insecticides has caused allergic alveolitis in one individual.[120]

Finally, many lists include smallpox handler's lung as an allergic alveolitis. Follow-up of the original patients with this, it is to be hoped, now extinct disease suggested that it was a smallpox pneumonia modified by vaccination[121] (see Chap. 21).

SYNDROMES RELATED TO ALLERGIC ALVEOLITIS

Mycotoxicosis

Mycotoxicosis is a term used to describe disease due to fungal toxins, usually when they have been ingested. However, the name has also been applied to a particularly acute form of farmer's lung occurring in workers clearing fungi from the tops of silage.[122] It is characterized by fever, cough, malaise, and dyspnea beginning four to six hours after exposure to massive numbers of fungal spores. The clinical and laboratory findings resemble farmer's lung except that precipitins cannot be demonstrated. Pathological changes are those of an acute bronchiolo-alveolitis with predominant neutrophil infiltration. Fungal spores can be demonstrated by methenamine silver stains. The condition seems to resolve spontaneously, though in some cases corticosteroids have been used.

It seems likely that this disease differs slightly in its etiological mechanisms from farmer's lung, though it is doubtful if it merits a separate name, in view of the several different mechanisms that undoubtedly contribute to the spectrum of disease known as allergic alveolitis. It has been suggested that mycotoxicosis is the result of activation, by dust containing fungi, of the alternative pathway of complement in unsensitized individuals, rather than a direct effect of fungal toxins.[18]

Humidifier Fever

Inhalation of organic material suspended as an aerosol in fine water droplets has been recognized for many years as an important means of spread of infectious disease and has recently come into prominence again in association with legionnaires' disease (see Chap. 21). There are many situations within workplaces in which the opportunity exists to inhale aerosols dispersed by humidifying systems or by processes that require the spraying of water. If that water is recycled through a sump, and this is often the case for reasons of economy or convenience, it will inevitably become contaminated by a food chain of microorganisms unless specific steps are taken to sterilize it.[123] The organisms grow in the sump or in any container in which water is allowed to lie. The precise species and their abundance presumably depend on the basic substance in the water and on conditions of temperature, pH, presence or absence of sunlight, and so on. It is not surprising therefore that a number of different syndromes have been described in association with humidifiers and that several different microorganisms have been shown to produce symptoms. The syndromes range from a dramatic and sometimes fatal pneumonia when *Legionella pneumoniae* is the predominant organism, through typical allergic alveolitis provoked by thermophilic actinomycetes,[32-34] to an ill-defined feeling of malaise, fever, cough, and myalgia with a tendency to be worse at the beginning of the working week, a syndrome that has been called humidifier fever.[123]

The first reports of humidifier fever came from Switzerland and Britain.[124, 125] Apparently similar occurrences in the United States were subsequently shown to be a form of allergic alveolitis caused by *Thermoactinomyces vulgaris*, *T. candidus*, *Micropolyspora faeni*, *Aureobasidium pullulans*, and *Aspergillus fumigatus*, among other theromophilic and mesophilic organisms. Sources of the aerosol included industrial humidifiers and air conditioners, home central heating and humidifiers, and a cool-mist domestic vaporizer. The clinical, radiographic, immunological, and histological features of these diseases were all typical of allergic alveolitis. Curiously, however, when the condition in Britain was investigated, a different pattern was observed.[126-128] Although the symptoms of malaise, myalgia, fever, cough, and chest tightness were similar to those of allergic alveolitis, the occurrence of symptoms early in the week with improvement as the week went on and the absence of radiological abnormalities suggested that this was a different disease. Furthermore, no consistent pattern of sensitization to thermophilic actinomycetes emerged on challenge testing, although precipitins were frequently found in the blood of patients. The workplaces in which outbreaks occurred in Britain were a printing works, a rayon factory, and a stationery factory, all of which employed cellulose as a substrate, and a hospital operating room.

Even in this small group of outbreaks, different patterns were described. Challenge testing with the contaminated water sometimes caused

fever and a fall in diffusing capacity[127] and sometimes only systemic symptoms with only a slight fall in vital capacity alone.[130] A possible clue as to etiology has come from the demonstration of amoebae, *Naegleria grubei* and *Acanthamoeba*, in the water from all outbreaks and of antibodies to these amoebae in the blood of exposed individuals.[131] These organisms live on gram-negative bacteria, and it is possible that inhalation of amoebal or bacterial antigen is the cause of the syndrome of humidifier fever. It has not so far proved possible to perform challenge tests with pure amoebal extracts, but tests with humidifier water have shown the reaction to be immunological rather than due to endotoxin, and yet not mediated by complement activation.[130] The last chapter in this interesting story has yet to be written.

In the investigation of outbreaks of febrile illness in the workplace, care should be taken to consider all the possible mechanisms of disease. Moreover, it is reasonable to suppose that other organisms causing similar syndromes will be identified in the near future. Humidifier fever may be diagnosed from the clinical history, the presence of precipitins to extracts of the water or sludge from sumps or baffle plates, and, if necessary, the reproduction of symptoms by challenge testing, by exposure to the suspected water either at work after a break or in the laboratory. As far as is presently known, typical humidifier fever is not progressive and does not cause chronic lung disease. It is preventable by stopping exposure, ideally by changing the system so that water does not recirculate or by injection of steam rather than cold water into humidifiers.[123] These solutions may often be expensive, and investigations of biocidal agents and the use of ultraviolet light are under way. The efficacy of preventive measures may be monitored by testing the water for antigen against the serum of patients known to contain antibody.

Sewage Sludge Fever

A disease similar to humidifier fever has been described in workers in sewage treatment plants.[132, 133] The symptoms of fever, malaise, and myalgia followed by a general feeling of tiredness do not have any special periodicity, but follow unusually high exposures to aerosolized sewage sludge or dust of dried sludge. The sludge contains large numbers of gram-negative bacteria, and it has been suggested that the disease is a response to inhalation of bacterial endotoxin. To date, no long-term or specific pulmonary effects have been described.

Grain Fever

As pointed out in Chapter 16, exposure to grain dust involves inhalation of not only cereal matter but also bacteria, fungi, and antigenic material from mites, weevils, and even small mammals.[94] Asthma is well recognized in such workers, allergic alveolitis may well occur in appropri-

ate circumstances, and there is also much discussion as to whether chronic airways obstruction may also be a consequence of prolonged exposure, though to date the epidemiological studies have failed to separate the effects of dust from those of smoking. In addition to these possible problems, a syndrome of fever, myalgia, and malaise, known as grain fever, has been described in workers following massive exposure, particularly upon first working in an elevator or after a period off work.[134, 135] Whether this syndrome is related to inhaled endotoxin, complement activation, or some other mechanism has not yet been determined.

References

1. Pepys, J., Hypersensitivity Diseases of the Lungs due to Fungi and Organic Dusts. New York, S. Karger, 1969.
2. Boyd, G., Clinical and immunological studies in pulmonary extrinsic allergic alveolitis. Scot. Med. J., *23*, 267, 1978.
3. Davies, B. H., Edwards, J. H., and Seaton, A., Cross reacting antibodies to *Micropolyspora faeni* in mycoplasma pneumonia. Clin. Allergy, *5*, 217, 1975.
4. Boyd, G., Madkour, M., Middleton, S., Lynch, P., Effect of smoking on circulating antibody levels to avian protein in pigeon breeder's disease. Thorax, *32*, 651, 1977.
5. Morgan, D. C., Smyth, J. T., Lister, R. W., et al., Chest symptoms in farming communities with special reference to farmer's lung. Br. J. Ind. Med., *32*, 228, 1975.
6. Hapke, E. J., Seal, R. M. E., and Thomas, G. O., Farmer's lung. Thorax, *23*, 451, 1968.
7. Rankin, J., Kobayashi, M., Barbee, R. A., and Dickie, H. A., Pulmonary granulomatoses due to inhaled organic antigens. Med. Clin. North Am., *51*, 459, 1967.
8. Seal, R. M. E., Hapke, E. J., Thomas, G. O., et al., The pathology of the acute and chronic stages of farmer's lung. Thorax, *23*, 469, 1968.
9. Emanuel, D. A., Wenzel, F. J., Bowerman, C. I., and Lawton, B. R., Farmer's lung. Clinical, pathologic and immunologic study of 24 patients. Am. J. Med., *37*, 392, 1964.
10. Barrowcliff, D. E., and Arblaster, P. G., Farmer's lung: a study of an early acute fatal case. Thorax, *23*, 490, 1968.
11. Mullins, J., and Seaton, A., Fungal spores in lung and sputum. Clin. Allergy, *8*, 525, 1978.
12. Mullins, J., Harvey, R., and Seaton, A., Sources and incidence of airborne *Aspergillus fumigatus* (Fres). Clin. Allergy, *6*, 209, 1976.
13. Pepys, J., Riddell, R. W., Citron, K. M., et al., Clinical and immunologic significance of *Aspergillus fumigatus* in the sputum. Am. Rev. Respir. Dis., *80*, 167, 1959.
14. Grant, I. W. B., Blythe, W., Wardrop, V. E., et al., Prevalence of farmer's lung in Scotland: a pilot study. Br. Med. J., *1*, 530, 1972.
15. DoPico, G. A., Reddan, W. G., Chonelik, F., et al., The value of antibodies in screening for hypersensitivity pneumonitis. Am. Rev. Respir. Dis., *113*, 451, 1976.
16. Burrell, R., and Rylander, R., A critical review of the role of precipitins in hypersensitivity pneumonitis. Eur. J. Respir. Dis., *62*, 332. 1981.
17. Boyd, G., McSharry, C. P., Banham, S. W., and Lynch, P. P., A current view of pigeon fancier's lung. A model for extrinsic allergic alveolitis. Clin. Allergy, *12* (Suppl), 53, 1982.
18. Edwards, J. H., Wagner, J. C., and Seal, R. M. E., Pulmonary responses to particulate materials capable of activating the alternative pathway of complement. Clin. Allergy, *6*, 155, 1976.
19. Roberts, R. C., and Moore, V. L., Immunopathogenesis of hypersensitivity pneumonitis. Am. Rev. Respir. Dis., *116*, 1075, 1977.
20. Neilsen, K. H., Parratt, D., Boyd, G., and White, R. G., Use of a radiolabelled antiglobulin for quantitation of antibody to soluble antigens rendered particulate; application to pigeon fancier's lung syndrome. Int. Arch. Allergy Appl. Immunol., *47*, 339, 1974.

21. Hendrick, D. J., Marshall, R., Faux, J. A., and Krall, J. M., Positive "alveolar" responses to antigen inhalation provocation tests: their validity and recognition. Thorax, *35*, 415, 1980.
22. Warren, C. P. W., Tse, K. S., and Cherniack, R. M., Mechanical properties of the lung in extrinsic allergic alveolitis. Thorax, *33*, 315, 1978.
23. Evans, W. V., and Seaton, A., Hypersensitivity pneumonitis in a technician using Pauli's reagent. Thorax, *34*, 767, 1979.
24. Bernardo, J., Hunninghake, G. W., Gadek, J. E., et al., Acute hypersensitivity pneumonitis: serial changes in lung lymphocyte subpopulations after exposure to antigen. Am. Rev. Respir. Dis., *120*, 985, 1979.
25. Godart, P., Clot, J., Jonquet, O., et al., Lymphocyte subpopulations in bronchoalveolar lavages of patients with sarcoidosis and hypersensitivity pneumonitis. Chest, *80*, 447, 1981.
26. Reynolds, H. Y., Fulmer, J. D., Kazmeirdwski, J. A., et al., Analysis of cellular and protein content of bronchoalveolar lavage fluid from patients with idiopathic pulmonary fibrosis and chronic hypersensitivity pneumonitis. J. Clin. Invest., *59*, 165, 1977.
27. Gourley, C. A., and Braidwood, G. D., The role of dust respirators in the prevention of recurrence of farmer's lung. Trans. Soc. Occup. Med., *21*, 93, 1971.
28. Hendrick, D. J., Marshall, R., Faux, J. A., and Krall, J. M., Protective value of dust respirators in extrinsic allergic alveolitis: clinical assessment using inhalation provocation tests. Thorax, *36*, 917, 1981.
29. Campbell, J. M., Acute symptoms following work with hay. Br. Med. J., *2*, 1143, 1932.
30. Fawcitt, R., Fungoid conditions of lung. I and II. Br. J. Radiol., *9*, 172 and 354, 1936.
31. Fuller, C. J., Farmer's lung, a review of present knowledge. Thorax, *8*, 59, 1953.
32. Banaszak, E. J., Thiede, W. H., and Fink, J. N., Hypersensitivity pneumonitis due to contamination of an air conditioner. N. Engl. J. Med., *283*, 271, 1970.
33. Fink, J. N., Banaszak, E. J., and Thiede, W. H., Interstitial pneumonitis due to hypersensitivity to an organism contaminating a heating system. Ann. Intern. Med., *74*, 80, 1971.
34. Fink, J. N., Banaszak, E. J., Barboriak, J. J., et al., Interstitial lung disease due to contamination of forced air systems. Ann. Intern. Med., *84*, 406, 1976.
35. Williams, J. V., Inhalation and skin tests with extracts of hay and fungi in patients with farmer's lung. Thorax, *18*, 182, 1963.
36. Pepys, J., and Jenkins, P. A., Precipitin (F.L.H.) test in farmer's lung. Thorax, *20*, 21, 1965.
37. LaBerge, D. E., and Stahmann, M. A., Antigens from mouldy hay involved in farmer's lung. Proc. Soc. Exp. Biol. Med., *121*, 463, 1966.
38. Pepys, J., Riddell, R. W., Citron, K. M., and Clayton, Y. M., Precipitins against extracts of hay and fungi in the serum of patients with farmer's lung. Acta Allergy, *16*, 76, 1961.
39. Barbee, R. A., Dickie, H. A., and Rankin, J., Pathogenicity of specific glycopeptide antigen in farmer's lung. Proc. Soc. Exp. Biol. Med., *118*, 546, 1965.
40. Pepys, J., Riddell, R. W., Citron, K. M., and Clayton, Y. M., Precipitins against extracts of hay and moulds in the serum of patients with farmer's lung, aspergillosis, asthma and sarcoidosis. Thorax, *17*, 366, 1962.
41. Pepys, J., Jenkins, P. A., Festenstein, G. N., et al., Farmer's lung: thermophilic actinomycetes as a source of "farmer's lung hay" antigens. Lancet, *2*, 607, 1963.
42. Wenzel, F. J., Gray, R. L., and Emanuel, D. A., Farmer's lung, its geographic distribution. J. Occup. Med., *12*, 493, 1970.
43. Madsen, D., Klock, L. E., Wenzel, F. J., et al., The prevalence of farmer's lung in an agricultural population. Am. Rev. Respir. Dis., *113*, 171, 1976.
44. Flaherty, D. K., Braun, S. R., Marx, J. J., et al., Serologically detectable HLA–A, B and C loci antigens in farmer's lung disease. Am. Rev. Respir. Dis., *122*, 437, 1980.
45. Braun, S. R., doPico, G. A., Tsiatis, A., et al., Farmer's lung disease: long-term clinical and physiologic outcome. Am. Rev. Respir. Dis., *119*, 185, 1979.
46. Buechner, H. A., Prevatt, A. L., Thompson, J., and Blitz, O., Bagassosis: review with further historical data, studies of pulmonary function, and results of adrenal steroid therapy. Am. J. Med., *25*, 234, 1958.
47. Hunter, D., and Perry, K. M. M., Bronchiolitis from industrial handling of bagasse. Br. J. Ind. Med., *3*, 64, 1946.

48. Hearn, C. E. D., and Holford-Strevens, V., Immunological aspects of bagassosis. Br. J. Ind. Med., 25, 283, 1968.
49. Weill, H., Buechner, H. A., Gonzalez, E., et al., Bagassosis: a study of pulmonary function in 20 cases. Ann. Intern. Med., 64, 737, 1966.
50. Miller, G. J., Hearn, C. E. D., and Edwards, T. H. T., Pulmonary function at rest and during exercise following bagassosis. Br. J. Ind. Med., 28, 152, 1971.
51. Bringhurst, L. S., Byrne, R. N., and Gershon-Cohen, J., Respiratory disease of mushroom workers. J.A.M.A., 171, 15, 1959.
52. Sakula, A., Mushroom worker's lung. Br. Med. J., 2, 708, 1967.
53. Riddle, H. F. V., Channell, S., Blyth, W., et al., Allergic alveolitis in a malt worker. Thorax, 23,271, 1968.
54. Grant, I. W. B., Blackadder, E. S., Greenberg, M., and Blyth, W., Extrinsic allergic alveolitis in Scottish maltworkers. Br. Med. J., 1, 490, 1976.
55. De Weck, A. L., Guttersohn, J., and Bütikofer, E., La maladie des laveurs de fromage, une forme particulière du syndrome du poumon du fermier. Schweiz Med. Wschr., 99, 872, 1969.
56. Schlueter, D. P., Cheesewasher's disease: a new occupational hazard? Ann. Intern. Med., 78, 606, 1973.
57. Tower, J. W., Sweaney, H. C., and Huron, W. H., Severe bronchial asthma apparently due to fungus spores found in maple bark. J.A.M.A., 99, 453, 1932.
58. Emanuel, D. A., Lawton, B. R., and Wenzel, F. J., Maplebark disease. N. Engl. J. Med., 266, 333, 1962.
59. Emanuel, D. A., Wenzel, F. J., and Lawton, B. R., Pneumonitis due to *Cryptostroma corticale* (maple-bark disease). N. Engl. J. Med., 274, 1413, 1966.
60. Wenzel, F. J., and Emanuel, D. A., The epidemiology of maple bark disease. Arch. Environ. Health, 14, 385, 1967.
61. Cohen, H. I., Merigan, T. C., Kosek, J. C., and Eldridge, F., A granulomatous pneumonitis associated with redwood sawdust inhalation. Am. J. Med., 43, 785, 1967.
62. Michaels, L., Lung changes in woodworkers. Can. Med. Assoc. J., 96, 1150, 1967.
63. Sosman, A. J., Schlueter, D. P., Fink, J. H., and Barboriak, J. J., Hypersensitivity to wood dust. N. Engl. J. Med., 281, 977, 1969.
64. Schlueter, D. P., Fink, J. N., and Hensley, G. T., Wood-pulp workers' disease. A hypersensitivity pneumonitis caused by Alternaria. Ann. Intern. Med., 77, 907, 1972.
65. Avila, R., and Villar, T. G., Suberosis. Respiratory disease in cork workers. Lancet, 1, 620, 1968.
66. Avila, R., and Lacey, J., The role of *Penicillium frequentans* in suberosis (respiratory disease in workers in the cork industry). Clin. Allergy, 4, 109, 1974.
67. Howie, A. D., Boyd, G., and Moran, F., Pulmonary hypersensitivity to Ramin (*Gonystylus bancanus*). Thorax, 31, 585, 1976.
68. Hunter, D., The Diseases of Occupations, 4th ed. London, English Universities Press, 1969, p. 1081.
69. Livingstone, J. L., Lewis, J. G., Reid, L., and Jefferson, K. E., Diffuse interstitial pulmonary fibrosis. Q. J. Med., 33, 71, 1964.
70. O'Brien, I. M., Bull, J., Creamer, B., et al., Asthma and extrinsic allergic alveolitis due to *Merulius lacrymans*. Clin. Allergy, 8, 535, 1978.
71. Rhudy, J., Burrell, R. G., and Morgan, W. K. C., Yet another cause of allergic alveolitis. Scand. J. Resp. Dis., 52, 177, 1971.
72. Strand, R. D., Neuhauser, E. B. D., and Sornberger, C. F., Lycoperdonosis. N. Engl. J. Med., 277, 89, 1967.
73. Plessner, M. M., Une maladie des trieurs de plumes: la fièvre de canard. Arch. Mal. Prof., 21, 67, 1960.
74. Pearsall, H. R., Morgan, E. H., Tesluk, H., and Beggs, D., Parakeet dander pneumonitis. Acute psittaco-kerato-pneumoconiosis. Report of a case. Bull. Mason Clinic, 14, 127, 1960.
75. Barboriak, J. J., Sosman, A. J., and Reed, C. E., Serological studies in pigeon breeder's disease. J. Lab. Clin. Med., 65, 600, 1965.
76. Reed, C. E., Sosman, A., and Barbee, R. A., Pigeon-breeder's lung. J.A.M.A., 193, 261, 1965.
77. Villar, T. G., Avila, R., and Araugo, J., O "pulmao dos criadores de pombos." A proposito de un case e de un plano. J. Soc. Ciencias Med. Lisboa, 130, 181, 1966.

78. Hargreave, F. E., Pepys, J., Longbottom, J. H., and Wraith, D. G., Bird breeder's (fancier's) lung. Lancet, *1*, 44, 1966.
79. Warren, C. P. W., and Tse, K. S., Extrinsic allergic alveolitis owing to hypersensitivity to chickens. Am. Rev. Respir. Dis., *109*, 672, 1974.
80. Boyer, R. S., Klock, L. E., Schmidt, C. D., et al., Hypersensitivity lung disease in the turkey raising industry. Am. Rev. Respir. Dis., *109*, 630, 1974.
81. Schlueter, D. P., Fink, J. N., and Sosman, A. J., Pulmonary function in pigeon breeder's disease. A hypersensitivity pneumonitis. Ann. Intern. Med., *70*, 457, 1969.
82. Allen, D. H., Williams, D. V., and Woodcock, A. J., Bird breeder's hypersensitivity pneumonitis: progress studies of lung function after cessation of exposure to the provoking antigen. Am. Rev. Respir. Dis., *114*, 555, 1976.
83. Christensen, L. T., Schmidt, C. D., and Robbins, L., Pigeon breeder's disease—a prevalence study and review. Clin. Allergy, *5*, 417, 1975.
84. Barboriak, J. J., Sosman, A. J., and Reed, C. E., Serological studies in pigeon breeder's disease. J. Lab. Clin. Med., *65*, 600, 1965.
85. Banham, S. W., McKenzie, H., McSharry, C., et al., Antibody against a pigeon bloom extract: a further antigen in pigeon breeder's lung. Clin. Allergy, *12*, 173, 1982.
86. Boyd, G., Dick, H. W., Lorimer, A. R., and Moran, F., Bird breeder's lung. Scot. Med. J., *12*, 69, 1967.
87. Newman Taylor, A. J., Taylor, P., Bryant, D. H., et al., False-positive complement fixation tests with respiratory virus preparations in bird fanciers with allergic alveolitis. Thorax, *32*, 563, 1977.
88. Faux, J. A., Hendrick, D. J., and Anand, B. S., Precipitins to different avian serum antigens in bird fancier's lung and coeliac disease. Clin. Allergy, *8*, 101, 1978.
89. Hood, J., and Mason, A. M. S., Diffuse pulmonary disease with transfer defect occurring with coeliac disease. Lancet, *1*, 445, 1970.
90. Berrill, W. T., Eade, O. E., Fitzpatrick, P. F., et al., Bird fancier's lung and jejunal villous atrophy. Lancet, *2*, 1006, 1975.
91. Hendrick, D. J., Faux, J. A., Anand, B., et al., Is bird fancier's lung associated with coeliac disease? Thorax, *33*, 425, 1978.
92. Carroll, K. B., Pepys, J., Longbottom, J. L., et al., Extrinsic allergic alveolitis due to rat serum proteins. Clin. Allergy, *5*, 443, 1975.
93. Korenblat, P., Slavin, R., Winzenburger, P., et al., Gerbil-keeper's lung—a new form of hypersensitivity pneumonitis. Ann. Allergy, *38*, 437, 1977.
94. Jiminez-Diaz, C., Lahoz, C., and Cento, G., The allergens of mill dust. Asthma in millers, farmers and others. Ann. Allergy, *5*, 519, 1947.
95. Frankland, A. W., and Lunn, J. A., Asthma caused by the grain weevil. Br. J. Ind. Med., *22*, 157, 1965.
96. Lunn, J. A., and Hughes, D. T. D., Pulmonary hypersensitivity to the grain weevil. Br. J. Ind. Med., *24*, 158, 1967.
97. Valléry-Radot, L., and Giroud, P., Sporomycose des pelleteurs de grains. Bull. Mém. Soc. Méd. Hôp. Paris, *52*, 1632, 1928.
98. Pimentel, J. C., Furrier's lung. Thorax, *25*, 387, 1970.
99. Mahon, W. E., Scott, D. J., Ansell, G., et al., Hypersensitivity to pituitary snuff with miliary shadowing in the lungs. Thorax, *22*, 13, 1967.
100. Butikoffer, E., De Weck, A. L., and Scherrer, M., Pituitary snufftaker's lung. Schweiz. Med. Wschr., *100*, 97, 1970.
101. Harper, L. O., Burrell, R. G., Lapp, N. L., and Morgan, W. K. C., Allergic alveolitis due to pituitary snuff. Ann. Intern. Med., *73*, 581, 1970.
102. Fuchs, S., and Valade, P., Étude clinique et expérimentale sur quelques cas d'intoxication par le Desmodur T. (Diisocyanate de toluylene 1–2–4 et 1–2–6.) Arch. Mal. Prof., *12*, 191, 1951.
103. Charles, J. M., Bernstein, A., Jones, B., et al., Hypersensitivity pneumonitis after exposure to isocyanates. Thorax, *31*, 127, 1976.
104. Fink, J. N., and Schlueter, D. P., Bathtub refinisher's lung: an unusual response to toluene diisocyanate. Am. Rev. Respir. Dis., *118*, 955, 1978.
105. Zeiss, C. R., Kanellakes, T. B., Bellone, J. D., et al., Immunoglobulin E–mediated asthma and hypersensitivity pneumonitis with precipitating anti-hapten antibodies due to diphenyl dimethane diisocyanate. J. Allergy Clin. Immunol., *65*, 346, 1980.
106. Malo, J.-L., and Zeiss, C. R., Occupational hypersensitivity pneumonitis after exposure to diphenylmethane diisocyanate. Am. Rev. Respir. Dis., *125*, 113, 1982.

107. Pimental, J. C., and Marques, F., Vineyard sprayer's lung: a new occupational disease. Thorax, *24*, 678, 1969.

108. Villar, T. G., Vineyard sprayer's lung. Clinical aspects. Am. Rev. Respir. Dis., *110*, 545, 1974.

109. Thomas, P., Seaton, A., and Edwards, J., Respiratory disease due to sulphasalazine. Clin. Allergy, *4*, 41, 1974.

110. Rosenow, E. C., DeRemee, R. A., and Dines, D., Chronic nitrofurantoin pulmonary reaction. N. Engl. J. Med., *279*, 1258, 1968.

111. Burgher, L. W., Cass, I., and Schenken, J. R., Pulmonary allergic granulomatosis: a possible drug reaction in a patient receiving cromolyn sodium. Chest, *66*, 84, 1974.

112. Sjögren, I., Hillerdal, G., Andersson, A., and Zetterström, O., Hard metal lung disease: importance of cobalt in coolants. Thorax, *35*, 653, 1980.

113. Newhouse, M. L., Tagg, B., Pocock, S. J., and McEwan, A. C., An epidemiological study of workers producing enzyme washing powders. Lancet, *1*, 689, 1970.

114. Franz, T., McMurrain, K. D., Brooks, S., and Bernstein, I. L., Clinical, immunologic and physiologic observations in factory workers exposed to *B. subtilis* enzyme dust. J. Allergy, *47*, 170, 1971.

115. Johnson, C. L., Bernstein, I. L., Gallagher, J. S., et al., Familial hypersensitivity pneumonitis induced by *Bacillus subtilis*. Am. Rev. Respir. Dis., *122*, 339, 1980.

116. Kohler, P. F., Gross, G., Salvaggio, J., and Hawkins, J., Humidifier lung: hypersensitivity pneumonitis related to thermotolerant bacterial aerosols. Chest, *69* (Suppl), 294, 1976.

117. Muittari, A., Kuusisto, P., Virtanen, P., et al., An epidemic of extrinsic allergic alveolitis caused by tap water. Clin. Allergy, *10*, 77, 1980.

118. Van den Bosch, J. M. M., van Toorn, D. W., and Wagenaar, S. S., Coffee worker's lung: Reconsideration of a case report. Thorax, *38*, 720, 1983.

119. Blackburn, C. R. B., and Green, W., Precipitins against extracts of thatched roofs in the sera of New Guinea natives with chronic lung disease. Lancet, *2*, 1396, 1966.

120. Carlson, J. E., and Villaveces, J. W., Hypersensitivity pneumonitis due to pyrethrum. J.A.M.A., *237*, 1718, 1977.

121. Ross, P. J., Seaton, A., Foreman, H. M., and Morris Evans, W. H., Pulmonary calcification following smallpox handler's lung. Thorax, *29*, 659, 1974.

122. Emanuel, D. A., Wenzel, F. J., and Lawton, B. R., Pulmonary mycotoxicosis. Chest, *67*, 293, 1975.

123. MRC Symposium, Humidifier fever. Thorax, *32*, 653, 1977.

124. Pestalozzi, C., Febrile Gruppener Krankungen in einer Modellschreinerei durch Inhalation von mit Schimelpilzen Kontaminierten Befeuchtewasser. Schweiz Med. Wschr., *89*, 710, 1959.

125. H. M. Chief Inspector of Factories, Annual Report 1969. London, H. M. Stationery Office, 1970, p. 72.

126. Pickering, C. A. C., Moore, W. K. S., Lacey, J., et al., Investigation of a respiratory disease associated with an air-conditioning system. Clin. Allergy, *6*, 109, 1976.

127. Friend, J. A. R., Gaddie, J., Palmer, K. N. V., et al., Extrinsic allergic alveolitis and contaminated cooling water in a factory machine. Lancet, *1*, 297, 1977.

128. Edwards, J. H., Microbial and immunological investigations after an outbreak of humidifier fever. Br. J. Ind. Med., *37*, 55, 1980.

129. Cockcroft, A., Edwards, J., Bevan, C., et al., An investigation of operating theatre staff exposed to humidifier fever antigen. Br. J. Ind. Med., *38*, 144, 1981.

130. Edwards, J. H., and Cockcroft, A., Inhalation challenge in humidifier fever. Clin. Allergy, *11*, 227, 1981.

131. Edwards, J. H., Griffiths, A. J., and Mullins, J., Protozoa as sources of antigen in "humidifier fever." Nature, *264*, 438, 1976.

132. Rylander, R., Anderson K., Belin L., et al., Sewage worker's syndrome. Lancet, *2*, 478, 1976.

133. Mattsby, I., and Rylander, R., Clinical and immunological findings in workers exposed to sewage dust. J. Occup. Med., *20*, 690, 1978.

134. Williams, N., Skonlas, A., and Merriman, J. E., Exposure to grain dust. I. A survey of the effects. *In* Dosman, J. A., and Cotton, D. S., eds., Occupational Pulmonary Disease. Focus on Grain Dust and Health. New York, Academic Press, 1980, p. 367.

135. Tse, K. S., Warren, P., Janusz, M., et al., Respiratory abnormalities in workers exposed to grain dusts. Arch. Environ. Health, *27*, 74, 1973.

20

TOXIC GASES AND FUMES

Anthony Seaton and W. Keith C. Morgan

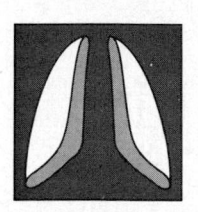

The danger to life of gases and fumes in mining has been appreciated since the earliest times. Pliny the Elder in Book 33 of his *Natural History* wrote: "But for that the vapour and smoke that ariseth from thence, by the means, may stifle and choke them within those narrow pits and mines, they are forced to give over such fire-work and betake themselves often-times to great mattocks and pickaxes."

This referred to the practice in gold mining of cracking rocks with fire. Silver miners were also at risk from naturally generated vapors: "And yet there is a damp or vapour breathing out of silver mines, hurtful to all living creatures and to dogs especially."

Apart from asphyxiation, it was appreciated that poisoning could occur from absorption of toxic matter from dust and fumes, and Pliny described the use of masks made from bladders for the prevention of mercury poisoning in vermilion workers. Agricola in Book 6 of *De re metallica* gave details of many poisonous fumes encountered in the mine atmosphere and described apparatus for minimizing the danger by ventilation.

PRINCIPLES OF ACTION

Harmful airborne material may be suspended in a molecular form as a gas or in a particulate form. A liquid particulate is called a mist, while a fine solid particulate, often formed by the vaporization and oxidation of a metal, is called a fume. A vapor is the gaseous form of a substance which is liquid if enclosed at normal temperature and pressure.

The behavior of such matter when inhaled depends on its physical and chemical properties. Gases are affected by Brownian movement, while particulates are affected more by gravity. The principles of deposition of particulate matter are outlined in Chapter 4. Large particles, of 15 to 20 microns in diameter, tend to be deposited in the nose, smaller ones in the

trachea and bronchi, and those between 1 and about 7 microns may be deposited in the alveoli. With particles below 0.5 microns very little deposition takes place, though even matter that is not deposited to any great extent may cause harm. In general, this occurs by one of four basic mechanisms. Table 20–1 lists the more commonly encountered toxic gases and fumes and their effects.

Asphyxiation

This may occur simply by displacement of oxygen from the inspired air, as occurs with nitrogen, carbon dioxide, and methane, or by chemical interference with the process of oxygen transport, as in poisoning by carbon monoxide or cyanides.

Local Irritation

Most toxic gases and fumes act in this way. Their site of action is related to their solubility, as a very soluble substance is absorbed onto the mucous membrane that it first contacts, namely, the nose and upper respiratory tract, while a less soluble substance exerts its harmful effects throughout the respiratory tract. Ammonia is an example of the former, while the oxides of nitrogen exemplify the latter.

Toxic Absorption

Absorption through the lungs of matter that has toxic effects either on the lung or elsewhere in the body is the case with carbon monoxide and cyanides, which are grouped as asphyxiants. Mercury and manganese may be absorbed this way to damage the nervous system. Beryllium and cadmium may cause progressive lung damage, and fluorides may harm the skeleton.

Allergy and Sensitization

This occurs with substances such as platinum compounds and iso-cyanates, and is discussed in Chapters 16 and 19.

ASPHYXIANT GASES

Carbon Dioxide

Carbon dioxide is heavier than air and is most commonly encountered in enclosed or ill-ventilated spaces, such as unworked mines, caissons, and tanks. In coal mines it is produced by the oxidation of contaminants of coal on unworked faces, and constitutes an important hazard when the

Table 20–1. TOXIC GASES AND FUMES

Agent	Principal Occupations Exposed	Main Mechanism of Injury	Time-Weighted Average*	IDLH Level†
Acrolein	Plastic, rubber, textile, resin making	Direct action on mucosa of the eye and respiratory tract, irritant effects	0.1 ppm	5 ppm
Acrylonitrile	Synthetic fiber, acrylic resin, rubber making	Asphyxiant	2 ppm	4 ppm
Ammonia	Fertilizer, refrigerator, explosive production	Direct action on mucosa of the eye and respiratory tract, tracheitis and pulmonary edema	50 ppm	500 ppm
Arsine	Smelting, refining	Systemic effects	0.05 ppm	6 ppm
Cadmium fumes	Ore smelting, alloying, welding	Acute tracheobronchitis, pulmonary edema	0.1 mg/m³ (40 μg/m³)	
Carbon dioxide	Foundry work, mining	Emphysema, renal effects	5000 ppm	50,000 ppm
Carbon disulfide	Degreasing, electroplating, sulfur processing	Asphyxiant	20 ppm (1 ppm)	500 ppm
		Systemic effects		
Carbon monoxide	Foundry work, petroleum refining, mining	Asphyxiant	50 ppm (35 ppm)	2500 ppm
Chlorine	Bleaching, disinfectant and plastic making	Direct action on mucosa of the eyes and respiratory tract, tracheitis and pulmonary edema. Possible chronic effect and airways obstruction?	1 ppm (0.5 ppm)	25 ppm
Copper fumes	Welding	Systemic effects	0.1 mg/m³	—
Formaldehyde	Disinfectant, embalming fluid use, paper and photography industry	Direct action on mucosa of the eyes and respiratory tract, dermatitis, and asthma?	3 ppm (1 ppm)	100 ppm

Table 20–1. TOXIC GASES AND FUMES *Continued*

Agent	Principal Occupations Exposed	Main Mechanism of Injury	Time-Weighted Average*	IDLH Level†
Hydrogen chloride	Refining, dye making, organic chemical synthesis	Direct action on mucosa of the eyes and respiratory tract, tracheobronchitis	5 ppm	100 ppm
Hydrogen cyanide	Electroplating, fumigant work, steel industry	Systemic effects	10 ppm	50 mg/m³
Hydrogen fluoride	Etching, petroleum industry, silk working	Direct action on mucosa of the eyes and respiratory tract, tracheitis	3 ppm	20 ppm
Hydrogen sulfide	Natural gas making, paper pulp, sewage treatment, tannery work, oil-well prospecting	Systemic and local effects, pulmonary edema, and asphyxia	20 ppm	300 ppm
Magnesium oxide fumes	Welding, alloy, flare, filament making	Systemic effects	15 mg/m³	—
Manganese fumes	Foundry work, battery making, permanganate manufacture	Systemic effects, possible predisposition to pneumonia	5 mg/m³	—
Mercury fumes	Electrolysis	Direct action on mucosa of eyes, GI tract, and lung. Interstitial pneumonitis, systemic effects	0.1 mg/m³	28 mg/m³
Methyl bromide	Fumigating, dye and refrigerant making	Direct action on mucosa of the eyes and respiratory tract	20 ppm	2000 ppm
Natural gas	Mining, petroleum refining, power plant work	Asphyxiant	—	—

			*	†IDLH
Nitrogen	Underwater work, mining	Asphyxiant	—	—
Nitrogen dioxide	Arc welding, dye and fertilizer making, farming	Irritant to respiratory tract, tracheitis, pulmonary edema, and bronchiolitis obliterans	5 ppm (1 ppm)	50 ppm
Osmium tetroxide fumes	Alloy making, platinum hardening	Direct irritation of respiratory tract	0.002 mg/m³	1 mg/m³
Ozone	Arc welding, air, sewage, and water treatment	Direct irritation of respiratory tract	0.1 ppm	10 ppm
Phosgene	Chemical industry, dye and insecticide making	Direct irritation of respiratory tract, pulmonary edema	0.1 ppm	2 ppm
Platinum, soluble salts (mist)	Alloy, mirror making, eletroplating, catalyst, and ceramic work	Asthmatic reactions	0.002 mg/m³	—
Sulfur dioxide	Bleaching, ore smelting, paper manufacture, refrigeration industry	Direct action on the respiratory tract, bronchitis, exceptionally pulmonary edema	5 ppm	100 ppm
Vanadium pentoxide fumes	Glass, ceramic, alloy making, chemical industry (catalysis)	Direct action on respiratory tract, bronchitis, asthma	0.1 mg/m³ (0.05 mg/m³)	70 mg/m³
Zinc chloride fumes	Dry cell making, soldering, textile finishing	Direct action on respiratory tract, irritant	1 mg/m³	200 mg/m³
Zinc oxide fumes	Welding	Systemic effects	5 mg/m³	—

*Figures in parentheses are National Institute of Occupational Safety and Health (NIOSH) recommendations.
†IDLH = immediately dangerous to life or health.

face is reopened. The symptoms of hyperventilation, headache, and sweating, and the signs of bounding pulse and loss of consciousness are familiar to most doctors in a nonindustrial setting. Management of the patient consists of removal from the gas and administration of oxygen. Mouth-to-mouth respiration should be carried out if breathing has ceased.

Carbon dioxide is detected by its ability to extinguish a flame. In mines, a safety lamp is needed, and in other situations, a naked flame is adequate. Once carbon dioxide has been detected, work should not be resumed without breathing apparatus until the gas has been displaced by air.

Nitrogen

Nitrogen constitutes almost 80 per cent of air, and when oxygen is removed in oxidative processes in mines the air remaining consists of nitrogen and carbon dioxide. As the content of oxygen falls, less is available for respiration. When the oxygen level drops to about 15 per cent, noticeable dyspnea occurs on exertion. At rest dyspnea may not occur until the oxygen level is 10 per cent, but below this there is serious danger of collapse and death on slight exertion. Again, detection depends on the atmosphere's gradually decreasing ability to support combustion, and treatment consists of removal of the subject, administration of oxygen, and artificial respiration, if necessary.

Methane

Methane, otherwise known as firedamp or marsh gas, is produced by decaying vegetable matter. Pockets of it occur in coal seams and can often be heard hissing or bubbling from the face. The two dangers associated with methane are asphyxiation and explosion. It is lighter than air and therefore has a tendency to accumulate in pockets at the top of a working. It is without taste or odor, so the first sign of its presence may be loss of consciousness. The danger of explosion is an important one, as methane forms an explosive mixture with air, and this was responsible for many mining disasters before the introduction of the Davy lamp to detect methane and of rock dusting to prevent coal dust explosions.

The Davy lamp was invented in 1816 by Sir Humphry Davy for the express purpose of detecting methane and thereby preventing explosions. Davy surrounded the flame by wire gauze, on the principle that the wire conducts away the heat of the flame and so prevents its spread outside the gauze. When the atmosphere contains methane, the flame in the lamp acquires a blue cap, thus warning the miner of the danger. Modern safety lamps have superseded the Davy lamp, but the principle is the same, the lamp being held close to the roof to detect accumulation of methane.

Depending on the fuel used and the height of the flame, a rough estimate of the concentration of gas can be obtained.

Carbon Monoxide

Carbon monoxide is a product of incomplete combustion of carbon-containing matter. It is odorless and somewhat lighter than air. It is formed in all fires and is an important cause of death in burning buildings and mines following explosions. While it is familiar as a hazard in garages and kitchens, in industry it may be encountered around blast furnaces and gasworks and in many other situations in which combustion takes place and leaks of exhaust gas can occur.

Carbon monoxide acts by combining with hemoglobin in such a way as to reduce the oxygen-carrying power of the blood, its combining power being some 200 times greater than that of oxygen. Moreover, increasing carboxyhemoglobin content of the blood shifts the oxygen dissociation curve to the left and depresses the upper part of the curve so that less oxygen is available to the tissues. Thus, although the oxygen content of blood (oxygen saturation) may be severely reduced by breathing relatively small concentrations of carbon monoxide, viz., around 0.5 per cent, the partial pressure of oxygen remains normal. As it is on this that the chemoreceptor response to hypoxia depends, breathlessness is not a feature of carbon monoxide poisoning.

Carbon monoxide poisoning causes rapid loss of consciousness with few premonitory symptoms. Cyanosis is not a feature, the subject generally looking pallid and often peaked. Headache and dizziness are variable symptoms. In patients who have recovered, extrapyramidal signs, due to degenerative changes in the basal ganglia, may develop. Alternatively, the tissue hypoxia may cause damage to any organ whose circulation was previously impaired by vascular disease, and death or permanent disability may result from myocardial or cerebral infarction.

The danger from carbon monoxide is related to its fractional concentration in the inspired air, the duration of the inhalation, and the oxygen requirements for exercise of the individual. Very low concentrations, of order of 0.5 per cent, if breathed for 1½ to 2 hours may cause death. An approximate calculation of the saturation of hemoglobin by carbon monoxide may be obtained from the formula $b = \dfrac{4ate}{100}$, in which b is the saturation, a the concentration in parts per million, t the exposure time in hours, and e an exercise factor, either a value of 1 for rest, 2 for walking, or 3 for working.[1] This formula is inaccurate for high concentrations or long exposures but may be useful for calculating the safety of a contaminated mine roadway.

Detection of carbon monoxide in mines has for the last century depended on the use of canaries, which usually respond to the gas by

falling off their perches before workers notice any ill effects. While this normally gives ample warning, occasionally in low concentrations of the order of 0.05 per cent carbon monoxide, the bird adapts to the gas and the worker may collapse while the bird remains well. More accurate methods of measurement are now available from simple detector tubes to highly accurate infrared analyzers, and these are used in situations in which accumulation of carbon monoxide is possible.

Management of a subject with carbon monoxide poisoning consists of removal from the gas and administration of oxygen. Whether this is given as 100 per cent oxygen or 93 per cent with 7 per cent carbon dioxide probably matters little, in spite of the theoretical advantages of producing increased ventilation and dissociation of carboxyhemoglobin with the carbon dioxide mixture. The essential element of therapy is prompt administration. The effect of oxygen is to speed the removal of carbon monoxide and until this occurs it has little effect on the oxygen content of the blood. In certain circumstances, however, if an appropriate hyperbaric chamber is available, removal may be achieved by increasing the oxygen dissolved in plasma at several atmospheres' pressure. This also speeds considerably the rate of dissociation of carboxyhemoglobin and is undoubtedly the most effective method of treatment. Such chambers should be available in all large works where carbon monoxide poisoning is an important hazard.

Useful information on carbon monoxide poisoning may be obtained from the proceedings of a conference on the subject at the New York Academy of Sciences.[2]

Cyanides

Cyanide may be encountered in industry as sodium or potassium cyanate or as acrylonitrile (vinyl cyanide). Exposure to the inorganic salts may occur in gold extraction, chemical and photographic laboratories, and electroplating, but cases of poisoning are relatively rare. Acrylonitrile is more important as an industrial hazard, since it is used in the production of synthetic rubber. Fumes of this substance may be inhaled or absorbed through the skin by workers loading or unloading tankers or those engaged in the industrial processes.

Cyanide acts as a poison of cellular respiration, by blocking the enzyme system cytochrome oxidase, and thus preventing the access of oxygen to the tricarboxylic acid cycle. Inorganic cyanides act by ionization in the blood, but acrylonitrile is much less ionized and has a direct toxic action also, perhaps by attacking cellular sulfhydryl groups. It has a direct neurotoxic action and may also be hepatotoxic.

Symptoms of poisoning initially consist of dizziness, nausea, and rapid breathing. Subsequently vomiting, abdominal and chest pains, irregular speech, and confusion herald the onset of loss of consciousness. Fortu-

nately, the rapid onset of symptoms, which occurs within seconds of exposure, warns the subject of the danger, and he is usually able to escape the vapor before absorbing a fatal dose.

Treatment of cyanide poisoning is based on attempts to compete with cytochrome oxidase for the cyanide ion. The body possesses an enzyme, thiosulfate transulfurase, that is capable of combining naturally occurring thiosulfate with cyanide to form relatively harmless thiocyanate. One of the principles of treatment has been to give intravenous or inhaled nitrite, which combines with hemoglobin to produce methemoglobin, followed by thiosulfate. The methemoglobin combines with cyanide to form a compound that then reacts with thiosulfate and the enzyme thiosulfate transulfurase to produce thiocyanate:

$$\text{sodium nitrite} + \text{hemoglobin} \longrightarrow \text{methemoglobin}$$

$$\text{methemoglobin} + \text{cyanide} \longrightarrow \text{cyanmethemoglobin}$$

$$\text{cyanmethemoglobin} + \text{thiosulfate} \xrightarrow{\text{thiosulfate transulfurase}} \text{thiocyanate}$$

A major drawback of this form of treatment has been the loss of oxygen-carrying power of the blood due to formation of methemoglobin. Moreover, it is not as effective in acrylonitrile poisoning as in poisoning by more fully ionized cyanide salts.

Cobalt has the ability to combine with cyanide, and this is now used in therapy. Hydroxycobalamine may be injected intramuscularly, but very large doses are required to neutralize appreciable amounts of cyanide. Moreover, cobalt ions are toxic in themselves. Chelated cobalt, dicobalt edetate, is therefore a more satisfactory therapy and it can be given in larger doses. One hundred and fifty milligrams of this substance contain sufficient cobalt to neutralize 40 per cent of an LD_{50} (50 per cent of lethal dose) of cyanide.

A patient poisoned by cyanide should therefore be removed from the area, any contaminated skin should be washed, and intramuscular hydroxycobalamine should be given by the first-aid worker. He may also be given amyl nitrite to inhale. If his condition is sufficiently severe (i.e., evidence of neurotoxicity, depression of respiration), the patient should be given 150 mg dicobalt edetate intravenously very slowly, and this may be repeated in 10 minutes. Oxygen should be given, as there is some evidence that high blood levels may speed the detoxification process, and artificial respiration and cardiac massage should be given if necessary until the antidotes work.

Obviously, great care is required in handling cyanides, and workers concerned with acrylonitrile should be protected by impermeable clothing. If there is any risk of vapor escaping, an independent air supply should be provided.

Hydrogen Sulfide

This gas is well known to schoolchildren on account of its unpleasant smell, a property which makes it useful as a means of irritating their elders with "stink bombs." It may occur in coal mines, gasworks, tanneries, and rubber works, but because its odor gives early warning poisoning is relatively rare. Accidental industrial exposure in the disposal of chemical wastes may occur,[3] and a number of fatal cases have been reported in the finishing and fishmeal industry,[4] where smells are presumably tolerated longer because of their universal occurrence. Hydrogen sulfide is also found in natural gas and constitutes a hazard in the oil and gas industry. Several fatalities have been reported in Alberta in which hydrogen sulfide, or as it is known "sour gas," has been emitted during drilling for natural gas and oil. It also accumulates occasionally in functioning oil and gas wells.

Conjunctivitis and keratitis may occur when hydrogen sulfide comes into contact with the eyes. Inhalation of the gas into the lungs may lead to pulmonary edema. Severe acute exposure causes a greenish discoloration of the face and chest. Coma and death due to central nervous system toxicity often ensue as a result of poisoning of the cytochrome oxidase system.[5] The gas binds iron, thereby inhibiting cellular respiration. Less acute exposure results in headache, dizziness, ataxia, nausea, and diarrhea. Treatment consists of removal of the victim and administration of artificial respiration if, as is usual, breathing is depressed. The time-weighted average for hydrogen sulfide is 20 ppm (30 mg/m^3), with a maximal allowable concentration of 50 ppm (75mg/m^3) for a maximum of 10 minutes.

IRRITANT GASES

Ammonia

Ammonia is an intensely irritant, highly soluble alkaline gas that is widely used in industry. Important uses include refrigeration, production of fertilizers and explosives, oil refining, and the making of plastics. Exposure to the gas occurs as a result of industrial accidents in which tanks or pipes fracture.

Since ammonia is very soluble, the brunt of its attack is borne by the skin, conjunctivae, and mucous membranes of the mouth and upper respiratory tract. On exposure to the gas, the worker feels intense pain in the eyes, mouth, and throat, and a sense of suffocation. The voice is lost and stridor develops. The patient is cyanotic, with bleeding, ulcerated mouth and nose, and aphonia. Continued exposure to high concentrations for a minute or less results in death from asphyxiation.

The pathology of the acute lesion comprises an acute inflammatory reaction, with edema, ulceration, and desquamation of mucous membranes. Edema of the larynx is the cause of death in most acute cases, supplemented by blockage of airways with desquamated epithelium. The lungs themselves may be the seat of an inflammatory reaction, with exudation of blood and edema fluid into alveoli, and this may be apparent radiographically as pulmonary edema.

Follow-up studies of survivors have shown that the initially severe airways obstruction gradually improves, though they may not recover fully for a year or more. There is little evidence that emphysema is an important complication, and it seems likely that in many cases the epithelial surface of the airways is able to regenerate almost completely.[6, 7] That is not to say that the patient does not occasionally suffer prolonged disability from his gassing, and Ziskind has reported two subjects with persistent chest symptoms following exposure to ammonia.[8] The symptoms were attributed to bronchitis and bronchiectasis. The possibility exists that with very severe exposure bronchiolitis obliterans may occur as a complication should the subject survive.

Management of the patient consists of his rapid removal from the area by rescuers wearing breathing apparatus, and administration of oxygen. Weakly acidic mouth and eye washes may give some symptomatic relief. Recovery will normally occur if the patient can be kept oxygenated for the critical 48 hours while airways obstruction is at its height. In severe cases this will require tracheostomy and, if parenchymal lung damage still prevents proper oxygenation, positive-pressure respiration with high inspired oxygen concentrations. Shock due to loss of fluid from burns may need to be treated and antibiotics should be administered. The value of steroids, bronchodilators, and digoxin is undetermined, though all tend to be used in the emergency situation.

Chlorine

Chlorine is a heavy irritating gas with a characteristic odor. It is used widely in industry in the manufacture of alkalis and bleaches and as a disinfectant. It is much less soluble than ammonia and is therefore more likely to affect the whole of the respiratory tract than to cause acute laryngeal edema. Chlorine is commonly stored and transported under pressure, and exposure occurs when tanks or pipes fracture or are damaged.

Exposure to chlorine causes choking, chest pain, and dyspnea. White or pink sputum is produced. The conjunctivae are sore and reddened. Coarse crackles and often wheezes are heard in the chest. Pulmonary edema may occur almost immediately or be delayed several hours. It is, however, a common occurrence with severe exposures and is related to

the greater degree of parenchymal damage than occurs with ammonia.[9] As a result of this, the acute illness after chlorine exposure is more prolonged, and measurements of blood and alveolar gas tensions have shown that hypoxemia with a high alveolo-arterial oxygen difference may persist for several days.[10] The radiograph typically shows the appearances of pulmonary edema (Fig. 20–1).

The pathological changes are of swelling and ulceration of the mucosa with desquamation into the bronchial lumen, and pulmonary edema with hemorrhage.

Treatment consists of removal from the gas and provision of oxygen. This may need to be given in high concentration by positive-pressure respiration in the case of severe pulmonary edema. The value of steroids is not established, but administration of antibiotics is a sensible precaution.

Most follow-up studies[11] have not shown any long-term effect on survivors, though airways obstruction would not be an unexpected sequel. Further observations over a 5-year period in the group of subjects described by Jones et al.[11] have not revealed permanent impairment of lung function.

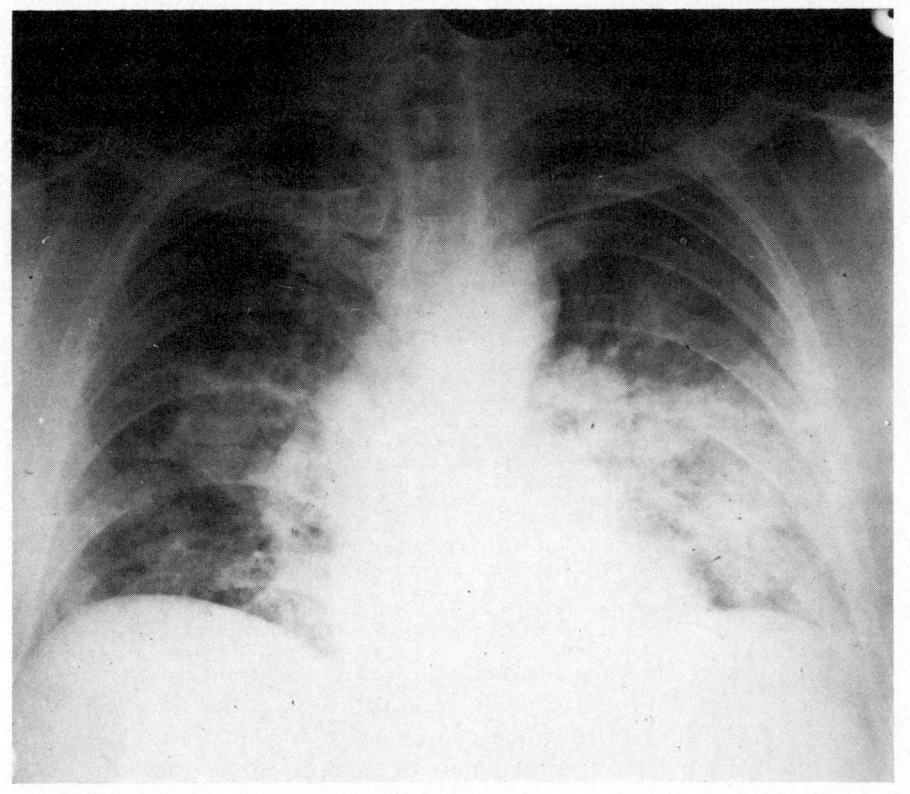

Figure 20–1. Portable chest radiograph of patient exposed to chlorine in an accident at a chemical factory, showing bilateral pulmonary edema. (Courtesy of Dr. F. X. M. Beach.)

Oxides of Nitrogen

Nitrogen forms four stable oxides. Nitrous oxide (N_2O) is an anesthetic; nitric oxide (NO) is oxidized in air to nitrogen dioxide, of which there are two forms, NO_2 and N_2O_4. These latter exist in equilibrium as a relatively insoluble, heavy, red-brown gas with an irritating odor. The oxides of nitrogen, and particularly the dangerous dioxide, may be met in several distinct situations in industry, including the handling of fresh silage, arc welding in a confined space, the combustion of nitrogen-containing material, and the production, use, and transport of nitric acid in the chemical industry.

Silo Filling. Ensilage is the agricultural process whereby green crops, particularly grass, alfalfa, and corn, are preserved in a nutritious state after cutting to be fed to livestock in the winter. The crops are packed in a tower or pit at a controlled temperature below 38°C. Oxygen is used up initially and the carbohydrates in the plant ferment, producing simple organic acids. A side reaction occurs whereby nitrates present in the silage, probably largely incorporated from soil treated with nitrogen-rich fertilizer, are oxidized to give off nitrogen dioxide. This process starts a few hours after filling of the silo, reaches a maximum in a few days, and generally ceases within a week or two. However, poisoning has been reported in a man exposed six weeks after filling.[12] Farm workers and their families are exposed to this hazard if they enter a silo in the first week after filling, and sometimes even if they approach closely. The disease was known to Ramazzini, who wrote: ". . . from grain which has been long conserved in a closed chamber, for example in underground places as is the custom of Tuscany, arises an exhalation so dangerous as to be sufficient to cause death to anyone who enters such a place to collect the grain, unless the pernicious air is first allowed to escape for a while."

Arc Welding. The very high temperature of an electric arc causes combination of oxygen and nitrogen from the atmosphere. Many other gases and fumes may be liberated and are normally dispersed by adequate ventilation. If the welder is working in a confined space, such as inside tanks, box girders, or ships' hulls, accumulation of nitrogen dioxide to toxic levels may occur.

Combustion of Nitrogen-Containing Material. The notorious example of this was an episode at the Cleveland Clinic, when accidental burning of radiographic film made of nitrocellulose resulted in over one hundred deaths among those exposed.[13] A more frequent occurrence is exposure to fumes from burning of dynamite or from shot-firing in coal and metal mines. Usually the ventilation of mines is adequate to remove the fumes rapidly, but injudicious early return to the face after firing may result in dangerous exposures. A more common cause of exposure to oxides of nitrogen underground nowadays is the exhaust fume of diesel locomotives. These fumes are a complex mixture of gases and particulates, but contain varying amounts of nitrogen dioxide (see p. 637).

Chemical Industry. The most frequent cause of nitrogen dioxide exposure occurs in the chemical industry, in the production, use, and transport of nitric acid. These exposures, as with chlorine and ammonia, usually result from rupture of containers with spillage of the nitric acid, which gives off fumes of nitrogen dioxide when it comes into contact with wood, paper, or other organic material. A risk of exposure may also occur in acid dipping of brass and copper, cleaning of aluminum and copper vats with nitric acid, handling of jet fuel, and nitration of organic compounds.

Clinical Features of Nitrogen Dioxide Inhalation

When inhalation of nitrogen dioxide occurs in the appropriate circumstances it is called silo filler's disease. The gas is not as intensely irritant as ammonia, and low concentrations may be tolerated with only mild upper respiratory tract symptoms. The worker, however, is often aware of the presence of the nitrogen dioxide from its distinctive color as well as from the cough it provokes. The immediate symptoms depend therefore on the concentration of the gas and vary from none to intense choking. Usually, however, they are sufficient to force the worker to leave the site rapidly. With sufficient dose there then follows an episode of coughing, mucoid or frothy sputum production, and increasing dyspnea. Within an hour or two the patient may be in frank pulmonary edema and cyanosed, with tachypnea, tachycardia, and fine crackles and wheezes throughout his lungs. Alternatively, the patient may simply suffer an increase in dyspnea and cough over several hours, with the symptoms then gradually improving over a two- to three-week period. At this stage, when all appears to be well, the disease may relapse rapidly. Fever and chills usher in the relapse, with increasing cyanosis, dyspnea, and generalized lung crackles.[14, 15]

Death from respiratory failure may occur either in the initial or the second stage of the disease. A severe second stage with death may occur even in the absence of a severe initial illness. If the patient survives the second stage, he gradually reverts to normal over two to three weeks. Whether long-term effects occur is not certain, though apparently almost complete recovery has occurred in most reported cases.

The radiographic features on the acute initial stage vary from normality to typical pulmonary edema (Fig. 20–2). Most reports mention a nodular component, however, even at the onset. The radiographic picture may then clear, only to show miliary mottling resembling hematogenous tuberculosis as the second stage commences (Fig. 20–3). In severe cases the mottling may become confluent in places.

Lung function tests in the acute stage show reduction in lung volumes and diffusing capacity, with a low arterial oxygen saturation. Similar findings are recorded in the second stage,[15] though generally they are more marked, and very high alveolo-arterial oxygen gradients may occur.

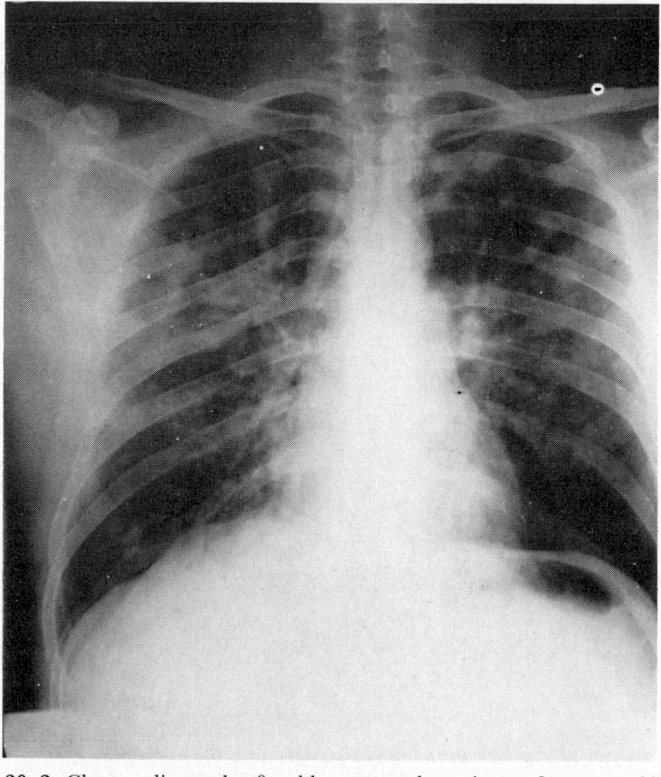

Figure 20–2. Chest radiograph of welder exposed to nitrous fumes working in a fuel tank, showing ill-defined, large nodular opacities throughout both lungs. The patient presented with signs of pulmonary edema and recovered with steroid treatment. (Courtesy of Drs. Glynne Jones and A. C. Douglas.)

Follow-up studies have shown varying results. Jones and colleagues[15] noticed an obstructive lesion with low diffusing capacity in one of their patients, with gradual improvement over two months, and Moskowitz[12] reported a slow increase in diffusing capacity in one patient over six months, whereas Becklake[16] found four of her seven patients to have developed symptoms of dyspnea associated with an obstructive pattern of lung function after recovery from the acute effects of exposure.

Pathological examination of the acute lesion shows extensive mucosal edema and inflammatory cell exudation. The alveolar capillaries are dilated, and edema fluid and blood cells fill the alveoli. The delayed lesion shows the appearance of bronchiolitis obliterans. Small bronchi and bronchioles are packed with an inflammatory exudate which organizes with fibrin, obliterating the whole lumen.[17] Serial lung biopsies in one patient[12] have shown that these lesions may resolve, leaving at six months some interstitial collagen and some associated alveolar dilatation.

In addition to a possible long-term effect following acute high-level exposures, it has been suggested that recurrent exposures to relatively low

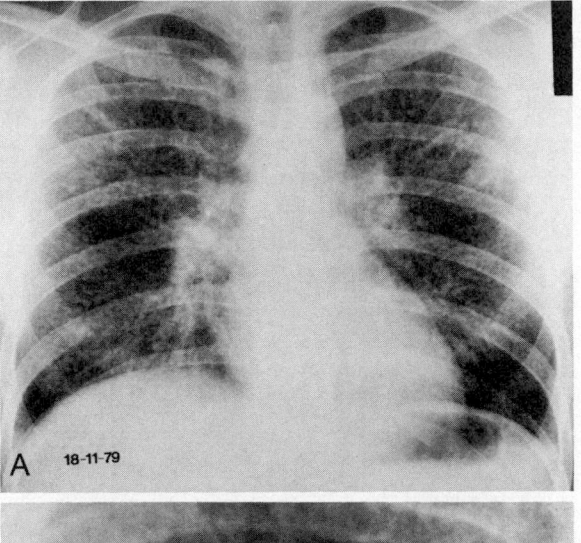

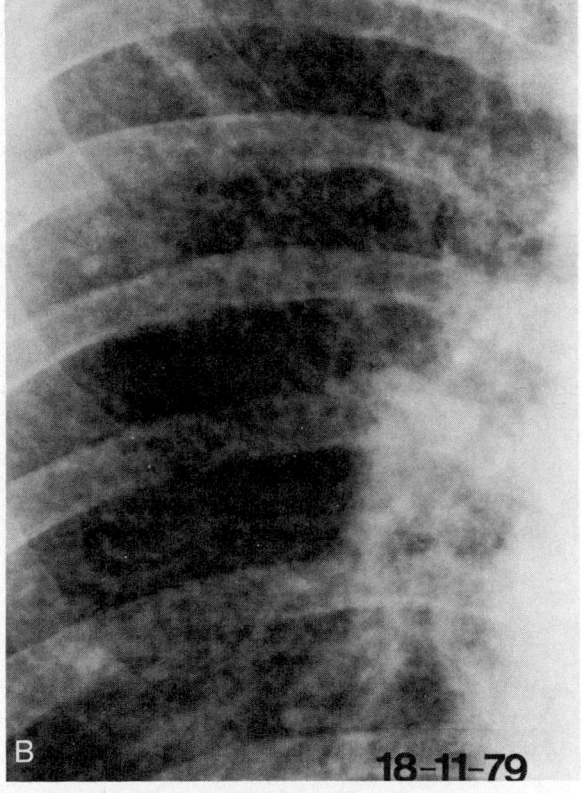

Figure 20–3. *A*, Chest radiograph of Ontario farmer 10 days after exposure to oxides of nitrogen following opening a silo. Bronchiolitis obliterans is present. The radiographic abnormalities subsequently completely cleared. (Courtesy of Dr. D. Ahmad.) *B*, Magnified view of *A*.

levels of nitrogen dioxide may cause emphysema. This followed the study by Kennedy,[18] who claimed that emphysema occurred in coal miners who had been shot-firing and had been exposed to high levels of gas. The study, however, was not controlled and took no account of factors, such as cigarette smoking and dust exposure, which could have caused the same long-term effects. Studies in animals have shown an emphysema-like lesion following prolonged exposure to nitrogen dioxide at levels above the threshold limit value (TLV),[19] and studies of children exposed to the gas from cookers and heaters at home have shown an increased prevalence of respiratory symptoms.[20] However recent studies in British coal mines have shown not only that exposures to nitrogen dioxide from shot-firing and diesel engines are relatively low, rarely exceeding the short-term limit value, but also that no excess of respiratory symptoms or of fall in FEV_1 can be found in the men with highest exposures compared to those with lowest exposures when matched for smoking habit and dust exposure.[21] It therefore seems likely that though long-term respiratory illness may occasionally follow acute high-dose exposures, intermittent low-dose exposures in fit working men carry little risk of permanent lung or airways damage.

Management

The disease can be prevented through the education of those likely to be exposed. Farm workers should be warned about approaching or entering recently filled silos, notices should be displayed on the silos, and fences should be provided to keep children away. Welders should not be allowed to work in poorly ventilated spaces. In chemical works where the risk obtains, the medical officer should educate workers to seek medical help even if the initial exposure was not very severe, in order to be alert to development of the later sequelae.

Management of the acute attack and of the later episode entails administration of oxygen, as judged by measurements of blood gases and if necessary given by respirator, and corticosteroids. Although the disease does not lend itself to the establishment of controlled trials, it is noteworthy that in most reports those subjects given steroids have improved rapidly from the time of administration, while those not so treated have often died. Antibiotics should probably be given to counter superinfection, but cardiac drugs are probably unnecessary. Bronchodilators may be helpful in the acute attack, though there are no objective studies to prove this.

Ozone

Ozone has achieved some importance recently following the demonstration of its presence in photochemical smog, in the cockpits of high-flying aircraft, especially of the supersonic type, and in the gas produced by arc welding. In the occupational setting, arc welders using inert gas–

shielded apparatus are the most likely to be affected by the gas, and their exposure is usually not complicated by the presence of other toxic substances.[22] Ozone is a respiratory irritant, which also causes headache and drowsiness. Cough, nose and eye irritation, and tightness in the chest are the main symptoms. Severe or fatal cases do not appear to have been reported, though animal studies have shown that high concentrations of gas may induce pulmonary edema. The subject has been comprehensively reviewed by Stokinger.[23] Management depends on recognition of the hazard and its removal by adequate ventilation.

Phosgene

Phosgene is a heavy, colorless gas that liquefies at 8°C. It has a faint odor of new-mown hay, but it is only slightly irritating, so it may be inhaled for prolonged periods without great discomfort. It was responsible for a high proportion of the deaths due to gassing in the First World War. It is now used as a chlorinator in the chemical industry, and it is from here that occasional cases of poisoning are reported.[24] Occasionally it may result from use of carbon tetrachloride fire extinguishers.[25]

Phosgene in poisonous doses acts directly on the pulmonary capillary. An exposed worker usually first develops a cough and after an hour or two becomes increasingly breathless. Crackles may be heard throughout the lungs, and hypovolemic shock may follow. The mechanism of death is pulmonary edema, though animal experiments suggest that very high doses may cause an ulcerative bronchitis and bronchiolitis. In survivors, the pulmonary edema gradually improves over a week, and there is no definite human evidence of long-term toxic effects.

Treatment of acute phosgene poisoning should be directed at oxygenating the patient adequately, by the use of a respirator if necessary, and maintenance of normal blood volumes. This can be achieved by measurement of central venous pressure and infusion of plasma expanders if necessary. Aminophylline may be useful on account of its ability to relax bronchial and pulmonary vascular smooth muscle, and steroids again may have a place, though the evidence for this is anecdotal.

Phosgene appears to have a reflex action on pulmonary vasculature, causing constriction by sympathetic paralysis. This results in massive transudation of fluid from the pulmonary capillaries into the lungs, and it is thought that this loss of fluid, in combination with the resultant hypoxemia, causes hypovolemic shock.[24]

Sulfur Dioxide

Sulfur dioxide is a heavy, irritating gas. It occurs chiefly as a general atmospheric pollutant, the result of combustion of coal and gasoline in

towns. Among its important effects are the causation of exacerbations of disease in patients with chronic bronchitis and the destruction of the limestone of historic buildings. However, it may also be encountered in industry in the production of paper, in refrigeration plants, in oil refining, and in fruit preserving.

It is a soluble gas, and as such the initial effect of breathing a high concentration is extreme irritation of the eyes and upper respiratory tract. This fortunately occurs instantaneously, thus allowing the subject to escape before severe damage is done. Immediate toxicity is therefore similar to that of ammonia and treatment is the same, with the exception that sodium bicarbonate solution or aerosol may be helpful in relieving local symptoms. Of more frequent occurrence than acute exposure is prolonged exposure to relatively low levels. There is some evidence that this may irritate or exacerbate chronic obstructive pulmonary disease, both in occupational and nonoccupational situations.[26, 27] However, a 10-year study of a group of paper workers in New Hampshire showed no increase in mortality from either respiratory or other diseases.[28] Neither was it possible to show that exposure to either sulfur dioxide or chlorine in the working environment had any significant effect on pulmonary function. There is a considerable body of physiological evidence that sulfur dioxide in low concentrations acts to increase airways resistance, and it is now clear that the combination of exercise and low concentrations of sulfur dioxide (0.5 ppm) may lead to an increase in airways resistance in asymptomatic asthmatics.[29]

IRRITANT AND TOXIC FUMES

Metal Fume Fever

Brass founders' ague, copper fever, brass fever, Monday morning fever, and metal fume fever are all names for a relatively common acute febrile illness. According to Hunter, it was first described by Potissier in 1822.[30] The condition results from the inhalation of minute particles of the oxides of various metals. While zinc, copper, and magnesium are the chief offenders, cadmium, iron, manganese, nickel, selenium, tin, and antimony are in some instances responsible. Metal fume fever occurs as a result of welding operations, and it is particularly common in shipbuilding yards where metal plates are being cut and then welded. The melting of copper and zinc in electric furnaces is also a frequent cause of this condition.[30, 31] Zinc smelting and galvanizing are other common causes of metal fume fever.

The condition can be reproduced in laboratory animals and in human experiments. It has been maintained that fresh fumes are necessary to produce the disease but most authorities feel that the particle size is the most important factor in the genesis of the condition. There is good

evidence to believe that the responsible particles are well below 1.5 microns in size and that most are in the range of 0.02 to 0.25 microns. Their high kinetic energy renders them particularly prone to come into contact with the alveolar walls.

The disease has an acute onset, and although there is no form of chronic metal fume fever, repeated bouts are quite common.[32, 33] It appears likely that resistance to the condition develops after a few days of exposure, but this wears off in a relatively short time, hence the term Monday morning fever. Metal fume fever may occur on the first day a new employee starts work, and there appears to be no latent period for sensitization to occur. The onset of metal fume fever in the absence of prior exposure argues compellingly against an immunological basis for the condition, and suggests that the fever and constitutional symptoms are likely to be due to chemotaxis of polymorphs, with these cells being responsible for the development of the febrile response.

The symptoms of the disease are the sudden onset of thirst and a metallic taste in the mouth. There is usually a 4- to 8-hour lag before these symptoms occur. Later the subject has rigors, high fever, muscular aches and pains, headaches, and a feeling of generalized weakness. He sweats profusely and the condition is often mistaken for influenza. Recurrent attacks have also been mistaken for malaria. The onset of the muscular pains and rigors may be delayed for 10 to 12 hours following exposure. A leukocytosis is often present. All the symptoms spontaneously subside within 24 to 36 hours.

The diagnosis of metal fume fever is entirely dependent on the history and signs. No specific tests exist for its identification. Most workers are able to recognize it, partly because it is relatively frequent and partly because they have seen their colleagues with repeated attacks, and the condition is well known to them. No treatment is known, and the usual folklore remedy of drinking milk is invariably associated with a satisfactory course and few harmful side effects.

Polymer Fume Fever

In 1951 Harris first described polymer fume fever.[34] This condition is characterized by a brief but sharp attack of chest tightness, choking, and a dry cough, and occasionally by rigors. Polymer fume fever is often known as "the shakes." The illness begins several hours after exposure to the heat-degraded polymer, polytetrafluoroethylene (PTFE), also known as Teflon or Fluon. Recovery is rapid and the condition bears a striking resemblance to metal fume fever. As in the latter condition, repeated attacks are common and do not seem to lead to permanent pulmonary damage.[35]

PTFE breaks down at a temperature of 250 to 300°C., and when it does it liberates a collection of aliphatic and cyclic fluorocarbon com-

pounds. Many are powerful irritants. Pernis and colleagues have suggested that the sublimate degranulates the leukocytes found in the lung and this liberates endogenous pyrogens.[36]

The smoking of PTFE-contaminated cigarettes is a factor common to most subjects who develop polymer fume fever. Thus, handlers of PTFE should be advised against smoking while handling the polymer.

Polyvinyl Chloride (PVC) Fumes

Polyvinyl chloride (PVC) fumes have been suggested as the cause of meat wrappers' asthma.[37] Polyvinyl chloride soft wrap is commonly used to package meat and other perishables. The wrap is dispensed as a pliable and transparent roll and is cut and sealed with a hot wire. Later a label is often attached to the meat package by placing a hot element on top of the label. The heating element has to have a temperature of around 150 to 200°C before the label adheres.

Sokol in 1973 described bronchoconstriction occurring in three meat wrappers.[37] Shortly thereafter the term meat wrappers' asthma came into existence and was used to describe the symptoms observed in a minority of meat wrappers. In 1975 Andrasch and Bardana described recurrent asthmatic attacks, prolonged cough, and other symptoms due to the inhalation of fumes which were generated during the affixing of the label to the meat package.[38] The price label adhesives which were used in this process were composed of co-polymers, elastomers, phthalic plasticizers, and sulfonamide compounds. A hypersensitivity reaction was postulated, but subsequent investigations have not confirmed that the price label adhesives are indeed the cause of the asthma.[39]

Since that time, a number of well-controlled epidemiological studies have been carried out, and these cast doubt on the specificity of so-called meat wrappers' asthma.[40, 41] Many of these studies included before and after shift measurements of ventilatory capacity and failed to detect a significant decline, or if a decline was present, it affected most subjects and was nonspecific. In some instances, meat wrappers have worked in refrigerated plants, and it has been suggested that their bronchoconstriction might have been induced by cold air, but there is little support for this suggestion.[41, 42] While there is some evidence that small airways obstruction of limited duration and severity may follow exposure to PVC fumes, this appears to be a nonspecific reaction and there is no evidence that it is in any way related to sensitization.[41, 42] Moreover, baseline values for ventilatory capacity in meat wrappers appear for the most part to be normal.[40–42] In a few subjects with known asthma, there may be an exacerbation brought on by exposure to PVC fumes, but the evidence suggests that this is nonspecific and is equally likely to be brought on by other factors such as exertion, cold, and other irritants.[39, 42] PVC fumes also lead to the development of conjunctivitis, rhinitis, and other nonspecific upper respiratory tract symptoms.

Osmium Bronchitis

Osmium is an element which is closely related to platinum and derives its name from the Greek word *osmē,* a smell. It is extremely dense and almost three times as heavy as iron. It is found as the ore osmiridium, a natural alloy of osmium and iridium. There are deposits of the ore in Russia, Canada, Colombia, Australia, and the Pacific Northwest in the United States.

The separation of osmium from the other metals with which it is found, such as platinum, is very difficult. Treatment with aqua regia is an essential part of the process. Osmium is used as a catalyst, as an alloy with iridium for the manufacture of nibs and compass needles, in photography, and as a stain for histological preparations.

While the metal itself is innocuous, osmic acid (osmium tetroxide) has very irritant effects similar to those of the halogen gases. Osmic acid is slowly formed when the metal is exposed to air. Osmium tetroxide causes intense conjunctivitis, tracheitis, and bronchitis.[43] Paroxysms of coughing and persistent lacrimation occur after exposure. Blindness following corneal damage can occur. Gastrointestinal disturbances including nausea and vomiting occur frequently following prolonged exposure.

Prevention depends on adequate ventilation and on storing osmium tetroxide in sealed containers.

Trimellitic Anhydride Pneumonitis

Relatively recently a hemorrhagic pneumonitis following exposure to epoxy resins has been described.[44, 45] The affected subjects had all been exposed to a powder containing a mixture of epoxy resin and trimellitic anhydride (TMA) in a poorly ventilated workplace. The application of heat or baking to the powder caused liberation of TMA fumes. Those affected complained of cough with repeated hemoptyses. Chest radiography sometimes showed patchy infiltrates, acinous in character and suggesting aspiration of blood. In addition, all subjects developed a hemolytic anemia. Pulmonary function testing revealed a marked hypoxemia and a reduction of the diffusing capacity, the latter being most prominent when the hemolytic anemia was severe. Earlier, before the anemia became evident, the DL_{CO} was occasionally increased owing to the soaking up of carbon monoxide by red cells sequestered in the alveoli. Pathologically there was a hemorrhagic pneumonitis with intra-alveolar hemorrhage and alveolar cell hyperplasia (Fig. 20–4). The cessation of exposure usually resulted in the rapid and striking improvement in the condition, with the recurrent hemoptyses disappearing within a few days.

TMA is used in a variety of industrial processes, including the manufacture of plasticizers, as a constituent of alkyl resins, and as a curing agent for epoxy resins. TMA is the anhydride of 1,2,4-benzene tricarbox-

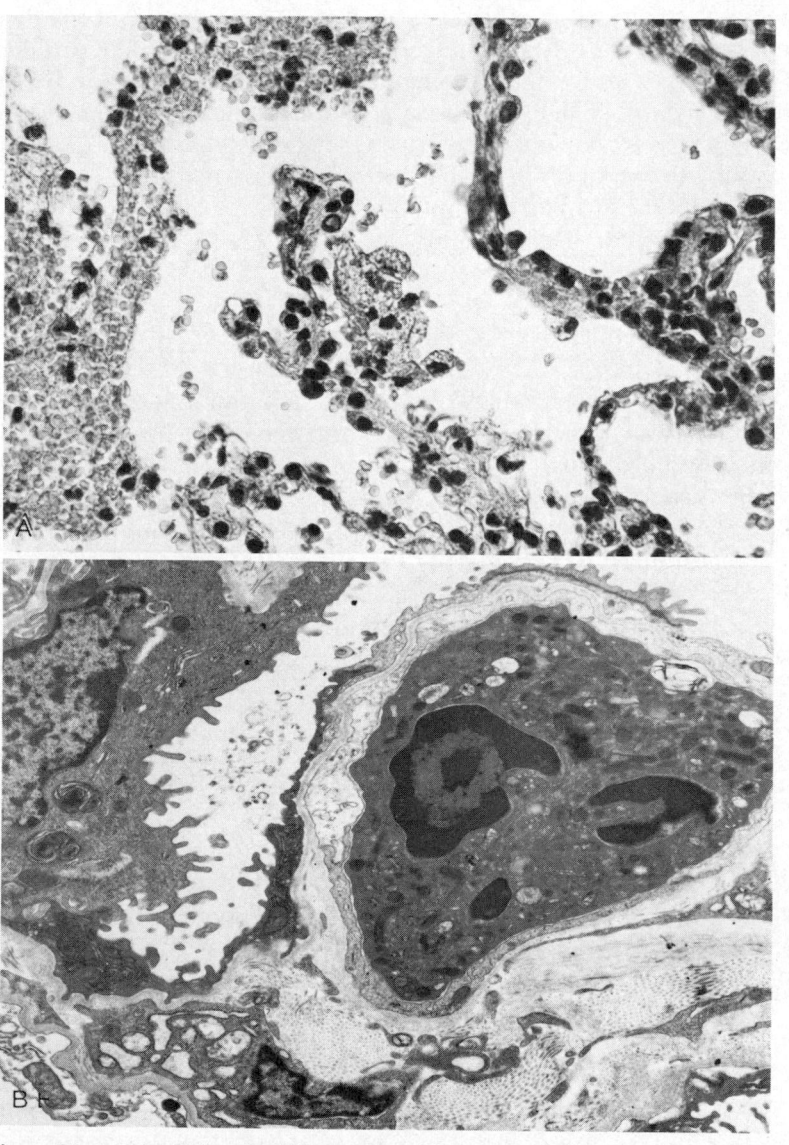

Figure 20–4. Trimellitic anhydride pneumonitis. *A,* Nonspecific alveolar wall injury with intra-alveolar hemorrhage, hemosiderin-laden macrophages, and hypertrophy of the type II pneumocytes. (Courtesy of Drs. A. Herbert and R. Orford.) *B,* Mild focal cytoplasmic edema of pulmonary endothelial cells suggesting endothelial injury.

ylic acid and leads to a variety of respiratory conditions including rhinitis; TMA flu, a late onset respiratory syndrome with systemic symptoms; asthma; and an irritative bronchitis.[46, 47] The asthma may be of the immediate type with IgE antibodies against TM protein, or of the delayed type characterized by IgG and IgA antibodies against TM protein.[48, 49] The subjects with TMA hemorrhagic pneumonitis were noted to have antibodies against TM human serum albumin and TM human erythrocytes. The levels of antibody activity resembled those of subjects with a late asthmatic response, in which systemic symptoms were present. IgE-specific antibody for TMA serum albumin was not found in the sera of subjects with hemorrhagic pneumonia.

Vanadium Bronchitis

Vanadium is a metal that is related to niobium and tantalum. It is a rare element and was discovered as a contaminant of iron ore. It occurs naturally as the ore patronite (vanadium sulfate) and also as descloizite (lead zinc vanadate). Desposits of the former are found in Peru and of the latter in South Africa. The metal is isolated by roasting patronite with coal. Vanadium is used in making certain steels, since it removes incorporated oxygen and nitrogen from the steel and it also increases its strength. Exposure to vanadium may also occur in the cleaning of boilers that have been used to heat oil, particularly from South America, that is contaminated by the metal.

Mining of the ore has not been noted to lead to harmful effects, and exposure to the metal itself is thought to be innocuous. However, vanadium pentoxide and ammonium metavanadate, both of which are used as catalysts, are definite respiratory hazards.[50, 51] The severity of the respiratory effects of vanadium compounds is related to their concentration in the ambient air.[52] Four workers from a vanadium pentoxide refinery have recently been noted to have developed asthma, a green tongue, and upper respiratory tract symptoms. They were nonatopic. In one subject the symptoms persisted for 8 weeks in the absence of further exposure.[52a] The duration of exposure is also important. Initially there is intense irritation of the eyes with excessive tear production, nasal irritation, a sore throat, coughing, and retrosternal discomfort and burning. Bronchitis and a patchy bronchopneumonia may occur. The tongue often becomes greenish. There appear to be no systemic effects from industrial exposure, but the metal is excreted in the urine and feces.

A detailed study of the effects of occupational exposure to vanadium pentoxide has been published recently.[53] Vanadium exposure increases the number of inflammatory cells in the nasal mucosa, presumably as a result of chemotaxis. Although wheezing occurs more frequently in vanadium pentoxide workers, lung function and chest radiography failed

to reveal any evidence of persistent pulmonary disease. A detailed account of all aspects of vanadium metabolism and exposure is to be found in the recent monograph.[53]

Prevention of vanadium bronchitis depends on adequate ventilation and preferably the process should be completely enclosed. This especially applies when the metal is being used as a catalyst. The wearing of masks and eye goggles is desirable in many circumstances.

Mercury Pneumonitis

Ramazzini, in his treatise *De morbis artificum diatriba,* commented on the association between lung disease and mercury exposure in the following words: "Those who make mirrors become palsied and asthmatic from handling mercury." The inhalation of mercury vapor may cause irritation of the respiratory tract with severe tracheitis, bronchitis, bronchiolitis, and pneumonitis. Mercury exposure is an uncommon industrial accident and has been described in extraction of the metal,[54] manufacture of tungsten-molybdenum wire,[55] production of thermometers,[56] and cleaning and repairing of tanks and boilers.[57, 58] It has also been described in a domestic setting, in attempts at alchemy, and in the use of mercury-containing paint on boilers.[59, 60] The common factor has been exposure to mercury vapor in an enclosed space.

The initial symptoms are tightness in the chest and breathlessness starting about an hour after exposure, followed quickly by paroxysmal cough, loss of appetite, fever, restlessness, rigors, and tremor.[58] With severe exposures the dyspnea may become extreme and death may occur. Otherwise, the symptoms last between a few hours and several days, presumably depending on the dose. With smaller repeated exposures, abdominal pain, diarrhea, and gingivitis may occur. Basal crackles may be heard in the lungs. The chest radiograph may show diffuse patchy changes of pulmonary edema, and lung function tests show a mixed restrictive and obstructive pattern, resolving quite quickly in accord with the patient's clinical improvement.[58] Though mercury may be detected in the serum and urine, initial levels may be surprisingly low, as the mercury is fixed in the tissues. Urinary excretion reaches a peak only one to three weeks after exposure.[58]

In fatal cases, a diffuse tracheobronchitis and associated acute toxic pneumonitis are found, with alveolar edema and hyaline membranes.[61] Some acute episodes may be followed by a patchy interstitial fibrosis and in infants pneumothorax and bronchiolitis have been reported as complications. Management of mercury vapor poisoning consists of administration of oxygen and corticosteroids, with general supportive measures if necessary.

Manganese Pneumonitis

Manganese is a silvery white metal that occurs naturally as pyrolusite. The latter is manganese dioxide and is a black ore found in Russia, India, Morocco, South Africa, and South America. Manganese is used as an alloy to harden steel in the manufacture of rails and mining equipment.

The effects of manganese on the nervous system have been recognized for many years, but some doubt exists as to whether the inhalation of the metal and its salts is harmful to the lungs. Following the construction of a manganese smelting plant in Norway, a tenfold increase in the mortality due to pneumonia was observed in the surrounding area by Riddervold and Halvorsen.[62] While such evidence is circumstantial, Lloyd-Davies described a high incidence of bronchitis and pneumonia in a group of men manufacturing potassium permanganate.[63] Manganese pneumonitis was slow to respond to treatment but apparently left no permanent damage. When mice were exposed to the oxides of manganese, there was a mononuclear interstitial infiltration of the lungs with necrosis and hemorrhage.[63] Further animal studies that tended to confirm the harmful pulmonary effects of manganese were later carried out by Lloyd-Davies and Harding.[64]

Cadmium Lung

Cadmium is a malleable bluish-gray metal which closely resembles zinc. The only naturally occurring cadmium ore is greenockite, but the metal is often present in small quantities in the ores of zinc, copper, and lead. The United States is by far the largest producer of cadmium. The metal is extracted mainly from zinc ores, but some is also obtained from certain lead and copper ores. Cadmium is recovered as a by-product of electrolytic zinc refining and from the fumes of lead and zinc smelting processes. The metal occurs in the form of its oxide, sulfate, or chloride, and subsequently has to be leached, electrolyzed, and precipitated before being cast into bars or anodes for electroplating.

Cadmium resists corrosion and hence is widely used for electroplating. It is also mixed with nickel and silver to form alloys, and is used in nuclear reactors and storage batteries and in the manufacture of jewelry. The ingestion of cadmium salts by mouth leads within 15 minutes to 2 hours to increased salivation, nausea, and vomiting. Later, diarrhea, tenesmus, and shock occur. However, recovery usually starts to take place within 5 to 10 hours.

Respiratory and Other Effects

The fumes of cadmium and its compounds are toxic to man. Exposure occurs mainly from the smelting of ores and from the firing and welding

of cadmium-plated metals and alloys. The recycling of metallic scrap containing cadmium is also hazardous.

Acute Exposure

Acute exposure is almost always a consequence of the inhalation of cadmium fumes or dust generated by heating or smelting. Concentrations in the ambient air of between 3 and 100 mg/m^3 have been reported.[65] The effects of acute respiratory exposure develop some 3 to 4 hours following exposure and have been well described by Beton and colleagues.[65] These authors reported on five subjects who were severely exposed while dismantling a frame of girders. The fumes were generated by melting cadmium-plated steel bolts with an oxyacetylene torch. Acute exposure is characterized initially by rhinitis, soreness of the throat, cough, a metallic taste in the mouth, and retrosternal discomfort. Later, malaise, rigors, and muscular pains develop in some subjects, along with dyspnea and hemoptysis. The symptoms are similar to those of metal fume fever. Physical signs are relatively nonspecific, but fever and tachypnea are usual. Cyanosis is common and patchy atelectasis with coarse or medium crackles is often present. The chest film shows either an appearance similar to that seen in pulmonary edema or, alternatively, vague infiltrates in the mid and lower zones.

The necropsy findings in fatal cases are limited mainly to the respiratory tract and kidneys. The trachea and bronchi are inflamed, while the lungs are heavy and filled with edema fluid. Histopathological study of the lungs shows congestion and intra-alveolar hemorrhages. The alveoli are crammed full of large cells showing a deep red cytoplasm when stained with hematoxylin and eosin. These cells are thought to be derived from the alveolar lining cells. Grossly, the kidneys are usually swollen and there is obvious cortical necrosis that is also microscopically evident. The glomerular vessels are often occluded by thrombi, and the tubules show widespread damage with the presence of proteinaceous and granular casts.

Chronic Effects of the Inhalation of Cadmium

Chronic exposure to cadmium fumes is felt by some to lead to the development of pulmonary emphysema[66, 67]; however, doubt exists as to whether this is really so. Most of the men in whom development of emphysema was reported had previously been exposed to heavy concentrations of cadmium fumes, viz., they had had a prior acute exposure, and this could account for any emphysema present. A definite answer as to the harmful effects of chronic cadmium exposure is not available, mainly because emphysema is difficult to recognize clinically and because the condition occurs in the normal population in the absence of bronchitis. The final answer must depend on appropriately controlled epidemiological studies.

Those who believe that prolonged cadmium exposure leads to emphysema feel that once the condition has developed, it may progress in the absence of further exposure. The symptoms of the cadmium emphysema are cough and gradually increasing shortness of breath. The cough is not as productive as that which usually occurs in naturally occurring bronchitis; in fact, bronchitis is reported to be unusual in cadmium emphysema.[66] Physical signs are pertinent to the presence of emphysema, namely, an overdistended and hyperresonant chest with a few scattered wheezes. Anosmia is frequent, as is nasal ulceration. There is often a yellowish band on the incisor and canine teeth; how it originates is not known, but both local and systemic mechanisms have been invoked.

Proteinuria is common and occurs in over 80 per cent of the workers who have been exposed to cadmium for 10 years or more. The protein has a molecular weight of around 20,000 to 30,000. Aminoaciduria has also been reported.[66, 68]

Pulmonary function tests may reveal airways obstruction. The annual decrement in FEV_1 and forced vital capacity is increased in exposed workers.[66] Although chronic cadmium exposure is thought to lead to emphysema, Smith and colleagues found a restrictive defect in a group of heavily exposed cadmium workers. Five of the 17 showed radiographic evidence of pulmonary fibrosis.[69]

Pathological examination of the lungs reveals the presence of marked emphysema in the absence of bronchitis.[70] Unfortunately, there is no unanimity concerning the type of emphysema—i.e., panacinar or centrilobular—that is meant to be associated with chronic cadmium poisoning, and this is one of the factors that argue against chronic exposure leading to the development of emphysema. In this regard, perhaps of significance is the report of an increased cadmium content in emphysematous lungs. The cadmium was thought to originate from the cigarettes that the subjects had smoked, although no claim was made for a cause-and-effect relationship.[71] While Snider et al. have induced centrilobular emphysema in rats by exposing them to cadmium chloride, their experiments provide evidence only that acute cadmium exposure may produce emphysema.[72] The disease model used by these workers differs greatly from naturally occurring emphysema, in that the latter condition develops insidiously over many years.

The changes found in the kidneys in chronic cadmium poisoning vary from no morphological change to severe tubular degeneration. In general, however, renal changes are minor. Much the same can also be said of the liver, despite the fact that cadmium accumulates in the liver and kidneys. Nevertheless, liver damage has been reported,[73] and anemia and bone marrow depression may also occur.[74] Finally, no specific treatment is known for either acute or chronic cadmium poisoning, and both British antilewisite (BAL) and ethylenediamine tetra-acetic acid (EDTA) are felt to be contraindicated.

Diesel Emissions

The acute and chronic effects of diesel emissions have recently been the subject of a number of investigations. Concern has been raised in regard to the carcinogenicity of diesel fumes and also as to whether they are a cause of chronic air flow obstruction. Diesel emissions contain a number of particulates and gases, including carbon monoxide, carbon dioxide, sulfur dioxide, formaldehyde, and nitrogen dioxide. In conditions of poor ventilation or if the engine is working inefficiently, levels may exceed the relevant standards. Moreover, sometimes locomotive exhaust fumes may be directed into cabin ventilation intakes, causing locally high concentrations.

A recent study of the acute effects of diesel fumes in coal miners showed no significant shift decrease in either the FEV_1 or the FEF_{50}.[75] Smokers in both the controlled and exposed groups showed a decline in ventilatory capacity over the shift, presumably an effect of exposure to coal dust. Similarly, Battigelli was unable to show any significant effect on a group of railway workers exposed to short-term diesel exhaust.[76] A well-conducted study in Swedish iron ore workers showed no effect on lung function from continued exposure to diesel emissions; however, bronchitis was found more frequently in the underground diesel workers.[77] Cigarette smoking had a far greater effect in producing symptoms of bronchitis.

In spite of the generally reassuring findings in studies of chronic exposure, complaints of acute respiratory effects should always be taken seriously, as different engines and different working conditions result in different concentrations of gases. The authors have recently investigated episodes in which the exhaust fumes containing high levels of aldehydes, and causing intense eye and respiratory irritation, were being directed into vehicle cabs. Proper occupational hygiene investigation of such complaints is essential.

OTHER NOXIOUS AGENTS

A variety of other agents may cause an acute rhinitis, tracheitis, and bronchitis when inhaled. Worth special mention as occupational hazards are the hexavalent chromium compounds. These lead to nasal ulceration and perforation, but when inhaled in high concentration may induce a severe tracheobronchitis and pneumonia. The pulmonary effects are usually short-lived, but secondary infection can occur.[78]

Hydrofluoric acid can also induce a severe tracheobronchitis when inhaled. This agent is used as a catalyst, in etching, and in the refining of metals. Zinc chloride, used in the manufacture of dry cells and in galvanizing iron, may have similar effects. Chemical bronchitis and pneu-

monitis should be treated symptomatically. Oxygen is occasionally necessary, and antibiotics often help to prevent secondary infection.

Paraquat

A note should be made of paraquat as an occupational hazard. This highly effective herbicide is used throughout the world in agriculture. It becomes inactive on contact with soil, being adsorbed by clays, and this property is made use of in the management of poisoning by administering Fuller's earth. Until recently all reports of poisoning were of accidental or suicidal ingestion of the liquid, but several cases have been reported of lung damage in agricultural workers spraying paraquat.[79, 80] It is almost certain that the poison is absorbed through the skin rather than through the lungs as an aerosol, and paraquat therefore constitutes a unique occupational lung hazard. However, there is one report of apparent absorption by aerosol.[81]

The clinical effects of acute oral ingestion are well known, with the lung involved by a progressive fibrosis in fatal cases, although individuals may survive smaller doses with few or no permanent lung sequelae.[82] Cutaneous absorption from leaking cylinders or from heavy contamination by spray results in skin inflammation and, some days later, pulmonary infiltration, breathlessness, and death from what appears to be pulmonary edema. Smaller doses may be associated with no obvious evidence of disease other than a reduced diffusing capacity, but in such patients biopsies have shown obliterative changes in small pulmonary arteries and interstitial fibrosis.[80] Similar pathological changes have been produced in rats by painting their skins with paraquat.[80]

Prevention of this disease depends upon knowledge of the dangers and the use of protective clothing and boots as well as respirators. Treatment in the event of cutaneous absorption is supportive, including the use of corticosteroids.

Formaldehyde

Formaldehyde, a colorless inflammable gas that is slightly heavier than air, has many industrial uses. It is incorporated into resins such as urea formaldehyde and phenyl formaldehyde, both of which are used in the manufacture of textiles, paper, rubber, adhesives, and cosmetics and as foams for cavity wall insulation; urea formaldehyde foam has been extensively used as an insulating material in North America. Formaldehyde is also a constituent of cigarette smoke, is present in fumes from the internal combustion engine, and is encountered in high concentrations in poorly ventilated, crowded areas where large numbers of persons are smoking, such as bars and discotheques. Formalin, an aqueous solution of

between 40 to 50 per cent formaldehyde mixed with 10 to 15 per cent methyl alcohol, is frequently used in anatomy and pathology laboratories, and by morticians.

The smell of formaldehyde is clearly recognizable. Its irritant effects have been known about for many years.[83] Exposure to 3 to 5 parts per million (ppm), especially in previously unexposed persons, leads to tearing, nasal irritation, sneezing, soreness of the throat, constriction of the chest, and often headache. Continued exposure to such levels is usually followed by some attenuation of the effects and by decreased sensitivity, so that the symptoms become far less troublesome. Dermatitis is also quite common.

There is some evidence that formaldehyde may cause occupational asthma, but the evidence is far from convincing.[84] Animal experiments have shown that formalin in exceptionally high doses may induce nasal cancer; however, there is no evidence to indicate that it is a carcinogen in man.[85] Similarly, there is little or no indication to suggest that urea formaldehyde is a hazard when used as an insulating material.

The present TWA is 3 ppm, although the National Institute of Occupational Safety and Health (NIOSH), with characteristic but unjustified fervor, has endorsed a ceiling of 1 ppm for exposure for 30 minutes, a level that is exceeded in many poorly ventilated bars and discotheques.[86] Levels of formaldehyde up to 3 to 4 ppm are frequently encountered in dissecting rooms and anatomy and pathology laboratories.

References

1. Spencer, T. P., and Lawther, P. J., Mine gases. In Rogan, J. M., ed., Medicine in the Mining Industries. London, Heinemann, 1972.
2. New York Academy of Sciences, Conference on the Biological Effects of Carbon Monoxide. Ann. N.Y. Acad. Sci., *174*, 1, 1970.
3. Simson, R. E., and Simpson, G. R., Fatal hydrogen sulphide poisoning in association with industrial waste exposure. Med. J. Aust., *1*, 331, 1971.
4. Dalgaard, J. B., Decker, F., Fallentin, B., et al., Fatal poisoning and other health hazards connected with industrial fishing. Br. J. Ind. Med., *29*, 307, 1972.
5. Milby, T. H., Hydrogen sulphide intoxication. J. Occup. Med., *4*, 431, 1962.
6. Levy, D. M., Divertie, M. B., Litzow, T. J., and Henderson, J. W., Ammonia burns of the face and respiratory tract. J.A.M.A., *190*, 873, 1964.
7. Walton, M., Industrial ammonia gassing. Br. J. Ind. Med., *30*, 78, 1973.
8. Ziskind, M., Ellithorpe, B. D., and Wiles, H., The relationship of lung disease to air pollutants and noxious gases. In Baum, J. L., ed., Textbook of Pulmonary Disease. Boston, Little Brown and Co., 1974.
9. Joyner, R. E., and Durel, E. G., Accidental liquid chlorine spill in a rural community. J. Occup. Med., *4*, 152, 1962.
10. Beach, F. X. M., Jones, E. S., and Scarrow, G. D., Respiratory effects of chlorine gas. Br. J. Ind. Med., *26*, 231, 1969.
11. Jones, R. N., Hughes, J., Glindmeyer, H., et al., Longitudinal changes in pulmonary function following single exposure to chlorine gas. Am. Rev. Respir. Dis., *123* (Suppl), 125, 1981.
12. Moskowitz, R. L., Lyons, H. A., and Cottle, H. R., Silo filler's disease, clinical, physiologic and pathologic study of a patient. Am. J. Med., *36*, 457, 1964.
13. Nichols, B. H., The clinical effects of the inhalation of nitrogen dioxide. Am. J. Roent., *23*, 516, 1930.

14. Lowry, T., and Schuman, L. M., "Silo filler's disease"—a syndrome caused by nitrogen dioxide. J.A.M.A., *162*, 153, 1956.
15. Jones, G. R., Proudfoot, A. T., and Hall, J. I., Pulmonary effects of acute exposure to nitrous fumes. Thorax, *28*:61, 1973.
16. Becklake, M. R., Goldman, H. I., Bosman, A. R., and Freed, C. C., The long-term effects of exposure to nitrous fumes. Am. Rev. Tuberc., *76*, 398, 1957.
17. McAdams, A. J., Bronchiolitis obliterans. Am. J. Med., *19*, 314, 1955.
18. Kennedy, M. C. S., Nitrous fumes and coalminers with emphysema. Ann. Occup. Hyg., *15*, 285, 1972.
19. Dawson, S. V., and Schenker, M. B., Health effects of ambient concentrations of nitrogen dioxide. Am. Rev. Respir. Dis., *120*, 281, 1979.
20. Melia, R. J. W., Florey, C. du V., Altman, D. G., and Swan, A. V., Association between gas cooking and respiratory disease in children. Br. Med. J., *2*, 149, 1977.
21. Robertson, A., Dodgson, J., Collings, P., and Seaton, A., Exposure to oxides of nitrogen: respiratory symptoms and lung function in British coalminers. Br. J. Ind. Med. In press.
22. Challen, P. J. R., Hickish, D. E., and Bedford, J., An investigation of some health hazards in an inert-gas tungsten-arc welding shop. Br. J. Ind. Med., *15*, 276, 1958.
23. Stokinger, H. E., Ozone toxicity. A review of research and industrial experience: 1954–1964. Arch. Environ. Health, *10*, 719, 1965.
24. Everett, E. D., and Overholt, E. L., Phosgene poisoning. J.A.M.A., *205*, 103, 1968.
25. Seidelin, R., Inhalation of phosgene in a fire-extinguisher accident. Thorax, *16*, 91, 1961.
26. Skalpe, I. O., Long-term effects of sulphur dioxide exposure in pulp mills. Br. J. Ind. Med., *21*, 69, 1964.
27. Higgins, I. T. T., Effects of sulfur oxides and particulates on health. Arch. Environ. Health, *22*, 584, 1971.
28. Ferris, B. G., Puleo, S., and Chen, H. Y., Mortality and morbidity in a pulp and paper mill in the United States: a ten-year follow-up. Br. J. Ind. Med., *36*, 127, 1979.
29. Sheppard, D., Saisho, A., Nadel, J. A., and Boushey, H. A., Exercise increases sulfur dioxide induced bronchoconstriction in asthmatic subjects. Am. Rev. Respir. Dis., *123*, 486, 1981.
30. Hunter, D., Diseases of the Occupations, 6th ed. London, English Universities Press, 1978, p. 405.
31. Hamilton, A., and Johnstone, R. T., Industrial Toxicology. New York, Oxford Loose Leaf Medicine, 1945, p. 164.
32. Doig, A. T., and Challen, P. J. R., Respiratory hazards in welding. Ann. Occup. Hyg., *7*, 223, 1964.
33. Schiotz, E. H., Welding from the medical point of view. Acta Med. Scand., *121*, 557, 1945.
34. Harris, D. K., Polymer-fume fever. Lancet, *2*, 1008, 1951.
35. Williams, N., and Smith, F. K., Polymer-fume fever: an elusive diagnosis. J.A.M.A., *219*:1587, 1972.
36. Pernis, B., Cavagna, G., and Finulli, M., Phagocytosis in vitro of particles with pyrogenic action. Med. Lavoro, *52*, 649, 1961.
37. Sokol, W. N., Aelong, Y., and Beall, G. N., Meat wrappers' asthma—a new syndrome. J.A.M.A., *226*, 639, 1973.
38. Andrasch, R., and Bardama, E. J., Thermoactivated price label fume intolerance: a cause of meat wrappers' asthma. J.A.M.A., *235*, 937, 1976.
39. Vanderwort, R., and Brooks, S. M., Polyvinyl chloride film thermal decomposition procedures as in occupational illness. I. Environmental exposures and toxicology. II. Clinical studies. Occup. Med. *19*, 188 and 192, 1977.
40. Polakoff, P. L., Lapp, N. L., and Reger, R., Polyvinyl chloride pyrolysis products. Arch. Environ. Health, *30*, 269, 1975.
41. Jones, R. N., and Weill, H., Respiratory health and polyvinyl chloride fumes. J.A.M.A., *237*, 1826, 1977.
42. Krumpe, P. E., Finley, T. N., and Martinez, N., The search for respiratory obstruction in meat wrappers: studies on the job. Am. Rev. Respir. Dis., *119*, 611, 1979.
43. McLaughlin, A. I. G., Milton, R., and Perry, K. M. A., Toxic manifestations of osmium tetroxide. Br. J. Ind. Med., *3*, 183, 1946.

44. Ahmad, D., Morgan, W. K. C., Patterson, R., et al., Pulmonary haemorrhage and haemolytic anaemia due to trimellitic anhydride. Lancet, 2, 328, 1979.
45. Herbert, F. A., and Orford, R., Pulmonary hemorrhage and edema due to inhalation of resins containing trimellitic anhydride. Chest, 76, 546, 1979.
46. Zeiss, C. R., Patterson, R., Pruzansky, J. H., et al., Trimellitic anhydride induced airways syndromes: clinical and immunologic studies. J. Allergy Clin. Immunol., 60, 96, 1977.
47. Fawcett, I. W., Newman-Taylor, A. J., and Pepys, J., Asthma due to inhaled chemical agents. Clin. Allergy, 7, 1, 1977.
48. Patterson, R., Zeiss, C., Roberts, M., et al., Human anti-hapten antibodies in trimellitic anhydride inhalation reactions. J. Clin. Invest., 62, 971, 1978.
49. Patterson, R., Addington, W., Banner, A. S., et al., Antihapten antibodies in workers exposed to trimellitic anhydride fumes. Am. Rev. Respir. Dis., 120, 1259, 1979.
50. Symanski, H., Gewerbliche Vanadinschadigungen ihre Enstelung und Symptomatologie. Arch. Gewerbepath., 9, 295, 1939.
51. Williams, N., Vanadium poisoning from cleaning oil fired boilers. Br. J. Ind. Med., 9, 50, 1952.
52. Zenz, C., and Berg, B. A., Human responses to continued vanadium pentoxide exposure. Arch. Environ. Health, 14, 709, 1967.
52a. Musk, A. W., and Tees, J. G., Asthma caused by occupational exposure to vanadium compounds. Med. J. Aust., 1, 183, 1982.
53. Kiviluoto, M., Clinical study of occupational exposure to vanadium pentoxide dust. Act. Universitatis Oulensis Series D, Medica No. 72, Medica Publica No. 2. Finland, 1981.
54. Warren, V. A., Toxicology of mercury. Vet. Bureau Med. Bull., 6, 39, 1930.
55. Lewis, L., Mercury poisoning in tungsten-molybdenum wire and rod manufacturing industry. J.A.M.A., 129, 123, 1945.
56. Vroom, F. G., and Greer, M., Mercury vapour intoxication. Brain, 95, 305, 1972.
57. Milne, J., Christophers, A., and De Silva, P., Acute mercurial pneumoconitis. Br. J. Ind. Med., 27, 334, 1970.
58. Seaton, A., and Bishop, C. M., Acute mercury pneumonitis. Br. J. Ind. Med., 35, 258, 1978.
59. Hallee, T. J., Diffuse lung disease caused by inhalation of mercury vapor. Am. Rev. Respir. Dis., 99, 430, 1969.
60. Natleson, E. A., Blumenthal, B. J., and Fred, H. L., Acute mercury vapour poisoning in the home. Chest, 59, 667, 1971.
61. Matthes, F. T., Kirschner, R., Yow, M. D., and Brennan, J. C., Acute poisoning associated with inhalation of mercury vapour. Pediatrics, 22, 675, 1958.
62. Riddervold, J., and Halvorsen, K., Bacteriological investigations on pneumonia and pneumococcus carriers in Sauda, an isolated industrial community in Norway. Acta Pathol. Microbiol. Scand., 20, 272, 1943.
63. Lloyd-Davies, T. A., and Harding, H. E., Manganese pneumonitis, Br. J. Ind. Med., 3, 111, 1946.
64. Lloyd-Davies, T. A., and Harding, H. E., Manganese pneumonitis, further clinical and experimental observations. Br. J. Ind. Med., 6, 82, 1949.
65. Beton, D. C., Andrews, G. S., Davies, H. J., et al., Acute cadmium fume poisoning—five cases with one death from renal necrosis. Br. J. Ind. Med., 23, 292, 1966.
66. Bonnell, J. A., Kazantzis, G., and King, E., A follow-up study of men exposed to cadmium oxide fumes. Br. J. Ind. Med., 16, 135, 1959.
67. Lane, R. E., and Campbell, A. C. D., Fatal emphysema in two men making a copper cadmium alloy. Br. J. Ind. Med., 2, 118, 1956.
68. Clarkson, R. W., and Kench, J. E., Urinary excretion of amino acids by men absorbing heavy metals. Biochem. J., 62, 361, 1956.
69. Smith, T. J., Petty, T. L., Ridding, J. C., et al., Pulmonary effects of chronic exposure to airborne cadmium. Am. Rev. Respir. Dis., 114, 161, 1976.
70. Smith, J. P., Smith, J. C., and McCall, A. J., Chronic poisoning from cadmium fume. J. Pathol. Bact., 80, 287, 1960.
71. Hirst, R. N., Jr., Perry, H. M., Jr., Criz, M. G., and Pierce, J. A., Elevated cadmium concentration in emphysematous lungs. Am. Rev. Respir. Dis., 108, 30, 1973.
72. Snider, G. L., Hayes, J. A., Korthy, A. L., and Davis, G. P., Centrilobular emphysema

experimentally induced by cadmium chloride aerosol. Am. Rev. Respir. Dis., *108*, 40, 1973.

73. Friberg, L., Chronic cadmium poisoning. Arch. Ind. Hyg., *20*, 401, 1959.
74. Berlin, M., and Friberg, L., Bone-marrow activity and erythrocyte destruction in chronic cadmium poisoning. Arch. Environ. Health, *1*, 478, 1960.
75. Ames, R. G., Attfield, M. D., Hankinson, J. L., et al., Acute respiratory effects of exposure to diesel emission in coal miners. Am. Rev. Respir. Dis., *125*, 39, 1982.
76. Battigelli, M. C., Effects of diesel exhaust. Arch. Environ. Health, *10*, 165, 1965.
77. Jorgensen, H., and Svenson, A., Studies of pulmonary function in respiratory tract syndromes of workers in an iron ore mine where diesel trucks are used underground. J. Occup. Med., *12*, 348, 1970.
78. Bidstrup, P. L., Other industrial dusts. *In* Muir, D. C. F., ed., Clinical Aspects of Inhaled Particles. London, Wm. Heinemann, 1972, p. 162.
79. Jaros, F., Acute percutaneous paraquat poisoning. Lancet, *1*, 275, 1978.
80. Levin, P. J., Klatt, L. J., Rose, A. G., and Fergusson, A. D., Pulmonary effects of contact exposure to paraquat: a clinical and experimental study. Thorax, *34*, 150, 1979.
81. George, M., and Hedworth-Whitty, R. B., Non-fatal lung disease due to inhalation of nebulized paraquat. Br. Med. J., *280*, 902, 1980.
82. Fitzgerald, G. R., Barnville, G., Gibney, R. T. N., and Fitzgerald, M. X., Clinical, radiological and pulmonary functional assessment in thirteen long-term survivors of paraquat poisoning. Thorax, *34*, 414, 1979.
83. Health hazards in formaldehyde (Annotation). Lancet, *1*, 926, 1981.
84. Hendrick, D. J., Rando, R. J., Lane, D. J. et al., Formaldehyde asthma. J. Occup. Med., *24*, 893, 1982.
85. Albert, R. E., Sella Kumar, A. R., and Larkin, S., Nasal cancer in the rat induced by gaseous formaldehyde and hydrogen chloride. J. Natl. Cancer Inst., *68*, 597, 1982.
86. NIOSH criteria for a recommended standard for occupational exposure to formaldehyde. DHEW Publication 77–126. Washington, D.C., Government Printing Office, Dec. 1976.

21

INFECTIOUS DISEASES

Anthony Seaton

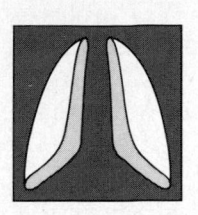

In general, infection is not an important cause of occupational disease, but there are certain occupations in which the chances of catching such a disease are increased, and in some cases these occupations may be recognized for compensation purposes. Physicians, nurses, and veterinary surgeons, medical and bacteriological laboratory workers, and farmers are groups whose contact with the infectious agent or its host may cause disease. In such cases the connection between occupation and infection is often clear, and preventive measures may normally be taken to avoid the disease.[1]

Infectious disease may also become an occupational hazard if the occupation in some way predisposes the worker to the disease, by means of selection, overcrowding, or unhygienic conditions or by the initiation of another disease that itself predisposes to infection. Illustrations of these mechanisms are the increase in morbidity due to tuberculosis that occurred in Britain at the onset of the industrial revolution and the increased susceptibility of silicotics to that disease.

Of all the infectious diseases associated with occupation, relatively few can be called strictly pulmonary, though some others may at certain stages affect the lung. This chapter is a brief review of such diseases.

TUBERCULOSIS

Tuberculosis may occur in three occupational situations. It is a true occupational hazard of physicians and nurses involved in the care of tuberculous patients and of laboratory workers concerned with the identification of the organisms. All such people should be protected by BCG inoculation if previously tuberculin-negative and should have annual chest radiographs. The risk of contracting infection with a resistant mycobacterium is also somewhat greater among medical personnel, as they have more frequent contact with such organisms. Nevertheless, treatment is

along standard lines, starting with triple therapy until the sensitivities are known. It is most unwise to bend the normal rules of therapy if one is treating a professional colleague.

A second group of workers who seem to contract tuberculosis more frequently than normal are those who work in bars (Fig. 21–1). Alcoholics are particularly susceptible to the disease; and it is probable that they play an important part in spread of the disease in public bars. The presence of crowds with a marked tendency to smoke and cough also probably plays a part. Overcrowding, be it domestic or industrial, is an important factor in the spread of tuberculosis and was probably the reason why the disease was so prevalent among the makers of boots and shoes in Britain in the 1940s.[2]

The third and numerically most important group of occupations in which there is an increased risk of tuberculosis is that in which silicosis occurs. These diseases occurred together so frequently that until the middle of the nineteenth century, when the pathological picture of

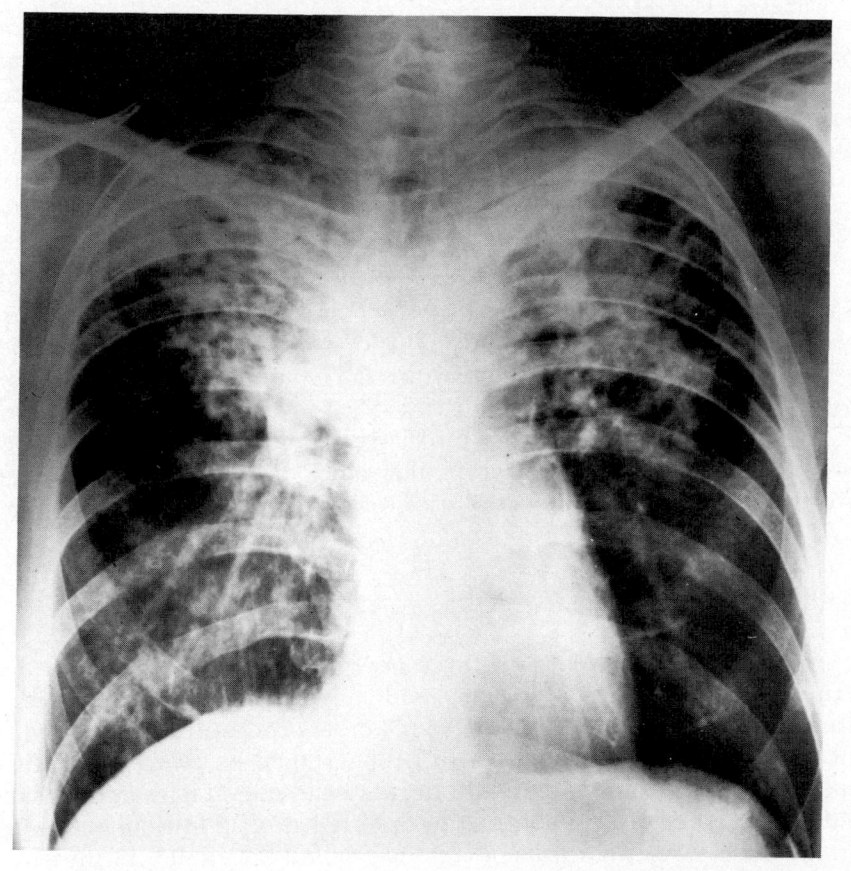

Figure 21–1. Bilateral upper lobe tuberculosis in 45-year-old bartender.

uncomplicated silicosis began to be outlined, a distinction between the diseases was not often made. Aside from any effect the dusty occupations may have had in causing overcrowding, poor living conditions, and so on, silica also acts by potentiating the effect of mycobacterial infection.[3] Even though increasing control of dust in these industries has reduced the prevalence of tuberculosis, the disease remains a not uncommon complication. The survey of United States metal miners in 1958 to 1961[4] showed radiographic signs of old or active tuberculosis in 5.3 per cent of silicotics as opposed to 0.6 per cent of nonsilicotics, while in the same period British slate workers were shown to have an 0.53 per cent prevalence of bacteriologically active disease.[5] British coal miners, by contrast, were shown to have a lower prevalence of the disease, around 0.14 per cent, although in the 1960s Enterline showed a raised mortality rate from tuberculosis among United States coal miners. More recent studies of slate miners in Britain,[7] metal miners in Sweden,[8] and sandblasters in the United States[9] have confirmed that the increased risk still exists among workers exposed to quartz, even in the era of chemotherapy.

The mechanism of the increased risk of tuberculosis in silicotics is probably related to the damaging effect of quartz on macrophages. Certainly, in vitro sublethal doses of quartz have been shown to allow mycobacteria to grow more rapidly in macrophage cultures.[3] In most cases, the disease process appears to be due to reactivation of an old primary infection rather than to new infection, and in developed countries it is expected that anti-tuberculosis campaigns will soon have nearly eradicated the risk.

Diagnosis of tuberculosis in patients with silicosis may be difficult because of pre-existing radiological changes. However, the disease should be suspected in the presence of systemic symptoms (although these may be a feature of accelerated or acute silicosis) and when rapid radiological change occurs. Features to look for are the rapid appearance of new infiltrates, the development of fluffy consolidation or pleural effusion, and cavitation. However, the mainstay of diagnosis is demonstration of the bacilli in sputum.

Treatment of tuberculosis in the presence of pneumoconiosis presents no special problems unless the pneumoconiosis is itself far advanced. The disease appears to respond as well, or almost as well, as uncomplicated tuberculosis to standard chemotherapy.[10–12] Nowadays, the combination of rifampicin with isoniazid and ethambutol for two months followed by seven months of rifampicin and isoniazid is the treatment of choice, though six-month regimens including rifampicin, pyrazinamide, isoniazid, and ethambutol are likely to prove equally effective.[13] Prevention of tuberculosis in silicotics is another matter, there being no consensus. Probably BCG vaccination in tuberculin-negative silicotics is to be avoided because of a risk of enhancing the silicotic process.[14] Moreover, in most developed countries the risk of infection of tuberculin-negative subjects is now very low. A sensible policy would be to treat tuberculin converters

with at least two drugs; many chest physicians, including the author, would use standard triple chemotherapy in these circumstances.

The possible role played by the tubercle bacillus is the etiology of massive fibrosis is discussed in Chapter 14. Most now take the view that this role is no longer important, though there is no doubt that silicosis may be accelerated by superimposed tuberculosis. In the past, treatment of massive fibrosis with antituberculous drugs has been shown to have no effect on the condition,[15] nor has there been any difference in tuberculin skin sensitivity between subjects with and without massive fibrosis.[16]

OPPORTUNIST MYCOBACTERIAL INFECTIONS

With the decline in tuberculosis, there appears to be a slow but real increase in the number of patients suffering from disease caused by opportunist or atypical mycobacteria.[17] The evidence for this comes mainly from Europe, where it has also been recorded that a high proportion of these patients work in dusty occupations (Fig. 21–2). In one study of 89 subjects with infection with *Mycobacterium avium-intracellulare*, almost half worked in coal mining or other dusty trades[18] and the same has been found true of subjects with *M. kansasii* infection.[19] A recent British study has shown that of individuals infected with *M. kanasasii*, a significantly higher proportion was working in dusty trades at the time of diagnosis than in nondusty trades,[20] while in a complimentary study comparing

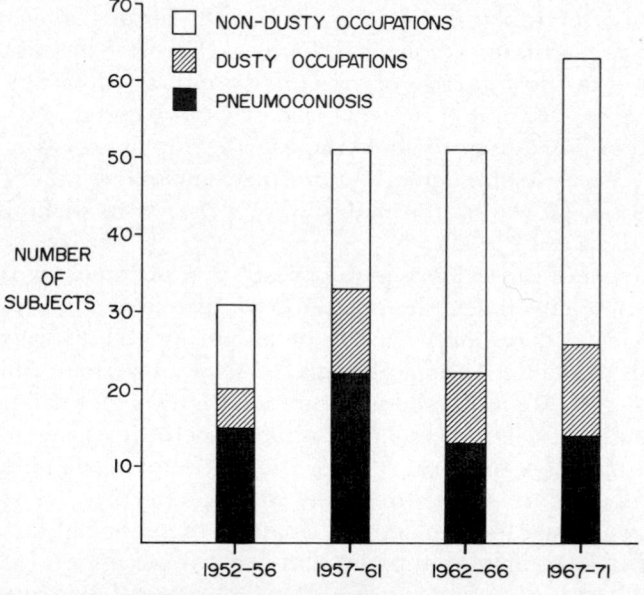

Figure 21–2. Number of patients with pulmonary disease from whom *Mycobacterium kansasii*, *M. avium*, and *M. intracellulare* were isolated. Wales 1952–71. (Data from Dr. J. Marks. Tuberculosis Reference Laboratory, Cardiff, Wales.)

patients with *M. kansasii* infection and controls with tuberculosis, the former had a higher frequency of dusty work.[21] It is not clear whether this means that the risk of infection is higher in certain trades or whether the dust load on the lungs impairs their defenses against these organisms.

Further evidence of the importance of opportunist mycobacteria in relation to dust exposure comes from studies of shotblasters in Louisiana and foundry workers in Wisconsin. Thirty-seven per cent of mycobacterial infections in the latter were reported to be due to opportunist organisms, mostly *M. avium-intracellulare,*[22] while in Louisiana (where *M. kansasii* is normally the pathogen in around 13 per cent of patients with mycobacterial disease[23]), 41 per cent of silicotic sandblasters with these diseases had *M. kansasii* infection.[9] There are clearly very striking geographical differences in the prevalence of these organisms, and much work still needs to be done on their epidemiology and mode of transmission.

The clinical picture of infection with these organisms mimics that of tuberculosis (Fig. 21–3). Treatment of *M. kansasii* infection should be with

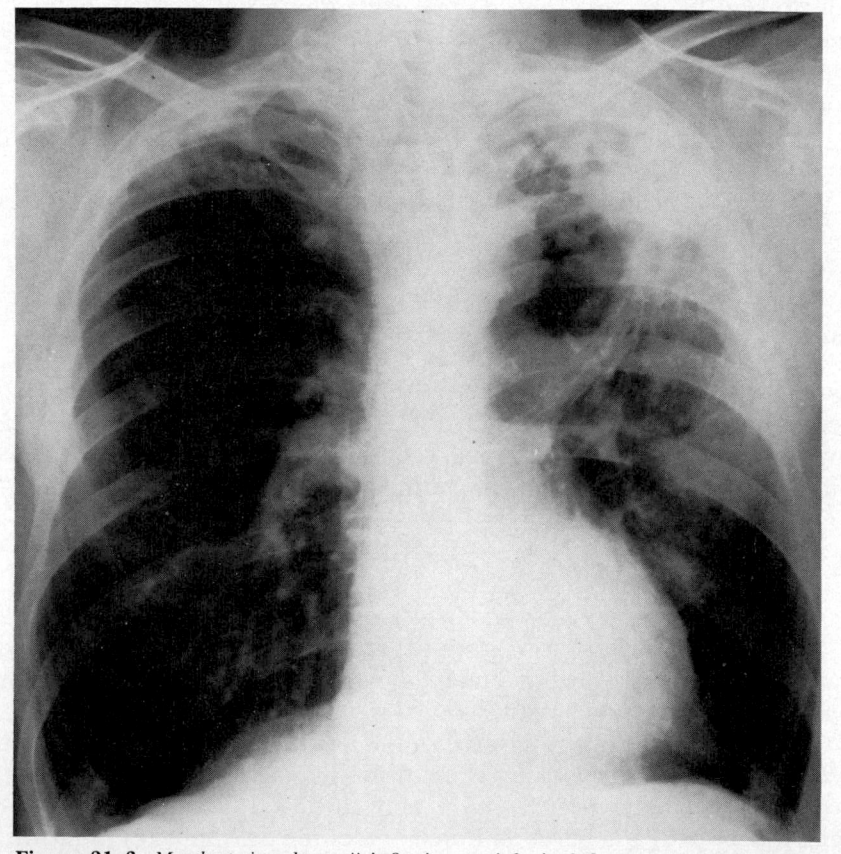

Figure 21–3. *Mycobacterium kansasii* infection mainly in left upper lobe of a chronic bronchitic who had a 30-year history of exposure to dolomite dust in a quarry crushing plant.

rifampicin, ethambutol, and another drug to which it is sensitive. It is usually resistant to streptomycin and isoniazid, but it responds well to treatment with appropriate drugs. *M. avium-intracellulare* is resistant to most drugs *in vitro* but nevertheless sometimes responds satisfactorily to standard three- or four-drug regimens.[24] In patients in whom the disease pursues a downhill course, surgical treatment may sometimes be necessary.

While these organisms do not normally spread directly to contacts of the patient, there is some anecdotal evidence of spread between pneumoconiotics. In this situation, therefore, contact tracing and radiography should be carried out as for tuberculosis.

Q FEVER

Q fever is an acute febrile illness transmitted by the microorganism *Coxiella burnetii*. The Q stands for "query," since when the disease was first described the organism isolated from the infected abattoir workers had not previously been recognized. The organism causes no clinical illness in animals, but is excreted in their milk and products of parturition. Man may be infected by ingestion or inhalation, and the disease affects predominantly farmers, veterinarians, and slaughterhouse workers.

The usual clinical picture is of a disease with a sudden, influenza-like onset, a fever of 38° to 40°C., and muscular aches. In half the patients a cough develops, and not uncommonly areas of consolidation may be seen on the chest radiograph. This consolidation may take up to a month to clear and occasionally is associated with a pleural effusion. Rarely the disease may be complicated by aseptic meningitis, jaundice, or bacterial endocarditis.[25]

The differential diagnosis is between influenza and other such respiratory viral diseases, brucellosis, and infectious mononucleosis. Diagnosis depends on the demonstration of a rising titer of complement-fixing antibodies. The disease is normally self-limiting, but responds to tetracyclines and to trimethoprim-sulfamethoxazole.

ANTHRAX

Bacillus anthracis, a large gram-negative rod, is the cause of a virulent disease of livestock which is endemic in the Middle East. The organism contaminates the bones, skin, and hair of dead animals and is liable to infect people who work with these substances. Such workers include those who are employed in making cloth from animal hair, in tanning, in the production of bone-meal fertilizer and glue, and in the importation of animal products. In almost all human cases the disease takes the form of a primary cutaneous sore associated with extensive edema.[26] The sore

starts as a pimple and develops a black central eschar with a ring of purplish vesicles around it. Occasionally, however, in workers exposed to large numbers of anthrax spores dispersed as an aerosol, inhalational anthrax or wool sorters' disease may develop. This is most likely to occur in the sorting and preparation of untreated wool or animal hair imported from the Middle East and India. One important outbreak has been reported in the United States in this century,[27] though the disease used to be more common in Britain in the last century. Most outbreaks are sporadic and associated with exposure to spores, the source of which may not be apparent; thus the diagnosis is often made postmortem. Recent examples are a man who worked next door to a factory processing middle-eastern goat hair[28] and a man who had been applying large amounts of bone-meal fertilizer to his garden.[29] Undoubtedly, workers may be exposed to large numbers of spores in the appropriate jobs, and it is surprising that more cases do not occur.[28]

Inhalational anthrax begins insidiously after an incubation period of about a week, with slight fever and malaise over a few days. There then develops a severe, short-lived, and usually fatal illness characterized by fever, profuse sweating, dyspnea with cyanosis, and often stridor. Crackles may be heard in the chest and a pleural effusion may occur. Shock ensues and the patient usually dies within 24 hours.[27] Pathologically, the disease appears not to be a pneumonia, the evidence indicating that the anthrax spores are engulfed by macrophages and carried to regional lymph nodes, where they germinate and cause a septicemia. The mediastinal nodes show acute inflammation and edema, and this spreads to the other mediastinal structures. Pulmonary edema and pleural effusion may occur.[30]

Anthrax may be controlled by disinfection of imported wool, as occurs in Britain, and by vaccination of exposed workers. Ideally such workers should carry a card warning their physician of the possibility of their contracting anthrax. The disease is diagnosed by examining fluid from a skin lesion or by culturing blood in the generalized disease. If the diagnosis is suspected, it is wise to treat the infection with a combination of penicillin and streptomycin. Severe anthrax septicemia will usually require other measures to combat shock and hypoxemia.

LEGIONNAIRES' DISEASE

Legionnaires' disease is so named because the outbreak that led to identification of the causative organism occurred at a convention of the American Legion in Philadelphia in 1976. On this occasion some 180 legionnaires contracted a severe form of the disease, of whom 29 died.[31] The event was sufficiently dramatic to attract national attention, and after the pursuit of several hares, the investigators tracked down a previously unknown bacterium, now called *Legionella pneumophila*.[32] The story of this

investigation will rank with other classics of epidemiology, such as John Snow's investigation of cholera in London in 1855; coincidentally, both the pump producing infected water in London and the hotel at which the legionnaires were staying in Philadelphia were situated on a Broad Street.[33]

Following identification of the organism, with the consequent ability of investigators to detect antibodies and culture Legionella from patients, many other outbreaks have been identified both subsequently and retrospectively. While sporadic cases occur, it has become clear that unexpected and unpredictable outbreaks, such as that in Philadelphia, are responsible for the bulk of cases. In particular, large hotels and institutions seem to be a frequent site of outbreaks, and investigation has often led to incrimination of water supplies as the carrier of the organism. In one particularly well-investigated episode, a large number of cases were found among patients, staff, and visitors at a large hospital at a time when a reserve cooling tower was being used for the air conditioning. Vapor containing the organism drifted from the tower into the entry ducts for the system.[34] Similar studies have pointed to showers as a source of infection, and bacteriological investigations of water in hospitals and hotels has shown Legionella to be widely distributed even in places where no recorded cases have occurred.[35] Why outbreaks occur in some circumstances and not in others is not clear, but the dose of the organisms delivered and their virulence may well be factors.

The disease itself varies considerably in severity, and judging from serological studies of hotel and hospital staff, subclinical infection may occur. An outbreak in Pontiac, Michigan, diagnosed retrospectively and previously known as Pontiac fever, was relatively mild and no fatalities occurred.[36] In cases coming to the hospital, the illness is typically severe, with 2 to 10 days of prodromal influenza-like symptoms, often including diarrhea, followed by a severe febrile illness, confusion, unilateral or bilateral pulmonary consolidation, abnormal liver function, and often hematuria. Almost any pattern of radiographic change, including pleural effusion, may occur. Sputum is usually scanty and nonpurulent, and this, together with the other clinical features and a white cell count not much above normal, often leads to a diagnosis of viral or mycoplasmal pneumonia. Diagnosis may be made by direct immunofluorescent staining of sputum or biopsy material or, after about a week, by serology. Treatment may not be successful, but the organism is sensitive to erythromycin and rifampicin.

The reason for including the disease among those of occupational etiology is that, like allergic alveolitis and humidifier fever, it may be transmitted by water systems in an occupational environment. Outbreaks may therefore be expected to occur among workers in hospitals and large office buildings where a source of warm water is available for bacterial growth and where the water may be circulated as an aerosol throughout the building. In such circumstances, preventive measures should be based on expert bacteriological advice.

OTHER INFECTIOUS DISEASES

Most of the other occupational infectious diseases are acquired either from contact with animals or in the laboratory.[37] Among these should be mentioned hydatid disease, glanders, brucellosis, psittacosis, and histoplasmosis.

Hydatid disease is relatively common among sheep farmers and their families. It is caused by a cestode organism, *Echinococcus granulosus,* which lives in the gut of dogs. Its ova, liberated in the animal's feces, may be ingested by the secondary host, usually a sheep but occasionally man. The embryo penetrates the intestinal wall and is trapped in the hepatic or pulmonary capillaries, where it produces the typical hydatid cysts (Fig. 21–4). These present as pulmonary opacities, slowly growing to a large size. Occasionally the cyst ruptures into bronchus or pleura. Anaphylactic reactions to the fluid have been described, but more commonly rupture

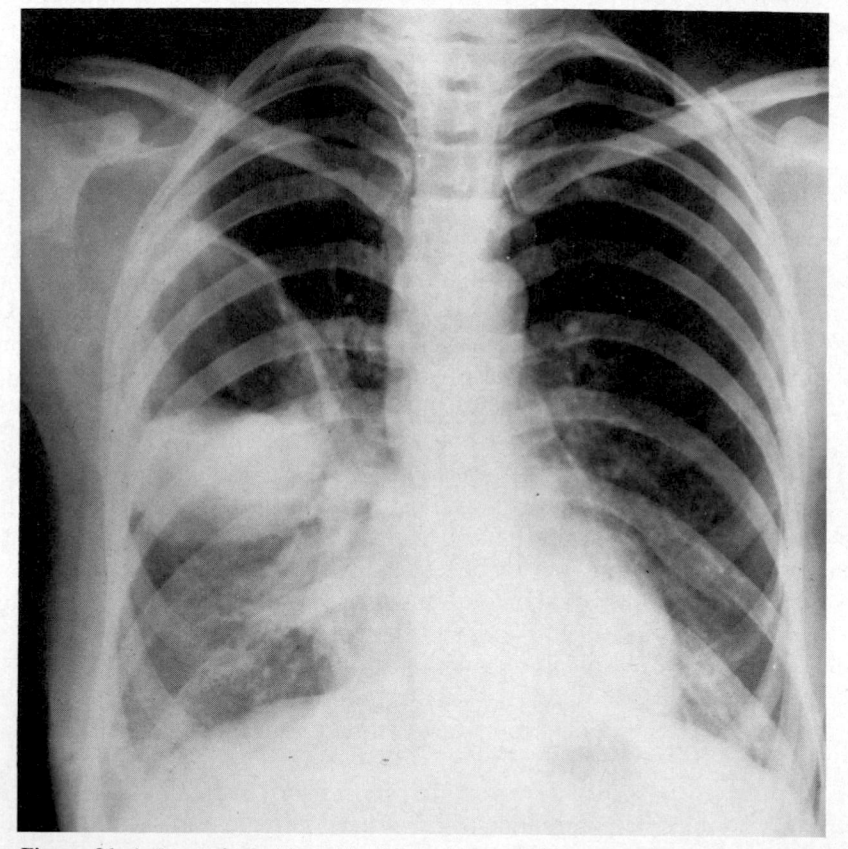

Figure 21–4. Large hydatid cyst in right midzone. Thirty-year-old farmer's wife. The patient had coughed up much of the fluid from the cyst, leaving the endocyst visible as a so-called "water lily" floating on the remaining fluid. Some aspirated fluid accounts for the shadowing in the right lower zone. (Courtesy of Dr. J. Meek.)

results in dissemination of the disease through the thoracic cavity. For these reasons, hydatid cysts should be removed surgically.

Glanders, caused by the organism *Pseudomonas mallei,* is a disease that used to be prevalent among those working with horses. It has now largely been eradicated. In 1947 a small epidemic was described among laboratory workers, to whom it poses an important hazard.[38] The clinical features are of an acute febrile illness with pneumonic consolidation and a tendency to cavitation. A severe disseminated form may occur. The organism in that outbreak was sensitive to sulfonamides.

Allied to glanders is melioidosis, caused by *Pseudomonas pseudomallei.* The disease, which is endemic in Southeast Asia, was significant as a cause of infection of soldiers in South Vietnam. It also can readily be acquired by laboratory workers handling the organism. It may cause a wide spectrum of illness, from an asymptomatic serological reaction to a toxic pneumonitis with formation of multiple lung and systemic abscesses. Melioidosis also responds to sulfonamides, though severe cases in Vietnam have required prolonged combination treatment with chloramphenicol, kanamycin, and novobiocin.[39, 40]

Brucellosis, a common disease among veterinarians and farmers, is acquired from dealing with the products of abortion in cattle or from drinking infected milk that has not been boiled. It is a generalized disease with multiple clinical manifestations, but cough occurs in approximately one third of those affected. Pneumonia is a very rare complication, occurring in severe cases.

Ornithosis, or psittacosis, is endemic in many birds and is an occupational hazard of those who handle them. Poultry farmers and those who deal with poultry carcassses as well as veterinarians are at particular risk.[41, 42] The illness varies from a mild influenza-like episode to a serious pneumonia with systemic symptoms. The disease may occasionally be fatal, but it normally responds to tetracycline.

Histoplasmosis is caused by a fungal intracellular parasite of the reticuloendothelial system, *Histoplasma capsulatum.* It affects a wide range of domestic and wild animals and is endemic in Ontario and in the Mississippi and Ohio valleys. Farmers in these regions, and particularly chicken farmers, are liable to be infected. Normally infection is either asymptomatic or self-limiting, but single or more often multiple miliary radiographic shadows occur (Fig. 21–5). These have a tendency to calcify. Epidemics of histoplasmosis may occur, producing an influenza-like illness associated with diffuse pulmonary mottling in those affected. Occasionally a disseminated infection, requiring treatment with amphotericin B, may occur.[43]

Leptospirosis is also occasionally seen as an occupational disease in stevedores, longshoremen, and farm workers.[44] Leptospirosis occasionally presents with a cough and blood-stained sputum. Radiographically there may be soft exudative parenchymal infiltrates.[45] This disease is contracted

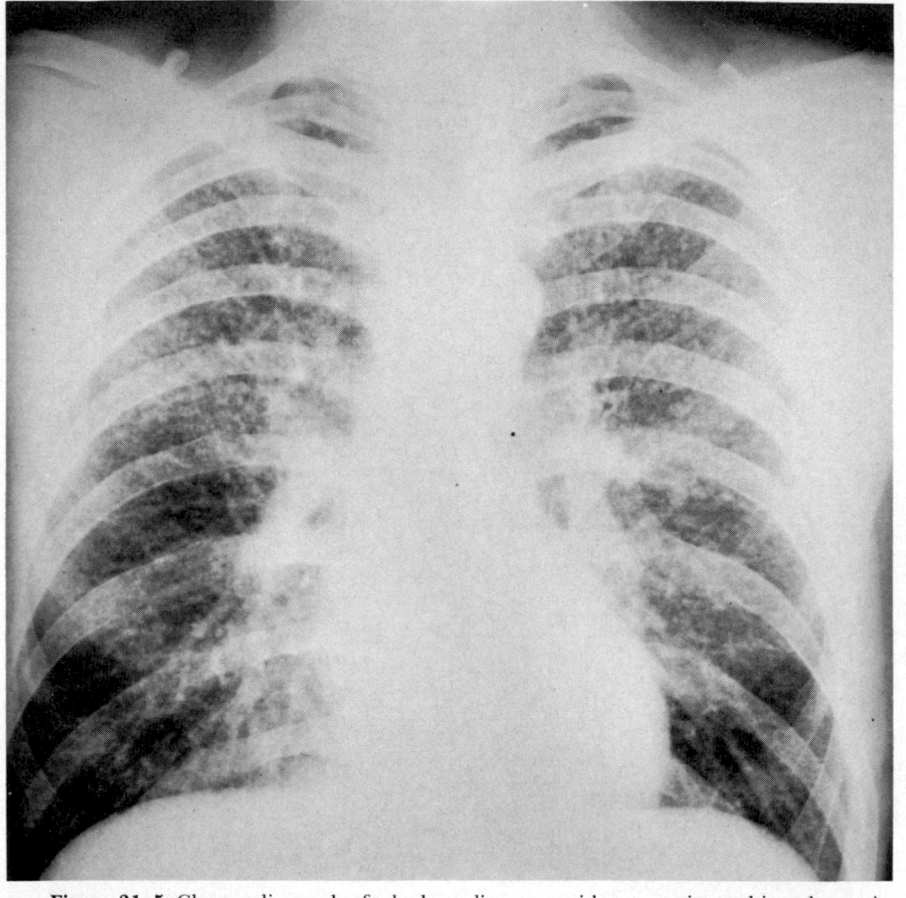

Figure 21–5. Chest radiograph of telephone linesman with acute primary histoplasmosis. The subject developed a high fever and myalgia 8 days after installing a telephone conduit in an attic infested by bats.

either from the usual carriers—rats, mice, and voles—or from cattle that have themselves been infected.

A final note should be recorded on smallpox handler's lung. This is an acute febrile illness occurring in recently immunized subjects who are in contact with smallpox patients. An outbreak was described in nurses during the last British epidemic of smallpox. The nurses were shown to have patchy pneumonic consolidation, and it was suggested that the disease was a form of allergic alveolitis.[46] However, follow-up of the patients showed miliary lung calcification (Fig. 21–6), and it now seems likely that the disease was an actual infection, attenuated by vaccination, with inhaled smallpox virus, producing radiographic changes analogous to those of chickenpox.[47]

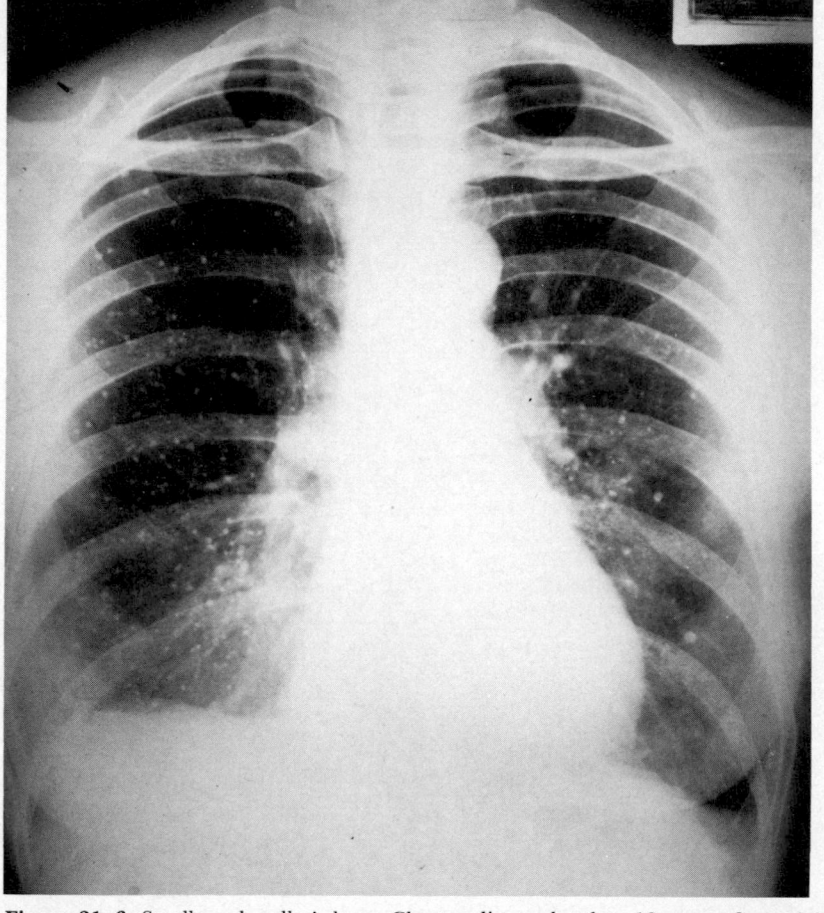

Figure 21–6. Smallpox handler's lung. Chest radiograph taken 10 years after original illness in nurse caring for smallpox patients. Discrete miliary calcification developed 6 years after that initial illness (Reproduced by permission from Ross, P. J., et al.: Pulmonary calcification following smallpox handlers' lung. Thorax, *29*, 659, 1974.)

References

1. Sulkin, S. E., and Pike, R. M., Survey of laboratory acquired infections. Am. J. Public Health, *41*, 769, 1951.
2. Stewart, A., and Hughes, J. P. W., Mass radiography in the Northamptonshire boot and shoe industry, 1945–6. Br. Med. J., *1*, 899, 1951.
3. Allison, A. C., and D'Arcy Hart, P., Potentiation by silica of the growth of *Mycobacterium tuberculosis* in macrophage cultures. Br. J. Exp. Pathol., *49*, 465, 1968.
4. Silicosis in the metal mining industry: a re-evaluation, 1958–61. Washington, D.C., U.S. Public Health Service, Department of Health, Education and Welfare, and Bureau of Mines, 1963, Chapter 5.
5. Jarman, T. F., Jones, J. G., Phillips, J. H., and Seingry, H. E., Radiological surveys of working quarrymen and quarrying communities in Caernarvonshire. Br. J. Ind. Med., *14*, 95, 1957.

6. Enterline, P. E., Mortality rates among coalminers. Am. J. Public Health, *54*, 758, 1964.
7. Glover, J. R., Bevan, C., Cotes, J. E., et al., Effects of exposure to slate dust in North Wales. Br. J. Ind. Med., *37*, 152, 1980.
8. Bruce, T., Silicotuberculosis. Scand. J. Respir. Dis. (Suppl), *65*, 139, 1968.
9. Bailey, W. C., Brown, M., Buechner, H. A., et al., Silico-mycobacterial disease in sandblasters. Am. Rev. Respir. Dis., *110*, 115, 1974.
10. Ramsay, J. H. R., and Pines, A., The late results of chemotherapy in pneumoconiosis complicated by tuberculosis. Tubercle, *44*, 476, 1963.
11. MRC/Miners' Chest Diseases Treatment Centre, Chemotherapy of pulmonary tuberculosis with pneumoconiosis. Tubercle, *44*, 47, 1963.
12. Dubois, P., Gyselen, A., and Prignot, J., Rifampicin combined chemotherapy in coalworkers' pneumoconio-tuberculosis. Am. Rev. Respir. Dis., *115*, 221, 1977.
13. British Thoracic Association, A controlled trial of six months chemotherapy in pulmonary tuberculosis. Second report: results during the twenty-four months after the end of chemotherapy. Am. Rev. Respir. Dis., *126*, 460, 1982.
14. Snider, R. E., The relationship between tuberculosis and silicosis. Am. Rev. Respir. Dis., *118*, 455, 1978.
15. Ball, J. D., Berry, G., Clarke, W. G., et al., A controlled trial of antituberculous chemotherapy in the early complicated pneumoconiosis of coalworkers. Thorax, *24*, 399, 1969.
16. Hart, J. T., Cochrane, A. L., and Higgins, I. T. T., Tuberculin sensitivity in coal workers' pneumoconiosis. Tubercle, *44*, 141, 1963.
17. Editorial, Opportunist mycobacteria. Lancet, *1*, 424, 1981.
18. Schaefer, W. B., Birn, K. J., Jenkins, P. A., and Marks, J., Infection with the Avian-Battey group of mycobacteria in England and Wales. Br. Med. J., *2*, 412, 1969.
19. Marks, J., and Jenkins, P. A., The opportunist mycobacteria—a 20-year retrospect. Postgrad. Med. J., *47*, 705, 1971.
20. British Thoracic and Tuberculosis Association, Opportunist mycobacterial pulmonary infection and occupational dust exposure: an investigation in England and Wales. Tubercle, *56*, 295, 1975.
21. Marks, J., Occupation and kansasii infection in Cardiff residents. Tubercle, *56*, 311, 1975.
22. Rosenzweig, D. Y., Silicosis complicated by atypical mycobacterial infection. *In* Transactions of the 26th V.A.–Armed Forces Pulmonary Disease Research Conference. Washington, D.C., U.S. Government Printing Office, 1967, p. 47.
23. Brown, M., Buechner, H. A., Bailey, W. C., and Ziskind, M. M., Atypical mycobacterial pulmonary disease at the New Orleans Veterans' Hospital and Metropolitan New Orleans (abstract). Am. Rev. Respir. Dis., *103*, 885, 1971.
24. Hunter, A. P., Campbell, I. A., Jenkins, P. A., and Smith, A. P., Treatment of pulmonary infections caused by mycobacteria of the *Mycobacterium avium-intracellulare* complex. Thorax, *36*, 326, 1981.
25. Brown, G. L., Clinical aspects of Q fever. Postgrad. Med. J., *49*, 539, 1973.
26. Christie, A. B., The clinical aspects of anthrax. Postgrad. Med. J., *49*, 565, 1973.
27. Plotkin, S. A., Brachman, P. S., Utell, M., et al., An epidemic of inhalation anthrax, the first in the twentieth century. I. Clinical features. Am. J. Med., *29*:992, 1960.
28. La Force, F. M., Bumford, F. H., Feeley, J. C., et al., Epidemiologic study of a fatal case of inhalation anthrax. Arch. Environ. Health, *18*, 798, 1969.
29. Seven, M., A fatal case of pulmonary anthrax. Br. Med. J., *1*, 748, 1976.
30. Albrink, W. S., Brooks, S. M., Biron, R. E., and Kopel, M., Human inhalation anthrax. A report of three fatal cases. Am. J. Pathol., *36*, 457, 1960.
31. Frazer, D. W., Tsai, T. R., Orenstein, W., et al., Legionnaires' disease: description of an epidemic of pneumonia. N. Engl. J. Med., *297*, 1189, 1977.
32. McDade, J. E., Shepard, C. C., Frazer, D. W., et al., Legionnaires' disease: isolation of a bacterium and demonstration of its role in other respiratory disease. N. Engl. J. Med., *297*, 1197, 1977.
33. Weill, H., and Sewell, E. M., In search of the pump handle, 1977. Am. Rev. Respir. Dis., *115*, 911, 1977.
34. Dondero, T. J., Rendtorff, R. C., Mallison, G. F., et al., An outbreak of legionnaires' disease associated with a contaminated air-conditioning cooling tower. N. Engl. J. Med., *302*, 365, 1980.

35. Tobin, J. O'H., Swann, R. A., and Bartlett, C. L. R., Isolation of *Legionella pneumophila* from water systems: methods and preliminary results. Br. Med. J., *282*, 515, 1981.
36. Glick, T. H., Gregg, M. B., Berman, B., et al., Pontiac fever. An epidemic of unknown etiology in a health department. I. Clinical and epidemiological aspects. Am. J. Epidemiol., *107*, 149, 1978.
37. Editorial, Occupational hazards for animal workers. Lancet, *2*, 789, 1981.
38. Howe, C., and Miller, W. R., Human glanders: report of six cases. Ann. Intern. Med., *26*, 92, 1947.
39. Patterson, M. C., Darling, C. L., and Blumenthal, J. B., Acute melioidosis in a soldier returning from South Vietnam. J.A.M.A., *200*, 447, 1967.
40. Cooper, E. B., Melioidosis. J.A.M.A., *200*, 452, 1967.
41. Editorial, Psittacosis. Br. Med. J., *1*, 1, 1972.
42. Palmer, S. R., Andrews, B. E., and Major, R., A common-source outbreak of ornithosis in veterinary surgeons. Lancet, *2*, 798, 1981.
43. Storch, G., Burford, J. G., George, R. B., et al., Acute histoplasmosis: description of an outbreak in Northern Louisiana. Chest, *77*, 38, 1980.
44. Crawford, S. M., and Miles, D. W., *Leptospira hebdomadis* associated with an outbreak of illness in workers on a farm in North Yorkshire. Br. J. Indust. Med., *37*, 397, 1980.
45. Poh, S. C., and Soh, C. S., Lung manifestations in leptospirosis. Thorax, *25*, 751, 1970.
46. Morris-Evans, W. H., and Foreman, H. M., Smallpox handler's lung. Proc. Roy. Soc. Med., *56*, 274, 1963.
47. Ross, P. J., Seaton, A., Foreman, H. M., and Morris-Evans, W., Pulmonary calcification following smallpox handlers' lung. Thorax, *29*, 659, 1974.

22

OCCUPATIONAL PULMONARY NEOPLASMS

Anthony Seaton

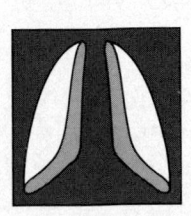

HISTORICAL ASPECTS

Cigarette smoking is by far the most important cause of bronchial carcinoma in the Western world.[1, 2] However, long before cigarettes became popular it was recognized that men in certain occupations had a tendency to die of lung disease that in retrospect seems likely to have been carcinoma. Paracelsus in the sixteenth century described the disease of metal miners at Schneeberg in the Erz mountains of Saxony, and Agricola shortly afterward suggested this was due to dust inhalation. The relative contributions of silicosis, tuberculosis, and lung cancer to the mortality were not clear at that time. Percival Pott,[3] in 1775, was the first to ascribe the development of carcinoma to a particular trade, in this case the scrotal cancer of chimney sweeps, and in the next century the recognition of skin tumors in Lancashire cotton workers, Scottish shale oil extractors, and German aniline dye workers gave a great impetus to the chemical theories of carcinogenesis. In 1879, Härting and Hesse[4] showed that a frequent cause of death in Schneeberg was tumor formation in the lungs, though the bronchogenic origin of these cancers was not recognized until somewhat later.

The Schneeberg mines have over the last five centuries produced copper, iron, and silver, and now bismuth, arsenic, and cobalt are being mined.[5] The air in the mines is radioactive, and this is the likely cause of the cancer hazard. These mines remained the only known source of occupational lung cancer until the same danger was recognized in uranium mines, first at Joachimsthal, also in the Erz mountains, and later in Colorado.[6] During the period 1940 to 1960 the risk of development of lung cancer in the use or production of arsenic, asbestos, chromates, iron ore, coal gas, and printing ink has been appreciated, and with the

increasing complexity of the chemical industry, new potential and actual hazards are still being recognized.

THE CURRENT PROBLEM

The chest physician, and especially the reader of this book who will be in the habit of taking a careful occupational history, may be struck by the contrast between his clinical practice, in which he only exceptionally sees a patient with lung cancer whose disease can realistically be attributed to occupational exposure, and those reports claiming that some 40 per cent of lung cancers can be so attributed.[7] In reality, the majority of lung cancers derive from their victims' addiction to that most widespread form of pollution, cigarette smoking. Nevertheless, it has been estimated that some 15 per cent of lung cancer in men and 5 per cent in women may be attributed to occupational factors and to asbestos exposure in particular.[8] In addition, since the number of chemicals used or produced in industry has been increasing almost exponentially and since those that are known to cause cancer have in the past largely been detected by astute clinical observations rather than in any planned way, it is likely that other carcinogens have been and are being introduced into the workplace unnoticed. There is therefore no more reason for complacency in this field than there is cause for panic. What is necessary is a sensible strategy for investigation of potential carcinogenic hazards combined with a policy by government and industry designed to reduce the exposure of workers to any new chemicals to the minimum level consistent with reasonable productivity.

How Much Respiratory Cancer is Attributable to Occupation?

Doll and Peto, in a monograph to which the reader is referred for a masterly exposition of the subject,[8] have pointed out that there is no current epidemic of cancer, with the exception of lung cancer. While the latter can almost entirely be attributed to cigarette smoking, a proportion of cases may fairly be blamed on asbestos (perhaps 5 per cent) and the other known occupational causes (coal combustion products, chromium, nickel, halo ethers, etc.) adding up to perhaps another 10 per cent of those tumors occurring in men. While these estimates may appear a bit high to the chest physician, they are based on a careful assessment of the epidemiological evidence. In this regard, it should be noted that such estimates consider the excess risk of cancer; thus they do not necessarily imply that in 15 per cent of people presenting with lung cancer the tumor is caused by workplace carcinogens, but that 15 per cent more people acquire the disease than would have been the case had there been no workplace exposures. In many, possibly most of these cases the individual

causes have been multiple, the separate causes adding up (or, as with asbestos and cigarettes, probably multiplying) to produce the disease in some who would not have otherwise contracted it if exposed to only one.

Whether the proportion of tumors due to occupational causes is rising or falling is unclear; certainly, as discussed in Chapter 13, there has been a rapid rise in pleural mesothelioma over the last decade and there is little doubt that this will continue over the next decade. However, this tumor is largely due to crocidolite and amosite and has a particularly long mean latent period. A stop to the use of these types of asbestos as soon as possible seems highly desirable. Whether the lung cancer peak has been reached is impossible to say. If the risk of asbestosis and the risk of lung cancer are approximately equal for a given dose of asbestos, then it could be argued from the British figures for asbestosis (see Chap. 13) that the peak of asbestos-induced lung cancer has now been passed and that exposures to asbestos in the workplace may now be insufficient to cause the great excess of tumors seen in the recent past. However, as just stated, asbestos and cigarettes inter-react and therefore exposure to both will cause cancer in some people who would not have got the disease had they only been exposed to one. Thus, even with further reductions in the asbestos hygiene standard, excess numbers of lung cancers are still likely to occur in that industry.

Apart from those involving exposure to asbestos, the other industries in which lung cancer has been shown to occur in excess can only be expected to contribute a small number of patients to the total. The largest group of men so exposed is probably that involved in coal combustion, though the United States industry in particular has made substantial progress in cleaning up the workplace. Smaller numbers of men are involved in exposure to radiation underground, and here again hygiene standards can be expected to have reduced their risks.

Investigation of a Suspected Lung Cancer Hazard

In the past, the detection of an association between exposure to a substance in the workplace and an excess risk of respiratory neoplasia has usually been the result of astute observation by a physician; for example, this was the case with asbestos and both lung cancer[9] and mesothelioma,[10] with nickel and lung and nasal cancer[11] and with furniture work and nasal cancer.[12] A notable recent example has been the discovery of hepatic angiosarcoma in men exposed to vinyl chloride.[13] However, in some cases the risk has first been detected in planned animal experiments, as was the case with chloromethyl ethers.[14] Apart from these methods, two others are available whereby a risk might be suspected: by chemical or physical analogy with known carcinogens and by *in vitro* carcinogenicity testing.

Investigation of a cancer hazard may therefore proceed in either of two broad directions—laboratory testing or epidemiological studies—

depending on the way in which suspicion is first aroused. If the first clue comes from knowledge that a substance to be liberated in the workplace is similar to one known already to be a carcinogen, either chemically or, in the case of fibers, physically, the appropriate route of investigation is by *in vitro* toxicity testing, proceeding generally to animal exposure studies. Such a pathway may also be appropriate in the test of new chemicals, for example, pharmaceuticals, to which people are likely to be exposed even if there is no *a priori* suspicion of carcinogenicity. If, on the other hand, the suspicion arises as a result of clinical observations, an epidemiological approach is desirable, since the advent of cases in a work force implies that human exposures have occurred and study of that population would be more fruitful than any number of tests on cells or animals.

Laboratory Testing

The mechanisms of carcinogenesis are incompletely understood. Nevertheless, most authorities now agree that at least two stages are usually involved: initiation, whereby a mutation is induced in the DNA of a target cell by a carcinogen, and promotion, in which increased cell multiplication results in expression of the disease.[15] Some workplace carcinogens may act directly as initiators, for example, irradiation, chloromethyl ethers, and mustard gas. These agents interact directly with DNA. Others, such as benzpyrene, are converted metabolically by the host organism to a substance that itself acts on DNA or, as in the case of nickel, interferes with the replication of DNA. Finally, some, like asbestos, seem to act as tumor promoters by a mechanism that depends on their physical properties.

With such an array of possible mechanisms of carcinogenesis, it is not surprising that laboratory tests can at best only be regarded as a rough guide to the relative potential harmfulness of substances. However, a number of tests have proved to be valuable, and it is probably sensible to view positive results from these not as a reason to ban substances outright so much as a means of setting priorities for the protection and surveillance of work forces and for further research.

Laboratory tests may be carried out on cells or on whole animals. Clearly the latter approximate the human response more closely, but the experiments are also more expensive and time-consuming. Animal experiments also raise ethical problems that researchers are required to take seriously. *In vitro* tests are cheaper and quicker, but only reach the stage of demonstrating effects of substances directly on DNA.[16] They can therefore be regarded as appropriate to the screening of new chemicals and possibly for ranking carcinogens in order of potency. Such tests include transformation in cultures of mammalian cells, usually fibroblasts; mutagenic changes in bacteria, such as the Ames test, which uses Salmonella; and direct tests on DNA. The relevance, if any, of cell tests to the

later stages, or promotion, of carcinogenesis is not clear, and this is an area of active research.[17]

Animal studies aimed at detecting a risk of lung cancer would normally involve exposing rats or other small rodents to airborne concentrations of the suspect material. Usually the concentrations are considerably higher than those existing in the workplace, in an attempt to compensate for the relatively short exposure time occasioned by the animal's life span. Extensive studies with asbestos have shown the rat to be a suitable animal for such studies in the testing, for example, of new manmade fibers.[18] Moreover, it has proved possible to use the rat as a model for mesothelioma, as intrapleural or intraperitoneal injection of asbestos results in a high incidence of that tumor.[19]

Epidemiological Investigations

It is important to remember that most known occupational carcinogens have been detected as a result of clinical and epidemiological observations. Of the 12 occupational exposures known to be related to the development of respiratory tract cancer (Table 22–1), all save one were detected first by observation of humans. In several cases the carcinogen has not yet been identified even though the workplace risk is known. The epidemiological methods used have been mortality studies of cohorts and case-control studies. In the former, a cohort known to have been employed in the suspect workplace some years before (the longer the better, in view of the long interval often occurring between first exposure and the development of cancer) is identified and the causes of death of those who have not survived are determined. This pattern of mortality may then be compared with the patterns in the community in general and

Table 22–1. KNOWN OCCUPATIONAL CAUSES OF RESPIRATORY TRACT CANCER

Cause	Occupation	Tumor Type
Asbestos	Mining, weaving, utilization	Lung cancer, serosal mesothelioma
Radioactivity	Uranium, metal, hematite, fluorspar mining	Lung cancer
Mustard gas	Manufacture	Lung cancer
Arsenic	Sheep-dip, metal refining	Lung, skin cancer
Nickel	Refining	Nasal sinus, lung cancer
Chromates	Extraction, production, and pigments	Lung cancer
Halo ethers	Chemical industry	Lung cancer
Isopropanol	Manufacture	Nasal sinus cancer
?	Furniture manufacture	Nasal sinus cancer
?	Shoe manufacture	Nasal sinus cancer
?	Coal carbonization	Lung cancer
?	Printing	Lung cancer

in those of similar social class and smoking habits. In addition, if data on exposure to possible carcinogens are available, internal comparisons may be made between workers with different levels of exposure. Such studies demand large resources and depend on the ability to obtain information in retrospect to identify a work force and determine its vital status and causes of death. Ideally, however, such studies hold the possibility of relating quantitative measurements of exposure to the actual risks of death from malignant disease. To approach this ideal, data must be available on which reasonable estimates of lifetime exposure may be based, and this is where such studies have almost always fallen short of perfection.

The case-control approach aims to identify individuals suffering from the disease under scrutiny and to compare them in terms of occupational exposures to controls, matched in various ways but suffering from some other unrelated condition. Ideally, the cases would be newly diagnosed patients with, for example, lung cancer from whom a detailed occupational and smoking history could be obtained. However, this technique has also been used to study asbestos levels in the lungs of subjects who have died of mesothelioma, in an attempt to identify the relative importance of different types of fiber.[20] A disadvantage of case-control studies in lung cancer is that, unless the cause is a very potent one (in which case it is unlikely to have remained undetected), large numbers of individuals have to be studied. It has been suggested that a large study, involving some 10,000 cases and 10,000 controls, would be an ideal method of obtaining an estimate of the proportion of lung cancer ascribable to occupational factors.[8, 21]

Finally, in the case of a rare tumor, such elaborate investigations may hardly be necessary. For example, adenocarcinoma of the nasal sinuses, pleural mesothelioma, and hepatic angiosarcoma are all rare tumors that occurred in unexpectedly high numbers among people exposed to toxic substances in workplaces. While epidemiological studies subsequently confirmed the clinical suspicions, these suspicions alone should have been sufficient as a basis for preventive action.

PREVENTION

Before discussing preventive measures, it is important to place occupational cancer in perspective. First, cancer is generally a disease of the elderly, and it has been calculated that if all forms of cancer were eradicated in the United States, average life expectancy would rise by only two years.[22] Second, there does not seem to be an epidemic of cancer, the only important type noted to be on the increase being bronchial carcinoma.[8] Third, any occupational factor in bronchial carcinogenesis pales in significance when compared with the effect of tobacco, which may be calculated to cause some 120,000 to 125,000 excess deaths from cancer each year in the United States, including an excess of about 80,000 to

85,000 lung cancers.[8] Fourth, while we do not live in a perfect society, industry nevertheless confers the benefits of employment and the production of the materials on which we rely for our high standard of living. Unrealistic pressures upon industry to prevent theoretical hazards may result in higher costs, loss of jobs, and reduced productivity, the net effect being to the disadvantage of society.

This is not to say that we should be complacent about occupational cancer, nor that the unnecessary death of an individual is not a tragedy to those close to him. It is, however, a hint that it might be wise to adjust our perspective at a time when outrage at cancer in the workplace seems to result more in filling the pockets of doctors and lawyers than in hastening the development by industry and government of sensible policies for prevention. Such policies must take account of the facts that man is exposed to some 60,000 chemicals in addition to many complex mixtures of unknown composition, that perhaps 2000 to 3000 of these are so far suspected carcinogens, but that only in 30 to 40 is there some human evidence of carcinogenicity. The resources required for detailed testing of all workplace chemicals would be enormous in terms of money, the time of scientists and technicians, and the lives of animals. Some balance must therefore be struck in investigation, and an appropriate starting point might be an *a priori* suspicion, based on chemical or physical analogy to a known carcinogen or on clinical hunch. Two appropriate actions could then follow: first, action could be taken to minimize human exposure and, second, laboratory or epidemiological studies could take place. If, as a result of this, evidence is produced that the substance is carcinogenic, decisions need to be made on what action to take. This should depend on an assessment of the risk, which is a function not only of the relative carcinogenic potency of the substance but also of the numbers of people likely to be exposed and the length and extent of their exposure.

Once a cancer hazard has been recognized, it is essential that exposures of humans should be reduced to the minimum possible. The primary aim should be to enclose processes and reduce fugitive emissions; personal protection of the work force by respirators is an important secondary step, particularly so when, as happens in all processes, accidents occur and workers have to venture into areas of high exposure. Industry's argument that men will not wear respirators is not convincing, though it is a convenient one for shifting responsibility onto the worker. Persuading workers to wear protective equipment does not seem to have been a problem in the nuclear industry.

Surveillance of the work force for lung cancer is a relatively unprofitable exercise. Large numbers of people have to have radiographs and sputum cytology performed for many years to pick up the *treatable* cases, for every one of whom many more will be found to have false-positive evidence of cancer, leading to unnecessary investigation and anxiety. The resources spent on such surveillance are therefore best kept to a minimum, with the surplus used in worker protection and health education. It should be recalled that routine surveillance implies that if a disease is found, it

can be cured. The evidence gained from attempts at early diagnosis of lung cancer does not yet clarify whether the return justifies the effort.[23]

MANAGEMENT

Once occupational bronchial carcinoma or mesothelioma has been diagnosed the treatment does not differ from that of the disease in a nonoccupational setting. (Management of mesothelioma is discussed in Chapter 13.) Bronchial carcinoma remains almost incurable, though surgical resection of early lesions affords a 20 to 30 per cent chance of surviving five years. Two factors combine to make the prognosis in occupational lung cancer even less favorable. First, many such tumors are of the adenocarcinoma or small-cell undifferentiated types, which are particularly resistant to treatment. Second, they often arise in lungs previously damaged by fibrosis, as in asbestos workers or hematite miners, thus reducing the possibilities of surgical resection.

If a reasonably clear association between occupational exposure and the tumor can be made, industrial injuries benefit or other legal compensation may be available to the victim or the dependants. This normally only applies where there is evidence of exposure to a known carcinogen for an appropriate period.

SPECIFIC OCCUPATIONAL CAUSES OF PULMONARY NEOPLASMS

Asbestos

The relationships between asbestos exposure and bronchial carcinoma and mesothelioma are discussed in Chapter 13.

Uranium and Radioactive Elements

The excess mortality in the Schneeberg metal miners due to lung carcinoma is very likely to be related, at least in part, to the radioactivity of these mines,[24] and knowledge of the existence of this mortality from respiratory causes dates back to the sixteenth century. Härting and Hesse[4] first showed that lung tumors were responsible for three quarters of the deaths of these miners, and it was later confirmed that these tumors were of bronchogenic origin.[25] In 1930, the uranium miners of Joachimsthal were also found to have an increased risk of developing lung cancer.[26, 27] Subsequently, a similar risk has been discovered in association with radioactivity in uranium mines in the United States, hard rock miners in the United States, hematite miners in Britain, and fluorspar miners in Canada.

Production and Use of Uranium

Uranium occurs as an oxide, as pitchblende, or as a compound oxide with vanadium and potassium known as carnotite. The ore contains amounts of silica varying from 5 to 50 per cent, and uranium mining often therefore entails a risk also of silicosis. It is mined chiefly in Czechoslovakia, the Colorado plain, Congo, Canada, and Australia. Both deep and surface mining is used, with drilling and blasting techniques similar to those in other forms of hard rock mining.

The crude ore is crushed at the mill, often on the site of the mine, and the uranium is then extracted in the form of a uranate known as yellowcake. This is packed into drums for transport to the user, and dust is liable to be liberated in these two processes. The uranium is then used principally in the production of atomic energy for peaceful and military purposes, but also to some extent in ceramics and in the chemical industry. Laboratory workers handling uranium are particularly at risk of toxic effects, which may include lung cancer or fibrosis.

Epidemiology

The most detailed study of the effects of uranium mining on the lungs is that carried out by the United States Public Health Service in Colorado and the mountain states between 1950 and 1967.[28] This study demonstrated a mortality from lung cancer among the miners of over six times that expected, the mortality being related to the calculated cumulative exposure to radiation expressed in working level months. A working level month is defined as an exposure for 170 working hours to a level of radon daughters in 1 liter of air resulting in the emission of 1.3×10^5 MeV of potential alpha energy. Even the group of miners with a relatively low exposure to one working level over 10 to 30 years experienced a fourfold increase in the risk of lung cancer. With the higher exposures, the risk was appreciably enhanced to the equivalent of seven or more working levels over 10 or more years.

Further suggestive evidence that radiation is to blame for this excess of lung cancer comes from another aspect of the same study,[29] in which it was shown that small-cell undifferentiated cancers became progressively more frequent with greater cumulative radiation exposure. This apparent association of radiation with small-cell carcinomas has been found also in Joachimsthal and among the fluorspar miners of Newfoundland, while a similar association has been observed with the radiomimetic agent mustard gas. Studies of uranium miners in Canada have also shown an increased proportion of small-cell tumors in workers with the highest exposures.[30]

Cigarette-smoking uranium miners in the United States are at greater risk than their nonsmoking co-workers.[31] However, the nonsmoking miners of Joachimsthal still have an increased risk of lung cancer, their tumors taking rather longer to develop. Archer has shown that the latent period prior to induction of lung cancer by alpha radiation is shorter the older

the miner when he starts mining, the more cigarettes smoked, and the greater the dose of radiation.[32]

Pathogenesis

Uranium generally represents only 0.5 per cent of the ore, though higher grade ores may occur, especially close to the surface. The uranium-238 decays to radium-226, and this in turn decays to radon-222. This substance is a gas and emits alpha radiation, as do three of its daughters, polonium-218, 214, and 210. These substances diffuse from the rock into the mine air, where they become attached to particles of dust or moisture on which they may be inhaled into the lungs. The alpha particles emitted have a range in tissue of between 40 and 70 microns, just sufficient for them to damage the nuclei of the basal cells of the bronchial epithelium by ionization. It is assumed that this damage may later lead to malignant change.

Prevention

Prevention of lung cancer in uranium miners depends on regular measurement of levels of radon daughters, usually by pumping air through a molecular filter and counting the alpha activity in a scintillation counter. Personal radiation badges are also being developed. Where levels are unacceptably high they should be reduced by ventilation, sealing off unused areas, and prevention of seepage of water containing dissolved radon. The individual exposures of miners should be monitored, and recent recommendations are that miners should not be exposed to more than four working level months in any year nor to more than two working level months in any three-month period. Medical supervision should involve exclusion of subjects with prior chest disease, annual or biennial chest radiography, and discouragement from smoking. As discussed above, cytological examination of sputum is probably not desirable, though it has its advocates.[33]

Other Hazards Associated with Uranium

The uranium miner is also at risk of silicosis, though the ventilation necessary to control the radiation hazard is sufficient also to control that from silica. There is some evidence that chronic irradiation may act with silica in producing generalized pulmonary fibrosis in a proportion of the miners.[34]

Workers in the uranium mill may be at risk of malignant disease of lymphatic and hemopoietic tissues, other than leukemia, one study having shown four deaths in a group of 104 workers, as against one expected.[35] Clearly these numbers are very small, and further study is required. Moreover, uranium is very toxic to the kidneys, causing chronic nephritis in animal experiments. Precautions must therefore be taken to prevent chronic absorption of uranium in the millers by enclosure of the process,

rotation of the workers from jobs involving exposure after a short period, and estimation of uranium levels in the urine.

A study of workers at a uranium processing plant involved in nuclear weapons production has so far shown no very convincing evidence of an excess cancer hazard.[36]

Fluorspar

This mineral, calcium fluoride, is used as a flux in steel making and in the production of aluminium, in ceramics, and as a source of fluorine in the chemical industry. While it is produced worldwide, important deposits have been worked in Newfoundland since the 1930s, and it was here that a detailed investigation of the health of the miners was carried out because of a suspected increased risk of lung cancer.[37] This study showed that fluorspar miners in this region had a death rate from lung cancer 29 times that anticipated from study of the unexposed population. This difference was not related to cigarette smoking or pneumoconiosis, and environmental investigation showed that the mine air was radioactive to a degree comparable to that found in uranium mines. No radioactive ore was present in the mines, and the activity was shown to emanate from radon daughters dissolved in water that had seeped into the mines.

Metal Mining

The pneumoconiosis of hematite miners is described in Chapter 15. The novelist A. J. Cronin[38] was one of the first to call attention to the high incidence of respiratory disease among these miners in the northwest of Britain. Subsequent pathological studies[39] suggested that lung cancer was a relatively common cause of death, apparently related to the presence of siderosilicosis. While it is possible that a combination of iron and silica is carcinogenic to the lungs, an alternative cause was discovered when a survey of radon in British mines revealed high levels in these same hematite mines.[40] Comparison of the mortality of hematite miners with that of coal miners and of the rest of the population in the same area of Britain showed an excess of deaths due to lung cancer of between 75 and 100 per cent.[41] Death rates among the miners could not be calculated because of unsatisfactory employment figures. This same study demonstrated that up to 40 per cent of these cancers were of the small-cell undifferentiated type, a similar proportion to that in uranium miners.[29] The source of radon in these mines is thought to be seepage of water, as in the fluorspar mines. If radiation is the carcinogen, a similar excess cancer mortality might not be expected in all hematite mines, but this has not yet been determined. Suggestive evidence, however, comes from a

Table 22–2. LUNG CANCER IN PERSONS EXPOSED TO RADIATION*

Population Group	Excess Lung Cancers per Year per WLM† per Million Persons	Excess per Year per Rem per Million Persons
U.S. uranium miners	1.8	0.3
Joachimsthal, Schneeberg miners	2.6	0.4
Newfoundland fluorspar miners	2.1	0.3
British hematite miners	5.9	1.0
U.S. hardrock miners	2.0	0.3
Danish thorotrast patients	4.0	0.7

*From Archer, V. E., Lung cancer among populations having lung irradiation. Lancet, 2, 1261, 1971.
†WLM, working level month.

comparison of excess lung cancers in different situations involving exposure to radiation, when correction of the cancer mortality for the calculated exposure produces closely similar figures (Table 22–2).[42]

Underground metal miners in the United States[43] and in Sweden[44] have been shown to have an increased lung cancer mortality, and this again appears to be associated with irradiation, though the possibility that traces of other carcinogens in the mine atmosphere play a part cannot be ruled out. Tin mines are another place where radon daughters might be expected, and raised levels of radiation have been found in British mines. A study of this work force has confirmed a small increase in lung cancer risk for underground miners.[45]

Mustard Gas

This substance, β,β' dichlorodiethyl sulfide, has effects on cells similar to those of radiation. It has been used as a weapon in warfare, a use that has led to its being suspected as a cause of bronchitis and lung cancer in veterans. During the Second World War, mustard gas was manufactured in Japan with few precautions to prevent exposure. Surveys of workers in this industry have shown a mortality from cancer of lung and upper airways at least 10 times that expected.[46] These tumors were either squamous or undifferentiated, no adenocarcinomas being found.

Arsenic

Arsenic has been suspected as a carcinogen since the mid-nineteenth century and was originally thought to be the agent responsible for the deaths of miners in Schneeberg.[4] Skin cancer has been shown to follow

prolonged treatment of psoriasis with arsenicals, and both skin and lung cancer were described in workers engaged in the manufacture of arsenical sheep-dip in 1934.[47] This industry was investigated in detail in Britain by Hill and Fanning,[48] who showed that workers involved in the chemical process itself had an increased risk of dying of cancer when compared both to other workers in the factory and to the socially comparable male population of the town. The excess of cancers in these men was due to an increase in those tumors involving the skin and respiratory tract. Investigation of the factory at that time[49] revealed an extremely dusty environment, with chemical evidence of arsenic absorption in the workers. Virtually all the process workers examined, moreover, showed clinical evidence of arsenic absorption, with increased pigmentation, hyperkeratosis, and warts.

The possible risks of arsenic poisoning and lung cancer have also existed among those involved in the preparation and use of arsenical insecticide sprays.[50, 51] All these substances have now largely been superseded, but arsenic may still be encountered in metal refining and the chemical industry, especially as a contaminant of sulfuric acid, and stringent precautions are necessary to prevent its inhalation or contact with skin.

Nickel

In 1900, Dr. Ludwig Mond opened his nickel refinery in Swansea, South Wales. The ore, then as now produced and concentrated in Canada, was shipped to Britain for extraction by Mond's carbonyl process, whereby the nickel was extracted by combination with carbon monoxide to form a gas, nickel carbonyl, which decomposes into its components on heating. After a period of some 40 years it became apparent that the workers in this refinery were showing an excessive death rate from cancer of the nose and lung, and these neoplasms were prescribed as industrial diseases among such workers in Britain in 1949. Doll studied the epidemiology of these conditions[52] and concluded that the risk of lung cancer among the workers was 5 times and that of nasal cancer 150 times that expected. However, by this time there had already been an appreciable decline in mortality, and Morgan[11] was able to show that the death rates had fallen to those expected by the 1930s. This he related to changes in the industrial process around the 1920s, when the levels of calcined nickel dust were reduced and sulfuric acid free of arsenical contamination was introduced for removal of copper in the ore.

Morgan's results have been confirmed in a more recent follow-up of the Mond workers,[53] though it appears the risk persisted a little longer than was first thought. Other studies of nickel workers in a Norwegian refinery,[54] in a Canadian sinter,[55] and in a South Pacific smelter[56] have shown an increased risk of lung cancer, especially in smokers, while a

study of workers making nickel alloys has shown no such increase.[57] The consensus now is that nickel subsulfide is the most likely carcinogen,[53] although an increased risk has also been found in a plant where exposures were predominantly to nickel sulfate and chloride.[58] One pathological study of the lungs of five cancer subjects failed to demonstrate the presence of arsenic.[59]

Chromates

Chrome ore is mined in the U.S.S.R., Turkey, and South Africa. Chromium is used principally in the production of alloys and electroplate but also in pigments, tanning, and the chemical industry. The main toxic effects of exposure to chrome salts are ulcers of the skin and perforation of the nasal septum, but early in this century cases of lung cancer in chrome workers were reported from Germany. In 1948 and 1950 similar findings were reported from the United States,[60, 61] and a death rate of 16 times that expected for lung cancer was recorded among chrome workers. Further confirmation of this increased predisposition to the disease has come from the United Kingdom,[62] in which a group of 723 workers in the bichromate-producing industry were followed up for six years, and 12 died of lung cancer during this period. This was three and a half times the expected figure. Furthermore, other cases of lung cancer were found during the survey but could not be included in the statistical analysis. This study has subsequently been extended to 2715 men, of whom only 298 were lost to follow-up. The observed to expected ratio of deaths from lung cancer was significantly elevated to 2.4, though this relative risk had fallen from 3.0 to 1.8 following modification of the plant to reduce exposures.[63] The results of several studies, showing differing relative risks of lung cancer, have been reviewed by Enterline.[64]

There is little doubt that exposure to chromium salts increases the risk of bronchial (and nasal) carcinoma. The risk seems to relate to exposure to hexavalent chromium compounds, such as in dichromates and chromium pigments,[65, 66] rather than to trivalent chromium.[67, 68] Chromium persists in the lungs long after the worker has ceased exposure, and is found especially in the upper lobes.[69] Prevention of the risk must depend on efficient dust extraction, enclosure of processes, and the use of effective respirators where exposure to dust or fume is inevitable. The TLV for chrome salts is 0.5 mg^{-3}.

Chloroethers

Chloroethers are alkylating agents and are used in industry as intermediates in organic syntheses, as bacteriocides, and as fungicides. Two important chloroethers, bischloromethyl ether and chloromethyl methyl

ether, are human carcinogens. These are so far unique among causes of human bronchial carcinoma in that their activity was first shown in animal experiments,[14] and this led to detailed hygiene and epidemiological studies which showed a considerably increased risk of oat cell carcinoma among the work force.[70, 71] This particularly applies to exposure to bischloromethyl ether,[72] and a dose-response relationship has been demonstrated with risk ratios exceeding 10 for the most heavy and prolonged exposures.[73]

Coal Carbonization

Exposure to the products of coal carbonization has been shown to increase the risks of bronchial carcinoma. In United States steelworkers, Lloyd showed that mortality from the disease was twice that expected among coke oven workers and increased 10 times among those employed full-time for five or more years on oven tops.[74] An association between estimates of exposure to coal tar pitch volatiles and risk of lung cancer has been described.[75] Renal, bladder, and scrotal cancers may also result from such exposures. Broadly comparable results were obtained in a prospective 12-year study of British gasworkers.[76] A recent detailed study of British coke workers has also shown an increased risk of death from lung cancer, though of a lower order than that found by Lloyd.[77] It seems clear that appropriate hygiene measures can go a long way towards reducing these risks.

Other Occupations in Which a Risk of Respiratory Cancer Has Been Suspected

In the chemical industry, carcinoma of the nasal sinuses and possibly of the lung appeared to occur unduly frequently in the manufacture of isopropanol.[78] In this industry, propylene gas reacts with arsenic-free sulfuric acid to produce isopropyl sulfates, which are then hydrolyzed to form isopropanol. Isopropyl oil, a volatile substance that is carcinogenic in animals, is given off, and this was suspected to be the offending agent. Measures have been taken to control exposure to this susbstance, and it is probable that the hazard has been removed.

Suspicion has also been raised that printing ink may be a lung cancer hazard, as studies in Denmark have shown a sixfold increase in risk in exposed workers,[79] while studies of British newspaper workers have shown a 30 to 40 per cent increase in risk.[80] A slight increase in lung cancer risk has also been suggested in foundry workers,[81] though the significance of such findings in the absence of information on smoking habits is open to debate.

It has been suggested that exposure to vinyl chloride monomer might entail an increased risk of lung cancer as well as of liver disease.[82] However,

another careful study, taking account of smoking histories, has not shown such an increase in risk.[83] Similarly, there are conflicting reports of an association of lung cancer with beryllium exposure, one showing an *inverse* relationship to length of exposure[84] and others a small excess risk.[85, 86] In none of the cases is convincing proof of human lung carcinogenesis yet established.

Finally, it should be noted that adenocarcinoma of the nasal cavity and sinuses, a rare tumor, has been shown to be associated with work with wood, principally in the furniture industry, and with leather in boot and shoe manufacture.[87]

References

1. Doll, R., and Hill, A. B., A study of the aetiology of carcinoma of the lung. Br. Med. J., 2, 1271, 1952.
2. Advisory Committee to the Surgeon General of the Public Health Service, Smoking and Health. Washington, D. C., Department of Health, Education and Welfare, 1964.
3. Pott, P., Chirurgical Works, Vol. 3. London, 1808, p. 177.
4. Härting, F. H., and Hesse, W., Der Lungenkrebs, die Bergkrankheit in der Schneeburger Gruben. Vjschr. Gerichtl. Med., 31, 102, 1879.
5. Doll, R., Specific industrial causes. In Bignall, J. R., Monographs on Neoplastic Disease, Vol. 1, Carcinoma of the Lung. Edinburgh, Livingstone, 1958.
6. Wagoner, J. K., Archer, V. E., Carroll, B. E., et al., Cancer mortality patterns among U.S. uranium miners and millers, 1950 through 1962. J. Natl. Cancer Inst., 32, 787, 1964.
7. Bridport, K., Deconfle, P., Fraumeni, J. F., et al., Estimates of the fraction of cancer in the United States related to occupational factors. Report prepared by NCI, NIEHS and NIOSH, 1978.
8. Doll, R., and Peto, R., The causes of cancer. J. Natl. Cancer Inst., 66, 1197, 1981.
9. Merewether, E. R. A., Asbestosis and carcinoma of the lung. In Annual Report of the Chief Inspector of Factories for the Year 1947. London, H. M. Stationery Office, 1949.
10. Wagner, J. C., Sleggs, C. A., and Marchand, P., Diffuse pleural mesothelioma and asbestos exposure in the North-West Cape Province. Br. J. Ind. Med., 17, 260, 1960.
11. Morgan, J. G., Some observations on the incidence of respiratory cancer in nickel workers. Br. J. Ind. Med., 15, 224, 1958.
12. Macbeth, R., Malignant disease of the paranasal sinuses. J. Laryng., 79, 592, 1965.
13. Creech, J. L., and Johnson, M. N., Angiosarcoma of liver in the manufacture of polyvinyl chloride. J. Occup. Med., 16, 150, 1974.
14. Nelson, N., Carcinogenicity of halo ethers. N. Engl. J. Med., 288, 1123, 1973.
15. Mastromatteo, E., Current concepts in occupational carcinogenesis. In Prevention of Occupational Cancer—International Symposium. Occupational Safety and Health Series No. 39. Geneva, International Labor Organization, 1982.
16. Griesemer, R. A., and Dunkel, V. C., Laboratory tests for chemical carcinogens. J. Environ. Pathol. Toxicol., 4, 565, 1980.
17. Slaga, T. J., Sivak, A., and Boutwell, R. K., eds., Carcinogenesis—A Comprehensive Survey, Vol. 2. New York, Raven Press, 1980.
18. Davis, J. M. G., The biological effects of mineral fibres. Ann. Occup. Hyg., 24, 227, 1981.
19. Wagner, J. C., and Berry, G., Mesotheliomas in rats following inoculation with asbestos. Br. J. Cancer, 23, 567, 1969.
20. McDonald, A. D., McDonald, J. C., and Pooley, F. D., Mineral fibre content of lung in mesothelial tumours in North America. In Walton, W. H., ed., Inhaled Particles V. Oxford, Pergamon Press, 1982, p. 417.

21. Peto, R., Considerations for designing a large case-control lung cancer study to explore occupational cancer risks. *In* Peto, R., and Schneidermann, M., eds., Banbury Report 9, Quantification of Occupational Cancer. Cold Spring Harbor Laboratory, 1981.
22. Cairns, J., Cancer, Science and Society. San Francisco, W. H. Freeman and Co., 1978.
23. Fontana, R. S., Early diagnosis of lung cancer. Am. Rev. Respir. Dis., *116*, 399, 1977.
24. Lorenz, E., Radioactivity and lung cancer: a critical review of lung cancer in the miners of Schneeberg and Joachimsthal. J. Natl. Cancer Inst., *5*, 1, 1944.
25. Rostoski, Saupe and Schmorl, Die Bergkrankheit der Erzbergleuter in Schneeberg in Sachsen. Zeit. für Krebsforschung, *23*, 360, 1926; abstract in J. A. M. A., *87*, 289, 1926.
26. Lowry, J., Über die Joachimsthaler Bergkrankheit. Med. Klin., *25*, 141, 1929.
27. Sikl, H., Über den Lungenkrebs der Bergleuter in Joachimsthal. Zeit. für Krebsforschung, *32*, 609, 1930.
28. Lundin, F. E., Lloyd, J. W., Smith, E. M., et al., Mortality of uranium miners in relation to radiation exposure, hard rock mining and cigarette smoking—1950 through September 1967. Health Physics, *16*, 571, 1969.
29. Saccomanno, G., Archer, V. E., Auerbach, O., et al., Histologic types of lung cancer among uranium miners. Cancer, *27*, 515, 1971.
30. Chovil, A., The epidemiology of primary lung cancer in uranium miners in Ontario. J. Occup. Med., *23*, 417, 1981.
31. Archer, V. E., Wagoner, J. K., and Lundin, F. E., Uranium mining and cigarette smoking effects on man. J. Occup. Med., *15*, 204, 1973.
32. Archer, V. E., Health concerns in uranium mining and milling. J. Occup. Med., *23*, 502, 1981.
33. Saccomanno, G., Saunders, R. P., Archer, V. E., et al., Cancer of the lung: the cytology of sputum prior to the development of carcinoma. Acta Cytöl., *9*, 413, 1965.
34. Trapp, E., Renzetti, A. D., Kobayashi, T., et al., Cardiopulmonary function in uranium miners. Am. Rev. Respir. Dis., *101*, 27, 1970.
35. Archer, V. E., Wagoner, J. K., and Lundin, F. E., Cancer mortality among uranium mill workers. J. Occup. Med., *15*, 11, 1973.
36. Polednak, A. P., and Frome, E. L., Mortality among men employed between 1943 and 1947 at a uranium processing plant. J. Occup. Med., *23*, 169, 1981.
37. de Villiers, A. J., and Windish, J. P., Lung cancer in a fluorspar mining community. I. Radiation, dust and mortality experience. Br. J. Ind. Med., *21*, 94, 1964.
38. Cronin, A. J., Dust inhalation by haematite miners. J. Ind. Hyg., *8*, 291, 1926.
39. Faulds, J. S., and Stewart, M. J., Carcinoma of the lung in hematite miners. J. Pathol. Bact., *72*, 353, 1956.
40. Duggan, M. J., Soilleux, P. J., Strong, J. C., and Howell, D. M., The exposure of United Kingdom miners to radon. Br. J. Ind. Med., *27*, 106, 1970.
41. Boyd, J. T., Doll, R., Faulds, J. S., and Leiper, J., Cancer of the lung in iron ore (haematite) miners. Br. J. Ind. Med., *27*, 97, 1970.
42. Archer, V. E., Lung cancer among populations having lung irradiation. Lancet, *2*, 1261, 1971.
43. Wagoner, J. K., Miller, R. W., Lundin, F. E., et al., Unusual cancer mortality amongst a group of underground metal miners. N. Engl. J. Med., *269*, 706, 1963.
44. Axelson, O., and Rehn, M., Lung cancer in miners. Lancet, *2*, 706, 1971.
45. Fox, A. J., Goldblatt, P., and Kinlen, L. J., A study of the mortality of Cornish tin miners. Br. J. Ind. Med., *38*, 378, 1981.
46. Wada, S., Miyanishi, M., Nishimoto, Y., and Kambe, S., Mustard gas as a cause of respiratory neoplasia in man. Lancet, *1*, 1161, 1968.
47. Henry, S. A., Industrial Maladies. London, Legge, 1934.
48. Hill, A. B., and Fanning, E. L., Studies in the incidence of cancer in a factory handling inorganic compunds of arsenic. I. Mortality experience in the factory. Br. J. Ind. Med., *5*, 1, 1948.
49. Perry, K., Bowler, R. G., Buckell, H. M., et al., Studies in the incidence of cancer in a factory handling inorganic compounds of arsenic. II. Clinical and environmental investigations. Br. J. Ind. Med., *5*, 6, 1948.
50. Mabuchi, K., Lilienfeld, A. M., and Snell, L. M., Cancer and occupational exposure to arsenic: a study of pesticide workers. Prev. Med., *9*, 51, 1980.
51. Oh, M. G., Holder, B. B., and Gordon, H. L., Respiratory cancer and occupational exposure to arsenic. Arch. Environ. Health, *29*, 250, 1974.

52. Doll, R., Cancer of the lung and nose in nickel workers. Br. J. Ind. Med., *15*, 217, 1958.
53. Doll, R., Mathews, J. D., and Morgan, L. G., Cancers of the lung and nasal sinuses in nickel workers: a reassessment of the period of risk. Br. J. Ind. Med., *34*, 102, 1977.
54. Kreyberg, L., Lung cancer in workers in a nickel refinery. Br. J. Ind. Med., *35*, 109, 1978.
55. Chovil, A., Sutherland, R. B., and Halliday, M., Respiratory cancer in a cohort of nickel sinter plant workers. Br. J. Ind Med., *38*, 327, 1981.
56. Lessarol, R., Reed, D., Maheux, B., and Lambert, J., Lung cancer in New Caledonia, a nickel smelting island. J. Occup. Med., *20*, 815, 1978.
57. Cox, J. E., Doll, R., Scott, W. A., and Smith, S., Mortality of nickel workers: experience of men working with metallic nickel. Br. J. Ind. Med., *38*, 235, 1981.
58. Pedersen, E., Høgetveit, A., and Andersen, A., Cancer of respiratory organs among workers at a nickel refinery in Norway. Int. J. Cancer, *12*, 32, 1973.
59. Jones Williams, W., The pathology of the lungs in five nickel workers. Br. J. Ind. Med., *15*, 235, 1958.
60. Machle, W., and Gregorius, F., Cancer of the respiratory system in the United States chromate-producing industry. Pub. Health Rep., *63*, 1114, 1948.
61. Baetjer, A. M., Pulmonary carcinoma in chromate workers. Arch. Ind. Hyg., *2*, 487 and 505, 1950.
62. Bidstrup, P. L., and Case, R. A. M., Carcinoma of the lung in workmen in the bichromates-producing industry in Great Britain. Br. J. Ind. Med., *13*, 260, 1956.
63. Alderson, M. R., Ratton, N. S., and Bidstrup, L., Health of workmen in the chromate-producing industry in Britain. Br. J. Ind. Med., *38*, 117, 1981.
64. Enterline, P. E., Respiratory cancer among chromate workers. J. Occup. Med., *16*, 523, 1974.
65. Langård, S., and Norseth, P., A cohort study of workers producing chromate pigments. Br. J. Ind. Med., *32*, 62, 1975.
66. Ohsaki, Y., Abe, S., Kimura, K., et al., Lung cancer in Japanese chromate workers. Thorax, *33*, 372, 1978.
67. Langård, S., Andersen, A., and Gylseth, B., Incidence of cancer among ferrochromium and ferrosilicon workers. Br. J. Ind. Med., *37*, 114, 1980.
68. Axelsson, G., Rylander, R., and Schmidt, A. Mortality and incidence of tumours among ferrochromium workers. Br. J. Ind. Med., *37*, 121, 1980.
69. Tsuneta, Y., Ohsaki, Y., Kimura, K., et al., Chromium content of lungs of chromate workers with lung cancer. Thorax, *35*, 294, 1980.
70. Figueroa, W. G., Razzkowski, R., and Weiss, W., Lung cancer in chloromethyl ether workers. N. Engl. J. Med., *288*, 1096, 1973.
71. Lemen, R. A., Johnson, W. M., Wagoner, J. K., et al., Cytologic observations and cancer incidence following exposure to BCME. Ann. N. Y. Acad. Sci., *271*, 71, 1976.
72. Nelson, N., The chloroethers—occupational carcinogens: a summary of laboratory and epidemiology studies. Ann. N. Y. Acad. Sci., *271*, 81, 1976.
73. Pasternak, B. S., Shore, R. E., and Albert, R. E., Occupational exposure to chloromethyl ethers. J. Occup. Med., *19*, 741, 1977.
74. Lloyd, J. W., Long-term mortality of steelworkers. V. Respiratory cancer in coke plant workers. J. Occup. Med., *13*, 53, 1971.
75. Mazumdar, S., Redmond, C., Sollecito, W., and Sussman, N., An epidemiological study of exposure to coal tar pitch volatiles among coke oven workers. J. Air Pollut. Control. Assoc., *25*, 382, 1975.
76. Doll, R., Vessey, M. P., Beasley, R. W. R., et al., Mortality of gasworkers—final report of a prospective study. Br. J. Ind. Med., *29*, 394, 1972.
77. Hurley, J. F., Archibald, R. McL., Collings, P.L., et al., The mortality of coke workers in Britain. Am. J. Ind. Med., *4*, 691, 1983.
78. Weil, C. S., Smyth, H. F., and Nale, T. W., Quest for a suspected industrial carcinogen. Arch. Ind. Hyg., *5*, 535, 1952.
79. Ask-Upmark, E., Bronchial carcinoma in printing workers. Dis. Chest, *27*, 427, 1955.
80. Moss, E., Scott, T. S., and Atherley, G. R. C., Mortality of newspaper workers from lung cancer and bronchitis, 1952–66. Br. J. Ind. Med., *29*, 1, 1972.
81. Egan-Baum, E., Miller, B. A., and Waxweiler, R. J., Lung cancer and other mortality patterns among foundrymen. Scand. J. Work Environ. Health, 7 (Suppl.), 147, 1981.

82. Buffler, P. A., Wood, S., Eifler, C., et al., Mortality experience of workers in a vinyl chloride monomer production plant. J. Occup. Med., *21*, 195, 1979.
83. Theriault, G., and Allard, P., Cancer mortality of a group of Canadian workers exposed to vinyl chloride monomer. J. Occup. Med., *23*, 671, 1981.
84. Mancuso, T. F., Relation of duration of employment and prior respiratory illness to respiratory cancer among beryllium worker. Environ. Res., *3*, 251, 1970.
85. Mancuso, T. F., Mortality study of beryllium industry workers' occupational lung cancer. Environ. Res., *21*, 48, 1980.
86. Infante, P. F., Wagoner, J. K., and Sprince, N. L., Mortality patterns from lung cancer and non-neoplastic respiratory disease among white males in the Beryllium Case Registry. Environ. Res., *21*, 35, 1980.
87. Acheson, E. C., Cowdell, R. H., and Rang, E., Adenocarcinoma of the nasal cavity and sinuses in England and Wales. Br. J. Ind. Med., *29*, 1, 1972.

Index